THE PREVENTION OF ORAL DISEASE

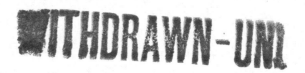

THE PREVENTION OF ORAL DISEASE

Third Edition

◆

Edited by

J.J. MURRAY

Professor of Child Dental Health,
University of Newcastle upon Tyne

Oxford New York Tokyo
OXFORD UNIVERSITY PRESS
1996

Oxford University Press, Walton Street, Oxford OX2 6DP

Oxford   New York
Athens   Auckland   Bangkok   Bombay
Calcutta   Cape Town   Dar es Salaam   Delhi
Florence   Hong Kong   Istanbul   Karachi
Kuala Lumpur   Madras   Madrid   Melbourne
Mexico City   Nairobi   Paris   Singapore
Taipei   Tokyo   Toronto
and associated companies in
Berlin   Ibadan

Oxford is a trade mark of Oxford University Press

Published in the United States
by Oxford University Press Inc., New York

A catalogue record for this book is available from the British Library.

Library of Congress Cataloging in Publication Data
The prevention of oral disease/edited by J.J. Murray.—3rd ed.
    p.   cm.
Rev. ed of: The prevention of dental disease. 2nd ed. 1989.
Includes bibliographical references and index.
ISBN 0–19–262457–1 (pbk.).—ISBN 0–19–262456–3 (hbk.)
1. Preventive dentistry.   I. Murray, John J.   II. Prevention of
dental disease.
[DNLM: 1. Preventive Dentistry.   2. Peridontal Diseases—
prevention & control.   3. Tooth Diseases—prevention & control.®]
RK60.7.P7113   1995
617.6′01—dc20
DNLM/DLC
for Library of Congress   95–15492
                                                                        CIP

ISBN 0 19 2624563 (Hbk)
ISBN 0 19 2624571 (Pbk)

Typeset by EXPO Holdings, Malaysia
Printed in Great Britain by The Bath Press, Bath, Avon

PREFACE TO THE THIRD EDITION

WHEN the idea of this book was first suggested in the early 1980s its main aim was to concentrate on the prevention of dental caries and periodontal disease. One reviewer, although complimentary overall, suggested that the book would have been improved by including a chapter on the prevention of trauma. I rejected this idea immediately—as I felt the reviewer had not understood the main purpose of the book.

The second edition reflected developments in the field of prevention, chapters on dental health education, root caries, and other problems affecting the dentition in middle and old age, and the difficulties in preventing dental disease in handicapped persons were added.

In planning the third edition it became obvious that if more chapters were to be added, then considerable revision of existing material was required. Professor Crispian Scully kindly agreed to write a chapter on the prevention of diseases of the oral mucosa. A chapter by Dr Richard Welbury on the prevention of trauma has been included (the reviewer of the first edition, Professor Dennis Picton, obviously had a clearer idea of where the book should be developing than I did!), and Professor Aubrey Sheiham has contributed a chapter on the prevention of oral disease from an international perspective. Dr Jimmy Steele, who has recently completed a study of the elderly in Salisbury, Darlington, and Richmondshire, provided a chapter on ageing in perspective. Unfortunately, Professor Emeritus J.R.E Mills died in January 1995 after a long illness. He suggested to me some time ago that a new author should review the topic 'Preventive orthodontics'. Dr Peter Gordon kindly agreed to prepare a chapter on 'The prevention of malocclusion'.

A final section has been added, looking briefly at the oral health needs in the twenty-first century.

In order to accommodate these changes, my chapter on 'Dental caries—a genetic disease?' has been omitted from the new edition. The sections on diet and fluorides and their effect on dental caries have both been reduced, partly by editing the text and partly by eliminating some of the references. For a fuller consideration of these topics the reader is referred to Andrew Rugg-Gunn's book, *Nutrition and dental health* or to the third edition of our book, *Fluorides in caries prevention*.

The title of the book has been changed slightly to *The Prevention of Oral Disease* to reflect the wider remit of the third edition.

The first edition was essentially a 'Newcastle' book in that a majority of contributors were either working in, or had worked at, Newcastle Dental School and Hospital. The present list of authors covers eight dental schools. I hope that this edition will be accepted as a 'British' contribution to our knowledge about the prevention of oral disease.

Newcastle-upon-Tyne   J.J.M.
March 1995

PREFACE TO THE SECOND EDITION

In the five years since the first edition was prepared the impetus for the prevention of dental disease has increased. Reviews of the book have been generally favourable, but in some cases pointed out areas that might have been included in a text on the prevention of dental disease. Most reviewers appreciated that the aim was not to provide details of clinical techniques but rather to concentrate on documented evidence. This general aim has been maintained: chapters on dental health education, root caries and other problems affecting the dentition in middle and old age, and the difficulties involved in preventing dental disease in handicapped persons have been added. The chapter on fissure sealants has been expanded so that the question of cost-effectiveness of preventive techniques can be considered in greater detail. The downward trend in dental caries in developed countries has been reviewed, together with a consideration of changes in child and adult dental health over the last 20 years, as found by results from national surveys. The implications of providing a preventively orientated service to deal with rapidly changing levels of oral disease are considered against a back-ground of dental services that have developed from a curative base.

I am most grateful to Mr J.R. McCarthy, Chief Dental Adviser, Dental Estimates Board, for providing me with details from the Board's Annual Reports, to Ms Diana Scarrott, Under Secretary, British Dental Association, for information on the General Dental Services, and most especially to Miss Sally Baldwin, who has been responsible for the secretarial work involved in compiling this second edition.

Newcastle-upon-Tyne   J.J.M.
September 1988

PREFACE TO THE FIRST EDITION

The Survey of Children's Dental Health in England and Wales in 1973 showed that over 90 per cent of our children leave school with untreated dental disease and over 50 per cent have had at least one general anaesthetic for dental treatment. This high level of dental disease seems to have been accepted with equanimity by the public at large, as though it were inevitable. It means that in adult life, at best a large amount of repair is required to maintain teeth in the mouth, at worst, that decayed teeth must be extracted. The extent of the problem can be judged by the fact that 30 per cent of all adults aged 16 years and over in Britain have no natural teeth at all.

And yet, and yet. Are things changing?

Over the last ten years there has been an increasing emphasis on good dental health and a number of encouraging reports, not only from Britain, but also from America, Australia, Scandinavia, and other European Countries that dental caries is decreasing in children. The idea is gaining round that dental disease is not inevitable, but preventable and that the possibility of keeping one's teeth for life is not just for the lucky few but is possible for almost everyone.

I was delighted to be given the opportunity of trying to draw together some of the main factors involved in the prevention of dental disease and am most grateful to my colleagues for agreeing to contribute the various chapters which make up this book. We do not attempt to cover all dental disease but concentrate on the prevention of dental caries and periodontal disease in order to draw together the available clinical and epidemiological information. In many instances we have referred to previous publications and have reproduced diagrams from other workers: due acknowledgement is made in the text. We would also like to thank our publishers for their help and encouragement. If our present knowledge could be translated into practice the impact on dental health would be immense and the practice of dentistry would change considerably. We hope that this book will help in some small way to encourage the movement towards prevention.

Newcastle-upon-Tyne   J.J.M.
January 1983

ACKNOWLEDGEMENTS

I would like to thank Oxford University Press for encouraging me to develop the theme of the prevention of oral disease. Preparing this edition has not been easy, because it was decided that, in order to accommodate new material, other chapters would have to be reduced to keep the book within reasonable bounds. I am most grateful to Georgina Klar, copy-editor, for her constructive comments on the manuscript and for her help in reducing mistakes in the text.

Part of the material on fluoride dentifrices was first published in the third edition of *Fluorides in caries prevention* and I thank Butterworth-Heinemann for permission to reproduce this material. Diagrams from the national surveys of child and adult dental health have been reproduced by kind permission of Miss Jean Todd and the Office of Population Censuses and Surveys. Our thanks go to the editors of *Archives of Oral Biology*, *British Dental Journal*, *Caries Research*, and the World Health Organization for permission to reproduce illustrations.

Finally, I thank all contributors and their secretaries for their help, and most especially Mrs Joan Smith, who has deciphered my handwritten notes with great skill and has been responsible for most of the secretarial work involved in compiling the current edition.

To provide the opportunity for everyone to retain a healthy functional dentition for life, by preventing what is preventable and by containing the remaining disease (or deformity) by the efficient use and distribution of treatment resources.

Aim of the Dental Strategy Review Group,
Towards Better Dental Health HMSO 1981

The retention throughout life of a functional, aesthetic natural dentition of not less that 20 teeth (shortened dental arch) and not requiring recourse to a prosthesis.

The Goal of Oral Health
WHO 1982

Oral Health is a standard of health of the oral and related tissues which enables an individual to eat, speak and socialize without active disease, discomfort and embarrassment and which contributes to general well being.

Oral Health Strategy Group 1994

CONTENTS

List of contributors   xiii

1. Introduction   1
   J.J. MURRAY

2. Diet and dental caries   3
   A.J. RUGG-GUNN

3. Fluorides and dental caries   32
   J.J. MURRAY and M.N. NAYLOR

4. Oral cleanliness and dental caries   68
   PHILIP SUTCLIFFE

5. Fissure sealants   78
   P.H. GORDON and J.H. NUNN

6. The carious lesion in enamel   95
   E.A.M. KIDD

7. Prevention of caries: immunology and vaccination   107
   W.M. EDGAR

8. The prevention and control of chronic periodontal disease   118
   W.M.M. JENKINS

9. Oral health promotion   139
   F.P. ASHLEY and C.D. ALLEN

10. The prevention of dental trauma   147
    R.R. WELBURY

11. The prevention of malocclusion   153
    P.H. GORDON

12. The prevention of oral mucosal disease   160
    CRISPIAN SCULLY

13. Prevention in the ageing dentition   173
    A.W.G. WALLS

14. Ageing in perspective   189
    J.G. STEELE

15. Preventing a dental handicap   200
    J.H. NUNN

16. Social factors and preventive dentistry   217
    J.F. BEAL

17. Oral health policy and prevention   234
    A. SHEIHAM

18. The changing pattern of dental disease   250
    J.J. MURRAY

19. Resources, treatment, and prevention   267
    J.J. MURRAY

20. Oral health for the twenty-first century   275
    J.J. MURRAY

Index   277

CONTRIBUTORS

C.D. ALLEN
Unit of Dental Public Health,
UMDS Guy's and St Thomas's Medical and Dental School,
London

F.P. ASHLEY
Professor of Periodontology and Preventive Dentistry,
UMDS Guy's and St Thomas's Medical and Dental School,
London

J.F. BEAL
Regional Dental Adviser
Northern & Yorkshire Regional Health Authority

W.M. EDGAR
Professor of Dental Science,
The University of Liverpool

P.H. GORDON
Department of Child Dental Health,
University of Newcastle upon Tyne

W.M.M. JENKINS
Department of Periodontology,
Glasgow Dental Hospital and School

E.A.M. KIDD
Department of Conservative Dental Surgery,
UMDS Guy's and St Thomas's Medical and Dental School,
London

J.J. MURRAY
Professor of Child Dental Health,
University of Newcastle upon Tyne

M.N. NAYLOR
formerly Professor of Preventive Dentistry,
UMDS Guy's and St Thomas's Medical and Dental School,
London

J.H. NUNN
Department of Child Dental Health
University of Newcastle upon Tyne

A.J. RUGG-GUNN
Professor of Preventive Dentistry,
Department of Child Dental Health,
University of Newcastle upon Tyne

CRISPIAN SCULLY
Dean and Director of Studies,
Eastman Dental Institute,
London

A. SHEIHAM
Department of Epidemiology and Public Health,
University College London Medical School,
London

J.G. STEELE
Department of Restorative Dentistry,
University of Newcastle upon Tyne

PHILIP SUTCLIFFE
Professor of Preventive Dentistry,
University of Edinburgh

R.R. WELBURY
Department of Child Dental Health,
The Dental Hospital,
Newcastle upon Tyne

A.W.G. WALLS
Professor of Restorative Dentistry,
University of Newcastle upon Tyne

1. Introduction

J.J. Murray

The mouth contains a number of different tissues, some of which, such as mucous membrane, connective tissue, blood vessels, nerves, muscle, and bone, are found throughout the body. Any of these tissues can suffer from infection, trauma, degeneration, or neoplastic change. Of overwhelming importance to the condition of the mouth are its two specialized tissues—the teeth and the periodontal structures. Indeed, dental caries and periodontal disease are so widespread that virtually everybody in the world, certainly every adult, has either one or both of these conditions.

About 2000 new cases of oral cancer occur in Britain each year, although in some countries, particularly in Asia, the prevalence of this disease is much higher. Treatment of oral cancer and other oral mucosal diseases requires specialist hospital services.

The cost of primary dental care in the General Dental Service in England and Wales has risen from £410 million in 1980 to just over £1 billion in 1992–3. The pattern of expenditure on various items of treatment has not changed dramatically over the last 12 years.

Almost half the cost is concerned with restoring teeth that had been attacked by dental caries and about £170 million in 1992–3 on the provision of dentures or bridges to replace teeth extracted, mainly because of dental caries or periodontal disease.

In addition, the cost of treatment carried out by dental practitioners, the cost of the Community Dental Services and the Hospital Dental Services, and to a much smaller extent the cost of dentistry in the Armed Forces and in industry, all of which are difficult to quantify, must be considered in any estimate of the total cost of treating dental disease in Britain, which must have reached £2 billion in 1995.

It has been reported that in terms of a single specific illness or disease the cost of dentistry is second only to the cost of mental illness and is greater than direct National Health expenditure on conditions such as pregnancy or the treatment of heart disease, bronchitis, or tuberculosis (Office of Health Economics 1969).

A considerable amount is known already about how to prevent both dental caries and periodontal disease. If put into practice this would affect dramatically their prevalence or at least would slow down the rate at which they progress, so that the vast majority of people would be able to keep their teeth in reasonable condition for the whole of their lives. At present, in Britain, only one adult in every thousand is caries-free, and 20 per cent of adults aged 16 years and over have no natural teeth at all—they have to rely on plastic dentures for the rest of their lives. This is, in part, due to attitudes of the general public to the importance of good dental health, and also to the attitudes of dentists in their management of dental disease.

Over the last 20 years marked reductions in the prevalence of dental caries in children have been observed in Britain, and in many other industrialized countries, and there is now strong evidence that this reduction in caries has resulted in improvements in the dental condition of young adults. This subject is considered further in Chapter 18.

Table 1.1. Cost of various items of dental treatment in the General Dental Services of the NHS in England and Wales (DEB 1985; DPB 1992–3)

	1980		1985		1987		1992–3	
	£m	%	£m	%	£m	%	£m	%
Examination and X-rays	65	16	101	15	125	17	155	15
Restoration of teeth	199	49	307	46	356	47	414	41
Dentures, bridges, etc.	69	17	122	18	136	18	170	17
Periodontal treatment	46	11	90	14	81	11	135	13
Extractions, other surgical treatment (except periodontal) and general anaesthetics	14	3	19	3	23	3	43	4
Orthodontic treatment	14	3	22	3	23	3	36	3.5
Other items	3	1	7	1	9	1	67	6.5*
Total	410	100	668	100	753	100	1020	100

* Includes domiciliary visits; weighted entry payments not available previously.

Although the prevalence of dental diseases and the provision of dental services varies in different countries, the same underlying general principles of prevention must apply throughout the world. The World Health Organization has pointed out that the potentially disastrous consequences of the rise in dental caries in developing countries (Fig. 1.1). The provision of dental treatment consumes economic resources and requires highly trained personnel. The only possible way forward in improving dental health for all is to reduce the prevalence of dental disease.

The aim of this book is to draw together the available epidemiological and clinical knowledge on the prevention of oral diseases in order to highlight the tremendous improvement in oral health which could be achieved if preventive measures were put into practice.

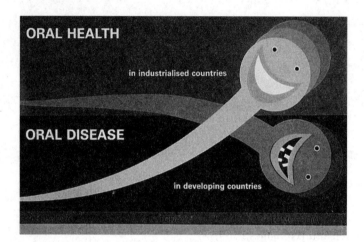

Fig. 1.1. 'Healthy mouths for all by the year 2000'—part of a World Health Education poster. (World Health Organization 1984.)

REFERENCES

Office of Health Economics (1969). *The dental services*, No. 29.
DEB (Dental Estimates Board) (1985).
DPB (Dental Practice Board) (1992–3). *Digest of statistics.*

2. Diet and dental caries

A.J. RUGG-GUNN

INTRODUCTION

Diet is one of the most important influences on oral health: it can affect the teeth in two ways—first, while the tooth is forming before eruption and, second, a local oral effect after the tooth has erupted into the mouth. On present evidence the post-eruptive local effect would seem to be very much more important and sugar the most important dietary factor in this local effect.

Various food items, other than sugar, have received attention such as starch, detersive (cleansing) foods, and the existence of various 'protective factors' in our diet. Since sugar, particularly sucrose, is so heavily incriminated as the major cause of caries, the search for alternative sweeteners has been active and evidence is now accumulating on their effect on caries and general health: this evidence will also be briefly reviewed. (For a full review of all aspects of this subject, the reader is referred to the textbook *Nutrition and dental health*, Rugg-Gunn 1993, published by Oxford University Press.)

PRE-ERUPTIVE EFFECT

In the years following the Second World War, advice about healthy eating often urged mothers to give their young children diets rich in calcium and vitamin D, so that they would form strong healthy bones and teeth: the inference was that these strong teeth would be less likely to decay. Although this is sound advice as far as the skeleton is concerned, there has always been little evidence to substantiate the view that good nutrition early in life helps to prevent dental decay by a systemic effect. This certainly does not mean that good nutrition should be discouraged, it merely reflects the current view that, in developed countries, diet has a much greater effect locally in the mouth on erupted teeth than it does pre-eruptively, while the teeth are still forming. Indeed, the Health Education Authority in the UK stopped giving advice concerning calcium, vitamin D, and strong healthy teeth many years ago, in order to concentrate the dietary aspect of dental health education on two uncontroversial messages: reduce sugar consumption and drink optimally fluoridated water. It should be emphasized that these remarks concerning the unimportance of nutrition (other than fluoride) while teeth are forming apply, at the present time, to developed countries where standards of nutrition are generally adequate—the same may not apply in countries with extensive malnutrition.

Although this section is entitled the 'pre-eruptive effect' of diet, it has often been difficult to be certain than an effect is purely pre-eruptive and, in some of the examples given, the possibility of some post-eruptive influence exists but cannot be adequately separated.

POSSIBLE MECHANISMS BY WHICH MALNUTRITION MIGHT INCREASE THE RISK OF DENTAL CARIES

Three mechanisms whereby malnutrition during tooth development could make teeth more susceptible to dental caries have been proposed, and they may well act together in many situations. The first, and the most widely discussed, is that malnutrition causes defectively formed teeth. The foremost proponent of the 'structural defect' theory was May Mellanby, whose work concerning vitamin D and hypoplasia and linking vitamin D and hypoplasia to dental caries, will be covered later.

The second mechanism has been proposed fairly recently by Alvarez and Navia (1989), although it is based on the observation, noted by a number of clinicians and epidemiologists, that the eruption of teeth is delayed in malnourished children.

One of the first clear indications of the late eruption of deciduous teeth in poorly nourished children was provided by Enwonwu (1973) (Fig. 2.1). In a study of 1292 children between the ages of 7 and 24 months, the 'optimum group' (well-nourished) children had, on average, 2–5 more teeth erupted than the malnourished children of a comparable age.

Alvarez and colleagues carried out a series of investigations into the nutritional status, times of exfoliation and eruption of teeth, and experience of dental caries, in Peruvian children. The children, living in a poor-class northern suburb of Lima, were classed as normal, wasted (acute malnutrition, assessed by height/weight ratio), or stunted (chronic malnutrition, assessed by height only). In the first survey of 285 children, 49 per cent were found to be stunted and 2 per cent wasted. The stunted children showed delayed exfoliation of deciduous teeth and delayed eruption of permanent teeth. Their study was expanded to include a total of 1481 children aged 1–13 years in Lima, Peru. The plot of dmft was, again, observed to be shifted to the right by about 2.5 years in the malnourished groups, compared with normal children. The authors concluded that malnutrition delayed tooth development, affected the age distribution of dental caries, and resulted in increased dental caries experience in deciduous teeth.

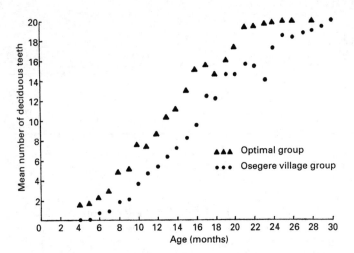

Fig. 2.1. The mean number of deciduous teeth erupted at various ages between 4 and 30 months in well-fed Nigerian children (optimum group) and in underprivileged, malnourished children (Osegere village group). All children were from the Yoruba tribe. (Reproduced from Enwonwu 1973, with permission of the editor *Archives of Oral Biology*.)

The third possible mechanism is that malnourishment can lead to an increased risk of dental caries, by affecting salivary glands so that the flow rate of saliva is reduced and its composition changed. However, since this is a nutritional effect on erupted teeth, it will be considered with other aspects of saliva and dental caries, later in this chapter.

VITAMIN D

The extensive work of May Mellanby, which showed that restriction of vitamin D intake caused hypoplasia of dental enamel in dogs is well accepted. However, Mellanby also postulated that vitamin D deficiency was responsible for the high prevalence of hypoplastic teeth in British children in 1920s, and that these teeth were more prone to decay, and thereby concluded that vitamin D deficiency was a factor in causing caries. Data given in Table 2.1 are taken from her examination of 302 deciduous teeth collected from 218 children aged 2–13 years in Sheffield. Nearly all of the hypoplastic teeth were carious, but only a quarter of the teeth without hypoplasia were carious.

Mellanby then embarked on a series of clinical trials in which the effect of giving 'abundant fat-soluble vitamins and

calcium with diminished oatmeal' to children was tested. (Oatmeal is rich in phytate which inhibits calcium absorption.) Some of the group sizes were unfortunately rather small but, nevertheless, the initiation and spread of dental caries was lower and the number of previously carious lesions which showed hardening was higher in the children who received the supplements. Some of the effect must have been post-eruptive, since the trials were too short to show any pre-eruptive effect and Mellanby did not fully explain this aspect of the mode of action of vitamin D.

There then followed a longer (2-year) trial carried out in three children's institutions in Birmingham. The children were in three groups, one in each institution, and received supplements of either treacle, olive oil (low in vitamin D), or cod-liver oil (high in vitamin D). At the start of the trial they were aged 9.5 years and were examined dentally every 6 months during the 2-year trial. The results showed that the children who received cod-liver oil had the smallest increment of dental caries (Table 2.2). A second trial was undertaken in which two groups of children, aged 10 years at the start of the trial, received either vitamin D or olive oil supplements for a period of 1.5 years. There was, again, a significant difference in favour of the vitamin D group for erupting permanent teeth, but not for teeth already erupted.

Not all dental workers in the 1930s and 1940s agreed with Mellanby's conclusions. Bunting and Jay, both working in the USA, stated quite clearly that they could not accept that

Table 2.2. The average caries figure (ACF) increments for permanent teeth observed in children participating in Mellanby's first Birmingham trial

Analysis by eruptive status	Groups		
	Treacle	Olive oil	Cod-liver oil
Teeth already erupted at start of trial	0.18	0.25	0.14
Teeth which erupted during the trial	0.29	0.22	0.16

* Statistically significant difference.

Table 2.1. Number of normal (good or sound) structured teeth or hypoplastic teeth, that were caries-free or were carious (Mellanby 1923)

Tooth type	No. teeth examined	Normal structure		Hypoplastic	
		Caries-free	Carious	Caries-free	Carious
Incisors	47	34	5	0	8
Canines	29	1	0	12	16
First molars	88	1	5	1	81
Second molars	138	0	1	0	137
Total	302	36	11	13	242

dental caries could be controlled by the addition of calcium, phosphorus, vitamins, or by altering the acid–base balance of the diet, although they carried out no experiments on these factors, and they considered dietary sugar was very much more important. In England, Weaver also found Mellanby's evidence unconvincing, criticizing the way she presented her data and indicating areas of her arguments which conflicted with other evidence. Subsequently, Mellanby modified her views on the beneficial effect of vitamin D, but still maintained that nutrition was 'a factor in resistance to dental caries', rather than '*the* factor'.

Despite the promising results obtained by Mellanby in the two trials of the use of cod-liver oil or vitamin D in the prevention of dental caries, only one other investigation on this subject seems to have been reported in the scientific press in English. The investigation by Bruszt and colleagues attempted to evaluate the effect of vitamin D_3 prophylaxis on dental caries in pre-school children living in Baja, Hungary, over the period of 1955–75. During this 20-year period, the mean dental caries experience of children aged 3–6 years increased from 3.8 dmft to 5.3 dmft. The authors concluded that 'vitamin D either does not possess a protective effect against caries or that the employed vitamin D doses are not sufficient to counteract the deleterious effect of the high carbohydrate diet'.

However, the issue is not completely dead in northern communities who experience little sunlight for several months of the year. Some schools in Alberta, Canada, have installed 'full spectrum' lighting in classrooms, and Hargreaves and Thompson (1989) reported a lower dental caries increment over 2 years in children who were exposed to this light (with high ultraviolet output), compared with children in classrooms with conventional lighting. The differences were substantial, and results of other studies are awaited with interest.

HARDNESS OF WATER

The possible influence of the hardness and calcium content of water on prevalence of dental caries has been suggested by many authors but investigated by only a few, mainly in the USA and South Africa. In the USA, Mills and East reported moderate inverse relationships between water hardness and dental caries experience in children, but the findings of Dean *et al.* (1942) were less impressive. Waters with appreciable levels of natural fluoride tend to be hard, leading most people to conclude that water hardness is of negligible importance compared with the fluoride content of the water. This conclusion seems justified when the data presented by Dean *et al.* (1942) are subjected to partial correlation analysis.

CALCIUM TO PHOSPHORUS RATIO

The ratio of Ca/P in the diet has been considered by some workers. Sobel and Hanok showed, in rats, that a massive decrease in the ratio of dietary P to Ca results in an increase in enamel carbonate and, some ten years later, Stanton (1969) published remarkable data suggesting that the optimum dietary Ca/P ratio (by weight) is 0.57 in man. As the subjects of Stanton's study were mainly adults, it is clear that he was principally interested in a post-eruptive effect. Stanton's hy-

pothesis was tested by Rugg-Gunn and colleagues using data from a study of diet and dental caries in 405 12–14-year-old English children. The range of Ca/P ratio in this study was 0.56 to 1.04, much narrower than the range reported by Stanton (0.24 to 1.05). Nevertheless, within this range, Rugg-Gunn *et al.* found no relationship between Ca/P ratio in the diets of adolescents and their caries prevalence or two-year increment.

FLUORIDE AND OTHER TRACE ELEMENTS

A very large number of studies have shown that fluoride has a substantial pre-eruptive caries preventive effect (see Chapter 3). On present evidence, fluoride is by far the most important trace element, dwarfing the observed effects of molybdenum, strontium, and lithium. These minerals have been associated, individually or in combination, with low caries prevalence in the UK, New Zealand, the USA, and in New Guinea. In contrast, selenium has been associated with higher caries prevalence. Foods (e.g. vegetables) are the main source of trace elements, and fluoride and strontium are alone in that water is the main dietary source. The evidence relating trace elements to caries prevalence has been reviewed in a book by Curzon and Cutress (1983).

In conclusion, on present evidence it would seem clear that fluoride is the most important dietary item influencing the caries resistance of the developing tooth. Other trace elements have a smaller effect. The pre-eruptive influence of Ca, P, Ca/P ratio and of vitamins is uncertain even after many years research, but their effect is unlikely to be great.

POST-ERUPTIVE EFFECT

The much greater post-eruptive effect of diet, than any pre-eruptive effect of nutrition, has been emphasized already. The post-eruptive effect of various classes of foods on dental caries are considered in turn below.

Foods differ in their ability to stimulate salivary flow which in turn can influence their intra-oral effect. The role of saliva in human health and well-being has received much less attention than it deserves. A much reduced salivary flow not only leads to very rapid progression of dental caries, but also makes speaking and eating, two importing functions in life, difficult. Our lack of interest in saliva in the past may have been because we felt unable to correct any failure in saliva functions or to enhance any favourable functions. With our increasing knowledge of saliva, this is no longer true, and the stimulation of salivary flow is now seen as an important factor in preventive dentistry. Chewing gums, in particular, have been advocated as 'good for teeth' because of their ability to stimulate salivary flow, and their effect upon caries development will be discussed during our consideration of non-sugar sweeteners.

In any consideration of diet and dental caries, it is important to consider all sources of evidence—these are human observational studies, human interventional studies, animal experiments, enamel slab experiments, plaque pH studies, and incubation experiments.

Diet and dental caries

HUMAN OBSERVATIONAL STUDIES

Epidemiology is concerned with observing the relationship between disease and social, environmental, and other factors. This information might then indicate possible causes and possible way of preventing disease. Epidemiological surveys are basically observational and should be distinguished from interventional studies in which factors are purposely altered and the effect on the pattern of disease observed.

World-wide epidemiology

At its crudest level, sugar intake and caries can be compared on a country basis. This type of comparison was undertaken by Sreebny (1982), who correlated the caries experience in the primary dentition (dmft) of 5- to 6-year-olds with sugar availability in 23 countries, and the caries experience of 12-year-olds (DMFT) with sugar availability in 47 countries. The data on sugar supplies were obtained from the Food and Agriculture Organization of the United Nations, and the caries data from the WHO Global Oral Epidemiology Bank. For both the primary and permanent teeth the correlation coefficients were positive, +0.31 for the primary dentition and +0.72 for the permanent dentition. Sreebny's data for the 47 countries are shown graphically in Fig. 2.2. On a linear regression, for each rise in sugar supply of 20 g/person/day,

caries increased by 1 DMFT. It should be appreciated that this type of epidemiological comparison is imperfect as sugar availability figures do not refer specifically to 5- or 12-year-olds, and both caries levels and sugar consumption will vary widely within each country. Sreebny published similar data comparing cereal availability and caries, and these results will be discussed on p. 19.

Caries experience in groups of people before and after increase in sugar consumption

The consumption of sugar is fairly recent phenomenon in many areas of the world. For one reason or another, isolated communities have become exposed to increased trade with 'westernized' countries and have subsequently adopted their high-sugar diet. In some of these communities, it is fortunate that the caries status of the population was recorded before as well as after the increase in the availability of sugar.

Eskimos

Numerous reports have stated that Eskimos living on their natural diet have low caries experience, but their dental health declined rapidly after exposure to a westernized lifestyle including a high-sugar western diet. Greenland has the largest group of people of Eskimo descent. Dental caries used to be virtually unknown but by 1977, the mean dmfs of 7-year-olds was 20 and the mean DMFS of 14-year-olds was 19. These figures are amongst the highest in the world.

Developing nations in Africa

Epidemiological data have been collected from several African countries over the past 60 years. These data tend to show low caries prevalence and severity when traditional, unrefined, low-sugar diets were consumed, but much higher caries experience after diets became more refined and consumption of sugar increased. One example is a study in Ondo State, Nigeria, which found that between the years 1977 and 1983, the mean dmft of 5-year-olds rose from 0.8 to 2.0, and the mean DMFT of 12-year-olds rose from 0.1 to 2.2. In both age-groups, the higher social-class children had substantially more dental caries than children from lower social classes. In a subsequent analysis of the diet of these Nigerian children, Olojugba and Lennon (1990) concluded that the sugar consumption patterns provided a plausible explanation for the changes in severity of dental caries.

The island of Tristan da Cunha

Tristan da Cunha is a remote, rocky island in the south Atlantic. 1500 miles west-south-west of Cape Town. The inhabitants, approximately 200, are of mostly European origin and have only occasional contact with the outside world. Because of a volcanic eruption, the islanders were evacuated to England between 1961 and 1963. Prior to 1940 their diet was very low in sugar, but since 1940 the island store has sold sugar and sugar-containing foods. The dramatic increase in consumption of imported sugary foods can be seen in Table 2.3. The dental health of the islanders have been recorded many times before and after the opening of the trading store in 1940. The results of the surveys (Fig. 2.3) show a very low caries experience in 1937 but a

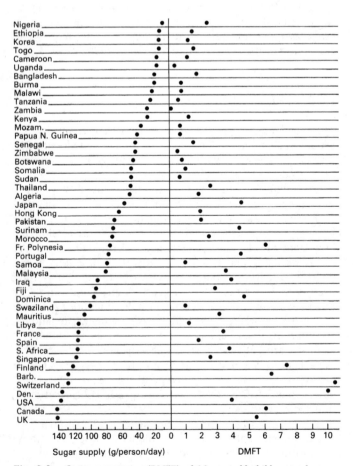

Fig. 2.2. Caries experience (DMFT) of 12-year-old children and sugar supply (g/person/day) in 47 countries. (Data from Sreebny 1982.)

Table 2.3. Consumption (g/person per day) of sugar- and flour-containing foods in Tristan da Cunha

	1938	1966
Sugar	1.8	150
Cakes and biscuits	0.5	24
Jam and condensed milk	0.2	20
Bread	1.7	
White flour		110
Sweets and chocolates	0	50

steady deterioration in their dental health since then; faster in the children than in the adults. The study is valuable in that it shows an increase in caries experience paralleling an increase in sugar consumption in the same population.

In conclusion, although many dental epidemiological surveys can be criticized because of poor response rates, different non-standardized examiners recording their findings over the years, and other technical reasons, it would be obdurate not to be impressed by the close parallel between the increase in consumption of sugar in many communities throughout the world and the increase in caries prevalence and severity. Some caries occurs in man in the absence of cane or beet sugar, but this is very small compared with the caries experience which occurs in population consuming the usual high-sugar, modern European diet.

Studies on groups of people eating low amounts of sugar

Several groups of people have habitually eaten low amounts of sugar and their dental status has been recorded. The following examples illustrate their lower caries experience.

Hopewood House

Hopewood House is a home in rural New South Wales, Australia, housing about 80 children of low socioeconomic background. Children enter the home soon after birth and remain under close supervision until about 12 years of age

when they can move to other accommodation but remain associated with the House. Dental examinations were conducted annually between 1947 and 1962, and thorough dietary surveys made. The diet could be classed as lacto-vegetarian. Only wholemeal flour was used to bake bread, biscuits and make porridge, and many of the vegetables were taken raw. Protein and vitamin levels exceeded the minimum recommended level. Sugar and white-flour products were virtually absent from the diet. On the other hand, their fluoride intake was estimated to be low and oral hygiene measures were virtually absent.

The dental surveys revealed a very low prevalence and severity of dental caries, much lower than children of the same age and socio-economic back-ground attending state schools in New South Wales, who were examined using the same methods (Fig. 2.4). Up to the age of 12 years caries prevalence was very low: 46 per cent of Hopewood House 12-

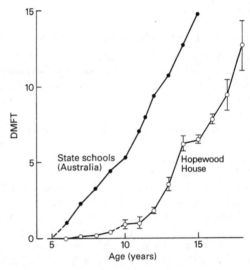

Fig. 2.4. Caries experience (DMFT) in children in Hopewood House (with SE of means) and children in state schools of South Australia. (Marthaler 1967, with permission of the editor *Caries Research*.)

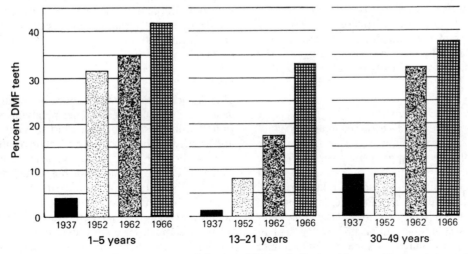

Fig. 2.3. Caries severity (per cent DMFT) in three age-groups of islanders of Tristan da Cunha at four examinations between 1937 and 1966.

year-olds being caries-free compared with only 1 per cent in the state schools. However, the rate of caries development increased in the Hopewood House children after 12 years of age (when their close supervision ended) to become virtually the same rate as observed in children in the state schools. This indicates that the diet received up until 12 years did not confer any protection from caries development in subsequent years.

Patients with hereditary fructose intolerance

This is a rare hereditary disease caused by an inborn error of metabolism, first recognized in 1956. These patients do not possess a liver enzyme (fructose 1-phosphate-splitting aldolase) and ingestion of foods containing fructose or sucrose (which contains fructose) causes severe nausea. On the other hand, starchy foods (not containing fructose) are well tolerated. Marthaler (1967) and Newburn (1978) have reviewed the dental state of 27 patients of age range 6 to 82 years. Their caries experience was very low—15 of the patients were caries-free.

Restrictions of sale of sweets in Australian schools

There have been two studies into the effect of selling sweets in school canteens on the caries increment of schoolchildren. Both studies were conducted in Australia and both showed that children had a lower caries increment in schools not selling sweets.

Fanning and colleagues recorded a 2-year increment of 10.9 DMFS in 981 children attending Adelaide secondary schools where sweets were sold, and 9.3 DMFS in 285 children attending schools not selling sweets; a difference of 1.57 surfaces or 14 per cent ($p < 0.05$). A few years later, in a further study in South Australia, Roder also recorded 2-year caries increments in children attending government or private schools. In half the schools of each type, sweets were not on sale. The 337 5- to 9-year-old children attending the government schools which did not sell sweets developed 0.9 DMFS, 16 per cent less caries ($p < 0.01$), than the same number of matched children in the schools which sold sweets. Similarly in the private schools, 314 7- to 13-year-old children in schools not selling sweets had 2.6 DMFS, 30 per cent less caries ($p < 0.01$) than matched children in the private schools selling sweets. Furthermore, the frequency with which the children attended the canteens was recorded and the frequent users of the canteens selling sweets had the highest caries increments. The profitability of the canteens not selling sweets was unchanged after removal of sweets.

War-time diets

A country at war usually experiences a reduction in availability of sugar. This was severe in Japan, for example, where sugar consumption fell from 15 kg/per person per year before the Second World War to 0.2 kg/person per year in 1946. In many countries attempts have been made to relate the level of sugar consumption before, during, and after war years to the caries prevalence in children over that period. The relation between sugar consumption and caries development in first permanent molars in children in Norway, Finland, and Denmark, is shown clearly in Fig. 2.5.

More recently, Alanen *et al.* (1985), using data collected in the 1979 Finnish National Dental Survey, suggested that the level of sugar consumption in the first few years after tooth eruption had a lasting effect upon caries experience. Sugar consumption reached a minimum in Finland in 1945. Caries experience of premolars and second permanent molars in people born in 1931–3 was significantly less than that in people born before or after these years, even after 40 years.

Groups of people with high sugar consumption

Sugar-cane chewers

There appear to have been six surveys of caries experience of people who habitually chew sugar-cane. An habitual chewer might chew 4 to 5 kg of cane per day, which could contain about 500 g of sugar. The results are equivocal. The two studies on Bantu workers in South African plantations reported very low caries experience. Thirty-seven per cent of the 98 adults examined by Harris and Cleaton-Jones were caries-free and their mean caries experience was 3.2 DMFT.

In contrast, the three Caribbean studies all reported higher caries experience in workers in sugar plantations in Cuba and Jamaica. The 147 adults (mainly white of Spanish background) in the study of Driezen and Spies had a mean DMFT of 15.1, which was similar to that reported by Kunzel (16.5 DMFT) for adult white workers in Cuba.

In Tanzania, the effect of sugar-cane chewing on dental caries was investigated by Frencken *et al.* (1989). The mean number of carious teeth in the 77 sugar-cane cutters was 3.5, compared with a mean of 2.0 carious teeth in the 68 control group of sisal cutters, leading the authors to conclude that chewing sugar-cane over a long period promotes dental caries.

Workers in the confectionery industry

There have been two studies comparing the caries experience of confectionery industry employees with similar groups of other workers. The caries experience of 722 Israeli confectionery workers was 71 per cent higher than the caries experience of 812 workers from textile factories. A further study confirmed previous results and, in addition, reported higher caries experience in production-line workers compared with non-production-line workers in the confectionery industry. The possibility that caries was caused by airborne sugar particles rather than by actual consumption should be borne in mind.

Phenylketonuria

This is a rare inherited metabolic defect in which there is a deficiency of the liver enzyme, phenylalanine hydroxylase. Unless a diagnosis is made within the first few weeks of life, and treated with special, high-carbohydrate diets which are low in phenylalanine, severe mental deficiency can occur. However, despite the fact that their diets from birth to 8 years contain about twice as much sucrose as is consumed by normal children. The caries experience of 105 phenylketonuric children in London and Liverpool was observed to be of the same order as that found in normal, similarly aged, London children. The reason for this lack of increase in caries experience following high sucrose ingestion is unclear.

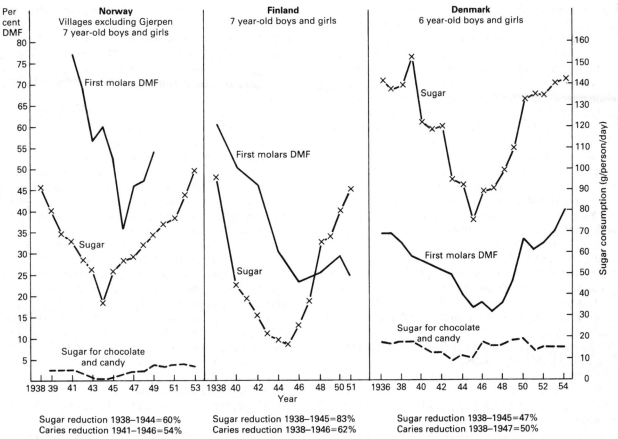

Fig. 2.5. Sugar consumption (g/person/day) in pre-war, war and post-war years, and the per cent of first permanent molars decayed, missing, or filled in 7- or 6-year-old children in Norway, Finland, and Denmark. (Reproduced from Toverud 1957.)

Children taking syrup medicines long-term

Paediatric medicines are conveniently given in syrup form: usually sucrose based. Roberts and Roberts (1979) compared the caries experience of 44 children, aged 9 months to 6 years (mean 47 months), who had been receiving syrup medicines for at least 6 months, with the caries experience of 47 similarly aged (mean 41 months) children who attended the same out-patient clinic but either did not take medicines or took tablets. Children receiving carbohydrates-controlled diets were excluded. There was no difference between the groups in the type of milk feeding they had received, use of dummies or other feeders, sweet or snack consumption, and the use of fluoride as tablets or toothpaste. The children taking the syrup medicines had much higher caries experience (5.6 defs) than the control children (1.3 defs).

Cross-sectional observational studies relating caries experience to the level of consumption of sugar and confectionery

There have been many cross-sectional observational studies in several countries. Interpreting results from these studies is often difficult as dietary information has been collected in a variety of ways: some reports have subdivided confectionery into type of sweets only some of which were significantly related to caries experience. Definitions of a 'sugary food'

were seldom given, which has frequently made interpretation of the correlation between caries and frequency of sugar intake difficult. Some studies have only looked at one aspect of sugar consumption, such as bedtime eating habits. In most of the studies, children were not selected for inclusion via their level of caries experience but, in some studies the eating habits of children at the two extremities of the caries experience distribution only were compared. It should be emphasized that in some studies, although significant correlations were found, the absolute differences in caries experience were small.

Several studies have investigated the effect of sugar in various methods of infant feeding on caries, particularly 'rampant caries' (or labial incisor caries) in the very young. Five British studies have all shown a strong relationship between labial incisor caries and sugared infant comforters, especially reservoir feeders. One study which did not show such a relationship was reported in South Africa. The world-wide use of comforters and their effect on oral health has been reviewed by Winter (1980).

Two studies by Granath and others are of particular interest because not only was the level of consumption of sugary foods compared with caries severity, but two other important confounding factors, fluoride supplementation and oral hygiene practices, were also considered. In both studies, diet was the most important of these factors in its relationship to dental caries and analysis showed that differences in caries experience between children with the highest and lowest between-meal sugar intake could not be explained by differences in fluoride supplementation or oral hygiene practices. The first study, on 6-year-olds, was small (179 children) and the higher levels of caries found in the children consuming more sugary foods between meals was not statistically significant. However, the second study, on 4-year-olds, was larger (515 children) and differences between the dietary groups were highly significant. When the effect of oral hygiene and fluoride were kept constant, the children with 'low between-meal sugar intakes' had 86 per cent less buccal and lingual caries and 68 per cent less approximal caries than children with a 'high between-meal sugar intake'.

The sensible approach, first used by Granath and co-workers, of attempting to quantify the importance of the three widely available methods of caries control (diet, tooth-cleaning, and fluoride) has been followed by other workers, almost all Scandinavian. Advanced statistical techniques have been used to identify clinically important aetiological factors, but one important criticism of all these studies is their cross-sectional nature: this aspect of study design will be discussed later.

Hausen and colleagues, in a study involving over 2000 Finnish children, aged 7–16 years, reported that water fluoride level, tooth-brushing frequency and sugar exposure were all important determinants of caries experience, although sugar exposure was the least important. Similarly, in another study in Finland, involving 543 children of three age-groups (5, 9, and 13 years), Kleemola-Kujala and Rasanen found the relation between poor oral hygiene and caries to be stronger than the relation between high sugar consumption and caries, although both were important. Again, very similar results were reported by Lachapelle-Harvey and Sevigny in a study of 159 12- to 16-year-old French Canadians. Holund and colleagues found that caries-active 14-year-old Danes consumed liquid sugar drinks more frequently than caries-inactive children.

Continuing the work begun by Granath in the 1970s, Schroder and Granath found that poor dietary habits and poor oral hygiene were both good predictors of high caries in 3-year-old Swedish children. A few years later, Schroder and Edwardsson reported that the predictive ability of diet and oral hygiene could be increased by additional tests involving counts of Lactobacilli and *Streptococcus mutans*. Another Swedish group also found *Strep. mutans* counts good predictors of caries experience in 13-year-old Karlstad children. They found no difference in caries between those who ate high, medium or low levels of sugar.

Stecksen-Blicks and others conducted a large survey of diet, tooth-brushing and caries experience in children of three age groups (4, 8, and 13 years) living in two northern and one southern community in Sweden. Children from the south had considerably more caries than children in the north in both deciduous and permanent teeth. The authors concluded that this difference was best explained by differences in tooth-brushing frequency and the age at which dental care started, and that the lack of observed differences in diet between north and south indicated that diet was an unimportant factor.

A large cross-sectional study in America looked specifically at the relation between the consumption of soft drinks and caries experience. Analyses of data from 3194 Americans aged 9–29 years revealed significantly positive associations between frequency of between-meal consumption of soft drinks and high DMFT scores. These associations remained even after accounting for the reported concurrent consumption of other sugary foods and other confounding variables.

Some studies have correlated caries experience with the dietary habits of the same person some years previously. In 275 Swedish children the consumption of sucrose-rich foods at 12 months of age was positively related to the presence of caries at 3 years of age. Both consumption of sugary foods and caries experience were linked to the educational status of the mother. The importance of social factors as determinants of eating habits and caries experience of young children has been highlighted in a number of studies, for example, caries and sugar-eating were much higher in children from socially deprived backgrounds in Edinburgh, Scotland.

Another study concerning past dietary experience was conducted in Hertford, England, where data were collected on infant feeding and caries status at the age of 3 years, and dietary habits and caries status at the age of 8–10 years, in 161 children. There was a positive relation between 'poor infant feeding' (including the use of sugared foods and drinks) and caries experience at 3 years and at 8–10 years. Children given sweetened drinks in bottles in infancy were more likely to be consuming sugar-containing snacks at the age of 8–10 years, supporting the idea that the development of a sweet tooth in infancy persists into later childhood.

While a few of the studies (e.g. those investigating sugar intake in infant feeding) attempted to assess life-long habits of sugar consumption, nearly all the studies tried to relate caries experience at one point in time to sugar or confectionery consumption at the same point in time or, at the most, over the previous 3 to 7 days. While this approach may be acceptable for young children whose teeth have only erupted and become carious over the preceding few years and whose sugar-eating habits may not have changed appreciably since the time dentition erupted, it may not be acceptable in older age groups.

It would seem, therefore, that there is a need for studies which assess sugar-eating habits over a defined period of time and relate this to dental caries which develops over the same period. Seven studies appear to have done this. In two of these only one-year caries increments were recorded and related to diet recorded at one point in time; despite this short period, significant relations were observed between sugar intake and dental caries increment.

The data collected in the two-year study of Rugg-Gunn *et al.* (1984) have been analysed fairly fully. The 405 children, initially aged 11–12 years, living in south Northumberland, UK, received annual dental examinations including bitewing radiographs. Diet was recorded by each child in a three-day diet diary, followed by an interview with a nutritionist on the fourth day. This was repeated on five occasions during the 2 years. The data were analysed in three ways; first, by correlating dental caries increment with dietary habits for all 405 subjects; secondly, by comparing the dental caries increments of children with the highest and lowest sugar intakes; and thirdly by comparing the diets of children who developed the highest or lowest dental caries increments. Correlations between diet and dental caries increments were generally low. The highest correlation was between fissure caries and weight of daily sugar intake (+0.146, $p < 0.01$). Multivariate analyses revealed that this relationship could not be explained by differences in sex, social class, tooth-brushing habits, or level of plaque as measured by gingival inflammation. The weight of sugar intake appeared to be more strongly related to dental caries than the frequency of intake. The 31 children who consumed the most sugar developed 56 per cent (0.9 DMFS/person/year) more dental caries than the 31 children who had the lowest sugar intake. When the diets of the children who developed no dental caries during the 2 years were compared with the diets of children with the highest caries increment, the former had lower intakes of confectionery ($p = 0.05$), sugared coffee, and drinking chocolate ($p = 0.05$), and higher intakes of unsugared tea ($p = 0.06$) and cheese ($p = 0.07$).

In 1988, Burt *et al.* (1988) reported results of a similarly designed study in Michigan, USA. Their study lasted 3 years and involved 499 children, initially aged 11–15 years. During the 3 years, diet was assessed by three or more 24-hour dietary recalls and dental caries increment was calculated from the results of examination at the beginning and end of the 3-year study period. Dental caries increments were low (mean of 2.9 DMFS) and 81 per cent of the increment occurred in fissure surfaces of posterior teeth. Children who consumed a higher proportion of their total energy intake as sugars had a higher increment of approximal caries, though there was little relation to pit and fissure caries. The average number of daily eating occasions was not related to dental caries increment, nor was the average number of sugary snacks (defined as foods with 15 per cent or more of sugars) consumed between meals, but the average consumption of between-meal sugars was related to the approximal caries increment. When children were categorized by high caries increment compared with no caries increment, a tendency toward more frequent snacks was seen in the high-caries children. The authors concluded that, in an age of generally declining dental caries, higher consumption of sugar was still a risk factor for children susceptible to approximal caries.

The quality of the diet of 11-year-old Canadian children was compared with dental caries development, over 20 months. There was a tendency for higher dental caries to occur in children with the poorest diet (assessed by one 3-day diary) (mean DMFS of 1.8), compared with those with the best quality diet (1.2 DMFS). Differences were not statistically significant, but the number of subjects in the latter group was only 19. Dental caries development was recorded in a group of Swedish children and a strong correlation found between dental caries incidence and consumption of sweets. The raw correlation was +0.25 ($p < 0.05$), but this increased to +0.51 ($p < 0.01$) in those with poor oral hygiene and decreased to +0.11 ($p < 0.05$) in those with good oral hygiene. The last incremental observational study to be discussed, was conducted in South Wales. The authors reported significant positive correlations between dental caries increments in posterior teeth of children and money spent on sweets. The children had been observed for 4 years between the ages of 11–12 and 15–16 years.

HUMAN INTERVENTIONAL STUDIES

The number of planned, interventional studies on human subjects in the field of diet and dental caries is few. This is because of the difficulties of placing groups of people on rigid dietary regimes for long periods of time. Some of the studies have involved providing daily sugar supplements to subjects—a practice which would now be considered ethically unacceptable. Nevertheless, these studies form an important contribution to our knowledge and so are discussed in some detail.

The Vipeholm studies

The Vipeholm study (Gustaffson *et al.* 1954) is probably the largest single study in the field of dental caries ever undertaken: it lasted from 1945 to 1953 and cost SwK 596 000 up until 1951. Previous studies had not provided an answer to whether caries was a deficiency disease or whether it was due to the local oral effect of diet.

The Vipeholm Hospital is situated near Lund in the south of Sweden and in 1951 contained 964 mentally disadvantaged patients from all parts of Sweden, supervised by about 700 staff. The patients were housed in 12 wards which were largely independent; about 80 per cent of the patients were male.

The main purpose of the study was to investigate how caries activity is influenced: (i) by the ingestion *at meals* of refined sugar with only a slight tendency to be retained in the mouth (non-sticky form), (ii) by ingestion *at meals* of sugar with a *strong tendency to be retained* in the mouth (sticky form, e.g. sugar-rich bread), and (iii) by the ingestion *between meals* of sugar with a *strong tendency to be retained* in the mouth (sticky form, e.g. toffees, etc.). There was one control group and six main test groups, although the 'bread' and '24-toffee' groups were both divided into separate male and female groups (Table 2.4). The groups lived in separate wards eliminating the possibility of exchange of diet between groups. Of the 633 patients examined in 1946, 436 completed the main study in 1951 (Table 2.4). In general, their caries experience was low—15.6 DMFT at the age of 32 years, compared with 18.4 DMFT found in 20-year-old Swedish army conscripts.

The dental examination system was developed during the preparatory period (1945–6) and examinations were conducted each year by the same two examiners. Five bitewing films were taken annually, together with models and photographs. Caries was diagnosed at two severity levels, including and excluding precavitation carious lesions.

It should be appreciated that individual patients were not randomly allocated to the different groups but rather that all suitable patients in a ward belonged to a group. This ensured minimum exchange of diet between groups (an important factor) but meant that the groups were likely to be imbalanced in certain factors which might influence caries susceptibility (e.g. age, number of sound tooth surfaces, initial caries experience). These imbalances can be seen in Table 2.4.

The study was in five parts: preparatory period (1945–6), vitamin period (1956–7), the first (1947–9) and second

Table 2.4. The Vipeholm study: Distribution of the 436 patients who completed the main study (1946–51) into the control and eight test groups

Group	No. of subjects		Age in 1946 (years)	Sound tooth surfaces in 1946	DMFT in 1946
	Male	Female			
Control	60		34.9	85.3	15.3
Sucrose	57		34.7	81.8	16.4
Bread—male	41		30.4	85.0	17.1
Bread—female		42	28.0	88.4	14.5
Chocolate	47		29.1	79.0	17.7
Caramel	62		35.6	87.3	15.5
Eight-toffee	40		26.3	96.9	11.7
24-toffee—male	48		31.0	88.1	15.1
24-toffee—female		39	31.1	89.1	14.1
Total	436		31.9	86.4	15.6

(1949–51) carbohydrate periods, and a post-study period (1951–3). The purpose of the vitamin trial was to find out whether differences in the amounts of vitamins ingested were capable of producing changes in caries activity. During this period all groups received an 'all-round-diet', which contained half the average level of sugar in Sweden (which was 37 kg/person per year in 1946), and the diet of different groups was supplemented with vitamins, calcium fluoride, calcium lactate, or bone meal. The caries activity in all groups was very low and unaffected by the additions, although the test period was too short for adequate evaluation (less than one year).

The basal diets during the two carbohydrate periods differed from each other. In the first period it was low in sugar and contained only 1800 kcal. but this was raised to 3000 kcal by sugar supplements in the test groups, and by 150 g margarine (on bread) in the control group. However, during the second carbohydrate period the basal diet was made as similar as possible to that of an ordinary Swedish household, but because the sugar supplements (40 g margarine for the control group) combined during this second period the subjects gained weight.

The changes in dental caries experience (DMFT) in each of the groups can be seen in Fig. 2.6, which is taken straight from the report.

Control group: these 60 males received a carbohydrate-poor, high-fat diet, practically free from sugar. Caries increment was almost nil.

Sucrose group: during the first carbohydrate period, these 57 males consumed about twice the national average level of sugar, but only at meals in solution. Sugar consumption was reduced in the second carbohydrate period to just over the national average and again only in solution at meals.

Bread groups: during the carbohydrates periods, the 41 males and 42 females consumed 345 g of especially sweetened bread (containing 50 g sugar) per day. Since the bread was fresh it had a sticky consistency. Nothing was consumed between meals. All the males ate all their ration, but one-third of the females did not. This may account for the higher caries activity in the last year of the study in the males compared with the females.

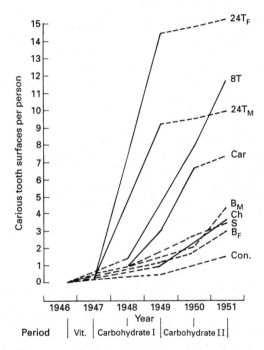

Fig. 2.6. Caries experience (DMFT) for the control group and eight test groups as recorded at the seven or eight examinations between 1946 and 1951. Solid line indicates that the subjects ate sugar both at and between meals; interrupted line indicates that subjects received sugar only at meals. (Gustaffson *et al.* 1954, with permission of the editor *Acta odontologica Scandinavica.*)

Chocolate group: during the first carbohydrate period, the 47 males consumed the same diet as the sucrose group. In the second period, the sugar in solution was reduced but supplemented by 64 g milk chocolate (30 g sugar) in four portions eaten between meals. Caries increment was low in the first carbohydrate period but increased in the second period.

Caramel group: the 62 males received stale sugar-rich bread during the first year of the first carbohydrate period. Caries increment was unchanged from that observed in the vitamin period. During the second year of the first period and most of the first year of the second period, they received 22 caramels (155 g containing 70 g sugar) per day: the caramels being issued between meals twice a day in the former year and four times a day in the latter. The consumption of caramels was accompanied by an increase in caries increment. This increase was so great that the caramels were withdrawn before the last year of the second carbohydrate period and replaced with an isocaloric quantity of margarine.

Eight-toffee group: during the first year of the first carbohydrate period, the 40 male patients received a low-carbohydrate, high-fat diet: caries activity was low. During the second year of the first carbohydrate period and the two years of the second carbohydrate period the diet was supplemented with eight toffees (60 g containing 40 g sugar) per day. During the first carbohydrate period the toffees were issued at breakfast and after lunch and were often eaten straight away; during the next two years the toffees were issued only between meals.

24-toffee groups: during the first carbohydrate period, the 48 males and 39 females received 24 toffees per day, which were available throughout the day. This was accompanied by a very marked rise in caries increment. Because of the very great increase in caries in these groups, issue of toffee was stopped just before the end of the first carbohydrate period and replaced by an isocaloric amount of fat.

Comment

The main conclusions of the Vipeholm study are:

1. Consumption of sugar, even at high levels, is associated with only a small increase in caries increment if the sugar is taken up to four times a day at meals and none between meals.
2. Consumption of sugar both between meals and at meals is associated with a marked increase in caries increment.

Other conclusions were:

(i) the increase in caries activity, under uniform experimental conditions, varies widely from person to person;
(ii) the increase in caries activity disappears on the withdrawal of the sugar-rich foods;
(iii) carious lesions occurred despite avoidance of sugar.

Both the study itself and the use of the findings of the study in dental health education have been criticized by a few authors. Criticisms are based largely on the fact that the subjects were mentally-deficient patients kept in unique conditions and fed abnormally high levels of sugary foods. The authors of the Vipeholm report point out that because the study was planned to be long-term and involved a large number of subjects, adults had to be used. The authors suggest that the subjects seemed to be more caries-resistant than the general population and that the greater caries resistance was found in the more mentally ill patient; therefore increases in caries in the Vipeholm patients might be even greater in normal subjects. In both the caramel and 24-toffee groups the increase in caries was so great that the between-meal sweet-eating was stopped before the end of the project.

Studies relating diet and dental caries are very difficult to conduct as caries is a chronic disease, and diet is infinitely

variable and very prone to strongly held personal preferences. It is very difficult to keep a large group of people on the same diet for a year or more, and this is only likely to be achieved in institutions. Mental institutions have a high staff: patient ratio (almost 1:1 at Vipeholm) and supervision of diet is likely to be more thorough. It would seem unreasonable, therefore, not to obtain as much information as possible from the Vipeholm study; despite its complicated nature and the abnormality of the subjects, the main conclusions appear to be valid.

The Turku sugar studies

By 1970, there was considerable evidence of variation in the rate of acid production from different sugars by plaque micro-organisms: for example, the sweet polyalcohols produced virtually no acid. In order to test whether the cariogenicity of sugars was also different in human subjects, a clinical study was conducted in Turku, Finland, between October 1972 and October 1974 (Scheinin and Mäkinen 1975). The object was to study the effect on dental caries increment of nearly total substitution of sucrose in a normal diet with either fructose or xylitol. Because full co-operation of the subjects in adhering to their diet was essential, and because it was planned that the subjects would undergo a wide range of biochemical and microbiological tests, it was decided to restrict the study largely to adults, most of whom were connected with the Turku dental or medical schools. Of the 125 adults who began the study, 115 remained after two years. Two-thirds of the subjects were female. The mean initial age of the subjects completing the study was 27.7 years, and although the age range was wide (12–53 years), 65 per cent of the subjects were initially aged 20–29 years.

The 125 subjects were allocated to three groups—sucrose (S), fructose (F), and xylitol (X). The caries examination was conducted blind by one person throughout the study; it was thorough, taking about 60 min per subject. In addition, two standardized bitewing radiographs were taken of each side of the mouth. Both pre-cavitation and cavitation lesions were recorded, for both primary and secondary caries. Because of the short duration of the trial (24 months), and because it was conducted in a largely adult population in whom low caries increment could be expected, the majority of caries results were expressed including the pre-cavitation caries grade.

The organization of the dietary regimes for the subjects in the three groups was very considerable. Virtually all foods which normally contained sucrose had to be manufactured with fructose or xylitol substituting for the sucrose. Altogether about 100 dietary items were especially manufactured by 12 food firms in Finland in order to ensure that as wide a variety of foods were available to subjects in the F and X groups as for the S group or normal subjects. Sugar and sugar-containing foods were provided free during the 2-year study. All subjects were asked to avoid sweet fruits such as dried figs, raisins, and dates, because the sugars in these foods could not be substituted. The fructose products presented no manufacturing problems, but some foods were more difficult to manufacture with xylitol, partly owing to its lower solubility and partly because it is not metabolized by yeast cells

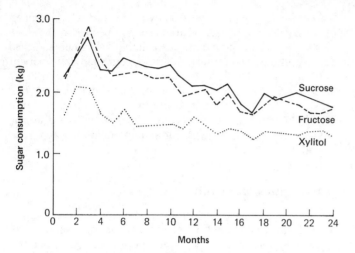

Fig. 2.7. The mean monthly sugar consumption by subjects in the three groups. This does not include sugar in manufactured items. (Scheinin and Makinen 1975, with permission of the editor *Acta odontologica Scandinavica*.)

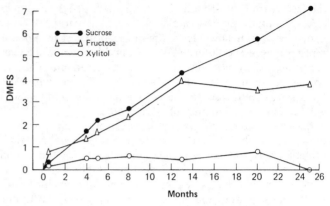

Fig. 2.8. The cumulative development of decayed, missing, or filled surfaces including cavitation and pre-cavitation carious lesions, diagnosed both clinically and radiographically, but not including secondary caries. At 24 months, differences between all groups were statisically significant ($p < 0.01$). (Scheinin and Makinen 1975, with permission of the editor *Acta odontologica Scandinavica*.)

used in making dough. Some products, though, were considered better tasting than their sucrose-containing counterparts. Participants kept a dietary diary for all 745 days of the study. From these, the consumption of sugars in the three groups during the 2-year study was obtained (Fig. 2.7.): consumption by the S and F groups was very similar but consistently higher than consumption by the X group. The advent of free food and initial curiosity resulted in higher consumption for the first few months.

Data analyses revealed that there were no substantial differences in baseline caries scores between the three groups (Table 2.5). The cumulative development of caries (DMFS), diagnosed both clinically and radiographically, is given in Fig. 2.8. These results include both precavitation and cavitation lesions. The 24-month DMFS increments were 7.2 in the S group, 3.8 in the F group, and 0.0 in the X group.

It was previously noted that the above DMFS score included precavitation lesions. Subsequently, Scheinin published DMFS increments for the three groups, excluding precavitation lesions. The 2-year mean DMFS increments for each group were: S group 3.33, X group 1.47, and F group 3.57. The 56 per cent reduction in the X group compared with the S group was statistically significant ($p < 0.01$). However, no difference between the S and F groups was observed, in fact the F group increment was slightly larger than the S group increment.

Table 2.5 The baseline conditions of the 115 subjects who completed the 2-year Turku sugar study

	Group		
	F	S	X
Total clinical and radiographic carious surfaces	13.9	11.0	13.4
Filled surfaces	29.4	27.3	29.8
DMFS	48.0	42.1	50.7
Number of subjects	35	33	47
Mean age (years)	26.2	27.2	29.1

Subsequently, the radiographs from the Turku study were re-examined in order to quantify changes in the size of approximal carious lesions. There was no difference in the mean size of the lesions in the X and S groups at baseline but at the end of the 2-year study the mean size was significantly smaller in the X group than in the S group ($p < 0.01$).

Analyses of the caries data over the 2-year study period indicated that substitution of xylitol for sucrose in a normal Finnish (high-sucrose) diet resulted in a very much lower caries increment of both carious cavities and precavitation lesions. While subjects in the S group developed more precavitation carious lesions than subjects in the F group, the F group subjects developed more carious cavities than subjects in the S group. The X diet was clearly less cariogenic than the S or F diet, but it cannot be concluded that the F diet was less cariogenic than the S diet.

Comprehensive biochemical and microbiological tests were carried out in parallel with the dental caries assessments. No adaptation by plaque organisms to produce acid from xylitol was observed during the 2-year study.

Results of serum analyses and liver-function tests indicated that neither dietary xylitol nor fructose altered metabolic parameters of liver function as compared with a normal sucrose diet. The only adverse side-effect of xylitol consumption appeared to be a raised incidence of osmotic diarrhoea. This was, however, less than had been expected and only one subject withdrew from the study for this reason. The occurrence of diarrhoea did not correlate well with the quantity of xylitol consumed as it was noted that 200 g of xylitol per day caused diarrhoea on some days, whereas the same or much higher doses led to no symptoms on other days.

In summary, the Turku sugar study required a considerable amount of careful planning and organization. Almost total substitution of sucrose by xylitol resulted in a substantial reduction in caries incidence. Although slight differences in amounts of sugars eaten and in frequency of intake, changes in salivary enzymes, the amount of plaque, and incidence of some micro organisms may have contributed to the observed results, the persistent inability of plaque organisms to metabolize xylitol to acids is likely to be the main explanation for its caries-preventive effect. The lack of any undesirable general metabolic processes, and the fairly low incidence of osmotic diarrhoea, indicates that xylitol is likely to be a suitable substitute for sucrose from the dental point of view. On the other hand, substitution of dietary sucrose by fructose did not lead to a clear-cut reduction in caries increment, and it cannot be concluded that substitution by fructose is a worthwhile caries-preventive measure.

Other studies

The Roslagen Study

Frostell *et al.* (1974) reported a study designed to investigate the effect upon dental caries increment of substituting sucrose in candies by Lycasin. Lycasin is a hydrogenated starch hydrolysate and was at that time made by the Lyckeby Co., Sweden. Since then an improved product has been made in France. Initially, 225 children, aged $2\frac{1}{2}$–4 years, took part in the study. They were allocated to a Lycasin and a control group, but it is uncertain whether this was random. Some 77 per cent of the children remained in the study after 1 year and 50 per cent after 2 years. Dental examinations were conducted 'blind'. Substitution of Lycasin for sucrose in candies was only partial but, from examination of the data, the authors seen justified in their conclusion that the reduction in caries increment in the Lycasin group was about 25 per cent.

Effect of pre-sweetened cereals on caries increment

The sugar content of breakfast cereals can be very high and there has been concern at their possible cariogenic potential.

Two studies, both in the USA, have reported caries increments in adolescent children who did or did not consume pre-sweetened cereals over a defined period of time. The first study lasted 2 years and the second for 3 years. The cereals were provided to the families *ad libitum*. In both studies no difference was found between the two groups of children. But, as Glass and Fleisch pointed out, these findings should not be construed to dilute in any way the evidence associating dental caries with sucrose in general. Some 94 per cent of the cereals were taken with milk, which will reduce acidogenicity, and cereals are usually eaten at meal times. It is also exceptionally difficult to test the importance of just one dietary item per day on caries because its effect is likely to go undetected amongst the many other sugar-containing foods and drinks.

Effect of acidulated carbonated beverages on caries increment

Steinberg and others conducted a study in which 119 institutionalized mentally subnormal patients, aged 8–21 years, consumed 6 oz of sugar-containing acidulated carbonated beverage at mid-morning and at bedtime each day for 3 years. At the same times, an age-matched control group (132 patients) in the same institution consumed 6 oz of water. The 3-year caries increment in the group receiving the sugared beverage (12.2 DMFS) was slightly higher than that for the control group (10.3 DMFS) but the difference was not statistically significant.

The consumption of soft drinks is increasing in many countries. Dental caries, caused by the presence of sugar, is not the only threat these pose to teeth. These drinks almost invariably have a low pH due to the presence of citric or phosphoric acid, which is considered to be an important cause of dental erosion.

Von der Fehr short-term caries experiments

Von der Fehr *et al.* (1970) reported on the development of an experimental caries system in which optical changes in enamel (similar to early carious lesions) were produced and subsequently reversed. It was hoped that this system could be used to test the cariogenicity of different sugars and diets, and the efficacy of various dietary additives or enamel pre-treatments in preventing lesion formation. In the experimental caries system, twelve dental students ceased oral hygiene for 23 days, and six of the 12 also rinsed nine times per day with 10 ml of 50 per cent sucrose solution. At the end of this test period, an increased 'caries index' score was observed in both groups, but the increase was more marked in the sucrose-rinse group (Fig. 2.9). As the authors pointed out, the control group did not refrain from sucrose intake, so the comparison is not between no sucrose and frequent intakes, but rather between different levels of sucrose intake.

Geddes and colleagues, using the same experimental system but with only 14 days of no oral hygiene and sucrose rinsing, also reported a greater increase in 'caries index' in the sucrose-rinsing group compared with a control group. In both experiments, the caries-like lesions were reversed by scrupulous oral hygiene in combination with fluoride rinsing.

Although this experimental caries model looked promising, because of the fairly high inter-subject variation in caries-index increments, the minimum sample size per treatment group has to be large, and it is unlikely that further studies will be undertaken using this method.

ANIMAL EXPERIMENTS

This section will only include discussion of animal experiments concerned with sugar and dental caries. Experiments concerned with pre-eruptive dietary effects have already been discussed; the cariogenicity of starch, the effect of adding phosphates to diets, and alternative sweeteners and caries

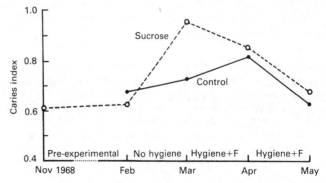

Fig. 2.9. Mean 'caries index' scores for buccal surfaces of canine, premolar, and maxillary incisor teeth in Danish dental students during the experimental caries study. (Von der Fehr *et al.* 1970, with permission of the editor *Caries Research*.)

Table 2.6 The mean number of carious lesions in rats fed a cariogenic diet either conventionally or by stomach tube. The salivary glands of some of the animals in each group had been removed. Number of animals in each group is given in parentheses

	Conventional	Tube fed
Intact	6.7 (13)	0 (13)
Desalivated	28.8 (4)	0 (3)

development will be considered later. The rat is the most commonly used animal, but hamsters, mice, and monkeys have also been used.

The importance of the local effect of sugar in the mouth was shown clearly by Kite *et al.* (1950) (Table 2.6). Apart from demonstrating this important fact, these animal experiments have been valuable at shedding light on the relevance of a number of aspects of sugar-eating and dental caries.

Frequency of feeding

The careful control of the frequency with which an animal could feed on a cariogenic diet became available when the Zurich Dental Institute developed an automatic feeding machine. Food could then be presented to animals at precisely controlled times and under-feeding ensured the animals ate all of the known quantity of foods. The results of the study by König *et al.* (1968) clearly showed a positive correlation between frequency with which animals ate a cariogenic diet and caries severity (Table 2.7). The group of rats feeding *ad libitum* consumed 11.7 g of food per day, nearly twice the 6 g consumed by the other groups. The level of caries severity in the groups indicates that frequency of eating a cariogenic diet is likely to be more important than the total amount of diet consumed.

Another relevant factor is the length of time interval between meals. Firestone and colleagues devised an experiment in which all animals ate a cariogenic diet 18 times a day: half the animals received their diet in three groups of 6 meals with no interval between the 6 meals in each group, but all the 18 meals consumed by the second group of animals were separated by intervals of 30 minutes. In both groups, each meal lasted 10 minutes. Caries development was greater in the latter group whose meals were spread out during the day, compared with the former group whose meals were bunched closely together.

Table 2.7. The mean caries severity, daily food intake, and weight gain in five groups of rats fed at different frequencies per day; six animals per group

Group	Eating frequency per day	No. of fissure lesions	Daily food intake (g)	Weight gain during experiment (g)
1	12	0.7	6.0	23
2	18	2.2	6.0	34
3	24	4.0	6.0	28
4	30	4.7	6.0	29
5	*ad libitum*	4.2	11.7	64

Concentration of sugar

Although a large number of experiments have shown that diets containing some sugar (e.g. about 10 per cent of the total diet) produce more caries in rats than diets with no sugar, further increases in caries have not always been observed when the sugar content is raised above 10 per cent. It would seem that differences in results have been due to, first, the type of diet used and, second, whether or not the rats were superinfected with cariogenic organisms. The composition of the non-carbohydrate part of the diet is also very important in determining how cariogenic a given amount of sugar will be. As little a 2–5 per cent sugar causes much caries in the presence of 50–70 per cent starch, while five times as much sugar is necessary in a high-fat diet.

A comprehensive study investigated two strains of rat, two basic diets (diet '2000' or 'DD') with up to five levels of sugar concentration, fed either *ad libitum* or fed 17 times/day by programmed feeding and found that in all cases caries was higher in animals receiving the 15 per cent compared with 0 per cent sugar. While caries increased linearly with dietary sugar concentration (0, 15, 30, and 56 per cent sugar) in Sprague–Dawley rats receiving the '2000' basic diet, those receiving the 'DD' basic diet showed no linear increase in caries for sugar concentrations above 15 per cent. Hefti and Schmid (1979) heavily superinfected their Osborne–Mendel rats with cariogenic *Strep. mutans* and *Actinomyces viscosus*. Their results (Fig. 2.10) showed that caries severity increased with increasing sugar concentration although the increase in severity fell with sugar concentrations above 40 per cent.

Types of sugar

Most animal experiments have used a basic starch diet and any added sugar has almost always been sucrose (usually as

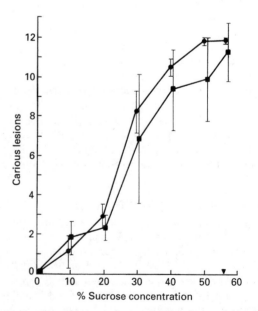

Fig. 2.10. Incidence of carious lesions (±SE) in fissures (●) and smooth surfaces (■) in rats fed *ad libitum*, diets containing 0, 10, 20, 30, 40, 50, and 56 per cent sucrose. (Hefti and Schmid 1979, with permission of the editor *Caries Research*.)

icing sugar). Dietary studies using rats suggested that the addition of 25 per cent glucose, fructose, lactose, or maltose did not produce significantly more caries than starch, while sucrose was much more cariogenic. However, all these animals were inoculated with a dextran-producing streptococcus. Other studies also found that sucrose was more cariogenic than glucose in gnotobiotic rats mono-infected with *Strep. mutans*. Some strains of streptococci utilize sucrose preferentially and do not thrive in its absence. Experiments, therefore, where the animals are superinfected with such organisms are likely to exaggerate differences between the cariogenicity of sucrose and other sugars. In three out of four experiments, sucrose was more cariogenic than glucose or fructose but the differences were small. There was no difference in the cariogenicity of glucose and fructose. Twenty per cent glucose syrup was less cariogenic than 20 per cent sucrose syrup when taken by rats in drinking water, the difference being particularly marked in smooth surface caries.

Colman and others studied the development of caries in monkeys fed diets containing either sucrose, glucose + fructose, or fructose alone. The sucrose and glucose + fructose diets were of almost equal cariogenicity, while fructose appeared to be slightly less cariogenic than sucrose. Their former finding does not support the view that sucrose is the most cariogenic of sugars, except that it is so widely present in our diet, but their latter finding supports the 24-month results of the Turku human studies where the analyses included precavitation carious lesions. These findings cast doubt on the theory that sucrose is uniquely cariogenic because it increases dextran formation in plaque. However, a different result was reported by Birkhed and colleagues who found that glucose + fructose (invert sugar) was less cariogenic than sucrose, but the significance of this is uncertain as the rats who received the sucrose diet were superinfected with *Strep. mutans* but the rats who received the invert sugar were not.

ENAMEL SLAB EXPERIMENTS

Intra-oral appliances have been made that can hold slabs of enamel. Plaque forms on the surface of the slabs, which remain in the mouth for 1 to 6 weeks. The experimental system is extremely flexible so that by using either sound or partially demineralized enamel, the cariogenic effect or the remineralizing effect of diets can be assessed.

Because of this flexibility of design, a variety of methods have been used. Some workers have used slabs made from bovine enamel; others have used human enamel. In some experiments the slabs have been covered with Dacron or terylene gauze to encourage plaque formation, but in others no gauze was used. Lesion formation has been measured by micro-hardness tests, micro-radiography, and iodine dye permeability.

An example of an appliance made to fit over mandibular teeth is shown in Fig. 2.11. There seems to be reasonably good agreement between results obtained by different methods of measuring lesion formation. Experiments have shown that sugars cause demineralization while non-fermentable non-sugar sweeteners aid remineralization. Increasing the concentration of sugars and the frequency of exposure to sugars increased demineralization.

Enamel slab experiments seem to have a number of advantages over *in vitro* incubation and demineralization experiments and *in vivo* plaque pH experiments, especially if the test foods are eaten with the appliance in place.

PLAQUE pH STUDIES

Methods of measuring plaque pH

There are four main methods of measuring plaque pH. First, metal probes (antimony, iridium, or palladium) which can be inserted *in situ* into plaque. Secondly, glass probes have been used and thirdly, a more complicated, but potentially more useful system employs a miniature glass electrode built into a

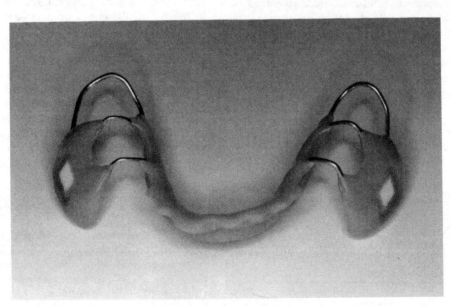

Fig. 2.11. An example of an acrylic resin appliance showing two buccal flanges each containing a terylene mesh-covered slab of enamel. (Illustration kindly supplied by E.I.F. Pearce; reproduced with permission of the editor *New Zealand Dental Journal*.)

partial denture that stays in the mouth for several days while plaque forms over the teeth and electrode. Recordings of pH are made either via wires coming from the mouth or by radio-telemetry, which avoids the possibility of wires interfering with eating. This system, which was developed in Zurich and has given consistent results for many years. The fourth method involves the removal of small samples of plaque from representative teeth and the measurement of the pH of this plaque on a small saucer-shaped glass ('one-drop') electrode outside the mouth. Each method has its advantages and disadvantages. However, regardless of methods used, there is reasonable agreement in the order in which foods and drinks are ranked according to their acidogenicity, although the methods differ in the absolute pH values recorded.

Snack foods and plaque pH

The largest survey of snack foods was carried out by Edgar *et al.* (1975) in America. They ranked 54 snack foods and drinks according to the value of the minimum pH reached by the plaque. This varied from pH 6.8 (virtually no pH depression) for 'sugarless' chewing-gum to pH 5.2 for a 'cherry sucker' (a hard fruit-flavoured sucrose sweet). Rugg-Gunn *et al.* (1978) ranked 22 British snacks and again found a boiled sweet gave the lowest pH minimum value. Sugared coffee and tea also gave low pH minimum values while peanuts tended to raise plaque pH. The availability of non-sucrose flavoured snacks and drinks has increased in recent years and Fig. 2.12 illustrates the difference in the acidogenicity of sucrose and non-sucrose containing snacks; diabetic chocolate is sweetened with sorbitol.

The indwelling glass electrode system tends to give an all-or-nothing response to foods. It has been very useful in demonstrating the non-acidogenic nature of non-carbohydrate foods but less useful at indicating the low acidogenicity of starchy foods such as bread. For example, one study reported that starchy foods (wheat-flakes and bread) produced deep pH responses, similar to those produced by sucrose, using the indwelling glass micro-electrode technique. The beneficial effect upon plaque pH of substituting sucrose or glucose by non-fermentable sweeteners in foods, drinks, and medicines will be discussed later in this chapter.

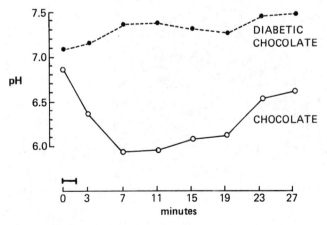

Fig. 2.12. Stephan curves produced by dark ('plain') chocolate (containing sugar) and 'diabetic' chocolate (containing sorbitol).

Different sugars and concentrations

Plaque pH studies have also been used to differentiate between the potential cariogenicity of different sugars and the different concentrations of sugar. Sucrose solutions in the range of 0.05–50 per cent have been tested by Frostell, and between 0.025 and 15 per cent by Imfeld. Their results (using different methods) are not in close agreement, for whereas Frostell found that rinses with 50 per cent solution produced a lower plaque pH than with 5 per cent solution, Imfeld observed deep and similar curves after rinses containing 2.5 per cent, 5 per cent, or 10 per cent sucrose. A fall in plaque pH of 1.5 units was also recorded after rinses with a very weak (0.025 per cent) sucrose solution, yet no comparable depression in the plaque pH was observed by Frostell. This may be an example of the all-or-nothing response of the indwelling glass electrode and it is therefore impossible to state, at present, a threshold concentration below which a sucrose solution may be considered safe.

Lactose (in both 10 per cent and 50 per cent solution) produced less severe falls in plaque pH than sucrose, glucose, or fructose. These results were confirmed by Imfeld, who also showed that galactose was of similar acidogenicity to lactose, and maltose of similar acidogenicity to sucrose, glucose, and fructose.

Meals and plaque pH

Although the effect of individual snacks has been investigated by many people, the acidogenicity of meals has not received much attention. Eating cheese after a sugary food (e.g. tinned pears in syrup) prevented the depression of plaque pH which otherwise would have been caused by the sugary food. Sugared coffee instead of the cheese further depressed plaque pH. The favourable action of cheese is likely to be due to (i) the high salivary flow rate induced by the strongly flavoured food; (ii) absence of fermentable carbohydrates. Peanuts and sugarless chewing-gum also have similar actions in raising the pH of plaque after it has been depressed by a sugary food. On the other hand, eating an apple was found to have little beneficial effect compared with peanuts.

The effect of the three-course 'breakfast' upon plaque pH has been described. The breakfast consisted of one sugary course (sugared coffee) and two non-sugary courses (a boiled egg, and crispbread and butter). The most favourable curve was produced when all three foods were taken together (curve F in Fig. 2.13); the fall in plaque pH being much less than when sugared coffee was taken alone (curve E). These experiments clearly show that one food can influence the acidogenicity of another.

INCUBATION EXPERIMENTS

These are simple tests and examine the ability of plaque micro organisms to metabolize a test food to acid. They are done outside the mouth and can be classed as 'test-tube experiments'. Saliva (which contains oral micro-organisms) or pure cultures of oral micro-organisms, have substituted for plaque. Rapid acid production is taken to indicate that the food under test is potentially cariogenic, while a slow rate of acid formation is likely to be of little clinical significance. To illustrate the point

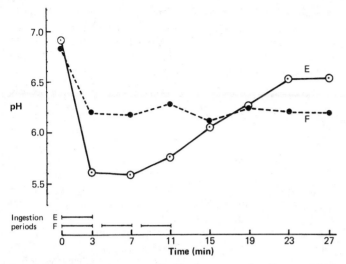

Fig. 2.13. Stephen curves produced when sugared coffee was taken alone (E) or taken together with the other two non-acidogenic foods (F). (Rugg-Gunn *et al.* 1981, with permission of the editor *Journal of Dental Research*.)

that all sugars can be fermented by plaque organisms, Bibby and Krobicka reported that the final pH reached after incubating 10 per cent solutions of sucrose, fructose, maltose, lactose, or raffinose, with plaque, were all below pH 4.5.

In some experiments, teeth, sectioned or powdered tooth enamel, or hydroxyapatite, were incubated with the test substance and organisms in order to simulate the dental caries process.

Extensive investigations of the potential cariogenicity of baby foods and drinks and other soft drinks have been reported. Potential cariogenicity was estimated from the amount of calcium and phosphorus released when the test products were incubated with hydroxyapatite and plaque organisms. Overall, the results indicate that sugars content was an important determinant of the amount of mineral dissolved, but other factors, such as the pH and buffering potential of the drink, were also relevant.

SUMMARY OF SUGAR AND DENTAL CARIES

The evidence relating diet and dental caries comes from several sources. It is important when reviewing the evidence to consider all these sources, although data from human studies should be considered the best type of data. From the evidence, the following conclusions can be made:

1. Sugar is the most cariogenic item in our diet.
2. Sucrose, glucose, fructose, and maltose are of similar cariogenicity. Lactose is less cariogenic.
3. Frequency of eating/drinking sugar is important. However, frequency of intake and weight of sugars consumed are closely correlated.

STARCHY FOODS AND DENTAL CARIES

It has been suggested that all carbohydrate foods should be considered cariogenic. The term fermentable carbohydrate

has been widely used as the dietary cause of dental caries; indeed, Miller (1890) launched the acidogenic theory of caries with his experiments on the incubation of starchy foods, saliva, and enamel. In Britain, as in many countries, current advice for healthy eating is to decrease consumption of fat, sugar, salt, and alcohol, and to increase consumption of starchy foods, fresh fruit, and vegetables. Because of this, it is sensible to consider the relative cariogenicity of starch compared with sugars as a separate issue. As with all aspects of cariogenicity, it is important to look at evidence from all sources and these will be discussed in turn.

HUMAN OBSERVATIONAL STUDIES

In two publications, Sreebny (1982, 1983) listed and correlated the caries status of 47 countries with the availability of sugar and cereals in those countries. The caries status was measured by the DMFT index for 12-year-old children, obtained primarily from the WHO Global Epidemiology Bank: data on sugar and grain availability were obtained from the food balance sheets compiled by the Food and Agricultural Organization of the UN. Cereal availability was quantified in two ways: (a) as the number of calories provided by the cereal per day: and (b) as the proportion of total energy intake provided by that cereal. Sreebny gave only bivariate correlations and showed that, while the correlation between sugar availability and DMFT was +0.72, the correlation between total cereals availability and DMFT was −0.25 (calculated as cal/day) and −0.45 (calculated as per cent of total energy). However, for wheat, positive correlations with DMFT were found (+0.45 and +0.30). Sreebny's data have been examined further, using partial correlation analyses (Table 2.8); this allows an examination of the caries versus cereal relationship, when the effect of differences in sugar availability is removed. It can be seen (in the right-hand column of Table 2.8) that all of the partial correlation between DMFT and sugar availability and DMFT are low and not statistically

Table 2.8. Correlations and partial correlations between DMFT (for 12-year-olds) and sugar or cereal availability in 47 countries. (Raw data taken from Sreebny 1982, 1983.)

		Bivariate correlation	Partial correlation, controlling for sugar availability
Total cereals	cal/day	−0.25	−0.03
	% of energy	−0.45***	−0.13
Wheat	cal/day	+0.45***	+0.05
	% of energy	+0.29	−0.03
Rice	cal/day	−0.07	+0.10
	% of energy	−0.09	+0.10
Maize	cal/day	−0.37*	−0.24
	% of energy	−0.40**	−0.26
Sugar	(g/day)	+0.70***	
	controlling for total cereal (cal/day)		+0.67***
	controlling for wheat (cal/day)		+0.60***

*** $p < 0.005$ ** $p < 0.01$ * $p < 0.05$

significant. On the other hand, it can be seen in the lower part of Table 2.8 that when the correlation between DMFT and sugar availability ($r = +0.70$, using Sreebny's data) was controlled for cereal availability, the correlation fell only slightly to $+0.67$ ($p < 0.001$) and $+0.60$ ($p < 0.001$) when controlling for the two measures of wheat availability. These findings suggest a much closer positive relation between DMFT and sugar availability than between DMFT and cereal availability.

Newbrun *et al.* (1980) compared diets and the dental status of 17 subjects with the rare disorder—hereditary fructose intolerance (HFI)—with 14 control subjects who were unaffected and mostly blood-relations. The mean ages were 29 years for the HFI subjects and 27 years for the control subjects. The respective mean DMFT scores were 2.1 and 14.3, and DMFS 3.3 and 36.1. The respective daily sucrose consumption was 3 g and 48 g, and the respective mean daily starch consumption was 160 g and 140 g. The nutrient, vitamin, and mineral contents of the diets of the two groups were similar. The finding that the HFI subjects consumed high levels of starch (higher than the control subjects) and yet developed minimal caries levels must indicate that starch is not particularly caries-inducive. Newbrun also concluded that while a diet with a high content and a high frequency of sucrose is cariogenic, a diet with an extremely low content of sucrose is non-cariogenic.

Although over 30 cross-sectional studies have correlated sugar-eating habits with dental caries experience, only a few of these have considered starch intake. In a comprehensive cross-sectional study of Swedish 14-year-old children, Martinsson compared the diet of children with high (H) caries experience (mean DFS = 37) with the diet of children with low (L) caries experience (DFS = 8). The H-group had a higher intake of sucrose, but this difference was statistically significant in the boys only. The intake of potatoes and bread was similar in the two groups, but the consumption of groats and flakes was higher in the caries-low children. The author stated that 'only the carbohydrate intake in the form of sucrose, especially between meals, was found to be significantly higher in the H-group than in the L-group', Hankin and colleagues reported the relationship between the dietary patterns and caries prevalence in Hawaiian schoolchildren. They found that the consumption of sugared gum and candy was strongly positively associated with DMFT ($p < 0.001$), but the consumption of breads and cereals was negatively associated with DMFT ($p < 0.05$). Kleemola-Kujala and Rasanen reported the dietary intake of low-caries and high-caries children of three different age groups (5, 9, and 13 years). While the total carbohydrate was similar in each pair of high- and low-caries groups, the intake of sugar was higher in each of the three high-caries groups, although the differences were statistically significant for the 5- and 13-year-old groups only. Calculated by subtraction, the intake of starch would have been higher in the low-caries groups.

A longitudinal observational study was conducted between 1979 and 1981 in northern England: 405 children initially aged 11.5 years completed the 2-year study. Sugars intake was positively correlated with DMFS increment ($p < 0.05$), but starch intake was not. When the starch versus caries correlations were controlled for sugars intake, they became negative, although not statistically significantly so. The children who had a high sugar/low starch diet developed 4.1 DMFS compared with 2.8 DMFS in the children who had a low sugar/high starch diet, although this difference of 1.3 tooth surfaces was not statistically significant.

HUMAN INTERVENTIONAL STUDIES

The main purpose of the Turku sugar studies (see p. 13 for detail) was to investigate the effect on dental caries of total substitution of dietary sugars with either fructose of xylitol. About 100 dietary items were especially manufactured by 12 food firms in Finland, in order to ensure that as wide a variety of foods as possible was available, Fructose or xylitol was substituted for sucrose but the starch content of the foods was not altered. The mean 2-year DMFS increments for the sucrose, fructose, and xylitol groups were 7.2, 3.8, and 0.0, respectively when precavitation carious lesions were included. When such lesions were excluded from the analyses and only cavities recorded, the 2-year increments were 3.33, 3.57, and 1.47 for the sugar, fructose, and xylitol groups, respectively. The trial showed that substitution of sucrose by xylitol resulted in a substantial reduction in caries incidence. As the starch intake was unaltered, dietary starch cannot have contributed significantly to caries development in these human subjects.

ANIMAL EXPERIMENTS

Animal experiments which have assessed the cariogenicity of starch have given variable results. Raw starches would appear to have very low cariogenicity, regardless of the method of feeding. In experiments where the animals were fed *ad libitum*, cooked starch caused caries, but the amount was less than that caused by sucrose: for example, in one study pre-gelatinized starch caused half as much caries as sucrose. Mixtures of starch and sucrose caused more caries than starch alone and the amount of caries developing was positively related to the amount of sugar in the starch/sugar food. Baking of starch/sugar mixtures increases their cariogenicity markedly. The oral flora of rats (or the amylase levels in the rat's salivary glands) did not adapt to metabolize starch more rapidly when several generations of rats were fed a starch diet.

In animal experiments where frequency of feeding was standardized, cooked starch or starchy foods (e.g. bread) were shown to be capable of causing caries but were less cariogenic than sucrose. Caries development increased as frequency of feeding starchy foods increased. A recently published study indicated that while sugars (excluding lactose) were positively correlated with caries development in rats, the correlation between starch intake and caries development was zero. When only the test foods were taken orally by the rats and the rest of the diet fed by stomach tube, a similar picture emerged with some caries developing when starchy foods were eaten but less than that caused by sucrose. The relevance of this type of feeding can be questioned as it is not the way foods are eaten in man, and there is no opportunity for foods to interact to influence caries development. Foods in animal experiments have to be given in a powdered form and not in the physical form in which they are consumed by humans. A further problem in extrapolation of findings on starch cariogenicity in the rat to its effect in man is that the buffering capacity of rat saliva is less than that of primates such as monkeys or humans. Clearly, animal experiments are useful in giving an indication of the cariogenicity of foods in man, but caution in their interpretation is necessary.

PLAQUE pH STUDIES

Plaque pH experiments investigate acidogenicity, not cariogenicity. Almost all of the plaque pH experiments with starch have been carried out using either the sampling method or the indwelling glass electrode method. The sampling method has tended to indicate that cooked starch or starchy foods are less acidogenic than sugar or high sugar foods. On the other hand, indwelling glass electrode experiments have shown that starch is capable of depressing plaque pH to below what is commonly called the 'critical pH' (pH 5.5) to a similar extent as sugar and, by these criteria, starch cannot be labelled 'safe for teeth'. These findings have led workers to conclude 'that the starch in foods may be a more important contributor to the acidogenicity of sugar-containing foods than generally is believed'. Whether this adequately reflects what occurs naturally in man has been questioned by others. They suggested that the indwelling glass electrode 'tends to give an all-or-nothing response to foods—any carbohydrate-containing food leading to a maximum drop in pH. This feature makes the application of the method to evaluating relative cariogenicity of normal snack foods difficult, as foods such as bread, judged to be of low relative cariogenicity by other methods, appear highly cariogenic, and the technique has mainly found favour in verifying the low cariogenicity of some sugar substitutes.'

ENAMEL SLAB EXPERIMENTS

There have been two reports of the effect of starchy foods upon the demineralization of enamel slabs worn in the mouth of volunteers; both indicated that starch is about one-quarter as 'cariogenic' as sugar.

INCUBATION EXPERIMENTS

Miller (1890) established, over a century ago, that when carbohydrate foods (such as bread) were incubated with oral organisms, acid was produced and this acidic incubate was capable of demineralizing tooth enamel. Since then many experiments have been conducted to elucidate the cariogenicity of foods, and these experiments have used a variety of methods.

Unlike sugars, starch is not transported across the cell membrane of plaque micro-organisms and must be split into sugars before it can be used by the cell and acid produced. This is achieved by amylase in saliva and plaque, but the rate at which it happens will vary, depending on salivary amylase levels and the nature of the starchy food. Solutions of starch are quickly degraded to sugars, but this is not the form in which starch is commonly eaten.

SUMMARY OF STARCH AND DENTAL CARIES

1. Cooked staple starchy foods, such a rice, potatoes, pasta, and bread would appear to be of very low cariogenicity in man.
2. If finely ground, heat-treated and eaten frequently, starch can cause caries but the amount is much less than that caused by sucrose.
3. The addition of sugar increases the cariogenicity of cooked starchy foods. Foods containing baked starch and substantial amounts of sucrose appear to be as cariogenic as a similar amount of sucrose.

FRUIT, FRUIT PRODUCTS, AND DENTAL CARIES

INTRODUCTION

Many reports have urged the population of the UK, and other industrialized countries, to increase its consumption of fresh fruit and vegetables in order to improve health. The Department of Health (1989) Committee on Medical Aspects of Food Policy (COMA) report on dietary sugars and human disease made this point strongly. It concluded, amongst other things, that 'fresh fruits, as eaten by humans, also appear to be of low cariogenicity' and 'In order to reduce the risk of dental caries, the Panel recommends that consumption of non-milk extrinsic sugars by the population should be decreased. These sugars should be replaced by fresh fruit, vegetables and starchy foods'.

The report stated clearly that consumption of *fresh* fruit and vegetables should be increased. Fruit juices were considered to contain extrinsic sugars, and the report stated that 'There is no reason to suppose that natural syrups (e.g. honey, maple syrup, concentrated fruit juices) are not cariogenic. Dried fruits (raisins, dates, and figs) were not specifically mentioned in the report with reference to dental caries, although it can be assumed that they were outside the definition of 'fresh fruit', and contain intrinsic rather than extrinsic sugars.

Thus, there are three aspects to consider in this chapter: first, the role of fresh fruit and vegetables, secondly, dried fruit and, thirdly, fruit juices. It should be appreciated that the amount of published information is small. This is especially true of vegetables, which have never been regarded as an important issue, except as a possible 'tooth-cleaner'.

HUMAN CLINICAL STUDIES

Observational studies

A number of local cross-sectional studies have compared fruit consumption with dental caries experience, but the most significant observational study was reported in South Africa which had the purpose of determining the effect of a high intake of either apples or grapes on dental caries experience and periodontal health of farm workers in the South Western Cape Province. The subjects were adults of both sexes, aged 15 years or more, who had lived on farms in three districts for a minimum of 8 years. These three districts grew predominantly apple, grape, or grain crops; the grain district served as a control area.

Table 2.9. Effect of high consumption of apples or grapes on experience of dental caries in South African adults

Farm workers	*n*(*n* males)	DMFT*	MT	DFT
Apple growers	95 (60)	24	20	4
Grape growers	109 (65)	17	13	4
Grain growers	50 (25)	10	4	6

MT: mean number of missing teeth per person.
DFT: mean number of decayed or filled teeth per person.
* Differences between groups were all significant ($p < 0.05$).

The results are given in Table 2.9. Dental caries experience (DMFT) was significantly higher in the adults from the apple-growing area than from the grape-growing area, and the dental caries experience of both these groups was significantly greater than that observed in the control (grain-growing) area. The authors state that workers in the apple area consumed at least eight apples per day during the picking period which lasted about 5 months; workers in the grape-growing area consumed at least eight bunches of grapes per day during a season which lasted 3 months. They concluded that 'the consumption of a high amount of apples and to a lesser degree, grapes, contributed to the development of dental caries'. One unexplained feature of the results can be seen in the two right-hand columns of Table 2.9, in that all the difference between groups was due to missing teeth (MT) and the number of decayed and filled teeth (DFT) did not differ between groups. No information is given on erosion of teeth, which would be expected to occur with such high intakes of fruit, and which can be difficult to distinguish from dental caries.

Interventional studies

Children living in National Children's Homes or Family Group Homes in Liverpool, UK, were offered 1 cm slices of crisp apple at the end of each meal and after any between-meal snacks. The children were divided into three age groups—under 6 years, 6–10 years, and 11–15 years—at the start of the 2-year trial. Development of dental caries in both primary teeth and permanent teeth was less in the apple group than in the control group, in all three age groups.

ANIMAL EXPERIMENTS

There have been a number of investigations into the cariogenicity of fruits in animals. The biggest series was carried out in the USA, more than 20 years ago. The experiments tested a total of 53 foods. Dental caries scores were considerably greater in the groups fed figs, apples, bananas, grapes, raisins, and dates, than the groups fed peanuts, citrus fruits, vegetables, and dried apricots, but all were less than the mean score of the sucrose group. The author stated that 'this finding fails to support the frequently voiced opinion that foods with naturally occurring sugars (sucrose, dextrose, fructose, or maltose), such as fruits, are non-cariogenic, or that fruits in general contain some unknown protective substances which presumably render them non-cariogenic'.

A rat study was reported where four groups of rats all received a basic diet by intubation: a positive control group received a cariogenic sucrose/starch (1:1 ratio) mixture, a negative control group was fed by intubation only, and the two test groups received either 'Milchschnitte' (a white cream-filled wafer snack) or apple. The total number of fissure lesions in the groups were: positive control 11.5, Milchschnitte 8.3, apple 6.8, and negative control 1.8.

Bananas and raisins were two of 22 snack foods tested using the rat caries model, which involves programmed feeding and feeding of essential nutrients by gastric intubation. The caries potential index was given as 1.1 for bananas and 1.2 for raisins, relative to a score of 1.0 for sucrose. It should be noted that peanuts gave a score of 0.4 in these experiments, while they have usually been classed as non-cariogenic by other workers.

PLAQUE pH STUDIES

One of the first investigations into the effect of eating foods upon plaque pH was reported by Ludwig and Bibby. Using the plaque sampling method, they found that apples 'gave rise to more acid than the ice-cream or potatoes' but considerably less than that produced by a 20 per cent glucose solution.

Using the indwelling micro-electrode system for monitoring, plaque pH fell to below 4.5 after eating half an apple, in experiments using both 1-day-old and 4-day-old plaque. No rise in pH was observed after 60 minutes. Subsequently experiments showed that the pH response to fresh fruit depended on its texture as well as its sugar content. Banana was classed as an 'acidogenic' food, since plaque pH fell to below 4.0 and remained low for at least 90 minutes. Apples were also classed as 'acidogenic', although the pH fell briefly to only 5.0, while oranges were 'hypoacidogenic', with plaque pH remaining above 6.0. Of the dried fruit tested, dates and raisins were acidogenic (low pH for a long period of time) while dried apricot and dried apple led to minimal falls in plaque pH.

More recently the acidogenicities of Milchschnitte and apple have been compared with a positive control (sucrose) and a negative control (sorbitol). Both Milchschnitte and apple were classed as 'acidogenic'.

INCUBATION EXPERIMENTS

Bibby has been a co-author of several published reports in this field. In 1951, he and colleagues listed 'decalcification potentials' for 96 foods. Apple gave a score of 4 (the lowest of any of the 96 foods), pineapple 22, peach 48, pear 130, grape 145, plum 167, banana 180, date 505, and fig 665; these can be compared with the score of sugar of 231. Vegetables tended to give low scores—carrot 4, lettuce 16, cucumber 25, and cabbage 43.

Bibby and Mundorff compared the degree of enamel demineralization which occurred when food and saliva were incubated with powdered enamel, for 180 American snack foods. Raisins produced twice as much (206 per cent) and apples produced slightly more (103 per cent) dissolution than sucrose, while bananas produced slightly less (92 per cent) and dates much less (29 per cent) dissolution than that produced by sucrose.

FRUIT JUICES, FRUIT FLAVOURED DRINKS, AND DENTAL CARIES

The relationship between the use of sugar in infancy and extensive (rampant) caries in the deciduous dentition was mentioned previously and the use of sugar most closely related to rampant dental caries in infancy is the provision of fruit, or fruit-flavoured, drinks with sugar added. This is an important cause of dental morbidity in young children, and the subject has been well reviewed by Winter (1980, 1988).

One of the earliest observations was made by Pitts, who concluded that the administration of dummies dipped into sugary liquids was the most important cause of caries of the deciduous incisor teeth. Syrrist and Selander, in a study of the incidence of dental caries and comforter habits of 1332 Swedish children, found a slight increase in the frequency of dental caries in the central and lateral incisors of the upper jaw in those children that had used a sweetened comforter. They described the unique labial caries picture most often observed in the sugar-comforter children.

James and colleagues supported those findings, stating that 'the occurrence of early labial caries of the deciduous incisors is strongly associated with local factors involving the retention of sweet, sticky and acid substances on the labial enamel surfaces. The most important vehicles were found to be sweetened comforters'.

In a survey of 110 pre-school children, the addition of sugar to bottles was observed to be an important factor in the occurrence of incisor caries. Very similar findings were reported in a survey of 100 pre-school children, who stated that the most important factor was 'the frequent and prolonged ingestion of milk, fruit juices or syrup which have been sweetened by the addition of sugar'. In a large survey of 6837 children, aged 1 and 2 years, gave 'propped bottles', 'infant feeders', and 'dummies dipped in vitamin syrup' as important causes of incisor caries.

Because of these reports, the Ministry of Health, London, UK, asked an expert panel to report on this issue. It did so in 1969 and the first four of its nine recommendations were:

(1) that reservoir feeders be abolished;
(2) that additional sucrose should not be added to welfare orange juice;
(3) that mothers be advised to use only plain dummies for comforting their babies; and
(4) that all vitamin supplements should carry cautions as to their use as comforting agents, as indeed some do now.

Since then, a series of three surveys of dental caries in pre-school children living in Camden, London, UK, have been undertaken by Winter, Holt, and colleagues. In the first survey (in 1966–68) 602 children, aged 12–60 months, were examined, and a prevalence of 8 per cent rampant dental caries was recorded. Prolonged bottle feeding and the use of sweetened comforters was clearly related to all forms of caries in the deciduous dentition. The authors reported that

The contents of the sweetened comforters and the cariogenic potential of each of the sweetening agents were assessed and compared with each other. With sweetened comforters in general, rose hip syrup and blackcurrant syrup appeared to be more significantly related to the prevalence of caries than any other of three sweetening agents ($p < 0.02$ and < 0.01). When comforter bottles were assessed alone not only did rose hip syrup and blackcurrant syrup appear to be most significantly related to caries ($p < 0.05$ and < 0.01) but the addition of sugar to the bottle was also seen to be significant factor ($p < 0.05$). When dummies and hollow feeders were assessed alone it was seen that sugar by itself was significantly more liable ($p < 0.05$) to cause decay than the other substances used.

The prevalence of dental caries was reported to be lower in the second survey in Camden in 1980, but by the third survey in 1986, the prevalence of dental caries had risen to the level previously observed in 1966–68: the percentage of children with rampant caries was 12 per cent, 9 per cent, and 11 per cent in the three studies, respectively. In all three surveys, the use of sweetened comforters was a major aetiological factor. The percentage of children using sweetened comforters, in the three surveys respectively, was 57 per cent, 19 per cent, and 46 per cent, respectively—a pattern broadly reflected by the proportion with rampant dental caries.

Silver also recorded a strong relationship between the use of a sweetened bottle and the prevalence of dental caries in 3-year-olds, and between the use of a sweetened bottle in early childhood and the consumption of sweet snacks at the age of 8 to 10 years.

SUMMARY OF FRUIT, FRUIT PRODUCTS, AND DENTAL CARIES

1. Fresh fruit, dried fruit, and fruit juices are capable of causing dental caries, but their role as a cause of dental caries in humans differs, as indicated below.
2. Sugared, fruit-flavoured drinks when used as a comforter are as significant cause of dental caries in young children. Virtually all the reports mention fruit-flavoured drinks (containing added sugars) and not pure fruit juices as a cause of dental caries. However, this may be due to the greater availability in the past of sugared fruit-flavoured drinks, compared with pure fruit juices.
3. As eaten by free-living people, fresh fruit appears to be of low cariogenicity. Citrus fruits have not been associated with the development of dental caries. Large consumption of apples and grapes can result in dental caries, but this has only been recorded in one study and such high consumption is outside usual levels in most countries. Bananas appear to have greater potential than citrus fruits or apples to cause dental caries, but this does not appear to have occurred in man.
4. High consumption of fruit or fruit juice is one cause of dental erosion.
5. On present evidence, increasing consumption of fresh fruit by the population in the UK, in order to decrease consumption of non-milk extrinsic sugars, as recommended by the Department of Health, is likely to decrease the level of dental caries in the population.

MILK, CHEESE, AND OTHER PROTECTIVE FACTORS

INTRODUCTION

Milk is one of the main sources of sugar in the human diet. For infants, it is the only source, and its importance declines after weaning, so by early adolescence the 12 g of lactose consumed per child per day contributes about 10 per cent of the total intake of sugars. In general, milk is not seen as a cause of dental caries, and the Department of Health (1989) COMA report on dietary sugars and human disease concluded that: 'Although lactose alone is moderately cariogenic, milk also contains factors which protect against dental caries, so that milk without added sugars may be considered to be virtually non-cariogenic'.

Various components of milk have been considered to be protective against dental caries, namely the minerals, casein, and other lipid and protein components. Cheese, a product of milk, has been the subject of much interest among dental scientists over the last two decades and it is considered by many to have substantial protective properties against dental caries.

Many components of plants are believed to help protect teeth against dental caries. More than 50 years ago, refining cereal and other plant foods was thought to remove some protective factor(s), and this lead to much work on the possible use of various phosphorus-containing compounds in prevention of dental caries. Cocoa contains a factor which may help to make chocolate less cariogenic than other sugar-containing confectionery, and liquorice also contains a caries-protective factor. The positive role of dietary fibre in maintaining oral health has been much discussed but little researched.

MILK AND CHEESE

Milk

Both human milk and cow's milk contain lactose, about 7 g/100 g in human milk and about 4.8 g/100 g in cow's milk (Table 2.10). These amounts could be sufficient to classify milks as cariogenic, but it should be remembered that lactose is the least cariogenic of the common dietary sugars. In addition, the high concentrations of calcium and phorphorus in milks will help to prevent dissolution of enamel (which is largely calcium and phosphate) and other factors may be protective as well. Thus, it is possible that milk could be caries-promoting (due to the lactose content), caries-preventing, or somewhere between these two. How the milk is taken—for example, the frequency and duration of exposure—is also important in determining in which direction the health-disease see-saw tilts. The amounts of calcium and phosphorus in human and cow's milk are quite different (Table 2.10); thus these two milks may have rather different cariogenic potentials.

There have been a few reports of dental caries being associated with 'on demand' breast-feeding and, more rarely, prolonged bottle-feeding with cow's or formula milk. Only seven reports of 13 specific cases relating prolonged breast-

Table 2.10. The average lactose, calcium, and phosphorus content of human and bovine (cow's) milk

	Lactose (g/100 ml)	Calcium (mg/100 ml)	Phosphorus (mg/100 ml)
Human milk	7.0	33	15
Bovine milk	4.8	125	96

feeding (at least 14 months and usually over two years) to rampant dental caries. Nine of these reports state that the children were fed 'at will', four children definitely suckled at night, four others slept with their mothers (with night-feeding implied), and another child was said to have suckled and slept alternatively. In four cases the suckling habit in relation to sleep was not reported. The food intake, apart from human milk, has probably not been adequately assessed in most of these cases, and more comprehensive reports would certainly be useful; nevertheless, the factors common to these reports appear to be prolonged breast-feeding and feeding at night.

Evidence from animal experiments not only indicates that cow's milk is non-cariogenic, but also strongly suggests an anti-cariogenic effect. Several studies have shown that the fall in plaque pH after drinking milk is negligible. In the studies of Rugg-Gunn *et al.* (1985) (Fig. 2.14), 14 volunteers rinsed their mouths with cow's milk, human milk, lactose solution, or sucrose solution. Sucrose solution caused substantial falls in plaque pH, while the milks depressed plaque pH only slightly.

Jenkins and Ferguson conducted *in vitro* comparisons of 4 per cent lactose solutions and cow's milk. They concluded that, within the limits of their experiments, their results 'gave no grounds for suggesting that milk has a local effect on the teeth which would favour caries', and suggested that the negligible fall in plaque pH was partly due to milk's high buffering power, and the low level of dissolution of test enamel was due to the protective action of milk's high levels of calcium and phosphate.

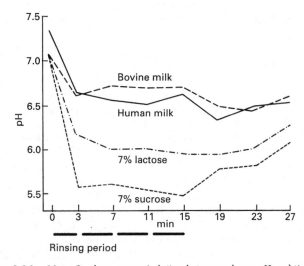

Fig. 2.14. Mean Stephan curves (relation between plaque pH and time) for 14 volunteer subjects who rinsed with bovine (cow's) milk, human milk, 7 per cent lactose or 7 per cent sucrose, four times during 15 minutes. (Reproduced from Rugg-Gunn *et al.* 1985, with permission of the editor *Caries Research*.)

Thus, in conclusion, milk can be considered non-cariogenic for practical purposes. Human milk is likely to have greater cariogenic potential, but dental caries in human infants due to breast-feeding is very rare and is always associated with prolonged, on-demand feeding.

Cheese

There is now strong evidence from a variety of sources that several types of cheese are not only non-cariogenic but also have anti-caries properties. One of the earliest reports of cheese's potential in prevention of dental caries showed that Emmental cheese reduced dental caries in rats when added to bread. This was followed by the plaque pH studies which demonstrated that eating cheese after a sugar-containing snack raised the pH of plaque back to a safe level.

Several mechanisms have been proposed to explain the anti-caries properties of cheese. These include: (1) the strong stimulation of salivary flow with its favourable properties; (2) raising the calcium concentration in plaque; (3) increasing the amount of basic substances in plaque; and (4) adsorption of protein (such as casein) on to the enamel surface, thereby physically slowing the caries process.

Cheese is a powerful sialogogue, as can be seen in Fig. 2.15. Although a bolus of cheese is initially acidic (pH 5.9 would be typical), within three minutes of ingestion the pH rises to 7.5 (Figure 2.15), thus favouring remineralization. Taking the evidence available from all sources, there are good grounds for recommending cheese as a caries-preventive food.

PROTECTIVE FACTORS DERIVED MAINLY FROM PLANT PRODUCTS

The observations of Osborn and his colleagues that South African Bantu have very low caries prevalence, despite a high-carbohydrate diet, began the search for factors in human diets which may protect teeth against dental caries.

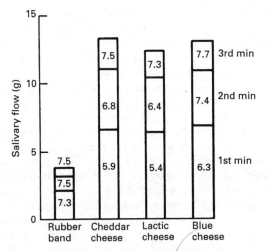

Fig. 2.15. Salivary flow produced during one minute periods (measured in g/min) upon chewing either a rubber band (mechanical chewing action only) or three types of cheese. Mean values for six subjects. pH values of the 'bolus' are given within the columns. (Reproduced from Rugg-Gunn *et al.* 1975, with permission of the editor *British Dental Journal.*)

As they also observed that less enamel dissolved from teeth incubated with 'unrefined' than with 'refined' foods, they suspected that these 'protective factors' act locally in the mouth rather than systematically via the developing tooth. However, it must be noted that the observed high-carbohydrate diets were low in sugar. Since then many possible 'protective factors', not necessarily normal constituents of food, have been studied, and their relevance in caries prevention will be discussed briefly. Some of the most widely studied of these 'protective factors' are inorganic phosphates and the cation is frequently calcium. This would seem logical because the caries process involves dissolution of enamel, which is very largely calcium and phosphate, and therefore any rise in the concentration of these two ions in plaque or saliva surrounding the tooth would, by the law of mass action, result in less enamel dissolving. The availability of calcium and phosphate during demineralization phases would also be increased aiding repair of the lesions. Phosphates have the additional advantage of being good buffers and their presence in plaque would therefore resist depression of plaque pH towards the 'critical pH'. Some organic phosphates have also been tested but, unlike inorganic phosphates, act mainly by binding to the tooth surface and reducing its solubility. The evidence concerning the effectiveness of protective factors comes principally from three sources, all important: animal experiments: laboratory experiments (largely enamel dissolution experiments in acid buffer or saliva incubates); and human clinical trials.

The categories of compounds investigated include: (1) inorganic phosphates, with sodium salts tending to be more caries-protective than the less soluble calcium salts, (2) trimetaphosphates, again with the sodium salt preferred, (3) calcium sucrose phosphate and calcium glycerophosphate, and (4) phytate. As a general rule, the inorganic phosphates are thought to act by increasing the phosphate levels in plaque and so helping to resist enamel dissolution through the law of mass action, while the organic compounds act by covering the enamel surface and physically slowing the dissolution process. Of all the compounds, phytate seemed to be most promising, but since it interferes with absorption of minerals from the gut, its use as a caries-preventive food additive seems unlikely.

Cocoa factor and liquorice

In the Vipeholm study (p. 11) the patients in the chocolate group developed less caries than other groups receiving similar sugar levels and frequency of eating. This led to speculation that chocolate might contain 'protective factors'. A subsidiary experiment to test this was, for various reasons, indecisive. Animal experiments also suggested that cocoa may have a caries-protective effect. Extraction is expensive and application of the cocoa factor as a method of caries prevention would be less efficient than the use of fluoride.

Likewise, the major constituent of liquorice—glycyrrhizinic acid—has potentially caries-preventive properties. Glycyrrhizinic acid acts in three ways: it reduces enamel dissolution in acid buffer/enamel systems, inhibits glycolysis, and increases plaque buffering power. However, it does have the undesirable properties of strong taste, dark staining, and, more importantly, it disturbs the body electrolyte balance. Its usefulness as a dietary additive may therefore be limited.

Fibre

There has been remarkably little research into the effect of fibre (now know by nutritionists as non-starch polysaccharide) and dental caries. For years, people have assumed that fibrous foods clean the teeth by their physical action, stimulate helpful salivary flow, and improve gingival health by exercising the jaws and stimulating the gingivae.

One of the few reviews of the effect of physical properties of foods on dental caries experience concluded that fibrous foods do not clean plaque from areas where dental caries commonly occurs in humans: secondly both liquids and solid foods cause dental caries and that stickiness may not be such an important factor in development of dental caries, as was initially concluded from the results of the Vipeholm study. The third aspect discussed was salivary flow, and it is this aspect which is likely to be the only positive anti-caries attribute of fibre.

SUMMARY OF PROTECTIVE FACTORS AND DENTAL CARIES

Some constituents of foods undoubtedly help to protect teeth against dental caries. Milk contains factors which are sufficient, in almost all circumstances, to counteract any cariogenic potential of lactose in milk. These factors— calcium, phosphorus, casein, and fats—have been studied fairly extensively in the search for possible caries-protective food additives. Cheese is very likely to be caries-protective, due to several favourable attributes; however, as yet, no clinical trials have been conducted to demonstrate the extent of the protection. Plants also contain factors which have been shown to protect against dental caries. The most thoroughly investigated factors have been the phosphates, which gave very promising results in rat experiments, but largely negative results in human clinical trials. Other constituents of foods—in cocoa, liquorice, and possibly tannins—may help to protect enamel from caries attack, but their practical potential in prevention of dental caries seems, at present, to be very limited. The role of dietary fibre is difficult to determine. On balance, it is likely to have caries-preventive properties, very largely because fibrous foods require more chewing than non-fibrous foods, and the increased salivary flow induced by chewing is beneficial.

NON-SUGAR SWEETENERS

TYPES OF SWEETENERS

Table 2.11 lists the more commonly discussed of the many sweet-tasting compounds. The number which are synthesized, rather than being naturally occurring compounds, has been steadily growing since the last century. Fluctuations in the price of natural sweeteners (e.g. sucrose) and their incrimination in the cause of disease such as caries, has accelerated

Table 2.11. Some sweet-tasting compounds

		Approx. sweetness relative to sucrose
Sugars	Glucose	0.7
	Fructose	1.2
	Sorbose	0.9
	Sucrose	**1.0**
	Lactose	0.3
	Maltose	0.4
Sugar compounds	Glucosylsucrose*	—
	Maltosylsucrose*	—
	Trichlorosucrose*	1000
	Sucralose	600
Sugar alcohols	Xylitol	1.0
	Sorbitol	0.5
	Mannitol	0.7
	Maltitol	0.75
	Lactitol	0.35
Complex	Hydrogenated glucose syrup*	0.75
	Isomalt*	0.5
Dipeptide	Aspartame*	180
Polypeptides	Monellin	3000
	Thaumatin	4000
Miscellaneous	Saccharin*	500
	Cyclamate*	50
	Stevioside	200
	Acesulfame potassium*	130
	Glycyrrhizin	50

* Not naturally occurring

the search for alternative sweeteners and, although many are at present expensive to manufacture, new technology and increased production will, no doubt, make them financially competitive. Not all the compounds give the same sweet taste. The slightly bitter after taste of saccharin is well known. Glycyrrhizin has a liquorice taste. Xylitol and other sugar alcohols have a negative heat of dissolution resulting in a cool taste when eaten. Polypeptides are known for their prolonged sweet taste. Sweetness relative to sucrose varies widely (Table 2.11); some of the compounds are not thermostable and are destroyed in food manufacture.

Although a very large number of sweet compounds are known, relatively few are permitted to be used in foods; those that are permitted will vary from country to country. In the United Kingdom, the list of permitted sweeteners was revised in 1982. Previously, only sorbitol and mannitol were permitted as 'bulk sweeteners', but the 1982 report recommended that three more—hydrogenated glucose syrup, isomalt, and xylitol—be permitted, in addition to sorbitol and mannitol. The report also recommended that three further 'intense sweeteners' be permitted: acesulfame potassium, aspartame, and thaumatin, where previously only saccharin was allowed. The bulk sweetener lactitol was permitted subsequently. It is hoped that this expansion of the list of permitted sweeteners will allow manufacturers, particularly of confectionery and soft drinks, to increase their range of 'sugarless' foods and drinks.

RELATIVE CARIOGENICITY OF NON-SUGAR SWEETENERS

Sorbitol and mannitol

Sorbitol and mannitol occur naturally in small quantities in a number of plants. Sorbitol is used extensively in foods manufactured for diabetics as the metabolism of sorbitol is insulin-independent. Sorbitol is commonly used as the sweetener in sugarless syrup medicines; mannitol is used mainly in chewing-gum and the amount consumed is very small compared with sorbitol.

Sorbitol and mannitol are fermented slowly by plaque organisms but the rate is very much slower than that of glucose or sucrose. Sorbitol and mannitol depress plaque pH only slightly (Fig. 2.16). When diets containing sorbitol were fed to rats or monkeys little caries developed in comparison with glucose or sucrose diets. *Strep, mutans* can adapt to metabolize sorbitol *in vivo* but only when sorbitol is the sole energy source and this is very unlikely to occur in man. In enamel slab experiments, sorbitol and mannitol gave rise to 45 per cent of the demineralization of enamel attributable to sucrose. Clinical trials of sorbitol have been limited to use in chewing-gum providing partial substitution of dietary sugars; these are discussed below.

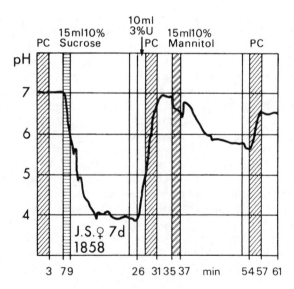

Fig. 2.16. Telemetrically recorded plaque pH after rinsing with (a) 15 ml of 10 per cent sucrose solution, (b) 15 ml of 10 per cent mannitol solution. (From Imfeld 1977, with permission of the editor *Helvetica odontologica Acta*.)

Xylitol

Xylitol also occurs naturally in foods in small quantities. Its use at present is confined to confectionery and toothpaste.

In all tests of cariogenicity it would appear to be non-cariogenic. Numerous incubation experiments have demonstrated that xylitol is fermented to acid very slowly (if at all) in comparison with glucose or even sorbitol. Plaque pH studies confirm the non-acidogenicity of xylitol and rat experiments have shown xylitol to be non-cariogenic. The Turku

sugar study showed that total substitution of dietary sugar by xylitol resulted in very low caries incidence; the use of xylitol chewing-gum is discussed below.

Hydrogenated glucose syrup

The hydrogenated glucose syrup approved for use in foods is manufactured by Roquette (France) and sold under the trade name Lycasin®. It contains less than 0.3 per cent free sugars, and is used in the manufacture of a variety of foods, drinks, and liquid medicines.

Lycasin is fermented slowly compared with sucrose and causes minimal depression of plaque pH when taken as a syrup or as a boiled sweet (Fig. 2.17). It is much less cariogenic than sucrose when fed to rats and does not contribute to the softening of enamel in intra-oral enamel slab experiments.

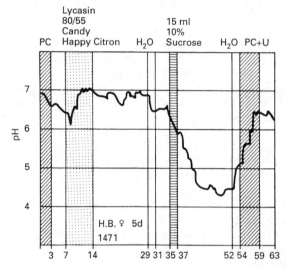

Fig. 2.17. Telemetrically recorded plaque pH after (a) eating a hard sweet containing Lycasin, (b) rinsing with 15 ml of 10 per cent sucrose solution. (From Imfeld 1977, with permission of the editor *Helvetica odontologica Acta*.)

Isomalt

Isomalt is, basically, a mixture of two polyols. It is manufactured in Germany and marketed under the trade name Palatinit®. It can be used in the manufacture of a number of foods and drinks. Isomalt causes little acid production when incubated with oral streptococci, and plaque pH is virtually unaffected after exposure to a 10 per cent solution. Isomalt's cariogenicity in rats is low.

Lactitol

Lactitol is a relative newcomer to the polyol scene but is now approved for use in foods in several countries. It is a 12-carbon polyol derived from lactose by the reduction of the glucose part of this disaccharide. It has only half the energy value of sucrose, but it is only a third as sweet as sucrose. Two animal experiments have shown lactitol to be of low cariogenicity and plaque pH studies have indicated only slight falls in plaque pH. Lactitol has a low cariogenic potential (greater than xylitol but less than other polyols) in incubation experiments. No clinical trials have been reported.

Intense sweeteners

Saccharin was discovered in 1879 and has been used widely as a food additive for more than 80 years. It has a bitter taste in concentrations over 0.1 per cent although the degree of appreciation of bitterness varies considerably between people. It is used as a 'table-top', sweetener and extensively in soft drinks, especially those marketed as 'low-calorie'.

Acesulfame K was discovered in 1967 in the laboratories of Hoescht AG. It has a clean, sweet taste. It is stable in aqueous solutions of wide-ranging pH, and can withstand moderately severe heat treatment. It is thought to have good potential as a sweetener, principally in 'reduced energy' soft drinks, but also in confectionery, chewing-gum, preserves and other foods.

Aspartame is a dipeptide, consisting of aspartic acid and phenylalanine. It is manufactured by GD Searle under the trade names Canderel® and NutraSweet®. It is moderately stable in solution although prolonged heat treatment and storage hastens its breakdown with subsequent loss of sweetness. It is now used extensively in soft drinks and chewing gum but is also thought to have potential for use in other foods, particularly in dried or frozen foods. Ingestion of aspartame should be avoided by phenylketonuric (PKU) persons (approximately 1 in 10 000 live births) who have a genetic defect of phenylalanine metabolism.

Thaumatin is a sweet-tasting protein extracted from a plant found in West Africa. Perception of sweetness is delayed and it has a slightly liquorice aftertaste. Thaumatin is reported to be used as a flavour enhancer in pharmaceutical products, and in combination with other sweeteners (e.g. saccharin) in soft drinks.

Cariogenicity of the intense sweeteners

Little is known of the effects of the intense sweeteners on caries development. Because of their composition, they are very unlikely to promote caries and research has been directed at investigating the caries-inhibitory properties of these substances. Saccharin has been reported to inhibit bacterial growth and metabolism, although its inhibitory effect on rat caries development was small. Because the intense sweeteners are used at low concentrations, possible direct effects (inhibitory or otherwise) on bacterial metabolism are likely to be less important than indirect effects on caries through salivary stimulation.

CONSIDERATIONS OF THE USE OF NON-SUGAR SWEETENERS

Role in caries prevention

On the positive side, non-sugar sweeteners can be considered 'safe for teeth' and provide manufacturers of foods, drinks, and medicines with a growing number of alternatives to sugars. If they are used as substitutes for sugars, dental health will benefit. On the negative side, most of the non-sugar bulk sweeteners (but not intense sweeteners) are more expensive than sugars and can cause laxation if consumed in large amounts. It should also be remembered that dietary goals for the population of the UK are to increase consumption of complex carbohydrates, i.e. staple starchy foods, fresh fruit and vegetables, rather than increasing consumption of bulk sweeteners. Nevertheless, as a substitute for cariogenic sugars, non-sugar sweeteners have a very useful role to play when it is not possible to reduce a liking for sweet-tasting foods, drinks or medicines. In this respect the initiative of the International Toothfriendly Association in identifying confectionery which is 'safe for teeth' is to be welcomed. This scheme developed from a Swiss idea and has lead to the establishment of similar, non-profit-making organizations in Germany, France, Belgium, the UK (where it is known as the British Association for Toothfriendly Sweets, or BATS), Italy, South Korea, and Japan.

Another aspect of the use of non-sugar sweeteners which is of considerable interest is whether they are anti-cariogenic as opposed to being just non-cariogenic. This is particularly relevant with sugar-free chewing gums, the trials of which will be discussed briefly.

Clinical trials of chewing gums containing sucrose, sorbitol and xylitol

A number of trials of chewing gum have been undertaken and these fall into three groups. First, trials which have compared the effect of giving subjects sugared gum, compared with subjects given no supplement: these test the effect of an additional 'sugar load' in the form of sugared gum. Secondly, trials which compared the effect of giving subjects sugar-free gum, compared with giving children sugared gum: these test the substitution of sugarless for sugared gum. Thirdly, trials which have compared the effect of giving subjects sugar-free gum, compared with subjects given no gum: these test any specific benefit of sugar-free gum. These trials are listed in Table 2.12. It can be seen that, in general, consumption of sugared gum increased dental caries increment, while consumption of sugarless gum (either in addition to the normal diet, or instead of sugared gum) decreased dental caries increment.

These conclusions are borne out by plaque pH studies: Fig. 2.18 illustrates the dramatic difference of the effect of the two gums. The rise in plaque pH when chewing the sugar-free gum is due to the induced increase in salivary flow being alkaline and raising the pH within the dental plaque.

SUMMARY OF NON-SUGAR SWEETENERS AND DENTAL CARIES

It would seem that sucrose, glucose, maltose, and fructose are the most cariogenic sugars, while lactose would seem to be less cariogenic. The bulk sweeteners sorbitol, mannitol, lactitol, hydrogenated glucose syrup, and isomalt are non-cariogenic or virtually so. Xylitol, saccharin, aspartame, acesulfame, and thaumatin are non-cariogenic. Effective caries prevention by sugar control includes (i) deciding which types of food or eating habits are the most harmful: substitution of sugar in these foods by less cariogenic sweeteners might then be cost-effective; (ii) development of new tech-

Table 2.12. Results of clinical trials testing the effect of sugar-containing or sugar-free chewing gums (based on a review by Edgar and Geddes 1990; see Rugg-Gunn 1993, for full references)

Comparison of sugared gum vs. no gum

	Increase in DMFS increment (%)
Volker (1948)	0
Toto *et al.* (1960)	0
Slack *et al.* (1972)	68
Baron (1981)	24
Glass (1981)	36

Comparison of sugar-free gum vs. sugared gum

	Decrease in DMFS increment (%)
Finn and Jamison (1967)	20
Scheinin *et al.* (1975, 1979)*	60

Comparison of sugar-free gum vs. no gum

	Decrease in DMFS increment (%)
Richardson *et al.* (1972)	0
Möller and Poulsen (1973)	10
Glass (1983)	12
Kandelman and Gagnon (1990)*	66
Isokangas *et al.* (1988)*	45

* Xylitol gum; all other gums were sorbitol.

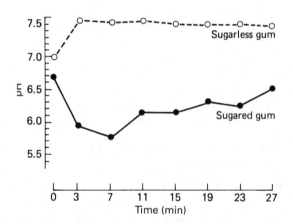

Fig. 2.18. Stephan curves produced by sugared and sugarless chewing-gum. (Rugg-Gunn *et al.* 1978, with permission of the editor *British Dental Journal*.)

nology to reduce the cost difference between sucrose, glucose, and fructose and other less cariogenic sweeteners; (iii) development of sweeteners free from adverse effects.

CONCLUDING COMMENTS

This chapter has provided a summary of the literature concerning diet and dental caries. It is not comprehensive and has not attempted to discuss the process of changing diet in individuals (patients) or communities. For a full discussion of the literature, dietary policy, and advice as well as a comprehensive list of references, the reader is referred to the textbook *Nutrition and dental health* (Rugg-Gunn 1993).

The scientific evidence clearly points to the need to reduce consumption of non-milk extrinsic sugars in the population in order to reduce the risk of dental caries. How this message is conveyed will depend on the target group. All non-commercial opinion supports this view and has done for many years. Many countries, including the UK, have nutrition policies which urge reductions in consumption of free (non-milk extrinsic) sugars. The sugar and sugar-related industries continue to dispute this message, although they now accept that dietary sugars are a factor in the development of dental caries. Most developed countries have enjoyed a marked decline in caries experience during the past 15 years which has been caused, almost certainly, by the widespread use of fluorides, particularly in toothpastes. However, dental caries still remains a serious problem for many children and adults. What is now needed is a policy which allows the optimum use of fluorides *as well as* sensible control of sugar consumption, in order to achieve dental health for all.

At the beginning of this chapter it was emphasized that our knowledge concerning the relation between diet and dental caries comes from many sources, largely because human dietary clinical studies are so difficult to carry out. Taking all these sources of evidence into account the following conclusions and comments can be made:

- In the development of dental caries, the influence of diet is much more important after a tooth has erupted into the mouth than any dietary influence on the forming tooth before its eruption. Sugar would appear to be the most important dietary item in caries aetiology and its presence around plaque-covered tooth surfaces essential for more than very limited caries development. Starch-containing foods, especially if finely-ground, cooked and eaten frequently, can cause some caries.

- Some sugars would appear to be more cariogenic than others. Sucrose is likely to be the most cariogenic sugar, although glucose, fructose, and maltose are virtually as cariogenic as sucrose. Lactose is less cariogenic than other dietary sugars. The alternative or non-sugar sweeteners (bulk and intense) are non-cariogenic or virtually so.

- Dietary sugars come from two sources—those naturally present in foods and those added by manufacturer, cook, or consumer. By far the majority of natural sugars come from milk and fruit. Milk can be considered non-cariogenic or virtually so. Fresh fruits, as eaten by man, are of low cariogenicity. Therefore, sugars naturally present in foods are of negligible importance as a cause of dental caries in man compared with non-milk extrinsic sugars.

- Cooked staple starchy foods, such as rice, potatoes, pasta, and bread, are of low cariogenicity in man. Refined, finely ground and heat-treated starch can cause caries but the addition of sugar increases the cariogenicity of cooked starchy foods.

- The frequency of sugar intake would appear to be a more important dietary variable than the total quantity of sugar eaten. However, frequently of eating sugar and total quantity of sugar consumed are closely correlated in many epidemiological surveys, so that as sugar becomes available to a population both total quantity of sugar eaten increases as well as the frequency with which it is eaten. The aim should be to decrease both the amount eaten and the frequency of intake.

- Dietary factors that protect tooth enamel from caries development during acid attack have been isolated. Phytate appears to be the most effective *in vitro* although inorganic and other organic phosphates also have an effect. Organic phosphates act primarily by forming a tightly bound protective layer on the enamel surface, whereas inorganic phosphates act mainly by a common ion effect. However, clinical studies have shown these compounds are less effective at caries prevention than might have been expected from animal and laboratory experiments.

- Although a large number of dietary compounds have been thought to influence a developing tooth's future caries susceptibility, only fluoride has been established to have any appreciable influence (see Chapter 3). Other trace elements may have a smaller effect, and the influence of calcium, phosphates, and vitamins A and D remains uncertain.

- Nutrition policy in the UK and other countries is now clearly directed towards decreasing consumption of dietary sugars. This policy is directed towards improving general and dental health. Control of dietary sugars and optimum use of fluorides together can considerably benefit dental health.

REFERENCES

Alanen, P., Tiekso, J., and Paunio, I. (1985). Effect of wartime dietary changes on dental health of Finns 40 years later. *Commun. dent. Oral Epidemiol.* **13**, 281–4.

Alvarez, J.O. and Navia, J.M. (1989). Nutritional status, tooth eruption, and dental caries: a review. *Am. J. clin. Nutr.* **49**, 417–26.

Burt, B.A., *et al.* (1988). The effects of sugars intake and frequency of ingestion on dental caries increment in a three-year longitudinal study. *J. dent. Res.* **67**, 1422–9.

Curzon, M.E.J. and Cutress, T.W. (1983). *Trace elements and dental disease*. Wright; PSG, Boston.

Dean, H.T., Arnold, F.A., and Elvolve, E. (1942). Domestic water and dental caries V. *Publ. Hlth Rep.* **57**, 1155–79.

Department of Health (1989). *Dietary sugars and human disease. Report on health and social subjects 37*. HMSO, London.

Department of Health (1991). *Dietary reference values for food energy and nutrients for the United Kingdom. Report on health and social subjects 41*. HMSO, London.

Edgar, W.M., Bibby, B.G., Mundorff, S., and Rowley, J. (1975). Acid production in plaques after eating snacks: modifying factors in foods. *J. Am. dent. Ass.* **90**, 418–25.

Edgar, W.M. and Geddes, D.A.M. (1990) Chewing gum and dental health; a review. *Br. dent. J.* **168**, 173–7.

Enwonwu, C.O. (1973). Influence of socio-economic conditions on dental development in Nigerian children. *Archs. oral. Biol.* **18**, 95–107.

Frencken, J.E., Rugarabamu, P., and Mulder, J. (1989). The effect of sugar cane chewing on the development of dental caries. *J. dent. Res.* **68**, 1102–4.

Frostell, G. Blomlöf, L., Blomqvist, T., Dahl, G.M., Edward, S., Fjellstrom, A., Henrikson, C.O., Larje, O., Nord, C.F., and Nordenvall, N.J. (1974). Substitution of sucrose by Lycasin in candy: the Roslagen study. *Acta odont. Scand.* **32**, 235–54.

Gustaffson, et al. (1954). The Vipeholm dental caries study. The effect of different levels of carbohydrate intake on caries activity in 436 individuals observed for five years. *Acta odont. Scand.* **11**, 232–364.

Hargreaves, J.A. and Thompson, G.W. (1989). Ultra-violet light and dental caries in children. *Caries Res.* **23**, 389–92.

Hefti, A. and Schmid, R. (1979). Effect on caries incidence in rats of increasing dietary sucrose levels. *Caries Res.* **13**, 298–300.

Imfeld, T. (1977). Evaluation of the cariogenicity of confectionery by intraoral wire telemetry. *Helv. Odont. Acta*, **21**, 1–28.

Kite, O.W., Shaw, J.H., and Sognnaes, R.F. (1950). The prevention of experimental tooth decay by tube-feeding. *J. Nutrit.* **42**, 89–103.

König, K.G., and Schmid, P., and Schmid, R. (1968). An apparatus for frequency-controlled feeding of small rodents and its use in dental caries experiments. *Archs. oral Biol.* **13**, 13–26.

Marthaler, T.M. (1967). Epidemiological and clinical dental findings in relation to intake of carbohydrates. *Caries Res.* **1**, 222–38.

Mellanby, M. (1923). The relation of caries to the structure of teeth. *Br. dent. J.* **44**, 1–13.

Miller, W.D. (1890). *The micro-organisms of the human mouth.* (ed. K. Konig). Karger, Basel.

Newbrun, E. (1978). *Cariology.* Williams and Wilkins, Baltimore.

Newbrun, E., Hoover, C., Mettraux, G., and Graf, H. (1980). Comparison of dietary habits and dental health of subjects with hereditary fructose intolerance and control subjects. *J. Am. dent. Ass.* **101**, 619–26.

Olojugba, O.O. and Lennon, M.A. (1990). Sugar consumption in 5- and 12-year-old schoolchildren in Ondo State, Nigeria in 1985. *Commun. dent. Health*, **7**, 259–65.

Roberts, I.F. and Roberts, G.J. (1979). Relation between medicines sweetened with sucrose and dental disease. *Br. med. J.* ii, 14–16.

Rugg-Gunn, A.J. (1993). *Nutrition and dental health*. Oxford University Press, Oxford.

Rugg-Gunn, A.J., Edgar, W.M., Geddes, D.A.M., and Jenkins, G.N. (1975). The effect of different meal patterns upon plaque pH in human subjects. *Br. dent. J.* **139**, 351–6.

Rugg-Gunn, A.J., Edgar, W.M., and Jenkins, G.N. (1978). The effect of eating some British snacks upon the pH of human dental plaque. *Br. dent. J.* **145**, 95–100.

Rugg-Gunn, A.J., Edgar, W.M., and Jenkins, G.N. (1981). The effect of altering the position of a sugary food in a meal upon plaque pH in human subjects. *J. dent. Res.* **60**, 867–72.

Rugg-Gunn, A.J., Hackett, A.F., Appleton, D.R., Jenkins, G.N., and Eastoe, J.E. (1984). Relationship between dietary habits and caries increment asssessed over two years in 405 English adolescent schoolchildren. *Archs. oral Biol.* **29**, 983–92.

Rugg-Gunn, A.J., Roberts, G.J. and Wright, W.G. (1985). The effect of human milk on plaque *in situ* and enamel dissolution *in vitro* compared with bovine milk, lactose and sucrose. *Caries Res.* **19**, 327–34.

Scheinin, A. and Mäkinen, K.K. (1975). Turku sugar studies. I-XXI. *Acta odont. Scand.* **33**, Suppl. 70, 1–349.

Sreebny, L.M. (1982). Sugar availability, sugar consumption and dental caries. *Commun. Dent. oral Epidemiol.* **10**, 1–7.

Sreebny, L.M. (1983). Cereal availability and dental caries. *Commun. Dent. oral Epidemiol.* **11**, 148–55.

Stanton, G. (1969). Diet and dental caries: the phosphate sequestration hypothesis. *NY St. dent. J.* **35**, 399–407.

Toverud, G. (1957). The influence of war and post-war conditions on the teeth of Norwegian schoolchildren II and III. *Millbank Mem. Fund Q,* **35**, 127–96; 373–459.

Von der Fehr, F.R., Löe, H., and Theilade, E. (1970). Experimental caries in man. *Caries Res.* **4**, 131–48.

Winter, G.B. (1980). Problems involved with the use of comforters. *Int. dent. J.* **30**, 28–38.

Winter, G.B. (1988). Prediction of high caries risk—diet, hygiene and medication. *Int. dent. J.* **38**, 227–30.

3. Fluorides and dental caries

J.J. MURRAY and M.N. NAYLOR

INTRODUCTION

The first suggestion of a possible connection between the fluoride ion and the prevalence of dental caries occurred towards the end of the nineteenth century when in 1892 Sir James Crichton-Browne addressed the Annual General Meeting of the Eastern Countries Branch of the British Dental Association in Downing College, Cambridge. He suggested that the specific cause of the increase of dental caries was a change in the type of bread eaten.

In as far as our own country, at any rate, is concerned, this is essentially an age of white bread and fine flour, and it is an age therefore in which we are no longer partaking to anything like the same amount that our ancestor did of the bran or husk parts of wheat, and so are deprived to a large degree of a chemical element which they received in abundance namely fluorine...I think it well worthy of consideration whether the reintroduction into our diet of child-bearing women and of children, of a supply of fluorine in some suitable natural form...might not do something to fortify the teeth of the next generation.

It is now over 100 years since Crichton-Browne's prophetic remarks were delivered. Today the dental literature groans under the weight of the enormous number of studies concerned with fluorides and caries. They can be divided into two main sections: the effect of fluoride taken systemically by water, or in the form of tablets and drops, or in enriched milk and salt; and the application of fluoride topically in the form of solutions, gels, mouth rinses, and toothpaste in much higher concentrations than found in water supplies. Dividing the literature into two in this way is simplistic in that those methods in the systemic group may also have a topical effect—for example, fluoride taken in the water supplies, in addition to being absorbed and incorporated into developing enamel, may also exert a topical effect both *pre-eruptively* by means of the tissue fluid contacting the maturing surface of the enamel and *post-eruptively* as the water washes over the tooth surface. Similarly, with 'topical methods'—for example, fluoride in toothpaste—as well as being brushed onto the surface of the tooth is ingested to a certain degree, particularly in young children, and so fluoride from this source can be incorporated into teeth still developing within the jaw.

In previous editions an attempt was made to give an outline of the historical background and to review the studies concerning each aspect of fluorides and dental caries. That information is now available elsewhere (Murray *et al.* 1991). In this chapter, starting with a short historical review concerning the effect of varying concentrations of fluorides into drinking water, a more selective approach will be adopted, concentrating on areas where new evidence has become available or where perceptions might have changed or developed in the last 10 years. The following topics will be considered.

1. An update on water fluoridation

2. Fluoride supplements—dosage recommendations

3. Developments in fluoride dentifrice formulations

4. Dental fluorosis

5. Reports from the World Health Organization

WATER FLUORIDATION: HISTORICAL BACKGROUND

Colorado stain

The man who had the greatest impact on the early history of water fluoridation was Dr Frederick McKay who arrived in Colorado Springs, Colorado in 1901, the year following his graduation from the University of Pennsylvania Dental School. He soon noticed that many of his patients, particularly those who had lived in the area all their lives, had a permanent stain on their teeth which was known to the local inhabitants as 'Colorado stain'. McKay checked his lecture notes but found nothing to describe such markings, nor could he find any reference to it in any of the available scientific literature. He called the stain 'mottled enamel', characterized by:

Minute white flecks, or yellow or brown spots or areas, scattered irregularly or streaked over the surface of a tooth, or it may be a condition where the entire tooth surface is of a dead paper-white, like the colour of a china dish (McKay 1916a).

McKay decided that, first, he needed help from a recognized dental research worker and, second, he needed to define the geographical area of the stain—the endemic area. To attain his first objective he approached one of America's foremost authorities on dental enamel, Dr Greene Vardiman Black, Dean of the Northwestern University Dental School in Chicago. At first Black thought that McKay was mistaking the stain for something else. He could scarcely believe there could be a dental lesion affecting so many people yet which remained unmentioned in the dental literature. Black asked that some of the mottled teeth be sent to him for examination

(Black 1916). He agreed to attend the Colorado State Dental Association meeting in July 1909, and promised to spend some weeks in Colorado Springs before the annual meeting.

In preparation for this visit, and as a first step in mapping out the entire endemic area, McKay and a fellow townsman, Dr Isaac Binton, examined the children in the public schools of Colorado Springs. In all they inspected 2945 children and discovered that 87.5 per cent of the children native to the area had mottled teeth (McKay 1916b). For the first time investigators had statistical data detailing the prevalence of the lesion in the community. This new information was given to Black when he arrived in Denver in June 1909, to tour the Colorado Springs area. Black addressed the State Dental Association meeting; he described his histological examination of the lesion and recounted his personal observations noted during the several weeks he had been touring the Rocky Mountain area. His interest together with his authority and prestige raised the study of the problem from the status of a local curiosity to that of an investigation meriting the earnest concern of all dental research workers. Black's histological findings were published in a paper: 'An endemic imperfection of the enamel of the teeth heretofore unknown in the literature of dentistry' (Black 1916).

Endemic areas of mottled teeth

Despite Black's involvement other dentists showed little enthusiasm for carrying on the investigation. It was left to McKay to sustain the study by his persistent interest. His Colorado Springs survey had shown that almost nine out of ten of the native children had mottled teeth; he began searching for other endemic areas. His travels took him up and down the creek valleys of the mountainous region and out onto the nearby plains. He examined children living in Pueblo, Maniton, La Junta, Cripple Creek, Woodland Park, and Green Mountain Falls. A few trips convinced McKay that the phenomenon called 'mottling' was much more widespread than he had thought. Slowly too, McKay began to get help from dentists in other parts of the country.

The horizons were broadened still further when, in 1912 McKay discovered that people from parts of Naples in Italy also had stained teeth. He came across an article written in 1902 by Dr J.M. Eager, a United States Marine Hospital Service Surgeon stationed in Italy, who reported that a high proportion of certain Italian emigrants embarking at Naples had a dental peculiarity known locally as denti di Chiaie (Eager 1902). Some of these Italians had ugly brown stains on their teeth; others had a fine horizontal black line crossing the incisor teeth. McKay heard that a young doctor, Dr J.F. McConnell from Colorado Springs, was planning a holiday in Italy, and asked him to examine some Naples children and report back. The doctor was familiar with the stain in Colorado Springs and wrote back from Naples that there was no doubt that the mottled teeth in Naples were the same as those being investigated by McKay (1916b).

Throughout this period the energy and enthusiasm which kept McKay going was generated by a desire to find out the cause of mottling so that some means might be found of preventing the unsightly stains on people's teeth. However, throughout his investigations, McKay was struck by the fact that caries experience was no higher in mottled teeth. This contradiction must have been in the back of McKay's mind throughout the whole period of his research. He expressed it forcibly in a paper to the Chicago Society on 17 April 1928:

Mottled enamel is a condition in which the enamel is most obviously and unmistakably defective. In fact it is the most poorly calcified enamel of which there is any record in dental literature. If the chief determining factor governing the susceptability to decay is the integrity or perfection of the calcification of enamel, then by all the laws of logic this enamel is deprived of the one essential element for its protection....In spite of this the outstanding fact is that mottled enamel shows no greater susceptibility to the onset of caries than does enamel that may be considered to have been normally or perfectly calcified. This statement is made as a result of extensive observations and examination of several thousand cases during the past years.... My testimony has been supplemented by that of others, who report that these mottled enamel cases, in the various districts are singularly free from caries. One of the first things noted by Dr Black during his first contact with an endemic locality was the singular absence of decay, and it can hardly be said that this faculty for observations was superficial (McKay 1928).

Mottled enamel—aetiological factors

In the forefront of McKay's mind all the time was the desire to determine the cause of mottled enamel. He established that the occurrence of mottled enamel was localized in definite geographical areas. Within these endemic areas a very high proportion of children were affected; only those who had been born and lived all their lives in an endemic area had mottled enamel; those born elsewhere and brought to the district when two to three years of age were not affected. The condition was not influenced by home or environment factors; families whether rich or poor were affected. This observation tended to eliminate diet as an aetiological factor. McKay observed that three cities in Arkansas where mottling occurred, although separated from each other by some miles, all received their water supply from one source, Fountain Creek. This, together with many other reports, led him to believe that something in the water supply was responsible for mottled enamel.

Further evidence supporting the water supply hypothesis came from a dentist, Dr O.E. Martin, practising in Britton, South Dakota. On reading McKay's 1916 article in *Dental Cosmos*, he felt that McKay's description of mottling sounded suspiciously like the blemishes he had seen in certain local children and asked for McKay's advice. McKay visited Britton in October 1916. He discovered that in 1898 Britton had changed its water supply from individual shallow wells to a deep-drilled artesian well. Without exception, McKay found that all those who had passed through childhood prior to the changing of the water supply had normal teeth, while natives who had grown up in Britton since 1898 had mottling. He concluded that some mysterious element in the water supply was responsible (McKay 1918).

A similar occurrence was reported in the town of Bauxite, a community formed in 1901 to provide homes for employees of the Republic Mining and Manufacturing Company, a subsidiary of the Aluminium Company of America (ALCOA). The first domestic water supply to Bauxite came from shallow wells and springs, but in 1909 a new source of water was obtained from a 297-foot well. A practising dentist, Dr F.L. Robertson, of nearby Benton, reported to the State Board of Health that the younger citizens of Bauxite seemed to have badly stained teeth, whereas the children living in Benton had normal teeth. The State Health Office made a formal request to the US Public Health Service in Washington to examine the children living in Bauxite and Benton. In 1928 the US Public Health Service asked Dr McKay to accompany Dr Gromer Kempf, one of their medical officers, to carry out the examinations. They found that no mottling occurred in people who grew up on Bauxite water prior to 1909, but all native Bauxite children who used the deep well water after that date had mottled teeth. No individual whose enamel developed during residence in Benton had mottled teeth. They reported that the standard water analysis of Bauxite water 'throws little light whatever on the probably causal agent' (Kempf and McKay 1930). Another piece of evidence had been gathered, but McKay seemed no closer to the solution.

Mottled enamel and fluoride concentration in the drinking water

The answer was now close at hand. In New Kensington, Pennsylvania, the chief chemist of ALCOA, Mr H.V. Churchill, read Kempf and McKay's paper and was greatly disturbed. Certain people in the United States were condemning the use of aluminium-ware for cooking. ALCOA mined most of its aluminium supply from Bauxite; if the story of the stain in Bauxite got into the hands of those who claimed that aluminium cooking utensils caused poisoning, ALCOA would have to reply to the charge. When Churchill received a sample of Bauxite water he instructed Mr A.W. Petrey, head of the testing division of the ALCOA laboratory, to look for traces of rare elements—those not usually tested for. Petrey ran a spectographic analysis and noted that fluoride was present in Bauxite water at a level of 13.7 parts per million. Churchill wrote to McKay on 20 January 1931:

We have discovered the presence of hitherto unsuspected constituents in this water. The high fluorine content was so unexpected that a new sample was taken with extreme precautions and again the test showed fluorine in the water (Churchill 1931*a*).

He also asked McKay to send samples of water from other endemic areas with a 'minimum of publicity'. McKay quickly arranged for dentists in Britton, South Dakota, Oakley, Idaho, and Colorado Springs to send samples of the water in their areas. The results of these analyses were published in 1931 (Table 3.1). Churchill emphasized the fact that no precise cor-

relation between the fluoride content of these waters and the mottled enamel had been established. All that was shown was the presence of a hitherto unsuspected common constituent of the waters from the endemic areas (Churchill 1931*b*).

The work of H. Trendley Dean

The study of the relationship between fluoride concentration in drinking water, mottled enamel, and dental caries was given an impetus by the decision of Dr Clinton T. Messner, Head of the US Public Health Service, in 1931, to assign a young dental officer, Dr H. Trendley Dean, to pursue full-time research on mottled enamel. Dean was responsible for the research unit within the US Public Health Service and was the first dental officer of the service to be given a non-clinical assignment. His first task was to continue McKay's work and to find the extent and geographical distribution of mottled enamel in the United States. He reported that there were 97 localities in the country where mottled enamel was said to occur and this claim had been confirmed by a dental survey. There were a further 28 areas referred to in the literature where mottled enamel was said to be endemic but no confirmatory dental surveys had yet been carried out, and there were 70 areas which had been reported by questionnaires but which had not yet been confirmed by extensive surveys (Dean 1933).

Many of these confirmatory surveys were carried out by Dean himself. He developed a standard of classification of mottling in order to record quantitatively the severity of mottling within a community (Dean 1934) so that he could relate the fluoride concentration in the drinking water to the severity of mottling in a given area. His aim was to find out the 'minimal threshold' of fluorine—the level at which fluorine began to blemish the teeth. He showed conclusively that the severity of mottling increased with increasing fluoride concentration in the drinking water (Dean and Elvove 1936; Dean 1936). His results are expressed diagrammatically in Fig. 3.1.

Dean continued his studies into the relationship between the severity of mottled enamel and the fluoride concentration in water supplies. He presented additional evidence to show that amounts of fluoride not exceeding 1 ppm were of no public health significance. On 25 October 1938, in conjunction with Frederick McKay, he summarized the knowledge of mottled enamel in a paper to the Epidemiology Section of the American Public Health Association. He reported that in the United States there were now 375 known areas, in 26 states, where mottled enamel of varying degrees of severity were found. He also stated that the production of mottled enamel had been halted at Oakley, Idaho, Bauxite, Arkansas, and Andover, South Dakota, simply by changing the water supply, which contained high concentrations of fluoride, to one whose fluoride concentration did not exceed 1 ppm. This information was 'the most conclusive and direct proof that fluoride in the domestic water is the primary cause of human mottled enamel' (Dean and McKay 1939). The publication of this information brought to a successful conclusion McKay's search for the cause of mottled enamel which began in Colorado Springs in 1902 and lasted for almost 40 years.

Table 3.1. Fluoride analyses from Churchill (1931*a*)

Location of sample	Fluorine as fluoride (ppm)
Deep Well, Bauxite, Ark.	13.7
Colorado Springs, Colo.	2.0
Well near Kidder, S. Dak.	12.0
Well near Lidgerwood, N. Dak.	11.0
Oakley, Idaho	6.0

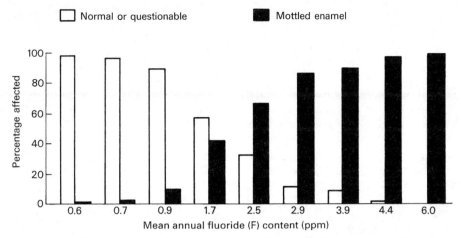

Fig. 3.1. The prevalence of mottled enamel in areas with differing concentrations of fluoride in the water supply. (From Dean 1936.) (Reproduced from *Fluoride drinking waters*, edited by F.J. McClure, by kind permission of the US Department of Health, Education and Welfare 1962.)

The story of fluoridation now entered a new and, from a public health point of view, a most important phase. Dean was aware of the reports from the literature that there may be an inverse relationship between the level of mottling and the prevalence of caries in a community. He knew of McKay's observations, first made in 1916, that mottled enamel was no more susceptible to decay than normal enamel. He had read Ainsworth's report in 1933 that caries experience in the high fluoride area was markedly lower than caries experience in all other district examined. During his study to determine the minimum threshold of mottling, Dean had, in some cities, also examined the children for dental caries. Taking a selected sample of 9-year-old children, he found that of 114 children who had continuously used a domestic water supply comparatively low in fluoride (0.6–1.5 ppm) only five, or 4 per cent, were caries-free. On the other hand, of the 122 children who had continuously used domestic water containing 1.7–2.5 ppm fluoride, 27 (22 per cent) were caries-free. He concluded: 'Inasmuch as it appears that the mineral composition of the drinking water may have an important bearing on the incidence of dental caries in a community, the possibility of partially controlling dental caries through the domestic water supply warrants thorough epidemiological-chemical study' (Dean 1938).

To test further the hypothesis that an inverse relationship existed between endemic dental fluorosis and dental caries, a survey of four Illinois cities was planned. The cities were Galesburg and Monmouth (water supply contained 1.8 and 1.7 ppm fluoride respectively), and the nearby cities of Macomb and Quincy (water supply contained 0.2 ppm F). Altogether 885 children, aged 12–14 years, were examined. The results were clear; caries experience in Macomb and Quincy was more than twice as high as that in Galesburg and Monmouth (Dean *et al.* 1939).

This study paved the way for a much larger investigation of caries experience of 7257 12–14-year-old children from 21 cities in four states. The results, (Fig. 3.2) show clearly the association between increasing fluoride concentration in the drinking water and decreasing caries experience in the population. Furthermore this study showed that near maximal reduction in caries experience occurred with a concentration

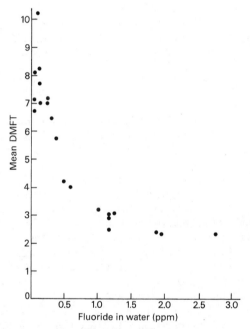

Fig. 3.2. The relation between caries experience of 7257 12- to 14-year-old white schoolchildren of 21 cities in the USA and the fluoride content of the water supply. (From Dean *et al.* 1942.) (Reproduced from *Fluoride drinking waters*, edited by F.J. McClure, by kind permission of the US Department of Health, Education and Welfare 1962.)

of 1 ppm F in the drinking water. At this concentration fluoride caused only 'sporadic instances of the mildest forms of dental fluorosis of no practical aesthetic significance' (Dean *et al.* 1942).

EFFECT OF VARYING CONCENTRATIONS OF FLUORIDE IN DRINKING WATER ON DENTAL CARIES

The work of Dean and colleagues demonstrating the relationship between caries experience and fluoride content of the

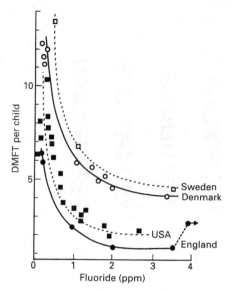

Fig. 3.3. Caries experience in 12- to 13-year-old children from Denmark, Sweden, and the USA in relation to concentration of fluoride in water supplies. (From Møller 1965.) (Reproduced with permission.)

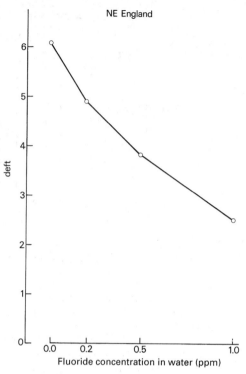

Fig. 3.4. The relationship between caries experience (deft) in 1038 5-year-old children living in four areas of NE England and the fluoride concentration in their drinking water. (Rugg-Gunn *et al.* 1981.) (Reproduced by courtesy of the editor *British Dental Journal*.)

water supply to 21 cities in the United States of America showed that near maximal reduction in caries occurred at approximately 1 and 2 ppm F. In addition, mottling of the teeth began to be noticeable when the fluoride concentration increased above 1.5 ppm. It was this work which formed the basis of the decision to fluoridate at 1 ppm in the United States of America. Dean's original observations have been substantiated by a number of investigators. Moller (1965) showed that data from Denmark and Sweden followed the same trend as that reported by Dean *et al.* (1942) (Fig. 3.3). In addition, studies in Great Britain, Hungary, Austria, Spain, and the United States show a decrease in caries experience with increasing fluoride content of the water supply up to about 2 ppm; this information is summarized in Table 3.2.

The relationship between caries experience in the deciduous dentition and the fluoride concentration in the drinking water was investigated by Rugg-Gunn *et al.* (1981). They examined 1038 5-year-old children from four areas in the north-east of England and showed a progressive decrease in caries experience with increasing concentration of fluoride in the water, up to 1.0 ppm (Fig. 3.4), thus following the same trend as that reported for the permanent dentition.

WORLD-WIDE STUDIES

The results of 113 studies in 23 countries have been compiled by Murray *et al.* (1991). A summary of that information showed that in 66 studies data were given for primary teeth and in 86 studies for permanent teeth.

Fifty-nine out of the 113 studies took place in the USA. The results for percentage caries reductions are given in Fig. 3.5; for primary teeth the modal caries reduction was 40–49 per cent (24 out of the 66 studies) and for permanent teeth 50–59 per cent (33 out of 86 studies). The results in Fig. 3.5 come from different types of study. They were carried out in different

countries and by different examiners, using different diagnostic criteria on subjects of different ages who were not always continuous residents in the communities investigated. In some areas, the caries prevalence was high and in others low. In general, factors such as these do not influence the validity of the results, since they affect the fluoridated and control communities equally. However, one factor which may influence the interpretation of the findings is the choice of a control group which can be either a 'self-control' or a 'control area' type. Just over half of the studies were self-control studies where the dental status of the community was measured before introduction of water fluoridation, and any change observed subsequently, after water fluoridation, was deemed to be caused by water fluoridation. This retrospective control design is satisfactory as long as no change in the underlying prevalence of the disease has occurred. This assumption is sometimes not justified, and, in some studies, fluoridation has been judged against a background rise or fall in caries prevalence.

A better design is to identify a control community similar to the fluoridated (or test) community, so that the test and control communities can be assessed in parallel. It is reasonable to assume that any rise or fall in background caries prevalence will occur in both communities equally and thus not influence assessment of the effectiveness of fluoridation.

Because of the possible influence of choice of control in fluoridation studies, Figs 3.6 and 3.7 were compiled: Fig. 3.6 for self-control studies only and Fig. 3.7 for control area studies only. There is a slight shift towards higher per cent caries reductions being recorded in self-control studies (Fig. 3.6), especially for permanent teeth. However, the modal

Table 3.2. Dental caries in 12- to 14-year-old children in communities with varying concentrations of fluoride in drinking water

Reference	Country	Town	F Supply	No. of children	Mean DMF
Dean (1942)	USA	Michigan City	0.09	236	10.37
		Elkhart	0.11	278	8.23
		Portsmouth	0.13	469	7.72
		Zanesville	0.19	459	7.33
		Middletown	0.2	370	7.03
		Quincy	0.13	330	7.06
		Lima	0.3	454	6.52
		Marion	0.43	263	5.56
		Pueblo	0.6	614	4.12
		Kewanee	0.9	123	3.43
		East Moline	1.2	152	3.03
		Colorado Springs	2.6	404	2.46
		Galesburg	1.9	273	2.36
		Waukegan	0.0	423	8.10
		Oak Park	0.0	329	7.22
		Evanstown	0.0	256	6.73
		Elgin	0.5	403	4.44
		Joliet	1.3	447	3.23
		Aurora	1.2	633	2.81
		Maywood	1.2	171	2.58
		Elmhurst	1.8	170	2.52
Arnold (1948)	USA	Nashville	0.0	662	4.6
		Key West	0.1	95	10.7
		Clarksville	0.2	60	4.6
		Vicksburg	0.2	172	5.87
		Escanaba	0.2	270	8.8
		Hereford.	3.1	60	1.47
Galagan (1953)[†]	USA	Yuma	0.4	29	2.45
		Tempe	0.5	45	2.82
		Tucson	0.7	167	3.48
		Chandler	0.8	42	2.45
		Casa Grande	1.0	22	2.00
		Florence	1.2	34	3.56
Nevitt et al. (1953)	USA	Low F	0.08–0.26	311	8.5
		Medium F	0.42–0.68	222	4.8
		High F	0.87–1.32	254	2.1
Lewis and Leatherwood (1959)	USA	Macon	0.11	1182	6.33
		Savanah	0.37	1188	5.22
		Moultrie	0.75	136	3.15
Gilooly et al. (1954)	USA	Low F	0.1–0.3	114	3.65
		Medium F	0.5	109	2.80
		High F	0.8–1.6	88	1.41
Klein (1948)	USA	Williamstown and Clayton	0.1	81	7.2
		Woodstown, Glassboro, and Pitman	1.3–2.2	176	1.9
Forrest (1956)	UK	Saffron Walden and district	0.1	145	6.6
		Stoneleign and Maldon West	0.1–0.2	114	6.1
		Slough	0.9	119	2.6
		Harwich	2.0	92	1.5
		Burnham-on-Crouch	3.5	62	1.4
		West Mersea	5.8	51	2.8
Adler (1951)	Hungary	Sarretudvari	0.20	166	4.25
		Öcsöd	0.21	222	2.09
		Bekesszentandras	0.21	177	2.43
		Biharnagybajom	0.33	143	3.06
		Kumszentmarton farms	0.72	86	1.29
		Szekszard	0.76	292	0.91
		Kunszentmarton village	0.99	283	1.02
		Komadi	1.09	343	1.31

Table 3.2.   *continued*

Reference	Country	Town	F Supply	No. of children	Mean DMF
Binder (1965)	Austria	Low F towns	0.0	90	4.9
		Umhansen, Silz. and Mallnitz	1.0–1.8	82	1.2
Sellman *et al.* (1957)	Sweden	Malmö	0.3–0.5	145	13.3
		Nyvang	1.0		
		Astorp	1.3	149	6.8
		Simrishamm	1.3		
Møller	Denmark	Vejen	0.05	148	12.5
		Aalestrup	0.2	52	12.2
		St. Heddinge	0.25	43	11.7
		Slagelse	0.34	424	11.2
		Naestved H	1.2	157	6.2
		Praestø	1.6	43	5.5
		Naestved N	1.8	42	5.2
		Naestved G	1.9	150	5.2
		Stroby Egede	2.0	12	4.9
		Tappernøje and Strøby By	3.4	14	4.2
Vines and Clavero (1968)*	Spain	Aezcoa	0.1	34	6.25
		Valle de Erro	0.1	22	6.02
		Tafalla	0.5	149	5.64
		Pitillas	0.7	21	5.14
		Pamplona	0.7	670	5.03
		Mueillo et Fruito	0.75	37	5.01
		Funes	0.65	66	4.91
		Falces	0.65	93	4.57
		Potasas	0.6	70	4.56
		Tudela	0.6	192	4.49
		Murcia	0.8	462	3.41
		Abanilla	1.5	47	2.35

* 10–12-year-old children.
† These studies were carried out in Arizona, which has a very high mean annual temperature.

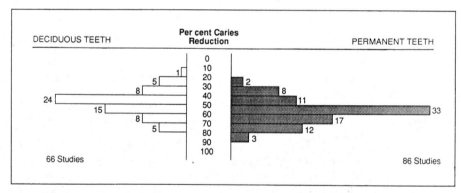

Fig. 3.5.   Per cent caries reduction in 113 studies into the effectiveness of artificial water fluoridation in 23 countries. Sixty-six studies gave results for the deciduous dentition, and 86 studies gave results for the permanent dentition. (From Murray *et al.* 1991, with permission.)

caries reductions are the same: 40–49 per cent for deciduous teeth and 50–59 per cent for permanent teeth.

PATTERN OF CARIES IN 15- TO 16-YEAR-OLD CHILDREN IN FLUORIDE AND LOW FLUORIDE AREAS

Studies in the north-east of England have provided considerable information concerning the relationship between caries experience and fluoride content of the drinking water.

The first study was carried out by Weaver (1944) in North and South Shields in 1941. He followed this up in 1949 with an investigation of 5-, 12-, and 15-year-old children living in Hartlepool. Twenty years later Murray (1969*a*, *b*) and Murray and Atkinson (1971) provided information on caries experience of 3800 Hartlepool children aged 2–18 years. In 1989–90 the caries experience in 1374 children aged 15–16 years from three towns in the north-east of England, with varying concentrations of fluoride in drinking water, was determined (Murray *et al.* 1991) (Table 3.3).

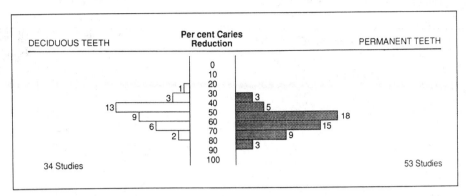

Fig. 3.6. Per cent caries reduction observed in studies of the effectiveness of artificial fluoridation. These studies were all self-control (or retrospective control) studies. (From Murray *et al.* 1991, with permission.)

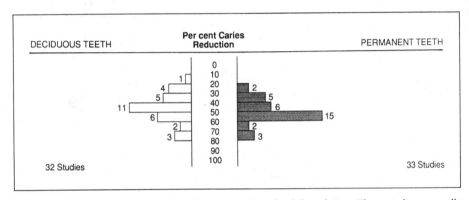

Fig. 3.7. Per cent caries reduction observed in studies of the effectiveness of artificial fluoridation. These studies were all control area (or parallel control) studies, (From Murray *et al.* 1991, with permission.)

The mean DMFT values for 15-year-old continuous residents was 1.7 in Hartlepool (natural F 1.0–1.3 ppm), 2.5 in Newcastle (F adjusted to 1.0 ppm), and 3.3 in Middlesbrough (F = 0.2 ppm). Forty per cent of Hartlepool 15-year-olds were caries free compared with 30 per cent in Newcastle and 24 per cent in Middlesbrough. DMF values were 32–35 per cent lower in Hartlepool children than in children living in fluoride-adjusted Newcastle, and values for Newcastle children were, in turn, 18–24 per cent lower than those obtained from Middlesbrough children (Table 3.4).

In theory, one might have expected results from Newcastle to be closer to those found in Hartlepool. Possible reasons for the lower results in Hartlepool are: (1) the natural fluoride concentration in Hartlepool is 1.0–1.3 ppm and has been as high as 2.0 ppm, and (2) fluoridation in Newcastle was suboptimal between 1977 and 1981 whilst a new water treatment plant was being built.

When the samples for each community were divided into continuous and non-continuous residents, it was found that DMF values for continuous residents were slightly lower in Hartlepool and Newcastle, but rather higher in Middlesbrough compared with non-continuous residents (Table 3.5). This confirmed the importance of continuous residence in a fluoride area to achieve maximal effect in reducing caries.

The patterns of decayed, missing, filled, and sound teeth for each tooth type are recorded in Figs 3.8–3.10. Included in

these figures are extractions for orthodontic reasons—hence the higher rate of missing first premolars in Hartlepool and Newcastle compared with Middlesbrough where there were

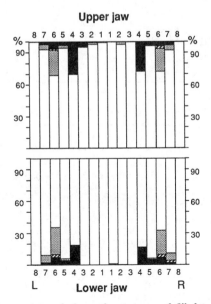

Fig. 3.8. Per cent sound, decayed, missing, and filled teeth, in each tooth type, in 15- to 16-year-old children in Hartlepool.

Table 3.3. Caries experience in continuous residents by age (Murray *et al.* 1991)

	Hartlepool	Newcastle	Middlesbrough
15-year-old children			
Number in group	254	227	259
Age, years			
Mean	15.6	15.7	15.6
SEM	0.01	0.01	0.01
DMFT			
Mean	1.7	2.5	3.3
SEM	0.13	0.16	0.26
DMFS			
Mean	2.9	3.5	6.1
SEM	0.26	0.27	0.46
Caries free, %	40	30	24
16-year-old children			
Number in group	107	122	115
Age, years			
Mean	16.1	16.2	16.2
SEM	0.01	0.01	0.01
DMFT			
Mean	1.9	3.0	3.6
SEM	0.20	0.24	0.29
DMFS			
Mean	2.9	4.1	6.4
SEM	0.37	0.38	0.70
Caries free, %	36	25	17

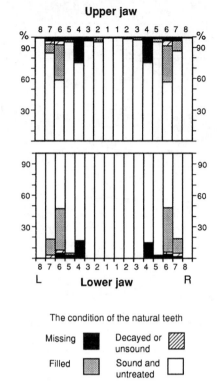

Fig. 3.9. Per cent sound, decayed, missing, and filled teeth, in each tooth type, in 15- to 16-year-old children in Newcastle.

Table 3.4. Per cent differences in DMFT/DMFS values for 15- to 16-year-old children in Hartlepool, Newcastle, and Middlesbrough (Murray *et al.* 1991)

	Hartlepool vs. Newcastle	Newcastle vs. Middlesbrough	Hartlepool vs. Middlesbrough
15-year-old children			
DMFT	32	24	45
DMFS	17	42	52
16-year-old children			
DMFT	35	18	46
DMFS	29	36	54

more extracted first permanent molars. The increasing amount of caries in first and second molars, as one moves from Hartlepool to Newcastle and on to Middlesbrough, is striking and shows where further preventive efforts need to be directed.

SECULAR CHANGES IN CARIES IN A NATURAL FLUORIDE AREA

A great deal has been written about the secular decline in caries in many countries in the 'developed' world, particularly since the 1970s. This secular decline in caries in fluoridated area has been noted in Britain, in Anglesey (Jackson *et al.* 1975, 1985) and in Newcastle (Rugg-Gunn *et al.* 1988).

Table 3.5. Caries experience in 15- to 16-year-old children (Murray *et al.* 1991)

	Hartlepool		Newcastle		Middlesbrough	
	Continuous residents	Non-continuous residents	Continuous residents	Non-continuous residents	Continuous residents	Non-continuous residents
Number in group	361	81	349	97	374	69
Mean age in group, years	15.8	15.8	15.8	15.8	15.8	15.8
DMFT						
Mean	1.7	2.1	2.7	2.7	3.4	3.1
SEM	0.11	0.31	0.13	0.29	0.16	0.32
DMFS						
Mean	2.9	3.7	3.7	4.1	6.2	5.0
SEM	0.21	0.69	0.22	0.56	0.38	0.74

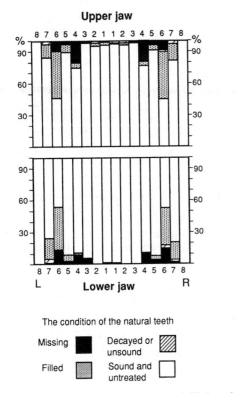

Upper jaw

Lower jaw

The condition of the natural teeth

Missing ■   Decayed or unsound ▨

Filled ▦   Sound and untreated □

Fig. 3.10. Per cent sound, decayed, missing, and filled teeth, in each tooth type, in 15- to 16-year-old children in Middlesbrough.

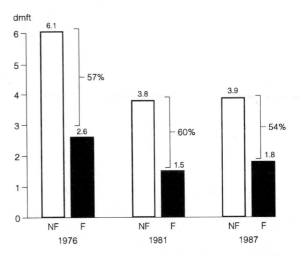

Fig. 3.11. Caries experience (mean dmft) of 5-year-old children in fluoridated (F; dark columns) and non-fluoridated (NF; open columns) areas of the North East of England in 1975, 1981, and 1987. (From Rugg-Gunn *et al.* 1988, with permission.)

Rugg-Gunn *et al.* (1988) have been involved in three surveys of 5-year-old children in fluoridated Newcastle and low-fluoride Northumberland. The results for this 1987 study are compared with the findings of the 1976 and 1981 surveys shown in Fig. 3.11. Caries experience fell in both areas between 1976 and 1981, but no further decline was noted between 1981 and 1987. In all three studies the difference between the two communities was 54–60 per cent.

Data for 5-, 12-, and 15-year-old Hartlepool children are available since the 1940s (Weaver 1950; Murray 1969*a, b*; Murray *et al.* 1991) and are summarized in Table 3.6. There are certain differences in epidemiological methods over the last 20 years. In 1969 a sharp probe was used, replaced or re-sharpened after every tenth examination. Nevertheless, if in doubt about a diagnosis, the surface was recorded as sound. The surveys carried out in 1989–90 based their criteria for diagnosis mainly on visual signs, using a ball-ended probe, diameter 0.5 mm in accordance with the national surveys. This difference in the level of diagnosis may be in

part responsible for some of the differences between the 1969 and 1989 surveys. A slight shift in diagnosis, or reduction in dental disease, can affect the per cent caries-free value quite markedly, in that it only takes one diagnosis of a 'sticky fissure' to a carious cavity to remove an individual from the caries-free group.

In spite of the secular changes in dental caries that have been referred to so often in the last few years, caries experience in Hartlepool remains one of the lowest recorded of any part of Great Britain.

PRE-ERUPTIVE EFFECT OF WATER FLUORIDATION

Marthaler (1979) reviewed the epidemiological evidence concerning the pre-eruptive effect of water fluoridation. His analysis of the Grand Rapids data (Table 3.7) provides evidence of a pre-eruptive effect. Permanent teeth do not usually erupt before 6 years of age, so that the difference between the DMF values of 13-year-old children first exposed to fluoridation at the age of 5 years (5.9 DMFT) and the figure for 13-year-old children exposed to fluoridation from birth (3.9 DMFT) can be taken as an indication of the benefit of exposure to fluoridation between birth and 5 years of age (a benefit of 2.0 DMFT). Marthaler (1979) found a similar benefit of pre-eruptive exposure to fluoridation on analysis of data from Kingston (USA), Oak Park (USA), Sarnia (Canada), and Hastings (New Zealand).

Table 3.6. Caries experience in Hartlepool children 1949–89 (Weaver 1950; Murray 1969*a, b*; Murray *et al.* 1991)

	5-year-old children			12-year-old children			15-year-old children		
	Weaver (1950)	Murray (1969*a, b*)	Murray *et al.* (1991)	Weaver (1950)	Murray (1969*a, b*)	Murray *et al.* (1991)	Weaver (1950)	Murray (1969*a, b*)	Murray *et al.* (1991)
Mean dmf/DMF	1.8	1.5	0.8	1.0	2.0	0.7	2.1	4.9	1.7
Per cent caries-free	54	51	67	60	30	59	37	26	39

Table 3.7. DMFT of 9- and 13-year-old children in Grand Rapids (USA) who were exposed to fluoridated water for different periods of time (Marthaler 1979; compiled Arnold *et al.* 1956, 1962)

	Year of exposure to fluoridation prior to examination			
	0	3	8	13
9-year-old children				
DMFT	3.9	3.1	2.0	–
Age at fluoridation, years	9	6	1	–
13-year-old children				
DMFT	9.7	8.5	5.9	3.9
Age at fluoridation, years	13	10	5	0

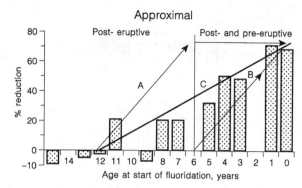

Fig. 3.13. Observed per cent reduction in approximal surfaces of first permanent molars in 15-year-old children who were at different ages at the onset of water fluoridation. Lines A and B indicate the theoretical curves of pure post- and pre-eruptive effects. Line C indicates similar pre- and post-eruptive effects. (From Groeneveld *et al.* 1990, with permission.)

The most thorough investigation into the relative importance of pre- and post-eruptive exposure to fluoride was undertaken by van Eck (1987). This author used the very extensive data collected during the Tiel–Culemborg Fluoridation Study in the Netherlands. Per cent caries reductions for approximal surfaces of premolars, molars, and upper incisors of 15-year-old children, in Tiel compared with Culemborg, are given in Fig. 3.12. The maximum caries reduction in these surfaces was about 65 per cent (fluoridation began 7 years before tooth eruption), whereas only about 30 per cent reduction was observed in teeth which erupted in the same year as fluoridation began and the teeth subjected to post-eruptive fluoride only. Van Eck (1987) concluded that fluoridated water consumed continuously from birth results in the greatest effect; pre- as well as post-eruptive consumption are both necessary to gain maximum benefit from water fluoridation. Since the publication of the thesis of van Eck (1987), Groeneveld *et al.* (1990) presented further evidence of the Tiel and Culemborg data and illustrated graphically the relative effectiveness of pre- and post-eruptive fluoride exposure (Fig. 3.13). The observed per cent reduction approximates to curve C, indicating the presence of both pre- and post-eruptive effects on the approximal surfaces of first permanent molars in 15-year-old children. Groeneveld *et al.* (1990) concluded:

'It is evident that fluoride has an important pre-eruptive effect on caries experience in all permanent dentition predilection sites. The maximum DMFS reduction in a fluoridated area at age 15 years was due about half to the pre-eruptive and about half to the post-eruptive effect of fluoride'.

EFFECT OF CESSATION OF FLUORIDATION

Mansbridge (1969) reported that after cessation of the fluoridation scheme in Kilmarnock, in 1962, the prevalence of caries increased in children aged 3–7 years. By 1968, the proportion of children free from decay approximated to the pre-fluoridation level of 1956 and to that of the control children in Ayr.

Stephens *et al.* (1987) reported the results of clinical and radiographic examinations of 5-year-old children who had been born and raised in the fluoridated town of Wick, compared with similar subjects 5 years after Wick water was de-fluoridated in 1979 because of a decision taken by Highland Regional Council. The results are summarized in Table 3.8 and show that a substantial rise in dental caries had occurred. The authors concluded that this localized caries increase, which is against all national, local, and social class trends, resulted from the 1977 decision to deprive Wick inhabitants of fluoridated water supplies.

Attwood and Blinkhorn (1988) reported on the effect of the decision to cease fluoridation in Stranraer. In 1980, a comparison had been made between the dental health of 10-year-old children in Stranraer, 10 years after the introduction of water fluoridation, and those in Annan which had a negli-

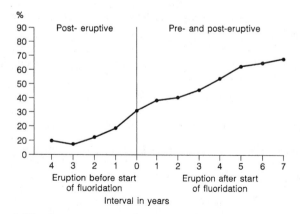

Fig. 3.12. Per cent caries reduction in approximal surfaces of premolars, molars, and upper incisors only in 15-year-old children, Tiel as compared with Culemborg.

Table 3.8. Caries experience in 5-year-old Wick children in 1979 and 1984 (Stephen *et al.* 1987)

	1979	1984	Percent increase (1979 base)
Number of children	106	126	
Clinical mean dmft	2.63	3.92	49
Clinical and radiographic dmfs	8.42	13.93	67

Table 3.9. Caries experience in 10-year-old children in Stranraer and Annan 1980–86 (Attwood and Blinkhorn 1988)

Study	Stranraer		Annan		Per cent reduction
	No. of children	Mean DMFT	No. of children	Mean DMFT	
1980	147	1.66	141	3.35	56
1986	127	1.72	105	2.81	39
Per cent difference		+4		−16	

gible concentration of fluoride in the public water supply. In 1986, the opportunity was taken to examine 10-year-old children again, employing the same diagnostic criteria and one of the examiners involved in the previous study. Only life-time residents were included in the analysis. The results (Table 3.9) show that whereas DMFT values had fallen by 16 per cent in Annan, they had risen by 4 per cent in Stranraer after fluoridation had been withdrawn. Although 10-year-old children in Stranraer may still have some residual benefit from earlier fluoridation, their study suggested that dental health had started to deteriorate.

FLUORIDATION AND THE LAW

Legislation authorizing water fluoridation is of two types. It may be mandatory, requiring a Ministry of Health or communities of a certain size to fluoridate their public water supplies, or the legislation may be permissive or enabling, giving the 'Ministry of Health' or a local government the authority to institute fluoridation. Such legislation does not automatically bring about fluoridated water supplies but paves the way for health officials or units of local government to act.

Mandatory laws requiring fluoridation of public water supplies that are fluorine-deficient have been enacted in Brazil, Bulgaria, Greece, Ireland, and five states of the United States of America.

Examples of countries with enabling legislation are several states of the USA, and also Australia, Israel, New Zealand, Canada, and United Kingdom (Roemer 1983).

THE STRATHCLYDE FLUORIDATION CASE

Background

In 1978 Strathclyde Regional Council, as a statutory water authority in Scotland, agreed to co-operate with local Health Boards by fluoridating water supplies for which they were responsible. Mrs Catherine McColl, a Glasgow citizen, applied for an interdict to restrain Strathclyde Regional Council from implementing its decision. The interdict was based on four main grounds:

1. Fluoridation would be *ultra vires*, i.e. beyond the legal powers of the Regional Council.

2. It would be a nuisance and, being a toxic substance, harmful to consumers, particularly in relation to cancer.

3. It would be a breach of the Water Act in that the Council would be failing in their duty to provide a supply of wholesome water.

4. It would be unlawful in that the Council would be providing a medicinal product for a medicinal purpose without having a product licence.

The hearings, held in the Court of Session, Edinburgh, commenced on 23 September 1980 and continued (after a few breaks) until 26 July 1982. The court sat on 201 days making it the longest and costliest case in Scottish legal history. The judge, Lord Jauncey, took almost 12 months to consider the massive evidence and gave his verdict on 29 June 1983. His judgment was contained in a 400-page document. He summarized his conclusions, in relation to the general topics which were canvassed in evidence, as follows.

Lord Jauncey's summary

'Before turning to consider the law it may be convenient to summarise my conclusions in relation to the general topics which were canvassed in evidence.

1. Fluoride at a concentration of 1 ppm is not mutagenic.

2. No biochemical mechanism has been demonstrated whereby fluoride at a concentration of 1 ppm is likely to cause cancer or accelerate existing cancerous growth.

3. No association between fluoridation of water supplies and increased CDRs (cancer death rates) in the consumers has been demonstrated.

4. There is no reason to anticipate that fluoride at a concentration of 1 ppm is likely to have an adverse effect upon the migration of leucocytes in the consumer.

5. There is no reasonable likelihood that CRF (chronic renal failure) patients drinking water fluoridated to 1 ppm will suffer harm.

6. Fluoridation of water supplies in Strathclyde would be likely to reduce considerably the incidence of caries.

7. Such fluoridation would be likely to produce a very small increase in the prevalence of dental mottling which would only be noticeable at very close quarters and would be very unlikely to create any aesthetic problems.

8. The present low levels of fluoride in the water supplies in Strathclyde do not cause caries.

I am not therefore prepared to make a finding that the present concentration of fluoride in the water in Strathclyde causes caries. However, I have no doubt that increasing the present concentrations to 1 ppm would considerably reduce the incidence of that disease.'

(Opinion of Lord Jauncey, pp. 326–63)

He then dealt with the four questions of Law. Namely, (1) *ultra vires*; (2) nuisance; (3) breach of the water (Scotland) Act 1980 and (4) breach of the Medicines Act 1968. He rejected the last three legal arguments but upheld that part of her case which claimed that water fluoridation was *ultra vires*.

The Judge's opinion on the legal point of *ultra vires* centred around the meaning of the word 'wholesome'. The relevant section of the Act provided 'it shall be the duty of every local authority to provide a supply of wholesome water in pipes to every part of their district where a supply of water is required for domestic purposes and can be provided at reasonable cost'.

The Judge considered in detail the judgment in the Lower Hutt Case in New Zealand, which had ruled in favour of fluoridation. He decided that:

the question is a narrow and difficult one but I consider that there are material differences between the circumstances in the Lower Hutt case and the present.... In my view the word 'wholesome' falls properly to be constructed in the more restricted sense advocated by the petitioner as relating to water which was free from contamination and pleasant to drink. It follows that fluoridation which in no way facilitates nor is incidental to the supply of such water is out with the powers of the respondents. The petitioner therefore succeeds on this branch of her case.

The UK Government's response

The Government's response was given by the Secretary of State for Social Services:

Fluoridation has been supported by successive Governments as a safe and effective public health measures and we consider that Lord Jauncey's opinion amply demonstrates that the Government should continue to support fluoridation as a positive means to promote good dental health. It is therefore the Government's intention, when the Parliamentary timetable permits, to bring forward legislation which will clarify the power of water authorities in Scotland to add fluoride to the water supply on the recommendation of the appropriate Health Boards.

The Fluoridation Bill was laid before Parliament in February 1985. It passed through its last stage 30 October 1985, supported by the leaders of all the main political parties, and received the Royal Assent. This legislation enables a health authority to make arrangements with a 'statutory water undertaker' to add fluoride to the water supply. The Bill requires the health authority, before implementing their proposal, to inform the public by publishing details in a newspaper and informing every local authority whose area falls wholly or partly within the area affected by the proposal.

Fluoridation and Cancer: A Review of the Epidemiological Evidence

A general review of the evidence on the health effects of the fluoridation of the water supplies was undertaken in the United Kingdom by the Committee of the Royal College of Physicians of London in 1976. The review concluded that fluoridation is safe, and in particular that there is no evidence that fluoride increases the incidence of mortality in any organ. Since the College Committee reported the results a number of new epidemiological investigations have become available, and the authors of some of the studies have claimed that increased cancer rates are associated with fluoridation. The Department of Health and Social Security set up a working party under the Chairmanship of Professor Knox 'to reappraise the published and other available data and conclusions on cancer incidence and mortality amongst populations whose drinking water is either artificially fluoridated or contains high levels of fluoride from natural sources.' The report was published in 1985 (Knox 1985).

The study reviewed data from 12 countries and concluded:

(1) We have found nothing in any of the major classes of epidemiological evidence which could lead us to conclude that either fluoride occurring naturally in water, or fluoride added to water supplies, is capable of inducing cancer, or of increasing the mortality from cancer. This statement applies both to cancer as a whole, and to cancer at a large number of specific sites. In this we concur with the great majority of scientific investigators and commentators in this field. The only contrary conclusions are in our view attributable to errors in data, errors in analytical technique, and errors in scientific logic.

(2) The evidence permits us to comment positively on the safety of fluoridated water in this respect. The absence of demonstrable effects on cancer rates in the face of long-term exposures to naturally elevated levels of fluoride in water: the absence of any demonstrable effect on cancer rates following the artificial fluoridation of water supplies: the large human populations observed: the consistency of the findings from many different sources of data in many different countries: lead us to conclude that in this respect the fluoridation of drinking water is safe.

FLUORIDE TABLETS AND DROPS

Effectiveness in Caries Prevention

During the 1950s, the value of water fluoridation as a way of preventing caries became clear. It was recognized, however, that water fluoridation was not always possible and that a sensible alternative might be to give children an equivalent amount of fluoride as a tablet. One of the first demonstrations of the value of fluoride tablets for caries prevention was given by Arnold *et al.* (1960). The authors concluded that: 'The results correspond with what has been observed in the use of drinking waters containing 1 ppm F'. Children over the age of 3 years received 1 mg F/day and this dose has formed the basis for further studies, and for individual and community prevention, for 30 years.

About 57 reports on the effectiveness of fluoride tablets or drops have appeared in the literature, although some of these are difficult to interpret because of the small size of the test group, the short experimental period or inadequate reporting. The remaining investigations fall into two groups: first, those where the fluoride supplements were given daily at home and were started before school age, and secondly, those where tablets have been distributed in school, on school days only, usually without additional supplementations during holidays or before school age. The effectiveness of the use of fluoride tablets at home is very much harder to investigate because it is difficult to choose a comparable control group and there is frequently a marked fall-off in co-operation; these difficulties do not usually arise in school-based trials. An excellent review of the effectiveness of fluoride tablets was given by Driscoll (1974), and Tables 3.10 and 3.11 are based on his report, but with additional recent data.

Primary teeth

Summaries of 21 trials into the effect of fluoride tablets on the primary dentition are given in Table 3.10. Thirteen were conducted in Europe, five in the USA and three in Australia. Sodium fluoride was used in all but one study (although the compound was not stated in one further study), sometimes in combination with vitamins.

The initial age of the subjects and the length of time the tablets were taken varied considerably, making it difficult to draw conclusions on effectiveness accurately. Nevertheless it would appear that a caries-preventive effect was observed consistently (about 50–80 per cent reduction) in studies where the initial age was 2 years or younger. In the three studies in which no effect was found, the children were initially aged 3 years or older. In a more thorough analysis of effectiveness in relation to the age at which ingestion of tablets began, Granath et al. (1978) suggested that while bucco-lingual surfaces may benefit if the commencement age is over 2 years, the effect on approximal surfaces is very much less if the commencement age is 2 years or over. This suggests that the topical effect is greater on the more exposed bucco-lingual surfaces than on the less accessible approximal surfaces.

The study of Hennon et al. (1977) is the only clinical trial of fluoride tablets conducted in an area with an almost optimal water fluoride level (0.6–0.8 ppm F), although the observations of Glenn (1979) and Glenn et al. (1982) were on children living in a fluoridated community. A substantial preventive effect was observed by Hennon and co-workers in the children taking fluoride tablets, in addition to the benefit that could be expected to be derived from living in an area with a moderate water fluoride level.

The practice of giving to young children, living in areas with optimal levels of fluoride in the water, additional fluoride dietary supplements has been criticized on the grounds that it substantially increases the risk of dental fluorosis (Schrotenboer 1981; Stookey 1981).

Permanent teeth

Summaries of the 34 investigations into the effectiveness of fluoride tablets in preventing caries in the permanent dentition are given in Table 3.11; again most of the studies are European. The initial age of the subjects and the duration of fluoride tablet intake varied widely. In only four of the studies (Hamberg 1971; Schutzmannsky 1971; Aasenden and Peebles 1974; Margolis et al. 1975) were fluoride tablets taken from birth for at least 7 years. Reductions ranged from

39 per cent in Schutzmannsky's trial to 80 per cent in the trial of Aasenden and Peebles. In the trial of Margolis and co-workers the children who started taking fluoride tablets at birth showed a 58 per cent reduction in DFT compared with only a 14 per cent reduction in the group of children who started at the age of 4 years, suggesting the importance of ingestion in the first few years of life, before the permanent teeth erupted.

Three of the 34 studies were conducted in the UK—all were school-based programmes and all reported substantial caries reductions. Stephen and Campbell (1978) reported an 81 per cent reduction in DMFS in a trial in Glasgow lasting 3 years, while Allmark et al. (1982) reported a reduction in DMFS of 61 per cent after 6 years' use in Portsmouth, and O'Rourke et al. (1988) reported a 48 per cent reduction in DMFT in Manchester children after 3 years.

Prenatal

Six trials have investigated the effectiveness of the ingestion of prenatal fluoride tablets, although results of only four of these are given in Tables 3.10 and 3.11, because in the remaining two (Feltman and Kosel 1961; Glenn 1979; Glenn et al. 1982) insufficient data were reported. In all these trials (Tables 3.10 and 3.11) the percentage caries reduction was greater in the children whose mothers received fluoride tablets in pregnancy. But in spite of the apparent greater benefit of prenatal fluoride, Hoskova (1968) concluded that fluoride administration should begin as soon after birth as possible, attributing the greater benefit to better home conditions in the prenatal group.

Dr Frances Glenn has written extensively on the benefits of prenatal fluoride supplementation (e.g. Glenn 1981; Glenn et al. 1982; LeGeros et al. 1985; Glenn and Glenn 1987). Glenn (1979) reported caries prevalence in children attending a private practice who had received prenatal fluoride supplements in addition to receiving an optimum water fluoride level. Nineteen of the 24 children aged 5–17 years who received prenatal supplements were caries-free.

Further data were presented at a symposium 'Perspectives on the use of pre-natal fluorides' (Glenn 1981) and again one year later (Glenn et al. 1982). The caries status of 492 children were reported: 97 per cent of the 117 children who received prenatal fluoride were caries-free, whereas only 15 per cent of the 375 children who did not receive prenatal fluoride were caries-free. Reasons put forward by Glenn for the very much better dental health of children who received prenatal fluoride included higher levels of fluoride in exfoliated primary teeth (enamel and dentine) and improved occlusal surface morphology. The recommended dose, according to Glenn and Glenn (1987), for mothers is between 1 and 4 mg F/day, for example, 2 mg F (4.4 mg NaF) per day, and this should be started by the twelfth week of pregnancy.

The clinical data upon which Frances Glenn based her recommendations have been criticized (Driscoll 1981; Schrotenboer 1981; Stookey 1981; Stamm 1981). These authors concluded that there was a lack of adequate data upon which to recommend the prenatal use of fluoride dietary supplements, but they agreed that properly controlled clinical studies should be undertaken. At present most countries

Fluorides and dental caries

Table 3.10. Caries-preventive effects of fluoride tablets/drops on deciduous teeth (based on Driscoll 1974 and Binder *et al.* 1978)

Study	F compound	Daily dosage (mg F)	Initial age of subjects (yr)	No. subjects in F group	Duration of F intake (yr)	Caries reduction (%) deft	defs	Statistical significance
Arnold *et al.* (1960)	NaF	0.5–1	Birth–6	121	1–12	'Comparable to water F'		NR
Pollak (1960)[5]	NaF + V	1	3	100	2	80		NR
	NaF + V	1	4	111	2	20		NR
Ziemnowicz-Glowaka (1960)[5]	NaF	0.8	3	139	2		26	S
Lutomska and Kominska (1962)[5]	NaF	0.6	3–4	154	2	'No significant effect'		NR
Kamocka *et al.* (1964)[5]	NaF	0.75[1]	3	64	3	0		NS
	NaF	0.75[1]	4	79	3	0		NS
Leonhardt (1965)[5]	NaF + V	1+	3	Not known	2	38		NR
	NaF + V	1+	4	Not known	2	30		NR
Hennon *et al.* (1966, 1967, 1970)	NaF + V	0.5–1	Birth–5½	85	3		63	S
	NaF + V	0.5–1	Birth–5½	54	4		68	S
	NaF + V	0.5–1	Birth–5½	60	5		66	S
Margolis *et al.* (1975)	NaF + V	0.5–1	Birth	149	4–6	76		S
	NaF + V	0.5–1	4	77	0–2	29		NS
Hoskova (1968)	NaF	0.25–1	Prenatal	78	4	93		S
	NaF	0.25–1	Birth–1	151	4	54		S
Kailis *et al.* (1968)	NaF	?	Prenatal	50	4–6	82		S
	NaF	?	Birth	92	4–6	56		S
Stolte (1968)[5]	?	1	3	130	3	11		NR
Prichard (1969)	NaF	?	Prenatal	176	6–8	70		S
	NaF	?	Birth	282	6–8	40		S
Hamberg (1971)	NaF + V (drops)	0.5	Birth	342	3	57		NR
	NaF + V (drops)	0.5	Birth	342	6	49		NR
Kraemer (1971)[5]	CaF$_2$	1	4	170	2	22		NR
	CaF$_2$	1	5	82	2	18		NR
Schützmannsky (1971)	NaF	1	Prenatal	100	<1	13		S
	NaF	0.25–1	Prenatal	100	9	30		S
	NaF	0.25–1	Birth	100	9	14		S
Aasenden and Peebles (1974)	NaF + V[2]	0.5–1	Birth	87	8–11		78	S
Fanning *et al.* (1975)	NaF	?	< 1	581	5	33		NR
Andersson and Grahnén (1976)	NaF	0.25–0.5	1	127	5[3]	31		S
Hennon *et al.* (1977)[4]	NaF + V	0.5–1	< 1	44	5		47	S
	NaF + V	0.5	< 1	47	5		37	S
Granath *et al.* (1978)	NaF	0.25–0.5	< 2	48	2–4		46 BL	NS
							51 AP	S
	NaF	0.25–0.5	2–3	123	1–2		33 BL	NS
							–1 AP	NS
O'Rourke *et al.* (1988)	NaF	1[1]	5	263	3	18		NS

V, Vitamins; S, Statistically significant; NS, Statistically non-significant; NR, No statistical test reported; BL, bucco-lingual; AP, Approximal surfaces.

[1] Tablets given only on school days.

[2] A NaF + V combination was given up to 3 years of age. Beyond this age, some children received NaF + V, while others received only NaF.

[3] Aged 8–10 at examination.

[4] In F area (0.6–0.8 ppm F).

[5] Quoted by Driscoll (1974).

Table 3.11. Caries-preventive effects of fluoride tablets on permanent teeth (based on Driscoll, 1974 and Binder *et al.* 1978)

Study	F compound	Daily dosage (mg F)	Initial age of subjects (yr)	No. subjects in F group	Duration of F intake (yr)	Caries reduction (%)		Statistical significance
						DMFT	DMFS	
Stones et al. (1949)	NaF	1.5	6–14	125	2	0		NS
Bibby et al. (1955)	NaF	1	5–14	133	1		Nil	NR
	NaF	1	5–14	119	1	Tentative finding: 'possible'		NR
Niedenthal (1957)[4]	NaF	1[1]	6–7	251	3	22		NR
Wrzodek (1959)[4]	NaF	1[1]	6–9	8381	3	21		NR
	NaF	1[1]	6–9	13 585	4	22		NR
Arnold et al. (1960)	NaF	0.5–1	Birth–6	121	1–15	'Comparable to water F'		NR
Krusic (1960)[4]	CaF$_2$	Not known	8–15	480	1–3	70		NR
Pollak (1960)[4]	NaF + V	1	6–7	300	2	38		NR
Ziemnowicz-Glowaka (1960)[4]	NaF	0.8[1]	3–6	704	2		33	S
	NaF	0.8[1]	5–6	204	3		28	S
Jez (1962)[4]	CaF$_2$	Not known	7–11	7200	2 1/2	0		NR
Krychalska-Karwan and Laskowa (1963)[4]	NaF	Not known	Grammar school	134	4		5	NR
Minoguchi et al. (1963)	NaF + V	0.25	Birth–6	75	6	36		NR
Grissom et al. (1964)	NaF	1[1]	6–11	178	2		34	S
Kamocka et al. (1964)[4]	NaF	0.75[1]	3	64	3	17		NS
	NaF	0.75[1]	4	79	3	60		S
Leonhardt (1964)	NaF	1	6	398	4	32		NR
	NaF	1	7	429	3	25		NR
Hippchen (1965)[4]	Not known	1	6	500	3	32		NR
Schützmannsky (1965)	NaF	0.75[1]	6	580	4		25	NR
	NaF	0.75[1]	6	197	6		27	NR
Berner et al. (1967)	NaF	0.5–1[1]	5–7	105	3		84 (except 1st molar)	NR
							33 (1st molar)	NR
	NaF	1[1]	7–9	158	4	16		NR
	NaF	1[1]	7–9	160	6	20		NR
	NaF	1[1]	7–9	109	7	24		NR
De Paola and Lax (1968)	APF	1[1]	6–8	130	2		23	S
Girardi-Vogt (1968)[4]	NaF	1	6	Not known	3	31		NR
Stolte (1968)[4]	Not known	1	3	150	3	69		NR
Marthaler (1969)	NaF	0.5–1[1]	7	450	1–8	36	47	S
Hamberg (1971)	NaF + V	0.5	Birth	342	7	70		NR
Schützmannsky (1971)	NaF	1	Prenatal	100	< 1	6		NS
	NaF	0.25–1	Prenatal	100	9	43		S
	NaF	0.25–1	Birth	100	9	39		S
Aasenden et al. (1972)	APF	1[1]	8–11	109	3		30	S
	NaF	1[1]	8–11	114	3		27	S
Plasschaert and Konig (1974)	NaF	1	7	208	2		38	S
Aasenden and Peebles (1974)	NaF + V[2]	0.5–1	Birth	100	8–11		80	S
Binder (1974)	NaF	0.25–1	Birth–14	3084	8–14	43		S
Margolis et al. (1975)	NaF + V	0.5–1	Birth	56	7–10	58		S
	NaF + V	0.5–1	4	31	3–6	14		NS

Table 3.11   *continued*

Study	F compound	Daily dosage (mg F)	Initial age of subjects (yr)	No. subjects in F group	Duration of F intake (yr)	Caries reduction (%)		Statistical significance
						DMFT	DMFS	
Anderssson and Grahnén (1976)	NaF	0.25–0.5	1	127	5[3]		40	S
Stephen and Campbell (1978)	NaF	1[1]	5 1/2	54	3		81	S
Driscoll *et al.* (1978)	APF	1[1]	6–7	150	6		28	S
	APF	2[1]	6–7	135	6		29	S
Allmark *et al.* (1982)	NaF	1[1]	6	124	6	59	61	S
O'Rourke *et al.* (1988)	NaF	1[1]	5	263	3	48		S

V, Vitamins; S, Statistically significant; NS, Statistically non-significant; NR, No statistical test reported.

[1] Tablets given only on school days.

[2] A NaF + V combination was given up to 3 years of age. Beyond this age, some children received NaF + V, while others received only NaF.

[3] Aged 8–12 at examination.

[4] Quoted by Driscoll (1974).

permit, but do not encourage, prenatal fluoride supplementation. A government sponsored trial of prenatal fluoride supplementation is currently in progress in the USA.

Fluoride–vitamin combination

Vitamin and fluoride supplementation has been combined in some preparations sold in the USA. This is convenient when both vitamins and fluoride are required. The results of trials listed in Table 3.10 and 3.11 seem to show that the effectiveness of fluoride drops/tablets is neither enhanced nor reduced by their combination with vitamins and minerals: Stookey (1981) came to the same conclusion. They are not at present marketed in the UK.

Type of fluoride compound

The results of the three trials testing CaF_2 compounds are very variable (0–70 per cent reduction); all were short-term trials. The impressive result of Krusic (1960) is surprising, since the insolubility of CaF_2 would obviate the likelihood of a topical effect comparable with NaF, and a systemic effect would be very unlikely to occur in this short trial in 8- to 15-year-old children.

From the three trials in which APF compounds were used, the effectiveness would appear to be no greater than that observed in the larger number of NaF trials. APF tablets are considerably more expensive than NaF tablets (Driscoll *et al.* 1978), but the greater salivary flow caused by the low pH of the APF tablets is likely to reduce the concentration of fluoride around the teeth and hasten its clearance from the mouth. It would appear that to ensure high and long-lasting salivary F levels, tablets should contain NaF rather than APF, disintegrate slowly in the mouth without being sucked, and possess as little flavour as possible, so long as the tablets are acceptable to children (McCall *et al.* 1981).

Although it is desirable that fluoride tablets dissolve slowly so that teeth are bathed in high levels of fluoride for a long time, it is important to appreciate that saliva does not flow extensively around the mouth. Weatherell *et al.* (1984) and

Primosch *et al.* (1986) have shown clearly that fluoride released from a tablet tends to remain highly concentrated at the site of tablet dissolution. There was very little mixing between the sides of the mouth or between vestibules of upper and lower arches. It would seem important, therefore, that the position of tablets in the mouth is changed regularly (Dawes and Weatherell 1990).

Effectiveness of fluoride tablets compared with other methods

Poulsen *et al.* (1981) compared the effectiveness of the daily use of a 1 mg F tablet and the fortnightly rinsing with 0.2 per cent NaF in a school-based programme in Denmark. The results (Table 3.12) indicated that caries increments were lower in the rinsing group than in the tablet group. This difference was seen in both age groups and was statistically significant in teeth erupted at baseline, but not in teeth erupting during the study. Holm *et al.* (1975) found no statistically significant difference in 2-year caries increments between a group of children who received fluoride tablets (0.42 mg F/day) and a group who rinsed fortnightly with 0.2 per cent NaF, although there was a statistically non-significant trend towards lower caries increment in the rinsing group.

Rather contrary results were reported by Heifetz *et al.* (1987). Two-year interim results from this American trial on children initially aged 5–6 years indicated that 331 children who received a 1 mg F tablet each school day developed an average of 2.06 dmfs, which was less than the average of 2.50 dmfs recorded for the 345 children who rinsed weekly in school with 0.2 per cent NaF. The difference was not statistically significant.

Summary of effectiveness of fluoride tablets and drops

From the results of published trials it would seem that there is no doubt that the use of fluoride tablets or drops is effective in preventing dental caries in both the deciduous and permanent dentitions. The effectiveness would seem to be greater

Table 3.12. Comparison of the effectiveness of daily use of 1 mg F tablets in school and fortnightly rinsing with 0.2 per cent NaF in school. Three-year mean DMFS data are given for children initially aged 7 years and for children initially aged 11 years (Poulsen *et al.* 1981)

Age at baseline (yrs)	Group	N	Teeth erupted at baseline	Teeth erupting during the study
			Mean (sd) DMFS	Mean (sd) DMFS
7	Tablets	124	1.65 (2.10)	0.30 (0.86)
	Rinses	125	1.09 (1.73)	0.22 (0.58)
11	Tablets	129	1.65 (2.52)	1.48 (1.68)
	Rinses	121	1.55 (2.79)	1.17 (1.58)

the earlier the child begins to take the fluoride supplement—from 40 to 80 per cent reduction being expected in both deciduous and permanent dentitions if supplementation is commenced before 2 years of age. For school-based schemes the effectiveness would appear to be slightly lower and more variable (30–80 per cent reduction) but still substantial. NaF would appear to be the compound of choice.

Results of the home-based trials have to be interpreted with caution, for the attitude to dental health of the mothers who gave their children supplements from birth is likely to be more favourable than mothers who began supplementation later or who formed the control group. Previous reviewers of the effectiveness of fluoride tablets have commented upon this problem of interpretation of results (Driscoll 1981).

It has to be admitted that daily administration of tablets at home from birth (or prenatally) requires a very high level of parental motivation, and campaigns to get parents to give their children fluoride supplements have not been successful in many countries.

DISCUSSION OF THE DOSAGE OF FLUORIDE TABLETS AND DROPS

At least 18 different dosage regimens for fluoride tablets and drops have been published. These range from the high dosage level recommended before 1976 in Australia of 0.5 mg F daily from birth to 12 months and 1.0 mg F from 1 year onwards (McEniery and Davies 1979), to the low dosage level in Denmark since 1978 of 0.25 mg F from 6 to 24 months and 0.5 mg F from 2 years onwards (Thylstrup *et al.* 1979). The recommended dosage regimen in Sweden is similar to the Danish schedule, except that the change form 0.25 to 0.5 mg F/day occurs at the age of 18 months (Widenheim 1985). In the UK, the dosage regimen used to be 0.5 mg F from birth to 2 years and 1 mg F from 2 years onwards (Silverstone 1973; Murray 1976), but in recent years there has been a trend to reduce the dosage of daily fluoride supplements in many countries.

In the UK, the current recommended dosage is 0.25 mg F from 6 months to 2 years, 0.5 mg F from 2 to 4 years and 1.0 mg F over 4 years. The schedule given in Table 3.13 is the same as that proposed by Dowell and Joyston-Bechal (1981), except that the commencement of fluoride supplementation is now delayed until 6 months of age. The schedule given in the British National Formulary (1990) does not give an upper age limit for fluoride supplementation and

Table 3.13. Fluoride supplements: age-related dosages (mg F/day) (from British Association for the Study of Community Dentistry 1988)

Age	Concentration of fluoride in drinking water (ppm F)		
	< 0.3	0.3–0.7	> 0.7
6 mos to 2 yrs	0.25	0	0
2–4 yr	0.50	0.25	0
4–16 yr	1.00	0.50	0

there is really no reason to stop or avoid supplementation in adulthood. Most regimens give sliding scales of dosages depending upon water fluoride levels (British Association for the Study of Community Dentistry 1988; Health Education Authority 1989; British National Formulary 1990). Since there is considerable disagreement between countries on the recommended dosage levels, it is pertinent to discuss the reasons for changes in dosage schedules.

The objective of any systemic fluoride administration is to obtain the maximum caries-preventive effect with a low risk of unacceptable enamel mottling. As far as water fluoridation is concerned this is achieved, in temperate climates, where drinking water contains 1 ppm F. In the past, fluoride tablet dosages have been calculated in an attempt to duplicate the fluoride intake which occurs in people receiving optimally fluoridated drinking water.

In this respect, it is necessary to make two comments. Arnold *et al.* (1960) estimated that the fluoride intake from public water supplies containing 1 ppm F was about 1 mg F/day in children over the age of 3 years and between 0.4 and 0.6 mg F/day in children less than 3 years. It is important to realize, however, that these were estimates (of older children drinking a litre of water per day) based on calculations published by McClure (1943), who in turn used figures of Adolph (1933), and were not based on epidemiological data. A review of the literature, covering the past 40 years, of water consumption by children, revealed that children drink considerably less (about 60–70 per cent less) water from public supplies that previously assumed (Rugg-Gunn *et al.*, 1987). Thus, the earlier estimates that children over 3 years ingest 1 mg F/day from water were almost certainly too high.

The second point is that fluoride from tablets is ingested and absorbed at one time of day and this is physiologically different from ingestion of fluoride from water where absorption is spread throughout the day. Animal experiments have shown that fluoride given once a day is more likely to cause fluorosis than the same amount of fluoride given intermittently throughout the day (Angmar-Månsson *et al.*, 1976) but it is unclear whether this applies to man. Because of these points, the balance between dosage of fluoride tablets and the occurrence of dental fluorosis need to be continually reassessed and considered separately from water-borne fluorides.

In 1991, a workshop on changing patterns of fluoride intake was held at Chapel Hill, U.S.A. (Bawden 1992) and agreed a new supplemental fluoride dosage schedule (mg/day) according to the fluoride concentration of drinking water (Table 3.14).

Table 3.14. Proposed supplemental fluoride dosage schedule (mg/day) (Newbrun 1992)

Weight/kg	Age	Concentration of fluoride in drinking water (ppm F)		
		< 0.3	0.3–0.7	> 0.7
3.14–12.4	Birth to 2 yrs	0.25	0	0
12.14–16.4	2–4 yrs	0.5	0.25	0
16.4–21.5	4–6 yrs	0.75	0.5	0
> 21.5	> 6	1.0	0.75	0

This schedule varies from the one given in Table 3.13 in that it recommends starting at birth rather than at six months and in the 2–6 year age group suggests a slightly higher dose schedule. An alternative view was put forward at a meeting convened by Colgate in Brussels a few months after the conference at Chapel Hill, in order to try to achieve a consensus European view of fluoride supplementation (Clarkson 1992). Delegates expressed concern over the complexity of the present dosage schedules. At the moment in Britain a parent with three children aged 5 years, 3 years, and 18 months is expected to administer daily three different dose regimes. This complexity precludes compliance by all but the most committed parents (whose children are probably the least at risk). From a risk-benefit point of view it was considered important to be able to state that no appreciable fluorosis to anterior teeth would occur if 0.5 mg/day were taken after the age of 3 years. It was acknowledged that some special risk infants would benefit from starting fluoride supplements before the age of 3 years (using a dose of 0.25 mg F), but this would be upon the advice of a dental practitioner. The participants agreed unanimously on the following recommendations for the use of fluoride supplements in Europe:

1. Fluoride supplements have no application as a public health measure.

2. A dose of 0.5 mg/day fluoride should be prescribed for at risk individuals from the age of 3 years.

3. Labelling should advise that fluoride supplements should not be used before 3 years of age unless prescribes by a dentist.

An expert working group of the World Health Organization also reviewed the current position of fluoride supplements (WHO 1994). The group acknowledged that there has been a general trend towards lowering the fluoride supplement dose, particularly in the early months of life, and reached the following conclusions.

1. Fluoride supplements have limited application as a possible health measure.

2. In areas with medium to low caries experience, a conservative prescribing policy should be adopted. A dose of 0.5 mg F/day should be prescribed for at risk individuals from the age of 3 years.

3. In areas where there is particular concern about caries in the primary and permanent dentitions, a regimen starting at 6 months of life, taking into account the fluoride content of the drinking water, should be used.

4. Prescribed supplements should be issued in 'child-proof' containers. The quantity of fluoride tablets issued at one time should not exceed 120 mg F.

OTHER METHODS OF FLUORIDE ADMINISTRATION

Fluoridized Salt

As a dietary vehicle for ensuring adequate ingestion of fluoride, domestic salt comes second to drinking water; Salt's enrichment with iodide already provides an effective means of preventing goitre. Indeed it was a medical practitioner concerned with prevention of goitre in Switzerland who, over 40 years ago, pioneered the addition of fluoride to salt as a caries-preventive measure (Wespi 1948,1950). Fluoridated salt has been on sale in Switzerland since 1955, and by 1967 three-quarters of domestic salt sold in Switzerland was fluoridated at 90 mg F/kg salt (or 90 ppm F). However, it was soon accepted that the original estimate of salt intake, upon which calculations of fluoride concentrations in salt were based, were too high and the ingestion of fluoride too low.

Since 1983, the amount of fluoride added to salt has been 250 mg F/kg salt (250 ppm F). This is available in 23 Swiss cantons with 5.5 million inhabitants and is used voluntarily by 70 per cent of the population (Marthaler 1983). In contrast to the situation in Switzerland, Toth (1976, 1980) suggested, on the basis of studies of urinary fluoride concentration, that the level of fluoride added in Hungary should be raised from 250 to 350 mg F/kg.

Despite the widespread use of fluoridated salt in Switzerland, its effectiveness is not easily measured since, in many Swiss communities, other preventive programmes (fluoride tablets or fluoride brushing) have been operating in many schools for over 20 years.

Interim results were published by Marthaler *et al.* (1977, 1978), from which they concluded that the caries-preventive

Table 3.15. Mean number of DMF sites per child living in the Canton of Vaud, Switzerland, which had received salt fluoridized to 250 ppm F since 1970, compared with children in a control area (de Crousaz *et al.* 1985)

Age (yrs)	Control					Test				
	1970	1974	1978	1982	% redn	1970	1974	1978	1982	% redn
8	3.7	2.5	3.3	1.9	49	2.2	1.9	1.6	1.8	17
10	7.4	6.0	4.4	4.4	40	5.4	3.7	3.6	4.3	19
12	15.4	11.2	8.5	8.2	47	10.4	7.3	6.6	5.0	52
14	—	—	—	—	—	16.2	12.6	10.5	8.2	49

effectiveness of fluoridized salt in Vaud was greater than the 25 per cent or so reduction observed following the addition of 90 mg F/kg in other Swiss cantons (Marthaler and Schenardi 1962). The results after 12 years are given in detail by de Crousaz *et al.* (1985). Dental examinations of 100–200 children in four age groups—8, 10, 12 and 14 years—were conducted on an examiner-blind basis in 1970, 1974, 1978, and 1982, although the numbers of children aged 14 years in the control area were too small to analyse. Results for DMF sites are given in Table 3.15. The authors concluded that: (a) there was a decline in caries experience in children in the control communities; (b) a similar decline occurred in 12- and 14-year-old children living in the test communities—this was not the case for 8- and 10-year-olds where a low caries prevalence already existed in 1970, probably due to earlier use of fluoride tablets; (c) caries experience was consistently lower in children who consumed salt fluoridized to 250 mg F/kg compared with children in the control communities. Caries experience of children in Vaud in 1982 was similar to those recorded for children in Basle who had consumed water fluoridated at 1.0 ppm F, and similar to children in Zurich Canton who had benefited from a school-based dental programme which had been operating for the past 16 years (Figure 3.14). The authors concluded that this study provides further evidence of substantial cariostatic effect of fluoride when added to salt.

The effect on the dental health of children after 9 years of salt fluoridization at 250 ppm F in the Canton of Glarus was reported by Steiner *et al.* (1986). Caries experience fell in Glarus more rapidly than in other areas, pointing to a cariostatic effect of fluoridated salt.

Toth (1976) reported the effectiveness of 250 mg F/kg salt fluoridized in Hungary after 8 years' use. The results (Table 3.16) indicated a reduction of 39 per cent in deft in 6-year-old children in the test community, while caries experience increased by 7 per cent in the control community children

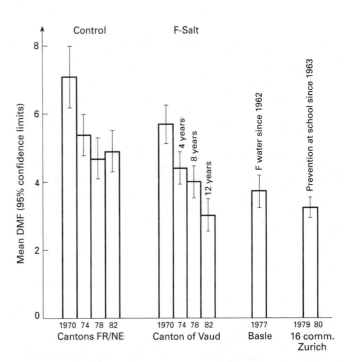

Fig. 3.14. Mean DMFT for 12-year-old Swiss children in the control Cantons of Fribourg and Neuchâtel; receiving salt fluoridized to 250 mg F/kg in Vaud; in fluoridized Basle; and in 16 communities in Zurich Canton. (After de Crousaz *et al.* 1985; reproduced with kind permission of editor, *Helvetica odontologica Acta*.)

Table 3.16. Caries experience (deft) for 6-year-old children living in test and control communities in Hungary after 8 years' salt fluoridization (at 250 mg F/kg) (from Toth 1976)

	Experimental	Control
1966	6.8	8.6
1974	4.1	9.2
Difference	−2.7 (−39.5%)	+0.6 (+7.1%)

over the same period. Although there was an imbalance in caries experience between the two communities at the start of the experiment in 1966, this alone could not explain the differences observed in 1974. After 10 years' exposure to salt fluoridation, Toth (1979) observed that 5- to 6-year-olds in the same test community had 2.8 deft, compared with 6.0 deft in the control community, and 1.4 deft in children of the same age living in an area with fluoridated water. These 10-year results indicated that a substantial caries reduction occurred after the introduction of salt fluoridization, but this was less than occurred with water fluoridation.

In 1964, a study was initiated in four Colombian communities (Mejia *et al.* 1976). In the village of Montebello, sodium fluoride was added to domestic salt (at 200 mg F/kg), while in Armenia calcium fluoride was added to domestic salt (at 200 mg F/kg), in San Pedro drinking water was fluoridated (at 1 ppm F) and Don Matias remained as the control community. At the end of the project, after 8 years, reductions in caries prevalence and experience in 8-year-old

Table 3.17. Caries experience (DMFT) for 8-year-old children living in three test communities and one control community in Colombia, South America, after 8 years (Mejia et al. 1976)

	NaF salt	CaF₂ salt	Water F	Control
1964	3.7	3.8	3.8	4.3
1972	1.4	1.1	0.8	3.8
Difference	2.3 (61%)	2.7 (72%)	3.0 (78%)	0.5 (13%)

children were large in the three communities receiving fluoride in salt or water, although a small reduction was also observed in the control town (Table 3.17). When all children aged 6–14 years were included in the data analyses, the reduction in DMFT between 1964 and 1972 was 50 per cent in Montebello (NaF in salt), 48 per cent in Armenia (CaF₂ in salt), 60 per cent in San Pedro (water F) and 5 per cent in the control town Don Matias.

Encouraging results were also reported after the addition of NaF to domestic salt in a closed children's institution in Pamplona, Spain (Vines 1971). Because of the high estimated salt intake, particularly in their special salt bread, the fluoride level was only 112 mg F/kg salt but, after 4 years, reductions in caries experience were observed in all ages in the range 8–13 years.

The average ingestion of salt amounts to 7–10 g/day per person in several developed countries: about 3–5 g comes from domestic salt, 2–3 g is naturally present in foods and 2–3 g is added during manufacture.

In summary, the caries-preventive effectiveness of fluoridized salt is substantial, approaching that of fluoridated water. This view is based on a comparatively small number of studies (compared with the data on water fluoridation) which have lasted for a maximum of 12 years. Since April 1983, the fluoride content of salt in Switzerland has been 250 ppm F. Urinary fluoride concentration studies have indicated that this concentration may be slightly less than optimal in children but sufficient in adults (Marthaler 1983). Salt appears to be a safe vehicle for fluoride administration.

FLUORIDIZED MILK AND FRUIT JUICES

Both bovine and human milk contain low levels of fluoride—about 0.03 ppm F (Ericsson and Ribelius 1971). Because milk is recommended as a good food for infants and children, it was considered, over 30 years ago, to be a suitable vehicle for supplementing children's fluoride intake in areas with fluoride-deficient water supplies. Ericsson (1958) showed that fluoride was absorbed in the gut just as readily from milk as from water, refuting the suggestion that the high calcium content of milk would render the fluoride unavailable. More recently, Villa et al. (1989) have shown that fluoride absorption from MFP in milk is as high as that from NaF in water. However, the binding of added fluoride to calcium or protein might reduce the topical fluoride effect in the mouth compared with fluoride in water (Duff 1981).

The results of five clinical trials of fluoridized milk and one trial of fluoridized fruit juice have been published. The study of Rusoff et al. (1962) involved 171 children aged 6–9 years from two schools in Louisiana, U.S.A. Children from one school received a half-pint of homogenized milk daily, fortified with 2.2 mg NaF (yielding 1 mg F). The fluoride was added in the form of 0.5 ml NaF solution to each half-pint before sealing. During the summer vacation, parents of children in the study group were given bottles of aqueous sodium fluoride solution so that 8 drops could be added to their 8 oz (225 ml) glass of milk per day. Children in the control group received homogenized milk without fluoride. This pilot study lasted 3½ years, when 65 children aged 9–12 years remained in the fluoride group and 64 children of similar age in the control group. Unfortunately the two groups were not well balanced with respect to first-molar caries experience at the beginning of the experiment. The DMFT in second molars and first and second premolars, after 3½ years' consumption of fluoridized milk, was 0.34 in the fluoride group and 1.70 in the control group. A difference was still apparent 18 months after cessation of the experiment. However, because of the considerable divergence in caries attack on first molars between groups before the study and the small size of the groups, the lower caries rate in the experimental children must be viewed with caution.

Ziegler (1962) reported his attempts to introduce fluoridized milk in Winterthur, Switzerland. At first, a sealed plastic bottle of 0.22 per cent sodium fluoride solution was made available to the public in pharmacies against a prescription. Each parent then added 1 ml of this fluoride solution to 1 litre of milk to produce 1 ppm F fluoridized milk. Thus the amount of fluoride ingested depended on the amount of milk consumed—a half-litre of milk contained 0.5 mg F. In 1955, school milk was fluoridized at the central dairy in Winterthur; initially 0.2 mg F was placed in 200 ml milk, but this was increased to 0.5 mg in 1961. A little later, the size of milk bottles was increased to 250 ml, which contained 0.625 mg F. The results of clinical surveys indicated that dental caries was lower in children who had consumed the fluoridized milk for 6 years, compared with control children (Wirz and Ziegler 1964, quoted in WHO, 1970).

Stephen et al. (1981, 1984) reported the results of a 5-year study of the effect on young Glasgow children of consuming fluoridized milk at school. Children entered the study in 1976 at age 4.5–5.5 years, and drank 200 ml of milk containing 1.5 mg F (7 ppm F) each school day (about 200 days per year).The control group drank milk without added fluoride. After 5 years, the 50 children in the test group had developed a mean of 3.8 DMFS compared with 6.6 DMFS in the 56 children in the control group—a difference of 43 per cent. When data analysis was restricted to permanent teeth which erupted during the study, the mean DMFS scores were 3.3 for the test group and 6.3 for the control group—a difference of 48 per cent. The milk was sucked through straws at least 15 minutes before the mid-morning break.

A 5-year trial was also conducted in Hungary (Banoczy et al. 1983, 1985) between 1979 and 1983. Children aged 3–9 in the children's city of Fót, north of Budapest, participated, and drank 200 ml of milk or cocoa-milk daily for about 300 days per year. Children aged 3–5 years received 0.4 mg F/day and children 6–9 years 0.75 mg F/day. Children living in another closed community formed a control group. They were similar to the children in the test group, with one exception— while the test group children used a fluoride toothpaste consistently, the control children used either a fluoride or non-fluoride toothpaste. Caries experience was reduced in the test group compared with the control group, both in the deciduous and permanent dentitions, but the beneficial effect was especially marked in first permanent molars in the youngest age group (85 per cent less caries), which received the fluoridized milk from 3 years of age.

The results of a study in Louisiana were more variable (Legett *et al.* 1987). Fluoridized chocolate-flavoured milk was given to young school children for 2 or 3 years. A statistically significant difference was observed in the group who consumed the fluoridized milk for 2 years but not in the group who participated for 3 years compared with the control groups. One explanation for this difference may be the breakdown of the equipment for 9 months in the middle of the trial. The composition of the control group was not clear from the report of this trial.

In warm climates, fluoridized fruit juices may be a practical alternative to fluoridized milk. Gedalia *et al.* (1981) have reported a 28 per cent reduction in DMFS increment in 6 to 9-year-old Israeli children who consumed 1 mg F in 100 ml of pure orange juice ($\equiv$ 10 ppm F) each school day for 3 years. The 111 test-group children developed 2.5 DMFS over 3 years compared with 3.5 DMFS in the 111 control children who had no beverage. However, interpretation of the results was complicated by the observation that a third group of similarly aged children, who consumed 100 ml of orange juice with no added fluoride, developed 2.9 DMFS over the 3-year period. It would appear, therefore, that the fluoride *per se* might have been responsible for only part of the difference between the fluoride drink group and the no-drink group.

In summary, all the reported trials have shown substantial caries-preventive effects, especially when milk consumption began before the eruption of permanent teeth. Clinical data are still limited, however. Milk fluoridation requires considerable logistic effort and, as yet, it has not been introduced on a community basis.

TOPICAL FLUORIDE THERAPY

Topical fluorides fall into two categories: those applied by the dentist in the surgery and those applied by the patient at home. In practice those employed by the dentist are of high fluoride concentration and are applied generally at regular but infrequent intervals, perhaps twice a year. Those used by the patient are of low fluoride levels and are applied at frequent intervals, often daily.

FLUORIDES APPLIED BY THE DENTIST

Such fluoride agents mainly include simple aqueous solutions of sodium fluoride and stannous fluoride, and low pH solutions and gels of an acidulated phosphate fluoride system. Other agents comprise fluoride prophylaxis pastes and fluoride-containing varnishes. Little change has occurred in this area in the last five years, and for that reason this topic will not be considered further in this chapter.

SELF-APPLIED FLUORIDE AGENTS: FLUORIDE DENTIFRICES

Without question the most widely used method of applying fluoride topically is by means of dentifrice. In countries where dentifrices are used over 95 per cent on sale contain a fluoride compound. Indeed, in Western countries it is only with difficulty that a non-fluoride dentifrice can be purchased. The first attempt to determine the value of a fluoride dentifrice was by Bibby (1945) who, in a 2-year study in which 0.1 per cent sodium fluoride was added to a conventional formulation and used unsupervised, failed to show any anticaries effect. No formulation details are given in Bibby's report, but it is reasonable to speculate that the fluoride added to the conventional paste combined with one or more of the original constituents and was thus inactivated. Indeed, one of the major problems in the manufacture of fluoride dentifrices is preventing the fluoride component reacting with other ingredients, notably the abrasive system. Because of the attractiveness in conveying fluoride to enamel surfaces by means of a dentifrice, considerable attention has been given to finding active fluoride compounds and compatible abrasive systems. The first fluoride dentifrice thus formulated contained 0.2 per cent sodium fluoride with an abrasive system comprising a heat-treated calcium orthophosphate (calcium pyrophosphate). The reductions reported (Muhler *et al.* 1955) were of neither clinical nor statistical significance. Other studies by Kyves *et al.* (1961) and Brudevold and Chilton (1966) failed to establish real clinical benefits.

During this time Ericsson and his colleagues in Sweden were actively studying the compatibility of a number of fluoride compounds with the various dentifrice constituents. They demonstrated that sodium fluoride was inactivated by calcium carbonate and calcium phosphate, both common abrasive systems. Following this work Torell and Ericsson (1965) tested a 0.2 per cent sodium fluoride-containing dentifrice in a sodium bicarbonate base and after 2 years showed a statistically significant reduction of questionable clinical relevance. In 1967 Koch reported an extensive clinical study of a dentifrice in which conventional abrasive systems were discarded and replaced by acrylic resin particles that were not only compatible with the fluoride compound but in addition conferred upon the formulation very low abrasiveness. The fluoride was the sodium salt at 0.22 per cent and over the 3-year period of study, in which the subjects brushed under supervised conditions, an overall reduction of 50–58 per cent were reported. In practical terms the cumulative reductions over 3 years represented 7 surfaces in the younger age group and 10 surfaces in the older ones.

Whilst the studies with dentifrices containing sodium fluoride were continuing, Muhler and his colleagues in Indiana were transposing to the dentifrice field their findings with topical applications of stannous fluoride. The final formulation was marketed first in 1955 under the brand name 'Crest' and contained 0.4 per cent stannous fluoride in a calcium pyrophosphate base into which was incorporated 1 per cent stannous pyrophosphate. After this formulation development, a formidable series of clinical trials ensued in which the dentifrice was tested using various age groups and

under differing conditions of usage. The design and conduct
of many of these studies are open to serious criticism by
present-day standards, but the validity of the findings were
sufficiently convincing for the Council of Dental Therapeutics
of the American Dental Association in 1964 to grant the dentifrice Grade A certification. This graded the formulation as
being of proven preventive value.

Studies carried out in other parts of the world, notably in
the United Kingdom, Australia, and Canada, have tested
stannous fluoride formulations. Some have involved the
'Crest' formulations as marketed whilst others have included
different abrasive systems including insoluble sodium meta-
phosphate. The findings of the United Kingdom studies have
been reviewed by Duckworth (1968). The difference in design
and method of conduct of these studies make valid comparison impossible. However, there can be no doubt that
regular usage led to a reduced caries experience though generally the reductions were less than those demonstrated in
the early United States studies.

Despite the undoubted clinical efficacy, stannous fluoride-
containing dentifrices have one major disadvantage in
that they lead to unsightly black/brown extrinsic staining of
tooth surfaces, especially around the margins of anterior
restorations. The enamel stain can easily be removed but the
discoloration of filling margins may often require replacement
of the restorations. The discoloration is probably due to precipitation on the acquired pellicle of oxides and sulphides of
tin. The original Crest formulation is now no longer on the
market, having been replaced by an entirely new formulation
containing sodium fluoride with an abrasive system based on
silicon dioxide. This means that no clinically tested and
proven stannous fluoride dentifrices is now available in the
marketplaces of the world. This new dentifrice is marketed as
'Crest +' and has been clinically tested by Beiswanger *et al.*
(1981) and Zacherl (1981), who demonstrated a significant
superiority over the previous stannous fluoride formulation.

Since sodium fluoride was introduced into Crest + in 1981
some investigations have compared sodium fluoride with
sodium monofluorophosphate (NaMFP) and also investigated
the effect of increasing the fluoride concentration in toothpaste. Lu *et al.* (1987) used three toothpastes (1100 ppm F as
NaF, 2800 ppm F as NaMFP, 2800 ppm F as NaF) in a 3-
year study of 4500 children, aged 7–15 years. The NaF
toothpaste at 2800 ppm F provided a significant 11 per cent
reduction in DMFS increment compared with the NaMFP
toothpaste (Table 3.18).

The authors claimed the NaF dentifrice was more effective
than the SMFP paste and that increasing the concentration of
NaF in a dentifrice from 1100 ppm F to 2800 ppm F resulted
in a statistically significant improvement in reducing new
carious lesions. However, the high F concentration used in
two of these test products was almost twice the limit set by
the EC cosmetics directive, and also higher than a study by
Hargreaves and Chester (1973), who used an MFP toothpaste
yielding 2200 ppm F.

By far the greatest number of dentifrices on sale in the
world today have as their active ingredient sodium
monofluorophosphate, the caries inhibitory value of which
was established over 30 years ago (Zipkin and McClure
1951). There is, however, uncertainty regarding its mode of

Table 3.18. Effect of high fluoride dentifrices on dental
caries in children (Lu *et al.* (1987))

Dentifrice	No. of children	3 year DMFS increment		
		Mean	SEM	Per cent reduction
1100 ppm F as NaF	703	4.40	0.195	—
2800 ppm F as SMFP	673	4.37	0.207	0.7
2800 ppm F as NaF	679	3.88	0.186	11.8

action. Ericsson (1963) on the one hand believes that the
MFP ion is incorporated into the hydroxyapatite crystal lattice
with a subsequent slower release of fluoride ion which then
replaces hydroxyl groups to form fluorapatite. On the other
hand it has been suggested by Ingram (1972) that it is the
MFP ion itself which is incorporated into the apatite crystal
by means of a substitution reaction with one or more of the
phosphate groups. This being the case, the transfer mechanism is not pH dependent. Apart from the fact that sodium
monofluoroposphate does not require an acid pH, it is also
compatible with the most commonly used chalk-based
abrasive systems.

A large number of clinical studies have been reported in
which MFP-containing dentifrices have been compared with
non MFP-containing control formulations. Virtually all
studies have demonstrated a clinically relevant anticaries
effect though, as in previous dentifrice studies, differences in
design of the trials make direct comparisons of findings
invalid. In general terms reductions in caries increments were
of the order of 30 per cent. MFP dentifrices have a neutral or
slightly alkaline pH, and do not stain enamel surfaces or the
margins of restorations.

DEVELOPMENT IN FLUORIDE DENTIFRICE FORMULATION: 1980–94

Fluoride dentifrices play an important part in the 'personal
care products' division of a number of multinational companies. It is an intensely competitive market and subject to
continuous developments. In the 1980s, research has been
concerned with: (a) changing the F concentration; (b) combining more than one fluoride agent; (c) comparing different F
formulations; (d) adding other 'active agents'; (e) the effect of
F toothpaste on root caries. The effect of the two behavioural
aspects, the frequency of toothbrushing and the ways in
which toothpaste is removed from the mouth after brushing,
have also been reported.

Fluoride concentration in dentifrice

The vast majority of fluoride dentifrice trials have involved
pastes yielding approximately 1000 ppm (either as 0.76 per
cent sodium monofluorophosphate, 0.24 per cent sodium
fluoride or 0.4 per cent stannous fluoride (See Table 3.19). A
directive from European Commission suggested an upper limit
of 1500 ppm F for toothpastes sold 'over the counter' without

prescription (*Directives Au Conseil* Vol. 78–768, 1977), although higher levels of fluoride in a dentifrice were formally recognized by the EC in 1982 (Council Directive 1982).

Koch *et al.* (1982) carried out a 3-year clinical trial in 12 to 13-year-old children to compare the caries prophylactic effect of two dentifrices containing 1000 ppm F and one containing 250 ppm F. The dentifrices were an MFP-based paste yielding 1000 ppm F (Colgate) and two sodium fluoride pastes yielding either 1000 or 250 ppm F. The results showed no statistical difference between the three pastes and the authors

Table 3.19. Three-year-mean DFS increments, clinical and radiographic data combined (Koch *et al.* 1982)

	ppm F		
	250 (NaF)	1000 (NaF)	1000 (MFP)
No. of children	96	96	96
Mean DFS	7.5	7.2	6.7

concluded that regular use of a low-fluoride paste was as effective in controlling caries as a 1000 ppm F paste.

Mitropoulos *et al.* (1984) compared the relative efficacy of a dentifrice containing 250 ppm F from sodium monofluorophosphate with a similar active control dentifrice containing 1000 ppm F in 725 15 to 16-year-old subjects over a 32-month period. Their results (Table 3.20) suggest that a dentifrice containing 250 ppm F, from sodium monofluorophosphate, would be significantly less effective in reducing dental caries than a dentifrice containing 1000 ppm F, and that it would be unreasonable to sacrifice efficacy by reducing the fluoride concentration available in the dentifrice.

A number of investigations have been carried out on toothpastes containing higher levels of fluoride.

Stephen *et al.* (1988) carries out a 3-year clinical trial on 3000 12-year-old children in Scotland involving sodium monofluorophosphate yielding 1000, 1500, and 2500 ppm F. The mean 3-year DMFS increments are recorded in Table 3.21 and show a trend to lower caries increments with increasing fluoride content of the toothpaste. The authors

Table 3.20. Mean DFS increment, clinical, and radiographic data combined (Mitropoulos *et al.* 1984)

	MFP level as ppm F	
	250	1000
No. of children	365	360
Mean DFS	4.29	3.61

concluded that, in the range of the 1000–2500 ppm F, every additional 500 ppm over and above 1000 ppm F would provide a cumulative 6 per cent reduction in caries increment. A similar trend was obtained by Conti *et al.* (1988), who evaluated the effectiveness of two MFP dentifrices yielding 1000 and 1500 ppm F in 2415 children aged 8–11 years who completed a 3-year daily supervised brushing pro-

Table 3.21. Three-year mean DMFS increments for fluoride groups, clinical and radiographic data combined (Stephen *et al.* 1988)

	MFP level as ppm F		
	1000	1500	2500
No. of in group	921	930	466
Mean DMFS	6.80	6.33	5.71

gramme (Table 3.22). A third study (Fogels *et al.* 1988) tested two MFP pastes delivering 1000 or 1500 ppm F in children aged 6–11 years. The results (Table 3.23) amounted to a benefit of 0.3 DMFS, over a 3-year period, for the higher fluoride dentifrice.

The longest study so far reported was by Triol *et al.* (1987), who determined the effect of three MFP dentifrices yielding 1000, 1450, and 2000 ppm F used by children initially aged 9.9 years, over a 4-year period. The results (Table 3.24) showed that the 1450 and 2000 ppm F pastes were significantly superior to the positive control paste.

Table 3.22. Three-year mean DMFS increments, clinical and radiographic data combined (Conti *et al.* 1988)

	MFP level as ppm F	
	1000	1500
No. of in group	1228	1187
Mean DMFS	2.39	1.87

Table 3.23. Three-year mean DMFS increments, clinical and radiographic data combined (Fogels *et al.* 1988)

	MFP level as ppm F	
	1000	1500
No. of children	950	963
Mean DMFS	2.36	2.02

The youngest age group involved in a toothpaste trial was studied by Winter *et al.* (1989). Their unique study involved children aged 2 years. A total of 2177 pre-school children were allocated to one of two groups, who used either conventional MFP paste yielding 1055 ppm F or a low-fluoride paste (0.209 MFP plus 0.060 NaF yielding 550 ppm F). The children were examined 3 years later (Table 3.25), and the authors concluded that the low-fluoride test toothpaste possessed similar anti-caries activity to the control paste and could therefore be recommended for use by young children.

Taking all these studies together, one conclusion can be drawn. In all studies the group using the paste with higher fluoride content showed the lowest caries increment. In Table 3.26, the percentage differences between each of the groups referred to in the above studies are summarized.

Table 3.24. Four-year mean DMFS increment (Triol *et al.* 1987)

	MFP level as ppm F		
	1000	1450	2000
No. of children	448	470	452
Mean DMFS	3.21	2.95	2.79

Table 3.25. Mean dmfs (caries-experienced) clinical and radiographic data combined (Winter *et al.* 1989)

	ppmf	
	550	1055
No. of children	477	428
Mean dmfs	2.52	2.29

Combining more than one fluoride agent

One of the first studies to use a mixed fluoride system was reported by Hodge *et al.* (1980). Two dentifrices, each containing 0.76 per cent MFP and 0.1 per cent NaF, one having an alumina and the other a dicalcium phosphate abrasive system, were compared with a positive control containing 0.76 per cent MFP in an alumina abrasive system and a non-fluoride negative control with an alumina abrasive system. In all, 799 children aged 14–15 years completed the 3-year clinical trial. The results (Table 3.27) showed that the mixed fluoride systems showed significant reductions in mean caries increments over the positive control. It is not clear from this study whether the improvement was due to the mixture of fluoride agents, or merely to the extra fluoride available from the two test pastes.

Table 3.27. Three-year DFS increment, clinical, and radiographic data combined (Hodge *et al.* 1980)

	ppm F			
	0	1000	1500	1500
No. of children	202	194	203	200
Mean DFS	7.83	7.31	5.94	6.08

A second study, by Mainwaring and Naylor (1983), tested a dentifrice containing 0.76 per cent MFP (1000 ppm F) against one in which half the MFP was replaced by sodium fluoride. A non-fluoride, calcium carbonate base dentifrice without other additives acted as a placebo, and a fourth group used 0.76 per cent MFP with 0.13 per cent calcium glycerophosphate. The results (Table 3.28) after 4 years showed that children using the mixed fluoride system had a lower caries increment than those using the MFP paste, although the differences were only statistically significant for smooth surfaces. The lower caries increment was found in the group brushing with MFP plus calcium glycerophosphate. In contrast to the two previous studies, Juliano *et al.* (1985) concluded there was no difference in efficacy between a NaMFP paste yielding 1000 ppm F or mixed MFP/NaF paste of the same F content. Furthermore, the report by Ripa *et al.* (1987) concluded that using a mixed fluoride dentifrice (NaF/MFP) at a standard 1000 ppm F concentration or at a 2.5 times standard did not provide superior

Table 3.28. Four-year mean DFS increments, clinical and radiographic data combined (Mainwaring and Naylor 1983)

	ppm F			
	0	1000 (MFP)	1000 (MFP + NaF)	1000 (MFP + CaGP)
No. of children	224	230	228	241
Mean DFS	11.00	9.30	8.46	8.17

Table 3.26. DMF increments and percentage differences reported in caries increments—studies involving mainly sodium monofluorophosphate dentifrices of different concentrations

Study	ppm F (approx.)				
	250	500	1000	1500	2000
Koch *et al.* (1982)	7.5[1] —	[13.4] →	6.7		
Mitropoulos *et al.* (1984)	4.29 —	[18.8] →	3.61		
Winter *et al.* (1989)		2.52[2] — [10.0] →	2.29		
Triol *et al.* (1987)			3.21 — [8.8] → 2.95		
			2.95 — [5.7] → 2.79		
Stephen *et al.* (1988)			6.80 — [7.4] → 6.33		
			6.33 — [10.9] → 5.71		
Conti *et al.* (1988)			2.39 — [27.8] → 1.87		
Fogels *et al.* (1988)			2.36 — [16.8] → 2.02		

[1] NaF dentifrice.
[2] 0.209 MFP + 0.060 NaF.
[ ] Percentage reduction.

Table 3.29. Two-year mean DMFS increment, clinical examination only (Ripa *et al.* 1987)

	ppm F		
	1000 (MFP)	1000 (MFP + NaF)	2500 (MFP + NaF)
No. of children	912	902	955
Mean DMFS	2.54	2.41	2.46

Table 3.31. Three-year mean DFS increments, clinical, and radiographic data combined (Edlund and Koch 1977)

	ppm F	
	1000 (MFP)	1000 (NaF)
No. of children	179	184
Mean DFS	3.2	2.7

caries inhibition compared with a conventional MFP paste containing 1000 ppm F (Table 3.29). Although the mixed NaF/MFP pastes showed the lowest caries increments, the reduction of approximately 5 per cent over the positive control was not significant. The authors pointed out that of the households interviewed, 52 per cent admitted that they were using commercial dentifrices for at least part of the time and so it was possible that any small differences in caries protection from the experimental pastes could have been diluted by the subject's use of other brands. A summary of the four trials in this section is given in Table 3.30.

Comparisons of different formulations

The previous section dealt with mixed fluoride systems. A number of research reports have been concerned with a direct comparison between sodium fluoride and sodium monofluorophosphate. Some care must be taken when comparing the various studies in this section. In some cases, experimental formulations have been tested which do not have direct relevance to products eventually launched commercially. A number of different abrasives have been used in formulating a dentifrice and it is essential that constituents do not react with the fluoride compound and reduce its bioavailability. Edlund and Koch (1977) were among the first workers to compare a conventional 1000 ppm F dentifrice (Colgate) with an experimental NaF paste. The results (Table

3.31) for children initially aged 9–11 years, who completed a 3-year supervised brushing programme, indicated that the group brushing with the sodium fluoride paste had the lower caries increment.

Lu *et al.* (1987) compared the anti-caries effects of three fluoride-containing dentifrices—1100 ppm F as NaF, 2800 ppm F as MFP, 2800 ppm F as NaF—in a 3-year trial involving initially 4500 schoolchildren aged 7–15 years. The results (Table 3.32) showed no significant differences between the 2800 ppm MFP group and the positive control (the 1100 ppm NaF dentifrice) at any point during the 3 years of the study.

The 2800 ppm NaF dentifrice showed significant reductions against the other two pastes after the third year of the study. The estimates of the percentage reductions for this 2800 ppm MFP paste versus the 2800 ppm NaF paste over the 1100 NaF positive control were 4 per cent and 15 per cent respect-

Table 3.32. Three-year mean DMFS increments, clinical, and radiographic data combined (Lu *et al.* 1987)

	ppm F		
	1100 (NaF)	2800 (NaF)	2800 (MFP)
No. of children	703	679	673
Mean DMFS	4.40	3.85	4.37

Table 3.30. Clinical trials of mixed fluoride dentifrices

Study	Fluoride (%)	Abrasive	Unsupervised (U) or supervised (S) use	Duration of trial (yrs)	No. carious surfaces saved per year	Reduction in carious surface increment (%)	Level of statistical significance
Hodge *et al.* (1980)	0.76 MFP + 0.1 NaF	Al$_2$O$_3$	S	3	0.6	22	0.01
	0.76 MFP + 0.1 NaF	DCP	S	3	0.6	24	0.01
Mainwaring and Naylor (1983)	0.39 MFP + 0.12 NaF	DCP	U	4	0.6	15	0.02
Juliano *et al.* (1985)	0.38 MFP + 0.11 NaF	DCP	S	2 yrs 7 mos	Positive control		
Ripa *et al.* (1987)	0.38 MFP + 0.11 NaF	SiO$_2$	U	2	Positive control	—	n.s. against positive control
	0.95 MFP + 0.28 NaF	SiO$_2$	U	2	Positive control	—	n.s. against positive control

ively. The authors concluded that their clinical findings were supported by laboratory data and emphasized by Stookey (1985), who related the advantage of NaF to its higher uptake by incipient lesions than that of MFP.

In contrast, Blinkhorn and Kay (1988) found no significant differences at the end of a 3-year study into three pastes all yielding 1450 ppm F. The positive control contained 0.76 per cent MFP and 0.10 per cent NaF; the other two pastes contained either 0.32 per cent NaF or 1.1 per cent MFP (Table 3.33).

Table 3.33. Three-year mean DMFS increments, clinical examination only (Blinkhorn and Kay 1988)

	ppm F		
	1450 (NaF)	1450 (MFP)	1450 (NaF + MFP)
No. of children	754	736	744
Mean DFS	4.72	4.76	4.52

Koch *et al.* (1988) carried out a study in 1035 11- to 12-year-old Icelandic children, involving five pastes. Three contained sodium fluoride yielding 1000 ppm F, the fourth contained 250 ppm F from sodium fluoride, and the positive control was an MFP paste yielding 1000 ppm F. The detailed results are not available, but the Abstract recorded that the paste containing 250 ppm was significantly less effective than the other pastes investigated. A test paste with sodium fluoride with a diphosphonic acid derivative (anti-tartar agent) showed the lowest caries increment, but there was no difference in effect between the 1000 ppm MFP paste and the 1000 ppm NaF paste without diphosphonates.

The penultimate paper to be reviewed in this section is by Beiswanger *et al.* (1989), who carried out a direct comparison of two pastes yielding 1100 ppm F with identical silica abrasive colour match and flavouring, one containing sodium fluoride (Crest) and the other 0.76 per cent sodium monofluorophosphate (Table 3.34). The authors concluded that their study demonstrated that sodium fluoride had greater cariostatic activity than sodium monofluorophosphate. In addition, they reported that the scientific literature contains no reports of clinical trials in which the use of MFP dentifrices resulted in significantly greater cariostatic activity. Furthermore, nine out of the 10 trials in which these two fluoride agents were compared found a numerical advantage in favour of sodium fluoride.

The latest study to compare the effect of sodium fluoride and sodium monofluorophosphate toothpastes gave informa-

Table 3.34. Three-year mean DMF increments, clinical, and radiographic data combined, 11- to 16-year-old children only (Beiswanger *et al.* 1989)

	ppm F	
	1100 (NaF)	1100 (MFP)
No. of children	257	262
Mean DMFS	3.95	4.58

tion on three-year caries increments (clinical examination only) in adolescents aged 11–13 years at baseline (Stephen *et al.* 1994). Six groups were involved: two SMFP toothpastes yielding 1000 and 1500 ppm F, two NaF toothpastes (1000 and 1500 ppm F), and two toothpastes using a combination of NaF plus sodium trimetaphosphate (1000 vs. 1500 ppm F). After three years clinical only data for 3517 children were available for the calculation of caries increments.

The mean three-year caries increments are recorded in Table 3.35 and show that subjects using a dentifrice containing NaF alone had a 6.4 per cent lower DMFS value than those using a dentifrice containing SMFP. The difference between the NaF plus TMP users and the SMFP users was 8.1 per cent. The authors concluded that in their clinical study NaF had been proven to be superior to SMFP when incorporated in well-formulated silica-based dentifrices.

The comparative efficacy of NaF and SMFP dentifrices in caries prevention has been the subject of heated debate recently involving the Procter & Gamble and Colgate companies, in particular. Johnson (1993) used meta-analysis in an 'overview' of all randomized controlled studies comparing NaF to SMFP dentifrices in the prevention of caries development. She concluded that, based on a pool of studies involving over 7000 subjects, NaF was associated with a significantly greater reduction of 6.4 per cent in caries development compared to SMFP over 2- to 3-year follow up period. This finding was supported by Stookey and co-workers (1993) in their review of the relative anticaries efficacy of NaF and SMFP dentifrices. They considered whether the difference in efficacy was clinically relevant:

Of course, in the absolute, any difference in efficacy (if real) between two therapeutic agents would be important, assuming that there are no increased risks, costs or other factors associated with using one therapy over another. However, in the real world, a number of factors complicate this judgment... It is our view that this difference must be considered as clinically relevant for several reasons. First the differences observed in the meta-analyses were derived from pooling several studies (eleven) and not from one or two individual studies. The second reason why

Table 3.35. Mean three-year DMFS increment (clinical examination only) 1000 ppm F (Stephen *et al.* 1994)

	1000 ppm F			1500 ppm F		
	SMFP	NaF	NaF+ TMP	SMFP	NaF	NaF+ TMP
No. of children	721	698	344	698	703	353
Mean DMFS	7.00	6.59	6.52	7.00	6.51	6.35

the difference in efficacy between NaF and SMFP should be considered clinically relevant involves consideration of the likely propagation of these differences over time, as suggested by the epidemiological assessment of Kingman (1993)... The third reason... involves the theoretical fact that NaF is chemically the most simple compound which ensures a maximum availability of fluoride, assuming an appropriate abrasive is employed in the dentifrices.

These views were disputed at an 'International Scientific Assembly on the Comparative Anticaries efficacy of Sodium Fluoride and Sodium Monofluorophosphate Dentifrices' held in London in August 1993 and published in a special issue of the *American Journal of Dentistry*, September 1993. A Consensus Position Statement was reached.

- It is the consensus of this International Scientific Assembly that the selection of studies and data included in a recently published meta-analysis comparing the anticaries efficacy of sodium fluoride and sodium monofluorophosphate dentifrices does not reflect an accurate view and should be called into question.

- The Assembly agreed that the published clinical studies available to date support the conclusion that sodium fluoride and sodium monofluorophosphate at similar concentrations (ranging from 1000 ppm F to 1500 ppm F) in commercially available dentifrices across the world provide equivalent anticaries effectiveness.

- The dental profession can confidently recommend either sodium fluoride or sodium monofluorophosphate dentifrices because the available evidence fails to support the superiority of one fluoride over the other.

There was obvious concern about the use of meta-analysis: 'In the biomedical area, however, meta-analysis should never be a substitute for well-designed, well-conducted, and well-analyzed trials of adequate size'.

Adding other 'active agents'

This section is concerned with the possible effect of other additives on the cariostatic action of fluoride in dentifrices.

The study by Mainwaring and Naylor (1983) has been referred to in a previous section. One of its conclusions was that including 0.13 per cent calcium glycerophosphate in a sodium MFP paste was associated with additional statistically significant reductions in caries increments.

In the early 1980s, Procter and Gamble directed attention to the possible effect of sodium pyrophosphate as an anti-calculus agent. Lu *et al.* (1985) tested a 0.243 per cent NaF paste with soluble pyrophosphate in Taiwanese children aged 8–15 years against a non-fluoride paste with no anti-calculus agent. After 1 year they reported (Table 3.36) that the experimental paste was effective against caries.

Although a number of studies have been reported on the effect of soluble pyrophosphate on dental calculus (Zacherl *et al.* 1985; Mallatt *et al.* 1985; Lu *et al.* 1988), no other studies on the effect of adding pyrophosphate to a fluoride paste on caries increments have been reported.

Table 3.36. One-year mean DMFS increments, clinical and radiographic data combined (Lu *et al.* 1985)

	ppm F	
	0	1100 (NaF)
No. of children	573	587
Mean DMFS (examiner 1)	3.78	2.80
No. of children	571	585
Mean DMFS (examiner 2)	1.22	0.59

Triol *et al.* (1990) compared the effectiveness, in a 3-year clinical trial, of four dentifrices:

1. 0.76 per cent MFP/silica (Colgate MFP Gel Toothpaste) (positive control).

2. 0.243 per cent NaF/3.3 per cent sol. pyro./1.0 per cent Gantrez/silica (Colgate Tartar Control Toothpaste).

3. 0.243 per cent NaF/2.0 per cent $ZnCl_2$/silica (experimental anti-tartar toothpaste).

4. 0.76 per cent MFP/1.25 per cent zinc oxide/silica (experimental anti-tartar toothpaste).

Final results indicated that there were no significant differences in caries increments among the four groups, suggesting that the experimental pastes were comparable in anti-caries efficacy to the clinically proven positive dentifrice.

The 3-year clinical trial by Stephen *et al.* (1988) confirmed that adding zinc citrate to MFP pastes (as an anti-plaque agent) had no effect on caries increment.

More recently, Colgate have launched a sodium fluoride paste containing triclosan, a non-ionic antibacterial agent and a copolymer polyvinylmethyl ether maleic acid (PVM/MA). The addition of the copolymer has been shown to enhance the retention of triclosan by plaque and saliva. A number of articles on the safety of triclosan and its effect on salivary bacterial counts (DeSalva *et al.* 1989; Addy *et al.* 1989) and plaque formation (Singh *et al.* 1989) have been reported, but no studies on caries increments have yet been published.

Effect of fluoride toothpaste on root caries

The vast majority of fluoride dentifrice trials have been carried out on children and adolescents. Little information is available on the effect of fluorides on root surface caries in adults, Jensen and Kohout (1988) carried out a double-blind clinical study of 810 healthy adults aged 54 years and older. Their results (Table 3.37) showed a statistically significant reduction in both coronal and root surface caries in favour of a sodium fluoride dentifrice (1100 ppm) over a placebo paste, after one year.

Effect of oral care habits on caries in adolescents

The effect of toothbrushing habits on caries increments was reported by Chesters *et al.* (1992). Four alternative rinsing methods were defined (Fig. 3.15).

Table 3.37.   Root surface caries in adults (Jensen and Kohout 1988)

	ppm F	
	0	1100
No. of adults	406	404
DFS (root surface)	1.24	0.73

Table 3.38.   Mean DMFS values for consistent brushers (Chesters *et al.* 1992)

	No. of children	Mean DMFS values baseline	3-year increment
Once per day or less	403	10.6	7.0
Twice per day or more	856	9.0	5.4

Table 3.39.   Rinsing method and caries data (Chester *et al.* 1992)

	No. in group	Mean DMFS	
		Baseline	3-year increment
Use brush	373	8.8	5.9
Head under tap	543	9.4	5.8
Use hand	150	10.0	5.5
Use beaker	1213	11.0	6.9

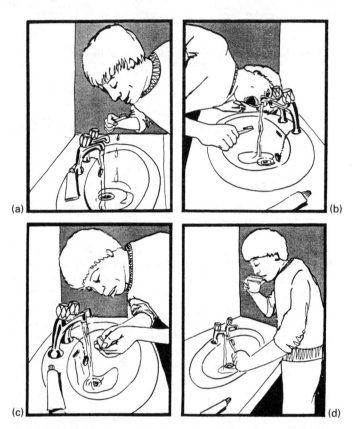

Fig. 3.15.   Sketches of alternative rinsing methods. (a) using a toothbrush to transfer water to the mouth; (b) putting the mouth under the tap; (c) transferring water using cupped hands; (d) using a beaker to transfer water to the mouth. (From Chesters *et al.* 1992.)

1. Using a toothbrush to transfer water to the mouth.

2. Putting the mouth under the tap.

3. Transferring water using cupped hands.

4. Using a beaker to transfer water to the mouth.

Information on toothbrushing frequency was also collected. Analysis of data for 'consistent brushers' (those who gave the same frequency response over a 2-year period) showed that twice-per-day brushers had lower caries levels (both prevalence and incremental) than once per day or less brushers (Table 3.38). The responses to the rinsing method showed a clear association between rinsing method and caries status, in terms of both prevalence at baseline and the 3-year increment (Table 3.39). Girls were more inclined to brush their teeth more frequently, and to rinse with a beaker, than boys, but it

was shown that the associations between caries and either brushing frequency or rinsing method were independent of gender (Table 3.40).

The 'best group' (non-beaker, brushed teeth at least twice a day) had a DMF increment of 5.1–5.2, compared with a DMF increment of 7.5–8.0 for the 'worst group' (beaker users, brushed teeth once per day or less).

DENTAL FLUOROSIS

Dental fluorosis is a hypoplasia or hypomaturation of tooth enamel or dentine produced by the chronic ingestion of excessive amounts of fluoride during the period when teeth are developing. The major cause of dental fluorosis is the consumption of water, containing high levels of fluoride, by infants and children during the first six years of life. Although both primary and permanent teeth may be affected by fluorosis, under uniform conditions of fluoride availability fluorosis tends to be greater in permanent teeth than primary teeth. This disparity may be due to the fact that much of the mineralization of primary teeth occurs before birth and the placenta serves as a barrier to the transfer of high concentrations of plasma fluoride from a pregnant mother to her developing fetus, thus controlling to a certain extent the delivery of fluoride to the developing primary dentition. Other reasons may be that the period of enamel formation for primary teeth is shorter than for permanent teeth and that the enamel of primary teeth is thinner than that of permanent teeth (Møller 1982; Horowitz 1986).

Interest in dental fluorosis has increased over the past 10 years or so, not only in areas like India and Kenya where there are communities with high levels of fluorosis associated with high concentrations of fluoride in the water supply, but also in temperate climates with optimal or low fluoridated water supplies where fluoride uptake from other sources, in particular fluoride supplements and fluoride toothpaste in early infancy, have resulted in an increase in the prevalence

Table 3.40. Effect of rinsing method, brushing frequency, and gender on caries (Chesters *et al.* 1992)

| Rinsing method | Brushing frequency | Gender | Mean DMFS | | |
			No. in group	Baseline	3-year increment
Non-beaker	≤ 1/day	F	134	9.9	6.4
		M	326	10.0	6.8
Non-beaker	≥ 2/day	F	358	9.0	5.1
		M	248	8.3	5.2
Beaker	≤ 1/day	F	187	13.5	7.5
		M	290	11.1	8.0
Beaker	≥ 2/day	F	500	10.6	6.2
		M	235	9.7	6.4

of enamel mottling. With the decline in caries, following fluoride therapy, increasing attention is now being given to levels of dental fluorosis (Fejerskov *et al.* 1988). In a sense, history is turning full circle, because the history of water fluoridation really started with attempts to ascertain the cause of 'Colorado stain' in the early 1900s.

In the last 10 years a number of workers have drawn attention to the possibility of an increase in the prevalence of dental fluorosis. For example, Osuji and Nikiforuk (1988) presented two cases which exhibited classical dental fluorosis in the permanent dentition, both of whom had receives more fluoride supplement than recommended in the dosage schedules. The first received 0.5 mg F/day from infancy and 1.0 mg F/day from the age of 2 to 6 years in an area that has a natural water fluoride concentration of 0.42 ppm. The second case received 1.0 mg F/day from birth to 7 years of age in an area with a natural water fluoride concentration of 0.1 ppm F.

Riordan (1993) called for a reconsideration of existing recommendations concerning fluoride supplements in order to reduce the risk of fluorosis. He proposed that fluoride supplements should be aimed only at identifiable high caries-risk individuals and should start at 6 months of age or later.

Pang and Vann (1992) quoted an NIDR sponsored international workshop on 'changing patterns of systematic fluoride intake', where it was agreed that the inadvertent ingestion of toothpaste could be a cause of increased dental fluorosis in children.

WHO Expert Working Group (1994) considered the appropriate levels of fluoride in drinking water. They noted that Dean's research over 50 years ago established 1.0 mg/l as the most appropriate concentration of F in drinking water. By 'most appropriate' he meant the concentration at which maximal caries reduction could be achieved without causing unacceptable levels of dental fluorosis. Because people in hot climates drink more water than those in moderate climates, this figure of 1.0 mg F/l was modified to a range of 0.7–1.2 mg F/l. By the 1990s, however, it was clear that these standards were not appropriate for all parts of the world, especially the subtropical areas of Africa and Asia. Hong Kong has reduced the fluoride concentration in its drinking water several times since water fluoridation began in 1961. It is now maintained at 0.5 mg/l.

In an editorial entitled 'Too much of a good thing?' Mason (1991) reported that:

The available evidence points to an increase in dental fluorosis in both fluoridated and non-fluoridated communities. Increased fluoride exposure from a variety of fluoride-containing dental products is the most likely source. In some cases, health professionals may be prescribing fluoride dietary supplements inappropriately, or failing to advise parents to teach their small children to spit out, not swallow, fluoride toothpaste. (In this regard, government regulations and the manufacturers of dental products need to look at the label instructions to see if they need to be more specific.) Increases in dental fluorosis are an indication that total fluoride exposure is increasing and may be more than necessary to prevent tooth decay. Prudent public health practice dictates using no more than the amount necessary to achieve a desired effect.

REPORTS FROM THE WORLD HEALTH ORGANIZATION

A conference in 1982 on the appropriate use of fluorides for human health, under the auspices of the International Dental Federation, the Kellogg Foundation, and the World Health Organization, reached the following conclusions and recommendations (WHO 1986).

1. The International Conference on Fluorides reviewed the findings of recent experimental, clinical and epidemiological research on the use of fluorides in promoting dental health. While welcoming the reports of declining caries experience in many developed countries, it was greatly concerned about the sharp increase in dental caries in some developing countries. As there is no possibility of treating so many decayed teeth with the dental resources at present available in the developing countries, the only hope is to contain the caries problem by preventive measures.

2. The Conference agreed that community water fluoridation is an ideal measure for the prevention of dental caries in countries with well-developed, centralized public water supplies. It was in agreement with the view of the FDI, WHO, and the medical and dental professions throughout the world that community water fluoridation is an effective, safe, and inexpensive preventive measure, which has the virtue of requiring no active compliance on the part of the persons benefited. The Conference recommended that community water fluoridation be introduced and maintained wherever possible.

3. Unfortunately, the vast majority of the world's population live in rural and urban areas with few large water installations. In these situations, community water fluoridation is not feasible and alternative strategies need to be adopted. There is evidence from three long-term studies in both developing and industrialized countries that fluoridized salt may be nearly as effective as water fluoridation in reducing the incidence of dental caries. Consequently, the Conference stressed the need for more long-term field trials of salt fluoridization.

4. There is no justification for using more than one systemic fluoride measure at any one time.

5. Various topical fluoride methods, or combinations of such methods, may be beneficial in communities that have a source of systemic fluoride that is used widely.

6. Wherever possible, when combinations of fluoride therapy are considered, it is best to choose those that are self-administered or group-administered because they are less expensive.

7. Professionally applied fluorides are particularly appropriate for individuals who have been identified as at high risk of dental caries.

8. The conference was concerned about the problems of dental fluorosis in areas with high concentrations of fluoride in the public water supply and urged research to develop effective, simple, and economical defluoridation methods for water supplies of varying sizes. It recommended that, in children under the age of 6 years, brushing with a fluoride toothpaste should be supervised in order to prevent excessive ingestion. For similar reasons, fluoride mouth rinsing should not be considered for children under 5 years.

9. Current knowledge of the effectiveness of various methods of using fluorides led the Conference to conclude that each country should review its own dental needs and take legislative action to adopt those methods of using fluorides that best suit its needs in different regions. In view of the proven value of fluorides in promoting dental health, their use should be extended without further delay to all populations throughout the world.

WHO considered the subject again in 1993. The expert working group made a number of recommendations, including the following.

- The effectiveness of all caries preventive programmes should be monitored on an ongoing basis.

- Community water fluoridation is safe and cost-effective and introduced and maintained wherever socially acceptable and feasible. The optimum water fluoride concentration will normally be within the range 0.5–1.0 mg/l.

- Salt fluoridization, at a minimum concentration of 200 mg/l F, should be considered as a practical alternative to water fluoridation.

- Encouraging results have been reported with fluoridization of milk but more studies are recommended.

- Fluoride supplements have limited application as a public health measure. In areas with medium to low caries experience a conservative prescribing policy should be adopted; a dose of 0.5 mg F/day should be prescribed for at risk individuals from the age of 3 years. In areas with high caries experience a regimen starting at 6 month of age, taking into account the fluoride content of the drinking water, should be used.

- Only one systemic fluoride measure should be used at any one time.

- Because fluoride toothpaste is a highly effective means of caries control, every effort must be made to develop affordable fluoride toothpastes for use in developing countries. Measures should be taken to exempt fluoride toothpastes from duties and taxation.

- Fluoride toothpaste tubes should contain advice that, for children under 6 years of age, brushing should be supervised and only a minimal amount (less than 5 mm) should be placed on the brush or chewing stick. Toothpastes with lowered levels of fluoride, manufactured especially for the use by children, should be fully studied.

- Toothpastes with candy-like flavours, and toothpaste containing 1500 ppm or more, are not recommended for use by children under 6 years of age.

- In low fluoride communities, school-based brushing and mouthrinsing programmes are recommended, but their adoption should be based on the cost of implementation and the caries status of the community. Fluoride mouthrinsing is contraindicated in children under 6 years of age.

- Further research on the effectiveness of fluoride on root surface caries is recommended.

- Dietary practices that increase the risk of infants and young children being over exposed to fluoride from all sources should be identified and appropriate action taken.

- Dental fluorosis should be monitored periodically to detect increasing or higher than acceptable levels of fluorosis. Action should be taken when fluorosis is found to be excessive by adjusting fluoride intake from water, salt or other sources. Biomarkers should be used to assess, where practical, current fluoride exposure to predict further risk of fluorosis.

CONCLUSIONS

The study of the systemic and topical effects of fluoride has produced a tremendous outpouring of research, particularly over the last 50 years, and our knowledge of dental epidemiology, clinical trials, community dental health, dental plaque, physiology, and biochemistry has increased enormously as a result. This chapter has concentrated on water fluoridation, fluoridization of salt and milk, fluoride supplements, fluoride dentifrices, and dental fluorosis. The incorporation of fluoride in it various forms as a caries-preventive agent for both the individual and the community, is one of the most important factors responsible for the decrease in dental caries in children observed in many industrialized countries.

REFERENCES

Aasenden, R. and Peebles, T.C. (1978). Effects of fluoride supplementation from birth on dental caries and fluorosis in teen-aged children. *Arch. oral Biol.*, **23**, 111–115.

Aasenden, R., De Paola, P.F. and Brudevold, F. (1972). Effects of daily rinsing and ingestion of fluoride solutions upon dental caries and enamel fluoride. *Arch. oral Biol.*, **17**, 1705–1714.

Addy, M., Jenkins, S. Newcombe. R. (1989). Toothpastes containing 0.3% and 0.5% triclosan. II Effects of single brushings on salivary bacterial counts. *Am. J. Dent.*, **2**, 215–219.

Adelph, E. F. (1993). The metabolism and distribution of water in body tissues. *Physiol. Rev.* **13**, 336–71.

Adler, P. (1951). The connections between dental caries experience and water-borne fluorides in a population with low caries incidence. *J. dent. Res.* **30**. 368–81.

Allmark, C., et al. (1982). A community study of fluoride tablets for schoolchildren in Portsmouth. *Br. dent. J.* **153**, 426–3.

Andersson, R. and Grahnén, H. (1976). Fluoride tablets in pre-school age—effect on primary and permanent teeth. *Swed. Dent. J.*, **69**, 137–143.

Angmar-Mänsson, B. and Whitford, G. M. (1982). Plasma fluoride levels and enamel fluorosis in the rat. *Caries Res.* **16**, 334–9.

Arnold, F.A. Jr. (1948). Fluorine in drinking waters. Its effect on dental caries. *J. Am. dent. Ass.* **36**, 28–36.

Arnold, F.A., McClure, F.J. and White, C.L. (1960). Sodium Fluoride tablets for children. *Dent. Prog.*, **1**, 8–12.

Attwood, D. and Blinkhorn, A.S. (1988). Trends in dental health of ten-year-old school children in south-west Scotland after cessation of water fluoridation. *Lancet* **ii**, 266–7.

Banoczy, J., et al. (1983). Effect of fluoridated milk on caries; three year results. *Commun. Dent. Oral Epidemiol.* **11**, 81–5.

Banoczy, J., et al. (1985). Effect of fluoridated milk on caries; five year results. *J. R. Soc. Hlth* **105**, 99–103.

Bawden, J. W. (1992). (Conference Editor). Changing patterns of fluoride intake. *J. dent. Res.* **71**, 1214.

Beiswanger, B.B., Lehnhoff, R.W., Mallatt, M.E., Mau, M.S. and Stookey, G.K. (1989). Clinical evaluation of the relative cariostatic effect of dentifrices containing sodium fluoride or sodium monofluorophosphate. *J. dent. Child.*, **56**, 270–276.

Berner, L. Fernex, E., and Held, A.J. (1967). Study on the anticarious effect of sodium fluoride tablets (Zymafluor). Results recorded in the course of 13 years of observation. *Schweiz. Monatsschr. Zahnheilkd.* **77**, 528–39.

Bibby, B.G. (1945). Test of the effect of fluoride-containing dentifrice on dental caries. *J. dent. Res.* **24**, 297–303.

Bibby, C. G., Wilkins, E., and Witol, E. (1955). A preliminary study of the effects of fluoride lozenges and pills on dental caries. *O. Surg., O. Med., O. Pathol.* **8**, 213–16.

Binder, K. (1965). Karies und fluorreiches Trinkwasser–kritische Betrachtung. *Osterr. Z. Stomat.* **62**, 14–18.

Binder, K. (1974). In *Cost and benefit of fluoride in the prevention of dental caries*, (ed. G. N. Davies). WHO Offset Publication No. 9, p. 64, Table 23. WHO, Geneva.

Binder, K. Driscoll, W.S. and Schützmannsky, G. (1978). Caries-preventive fluoride tablet programs. *Caries Res.*, **12**, suppl. 1, 22–30.

Black, G.V. (1916). Mottled teeth. *Dent. Cosmos* **58**, 129–56.

Blinkhorn, A.S. and Kay, E.J. (1988). A clinical study in children: comparing the anticaries effect of three fluoride dentifrices. *Clinical Prevent. Dentist.*, **10**(3), 14–16.

British Association for the Study of Community Dentistry (1988). *The home use of fluorides for pre-school children*. A policy statement BASCD, Cardiff.

British National Formulary (1990). *British National Formulary No. 19: 1990–92*, Section 9.5, British Medical Association, London

Brudevold, F. and Chilton, N.W. (1966). Comparative study of a fluoride dentifrice containing soluble phosphate and a calcium-free abrasive. Second year report. *J. Am. dent. Ass.* **72**, 889–94.

Chesters, R.K. Huntington E., Burchell, C.K., Stephen, K.W. (1922). Effects of oral care habits on caries in adolescence. *Caries Res.*, **26**, 299–304.

Churchill, H. V. (1931*a*). Letter to F. S. McKay in the McKay papers. Cited by McNeil (1957), p. 16.

Churchill, H.V. (1931*b*). Occurrence of fluorides in some waters of the United States. *Ind. Engng. Chem.* **23**, 996–8.

Clarkson, J. (1992). A European view of fluoride supplementation: meeting matters. *Br. dent. J.* **172**, 357.

Conti, A.J., Lotzkar, S., Daley, R., Cancro, L., Marks, R.G. and McNeal, D.R. (1988). A 3-year clinical trial to compare efficacy of dentifrices containing 1.14% and 0.76% sodium monofluorophophate. *Community Dent. Oral Epidemiol.* **16**, 135–138.

Crichton Browne, J. (1892). Address to the Annual General Meeting of the Eastern Counties Branch of the British Dental Association. *J. Br. dent. Ass.* **13**, 404–16.

Dawes, C. and Weatherell, J.A. (1990). Kinetics of fluoride in the oral fluids. *J. dent. Res.*, **69** (spec. issue), 638–644.

Dean, H.T. (1933). Distribution of mottled enamel in the United States. *Publ. Hlth. Rep.* **48**, 704–34.

Dean, H. T. (1934). Classification of mottled enamel diagnosis. *J. Am. dent. Assoc.* **21**, 1421–6.

Dean, H.T. (1936). Chronic endemic dental fluorosis (mottled enamel). *J. Am. med. Ass.* **107**, 1269–72.

Dean, H.T. (1938). Endemic fluorosis and its relation to dental caries. *Publ. Hlth. Rep.* **53**, 1443–52.

Dean, H.T. and Elvove, E. (1935). Some epidemiological aspects of chronic endemic dental fluorosis. *Am. J. publ. Hlth.* **26**, 567–75.

Dean, H.T. and McKay F.S. (1939). Production of mottled enamel halted by a change in common water supply. *Am. J. publ. Hlth* **29**, 567–75.

Dean, H.T., Jay, P., Arnold, F.A. Jr. and Elvove, E. (1939). Domestic water and the dental caries including certain epidemiological aspects of oral L. acidophilus. *Publ. Hlth Rep.* **54**, 862–88.

Dean, H.T., Arnold, F.A. Jr., and Elvove, E. (1942). Domestic water and dental caries, V. additional studies of the relation of fluoride domestic waters to dental caries experience in 4425 white children aged 12–14 years, of 13 cities in 4 states. *Publ. Hlth. Rep.* **57**, 1155–79.

de Crousaz, P., et al. (1985). Caries prevalence in children after 12 years of salt fluoridation in a Canton of Switzerland. *Schweiz. Mschr. Zahnmed.* **95**, 805–15.

De Paola, P. F. and Lax, M. (1968). The caries inhibiting effect of acidulated phosphate-fluoride chewable tablets: a two year double blind study. *J. Am. dent. Assoc.* **76**, 554–7.

DeSalva, S.J., Kong, B.M. and Lin, Y.J. (1989). Triclosan: a safety profile. *Am. J. Dent.*, **2**, 185–196

Dowell, T.B. andd Joyston-Bechal S. (1981). Fluoride Supplements—age related dosage *Br. dent. J.* **150**, 273–275.

Driscoll, W.S. (1974). The use of fluoride tablets for the prevention of dental caries. In *International workshop of fluorides and dental caries prevention*, (ed. D.J. Forrester and E.M. Schulz), pp. 25–111. University of Maryland, Baltimore.

Driscoll, W.S., Heifetz, S.B., and Korts, D.C. (1978). Effect of chewable fluoride tablets on dental caries in schoolchildren: results after six years of use. *J. Am. dent. Ass.* **97**. 820–4.

Driscoll, W.S. (1981). A review of clinical research on the use of prenatal fluoride administration for prevention of dental caries. *J. dent. Child.*, **48**, 109–117.

Duckworth, R. (1968). Fluoride dentifrices. A review of clinical trials in the United Kingdom. *Br. dent. J.*, **124**, 505–9.

Duff, E.J. (1981). Total and ionic fluoride in milk. *Caries Res.* **15**, 406–8.

Eager, J. M. (1902). Abstract: chiae teeth. *Dent. Cosmos.* **44**, 300–1.

Edlund, K. and Koch, G. (1977). Effect on caries of daily supervised toothbrushing with sodium monofluorophosphate and sodium fluoride dentifrices after three years. *Scand. J. dent. Res.* **85**, 41–5.

Erricsson, Y. (1958). The state of fluorine in milk. *Acta odont. Scand.* **16**, 51–77.

Erricsson, Y. (1963). The mechanism of monofluorophosphate action on hydroxyapatite and dental enamel. *Acta odont. Scand.* **21**, 341–58.

Ericsson, Y. and Ribelius, U. (1971). Wide variations of fluoride supply to infants and their effect. *Caries Res.* **5**, 78–88.

Fanning, E. A., Cellier, K. M., and Leadbetter, M. M. (1975). South Australian kindergarten children: fluoride tablet supplements and dental caries. *Aust. dent. J.* **20**, 7–9.

Fejerskov, O., et al. (1988). *Dental fluorosis—A handbook for health workers.* Munksgaard, Copenhagen.

Feltman, R. and Kosel. G. (1961). Prenatal and postnatal ingestion of fluorides—fourteen years of investigation—final report. *J. dent. Med.* **16**, 190–8.

Fogels, H.R., Meade, J.J. Griffith, J., Miragliuolo, R. and Cancro, L.P. (1988). A clinical investigation of a high-level fluoride dentifrice. *J. dent. Child.*, May–June, 210–215.

Forrest, J.R. (1956). Caries incidence and enamel defects in areas with different levels of fluoride in the drinking water. *Br. dent. J.*, **100**, 195–200.

Galagan, D.J. (1953). Climate and controlled fluoridation. *J. Am. dent. Ass.* **47**, 159–70.

Gedalia, I., Galon, H., Rennert, A., Biderco, I., and Mohr, I. (1981). Effect of fluoridated citrus beverage on dental caries and on fluoride concentration in the surface enamel of children's teeth. *Caries Res.* **15**, 103–8.

Gilooly, C.J., Heinz, H.W., and Eastman, P.W. (1954). A dental caries and fluoride study of 19 Nebraska cities. *J. Neb. dent. Ass.* **31**, 3–13.

Glenn, F. B. (1979). Immunity conveyed by sodium fluoride supplement during pregnancy: part II. *J. dent. Child.* **46**, 17–24.

Glenn, F.B. (1981). The rationale for the administration of a NaF tablet supplement during pregnancy and postnatally in a private practice setting. *J. dent. Child.*, **48**, 118–122.

Glenn, F. B., Glenn, W. D., and Duncan, R. C. (1982). Fluoride tablet supplementation during pregnancy for caries immunity: a study of the offspring produced. *Am. J. Obstet. Gynecol.* **143**, 560–4.

Glenn, F.B. and Glenn, W.D. (1987). Optimum dosage for prenatal fluoride supplementation (PNF): part IX, *J. dent. Child.*, **54**, 445–450.

Giradi-Vogt, J. (1968). Results of fluoridation in Darmstadt. Dissertation: Johan Wolfgang Goethe University, Frankfurt, Germany, p. 127.

Granath, L.E., Rootzen, H., Liljegren, E., Holst, K., and Kohler, L. (1978). Variation in caries prevalence related to combinations of dietary and oral hygiene habits and chewing fluoride tablets

in 4-year-old children. *Caries Res.* **12**, 83–92.

Grissom, D. K., et al. (1964). A comparative study of systemic sodium fluoride and topical stannous fluoride applications in preventive dentistry. *J. dent. Child.* **31**, 314–22.

Groeneveld A, van Eck AAML, Backer Dirks, O (1990). Fluoride in caries prevention. Is the effect pre- or post-eruptive? *J. dent. Res.*; **69** (special issue), 751–5.

Hamberg, L. (1971). Controlled trial of fluoride in vitamin drops for prevention of caries in children. *Lancet* **1**, 441–2.

Hargreaves, J. A. and Chester, C. G. (1973). Clinical trial among Scottish children of an anti-caries dentifrice containing 2% sodium monofluorophosphate. *Commun. Dent. oral Epidemiol.* **1**, 47–57.

Health Education Authority (1989). *The scientific basis of dental health education. A policy document*, 3rd edn, HEA, London.

Hennon, D. K., Stookey, G. K., and Muhler, J. C. (1966). The clinical anti-cariogenic effectiveness of supplementary fluoride–vitamin preparations. Results at the end of three years. *J. Dent. Child.* **33**, 3–12.

Hennon, D. K., Stookey, G. K., and Muhler, J. C. (1967). The clinical anti-cariogenic effectiveness of supplementary fluoride–vitamin preparations. Results at the end of four years. *J. Dent. Child.* **34**, 439–43.

Hennon, D. K., Stookey, G. K., and Muhler, J. C. (1970). The clinical anti-cariogenic effectiveness of supplementary fluoride–vitamin preparations. Results at the end of five and a half years. *J. Pharmacol. Ther. Dent.* **1**, 1–6.

Hennon, D.K., Stookey, G.K. and Beiswanger, B.B. (1977). Fluoride-vitamin supplements: effects on dental caries and fluorosis when used in areas with suboptimum fluoride in water supply. *J. Am dent. Assoc.*, **95**, 965–971.

Hippchen, P. (1965). Caries prevention with fluorides in Düsseldorf children. *Zahnaerztl. Mitt.* **55**, 897–8.

Hodge, H.C. Holloway, P.J., Davies, T.G.H. and Worthington, H.V. (1980). Caries prevention by dentifrices containing a combination of sodium monofluorophosphate and sodium fluoride. *Br. dent. J.*, **149**, 201–204.

Holm, G. B., et al. (1975). Fluoridsugtablett, nytt hjalpmedel: Kariesprofylakktiken. *Tandlakartidningen* **64**, 354–461.

Horowitz, H. S. (1986). Indexes for measuring dental fluorosis. *J. Publ. Dent. Hlth* **46**(4), 179–83.

Hoskova, M. (1968). Fluoride tablets in the prevention of tooth decay. *Cesk. Pediatr.* **23**, 438–41.

Ingram, G.S. (1972). The reaction of monofluorophosphate with apatite. *Caries Res.* **6**, 1–15.

Jackson, D., James, P.M.C., and Wolfe, W.G. (1975). Fluoridation in Anglesey, *Br. dent. J.* **138**, 165–71.

Jackson, D., James, P.M.C. and Thomas, F.D.: Fluoridation in Anglesey in 1983: A clinical study of dental caries, *Br. dent. J.* **158**, 45–49.

Jauncey, (1983). *Opinion of Lord Jauncey* in causa Mrs. *Catherine McColl against Strathclyde Regional Council.* The Court of Session, Edinburgh.

Jensen, M.E. and Kohout, F. (1988). The effect of a fluoridated dentifrice on root and coronal caries in an older adult population. *J. Am. dent. Assoc.*, **117**, 829–832.

Jez, M. (1962). Izledki mnozicne fluorizacij zobovja solske mladine. *Zobozdrav. Vest.* **17**, 113–18.

Johnson, M.F. (1993). Comparative efficacy of NaF and SMLP dentifrices in caries prevention: A meta-analysis overview. *Caries Res.* **27**, 328–336.

Juliano, G. F. et al. (1985). Clinical study comparing the anticaries effect of two fluoride dentifrices. Abstr. 131. IADR/AADR.

Kailis, D. G., *et al.* (1968). Fluoride and caries: observations on the effects of prenatal and postnatal fluoride on some Perth pre-school children. *Med. J. Aust.* **11**, 1037–40.

Kamocka, D., Sebastyanska, Z., and Spychalska, M. (1964). The effect of administration of 'Fluodar' tablets on the appearance of caries in children of pre-school age in Szczecin. *Czas. Stomatol.* **17**, 299–303.

Kempf. G.A. and McKay, F.S. (1930). Motted enamel in a segregated population. *Publ. Hlth. Rep.* **45**, 293–40.

Kingman, A. (1933). Methods of projecting long-term relative efficacy of products exhibiting short-term efficacy. *Caries Res.* **27**, 322–7.

Klein, H. (1948). Dental effects of accidentally fluoridated waters—dental caries experience in deciduous and permanent teeth of school age children. *J. Am. dent. Ass.* **36**, 443–53.

Knox, E.G. (1985). *Fluoridation of water and cancer: a review of the epidemiological evidence.* Report of a Working Party. HMSO, London.

Koch, G. (1967). Effect of sodium fluoride in dentifrice and mouthwash on the incidence of dental caries in school children. *Odont. Revy.* **18**, 48–71.

Koch, G., Petersson, L.G., Kling, E. and Kling, L. (1982). Effect of 250 and 1000 ppm fluoride dentifrice on caries: a three-year clinical study. *Swed. Dent. J.*, **6**, 233–238.

Kraemer, O. (1971). Results of two years of dental caries prophylaxis by oral administration of fluoride in Bonn kindergarten. Dissertation: Rheinische Friedrich Wilhelm University, Bonn, Germany.

Krusic, V. (1960). Our tests in fluoridation with the calcium fluoride 'Fluokalcia' (CaF$_2$). *Zobozdrav. Vest.* **15**, 27–31.

Krychalska-Karwan, Z. and Laskowa, L. (1963). Use of fluoride tablets in Polish children. *Czas. Stomatol.* **16**, 201–5.

Kyves, F., Overton, N.J., and McKean, T.W. (1961). Clinical trials of caries inhibitory dentifrices. *J. Am. dent. Ass.* **63**, 189–93.

LeGeros, R.Z., Glenn, F.B., Lee, D.D. and Glenn, W.D. (1985). Some physicochemical properties of deciduous enamel of children with and without pre-natal fluoride supplementation (PNF). *J. dent. Res.*, **64**, 465–469.

Leggett, B. J., *et al.* (1987). The effects of fluoridated chocolate-flavoured milk on caries incidence in elementary schoolchildren; two and three year studies. *J. dent. Child.* **54**, 18–21.

Leonhardt, H. (1965). Mulgatum and Mulgatum-fluoridation in pre-school children. *Therapie der Gegenwart* **104**, 118–33.

Lewis, F.D. and Leatherwood, E.C. Jr (1959). Effects of natural fluorides on caries incidence in three Georgia cities. *Publ. Hlth. Rep. Wash.* **74**, 127–31.

Lu, K.H. Ruhlman, C.D., Chung, K. and Adams, A. (1988). A clinical comparison of anticalculus dentifrices over 4 months of use. *J. Indiana dent. Assoc.*, **67**, 2.

Lu, K.H. Ruhlman, C.D., Chung, K.L., Sturzenberger, O.P. and Lehnhoff, R.W. (1987). A three-year clinical comparison of a sodium monofluorophosphate dentifrice with sodium fluoride dentifrices on dental caries in children. *J. dent. Child.*, July–Aug., 241–244.

Lu, K.H., Yes, D.J.C., Zacherl, W.A., Ruhlman, C.D., Sturzenberger, O.P. and Lehnhoff, R.W. (1985). The effect of a fluoride dentifrice containing an anticalculus agent on dental caries in children. *J. dent. Child.*, **52**, 449–451.

McCall, D., Stephen, K.W. and McNee, S.G. (1981). Fluoride tablets and salivary fluoride levels. *Caries Res.*, **15**, 98–102.

McClure, F.J. (1943). Ingestion of fluoride and dental caries. *Am. J. Dis. Child.*, **66**, 362–369.

McEniery, M. and Davies, G.N. (1979). Brisbane dental survey 1977: a comparative study of caries experience of children in Brisbane, Australia over a 20 year period. *Community Dent. Oral Epidemiol.*, **7**, 42–50.

McKay, F.S. (1916a). An investigation of mottled teeth (I). *Dent. Cosmos* **58**, 477–84.

McKay, F.S. (1916b). An investigation of mottled teeth (III). *Dent. Cosmos* **58**, 781-92.

McKay, F.S. (1928). The relation of mottled teeth to caries. *J. Am. dent. Ass.* **15**, 1429–37.

McNeil, D. R. (1957). *The fight for fluoridation.* Oxford University Press, New York.

Mainwaring, P.J. and Naylor, M.N. (1983). A four-year clinical study to determine the caries inhibiting effect of calcium glycerophosphate and sodium fluoride in calcium carbonate base dentifrices containing sodium monofluorophosphate. *Caries Res.* **17**, 267–76.

Mallatt, M.E., Beiswanger, B.B., Stookey, G.K., Swancar, J.R. and Hennon, D.K. (1985). Influence of soluble pyrophosphate on calculus formation in adults. *J. dent. Res.*, **64**(9), 1159–1162.

Margolis, F.J., Reames, H.R., Freshman, E., Macauley, J.C., and Mehaffey, H. (1975). Fluoride-ten year prospective study of deciduous and permanent dentition. *Am, J. Dis. Child.* **129**, 794–800

Mansbridge JN: The Kilmarnock Studies. Appendix to: *The fluoridation studies in the United Kingdom and results achieved after 11 Years.* London, HMSO, 1969.

Marthaler, T.M. (1969). Caries-inhibiting effect of fluoride tablets, *Helv. odontol. Acta.* **13**, 1–13.

Marthaler, T.M. (1979). Fluoride supplements for systemic effects in caries prevention. In *Continuing evaluation of the use of fluorides*, (ed. E. Johansen, D. R. Taves, and T. O. Olsen), pp. 33–59. AAAS, Washington, DC.

Marthaler, T.M. and Schenardi, C. (1962). Inhibition of caries in children after 5½ years use of fluoridated table salt. *Helv. odontol. Acta.* **6**, 1–6.

Marthaler, T.M., De Crousaz, Ph., Meyer R., Regolati, B., and Robert. A. (1977). Frequence globale do la carie dentaire dans le canton de Vaud, apres passage de la fluoruration par comprimes a la fluoruration du sel alimentaire. *Schweiz. Machr. Zahnheilk.* **87**, 147–58.

Marthaler, T.M., Mejia, R., Toth, K., and Vines, J.J. (1978). Caries-preventive salt fluoridation, *Caries Res.* **12**, Suppl. 1, 15–21.

Marthaler, T. (1983). Practical aspects of salt fluoridation. *Schweiz. Mschr. Zahnmed.*, **93**, 1197–1214.

Mason, J.O. (1991). Too much of a good thing? Editorial *J. Am. Dent. Assoc.* **122**, 93–94.

Mejia, D.R., Espinal, F., Velez, H. and Aguirre, S.M. (1976). Use of fluoridated salt in four Columbian communities VIII. *Bol. Sanit, Panam.*, **80**, 205–219.

Møller, I. J. (1965). *Dental fluorose og caries.* Rhodos International Science Publishers, Copenhagen.

Møller, I. J. (1982). Fluorides and dental fluorosis *Int. dent. J.* **32**, 134–7.

Muhler, J.C., Radike, A.W., Nebergall, W.H., and Day, H.G. (1955). A comparison between the anticariogenic effect of dentifrices containing stannous fluoride and sodium fluoride. *J. Am. dent. Ass.* **51**, 556–9.

Murray, J.J. (1969a). Caries experience of five-year-old children from fluoride and non-fluoride communities. *Br. dent. J.* **126**, 352–4.

Murray, J.J. (1969*b*). Caries experience of 15-year-old children from fluoride and non-fluoride communities. *Br. dent. J.* **127**, 128–31

Murray, J. J. (1976). *Fluorides in caries prevention* (1st edn). Wright, Bristol.

Murray, J. J. (1993). Efficacy of preventive agents for dental caries: systemic fluorides, water fluoridation. *Caries Res.* **27** (suppl. 1), 2–8.

Murray, J. J. and Atkinson, K. (1971). Caries experience of West Hartlepool children aged 2–18 years. *Dent. Pract. dent. Res.* **21**, 387–8.

Murray, J.J. Rugg-Gunn, A.J., and Jenkins G.N. (1991). *Fluorides in caries prevention*, 3rd edn. Wright, Butterworth Heinemann.

Nevitt, G.A., Difenbach, V., and Presnell, C.E. (1953). Missouri's fluoride and dental caries study. A study of the dental caries experience and the fluoride content of the drinking water of 3,206 white children in nine selected cities in Missouri. *J. Mo. State dent. Ass.* **33**, 10–26.

Newbrun, E. (1992). Current regulations and recommendations concerning water fluoridation, fluoride supplements and topical fluoride agents. *J. dent. Res.* **71**, 1255–65.

Niedenthal, A. (1957). Caries prophylaxis with sodium fluoride tablets in Offenbach school children. *Zahnaerztl. Mitt.* **45**, 576–87.

O'Rourke, C., Attrill, M. and Holloway, P.J. (1988). Cost appraisal of a fluoride tablet programme to Manchester primary school-children. *Commun. Dent. oral Epidemiol.*, **16**, 341–344.

Osuji, O.O. and Nikiforuk J. (1988). Fluoride supplements induced dental fluorosis—case reports. *Pediatric Dentistry* **10**, 48–52.

Pang, D. T. and Vann, W. F. Jr. (1992). The use of fluoride containing toothpastes in young children: the scientific evidence for recommending small quantity. *Paed. Dent.* **14**, 384–7.

Plasschaert, A. J. M. and Konig, K. G. (1974). The effect of information and motivation towards dental health and of fluoride tablets on caries in school children: I. Increment over the initial 2-year experimental period. *Int. Dent. J.* **24**, 50–65.

Pollack, H. (1960). Caries prophylaxis with Mulgatum F. Result of an investigation over a period of two years in Nordheim-Westphalia. *Dtsch. Zahnaerzteble* **14**, 363–5.

Poulsen, S., Gradegaard, E., and Mortensen, B. (1981). Cariostatic effect of daily use of a fluoride-containing lozenge compared to fortnightly rinses with 0.2% sodium fluoride. *Caries Res.* **15**, 236–42.

Primosch, R.E., Weatherell, J.A. and Strong, M. (1986). Distribution and retention of salivary fluoride from a sodium fluoride tablet following various intra-oral dissolution methods. *J. dent. Res.*, **65**, 1001–5.

Pritchard, J. L. (1969). The prenatal and postnatal effects of fluoride supplements on West Australian schoolchildren aged 6, 7, and 8, Perth, 1967. *Aust. dent. J.* **14**, 335–8.

Riordan, P. J. (1993). Fluoride supplements in caries prevention: a literature review and proposal for a new dosage schedule. *J. Publ. Hlth Dent.* **53**, 174–89.

Ripa, L.W., Leske, G.S. Sposato, A. and Varma, A. (1987). Clinical comparison of the caries inhibition of two mixed NaF-Na₂PO₃F dentifrices containing 1000 and 2500 ppmF compared to a conventional Na₂PO₃F dentrice containing 1000 ppmF: results after two years. *Caries Res.*, **21**, 149–157.

Roemer. R. (1983). Legislation on Fluorides and dental health. *Int. Dig. hlth. Legislation.* **34**, 3–31.

Rugg-Gunn, A. J., *et al.* (1981). Caries experience of 5 year old children living in four communities in N.E. England receiving different water fluoride levels. *Br. dent. J.* **150**, 9–12.

Rugg-Gunn, A. J., *et al.* (1987). The water intake of 405 Northumbrian adolescents aged 12–14 years. *Br. dent. J.* **162**, 335–40.

Rugg-Gunn, A.J, Carmichael C.L, Ferrell R.S. (1988). Effect of fluoridation and secular trend in caries in 5-year-old children living in Newcastle and Northumberland. *Br. dent. J.* **165**, 359–364.

Rusoff, L.L., Konikoff, B.S., Frye, J.B., Johnston, J.E. and Frye, W.W. (1962). Fluoride addition to milk and its effect on dental caries in school children. *Am. J. Clin. Nutr.*, **11**, 94–107.

Schrotenboer, G. (1981). Perspectives on the use of prenatal fluorides: a reactor's comments. *J. dent. Child.* **48**, 123–5.

Schützmannsky, G. (1965). Further results of our tablet fluoridation in Halle. *Dt. Stomatol.* **15**, 107–14.

Schützmannsky, G. (1971). Fluorine tablet application in pregnant females. *Dt. Stomatol.* **21**, 122–9.

Sellman, S., Syrrist, A., and Gustafson, G. (1957). Fluorine and dental health in Southern Sweden. *T. Odont. Tskr.* **65**, 61–93.

Silverstone, L.M. (1973). *Preventive dentistry: systemic fluoride* Part 2 Dental Update, **1**, 101–5.

Singh, S.M., Rustogi, K.M., Volpe, A.R., Petrone, M., Kirkup, R. and Collins, M. (1989). Effect of a dentifrice containing triclosan and a copolymer on plaque formation: a 6-week clinical study. *Am. J. Dent.*, **2**, 225–30.

Stamm, J.W. (1974). Fluoride uptake from topical sodium fluoride varnish measured by an *in vivo* enamel biopsy. *J. Can. dent. Ass.* **40**, 501–5.

Stephen, K.W. and Campbell, D. (1978). Caries reduction and cost benefit after 3 years of sucking fluoride tablets daily at school. *Br. dent. J.* **144**, 202–6.

Stephen, K.W., Campbell, D., and Boyle, I.T. (1981). A double-blind caries study with fluoridated school milk—five year data from a vitaman D deficient area. *Caries Res.* ORCA Congress, Erfurt, 1981, Abstr. 71.

Stephen, K. W., *et al.* (1984). Five year double-blind fluoridated milk study in Scotland. *Commun. Dent. oral Epidemiol.* **12**, 223–9.

Stephen, K. W., McCall, D. R., and Tullis, J. I. (1987). Caries prevalence in North Scotland before, and 5 years after, water defluoridation. *Br. dent. J.* **163**, 324–6.

Stephen *et al.* (1988). a 3-year oral health dose–response study of sodium monofluorophosphate dentifrices with and without zinc citrate: anti-caries results. *Commun. Dent. oral Epidemiol.* **16**, 321–5.

Stephen K.W., Chestnutt, I.G., Jacobson, APM, M'Call, D.R., Chesters, R.K., Huntington, E. and Schäfer, F. (1994). The effect of NaF and NaMFP toothpastes on 3 year caries increments in adolescent. *Int. Dent. J.* **44**, 287–95.

Steiner, M., Marthaler, T.M., Weisner, V. and Menghini, G. (1986). Kariesbefall bei Schuklindern des Kanton Glarus, 9 Jahre nach Einführung des höher fluoridierten Kochsalzes (250 mg F/kg). *Schweiz Mschr. Zahnmed.*, **96**, 688–699.

Stolte, G. (1968). Results of three years of caries prophylaxis by oral fluoride applications in Solingen kindergarten. *Zahnaerztl. Mitt.* **58**, 380–2.

Stones, H. H., *et al.* (1949). The effect of topical application of potassium fluoride and of the ingestion of tablets containing sodium fluoride on the incidence of dental caries. *Br. dent. J.* **86**, 264–71.

Stookey, G. K. (1981). Perspectives on the use of prenatal fluorides: a reactor's comments. *J. dent. Child.* **48**, 126–7.

Stookey, G.K., De Paola, P.F., Featherstone, J.D.B., Fejerskov, O., Möller, I.J., Rotberg, S., Stephen, K.W., and Welfel, J.S. (1993). A critical Review of the relative anticaries efficacy of sodium fluoride and sodium monofluorophosphate dentifrices. *Caries Res.* **27**, 337–360.

Thylstrup, A., Fejerskov, O., Brunn, C. and Kann, J. (1979). Enamel changes and dental caries in 7-year-old children given fluoride tablets from shortly after birth. *Caries Res.*, **13**, 265–276.

Torell, P. and Ericsson, Y. (1965). Two year clinical tests with different methods of local caries prevention. Fluoride application in Swedish school children. *Acta odont. Scand.* **16**, 329–41.

Toth, K. (1976). A study of 8 years domestic salt fluoridation for prevention of caries. *Commun. Dent. oral Epidemiol.* **4**, 106–10.

Toth, K. (1979). 10 years of domestic salt fluoridation in Hungary. *Caries Res.* **13**, 101 (abstr.).

Toth, K. (1980). Factors influencing the urinary fluoride level in subjects drinking low fluoride water. *Caries Res.* **14**, 168 (abstr.)

Triol, C.W., Graves, R.C., Webster, D.B. and Clarke, B.J. (1987). Anticaries effect of 1450 and 2000 ppm F dentifrices. *J. Dent. Res.*, **66** (Spec. Issue), 216 (Abstr. 879).

Van Eck, A.A.M.J. (1987). Pre- and post-eruptive effect of fluoridated drinking water on dental caries experience. Thesis, University of Utrecht (NIPG-TNO No. 87021).

Villa, A., *et al.* (1989) Fluoride bio-availability from disodium monofluorophosphate fluoridated milk in children and rats. *Caries Res.* **23**, 179–83.

Vines, J. J. (1971). Fluorprofilaxis de la caries dental a traves de la sal fluorurada. *Revta Clin. Esp.* **120**, 319–34.

Vines, J. J. and Clavero, J. (1968). Investigacion de la relacion entre la incidencia de caries y contenido del ion fluor en las agnas de abastecimiento. *Rev. San. E. Hig. Pub.* **42**, 401–31.

Weatherell, J.A., Robinson, C., Ralph, J.P. and Best, J.S. (1984). Migration of fluoride in the mouth. *Caries. Res.*, **18**, 348–353.

Weaver, R. (1944). Fluorosis and dental caries on Tyneside. *Br. dent. J.* **76**, 29–40.

Weaver, R. (1950). Fluorine and wartime diet. *Br. dent. J.* **88**, 231–9.

Wespi, H.J. (1948). Gedanke zuer Frage der optimalen Ernahrung in der Schwangerschaft. Salz and Brot als Trager zusatzlicher Nahrungsstoffe. *Schweiz. med. Wschr.* **78**. 153–5.

Wespi, H. J. (1950). Fluoriertes Kochsalz zur Cariesprophlaxe. *Schweiz. med. Wschr.* **80**, 561–4.

Widenheim, J. (1985). On fluoride tablets: a retrospective study of intake patterns and the pre-eruptive effect on occurrence of caries, restorations and fluorosis in teeth. Thesis. University of Lund, Malmo.

World Health Organization (1970). *Fluorides and human health.* WHO Monogr. Series No. 59. WHO, Geneva.

World Health Organization (1986). *Appropriate use of fluorides for human health.* WHO. Geneva.

World Health Organization (1992). *Recent advances in oral health.* WHO Technical Report Series No. 826. Geneva.

World Health Organization (1994). Fluorides and oral health. WHO, Geneva (in press).

Winter, G.B., Holt, R.D. and Williams, B.F. (1989). Clinical trial of a low-fluoride toothpaste for young children. *Int. Dent. J.*, **39**, 227–235.

Wrzodek, G. (1959). Does the prevention of caries by means of fluoride tablets promise success? *Zahnaerztl. Mitt.* **47**, 1–5.

Zacherl, W.A. (1981). A three-year clinical caries evaluation of the effect of a sodium fluoride-silica abrasive dentifrice. *Pharmacol.ther. Dent.* **6**, 1–7.

Ziegler, E. (1962). Milk fluoridation. *Bull. Schweiz. Akad Med. Wiss.* **18**.

Ziemnowicz-Glowaka, W. (1960). Prevention of caries by means of 'Fluodar' tablets. *Czas. Stomatol.* **13**, 719–28.

Zipkin, I. and McClure, F.J. (1951). Complex fluorides: caries reduction and fluoride retention in the bones and teeth of white rats. *Publ. Hlth. Rep.* **66**, 1523–32.

4. Oral cleanliness and dental caries

PHILIP SUTCLIFFE

This exploration of the relationship between oral cleanliness and caries begins with the widely accepted premise that dental caries occurs only after plaque has accumulated on susceptible tooth surfaces in individuals who eat sugar frequently. The process is slow and all three factors must occur together.

The interdependence of plaque, sugar, tooth susceptibility, and time has been well demonstrated in Tristan da Cunha and Hopewood House where susceptible populations with heavy accumulations of plaque remained relatively free from dental caries as long as only small amounts of sugar were eaten. In 1938 no one under the age of 20 years in Tristan da Cunha had a carious first permanent molar, even though the standard of oral cleanliness was poor. The average daily consumption of sugar, confectionery, preserves, and sweets totalled 2.5 g per person. By 1962 this had risen to 244 g (Fisher 1968) and 50 per cent of first permanent molars were found to be carious in a sample of 64 islanders aged between 6 and 20 years. The standard of oral cleanliness had remained poor (Holloway et al. 1963).

Hopewood House was established in New South Wales, Australia, to look after needy children. The diet, which was lactovegetarian, consisted mainly of uncooked vegetables and was notable for an almost complete absence of sugar. The food was adequate in essential nutrients and the general health of the children compared well with that of other children in New South Wales except for dental caries where the Hopewood House children were much better off. The standard of oral cleanliness was poor. Thirteen-year-olds in Hopewood House had a mean of 1.1 DMF teeth compared with 10.7 in children of similar age attending state schools (Sullivan and Harris 1958; Gillham and Lennon 1958).

Epidemiological corroboration of the relationship between plaque and caries lacks consistency and as a result the intrinsic value of oral hygiene practices against the initiation of caries has been vigorously challenged (Bibby 1966).

Studies of the relationship may be divided into four approaches: point-prevalence surveys of total caries experience and oral cleanliness; longitudinal retrospective studies of oral cleanliness and increments in caries experience; reported tooth-brushing frequency and total caries experience; and finally prospective studies of improved oral cleanliness and increments in caries experience. The latter is the most satisfactory method; the fundamental difficulty with the first three approaches is that good oral hygiene habits may be accompanied by other practices that help to preserve the teeth (Schou et al. 1990). It is extremely difficult to disentangle the

effect of these habits retrospectively and frequently this has not been attempted.

Fluoride has a proven effect against caries and fluoride dentifrices are becoming an increasingly important method of topical application. Except where a specific note is made the first, and main part of this review is confined to fluoride-free, unmedicated toothpastes. The final part of the chapter reviews the relationship between dental caries, brushing frequency and rinsing methods after using fluoride toothpastes.

POINT-PREVALENCE SURVEYS (Table 4.1)

Oral cleanliness is usually described by a qualitative plaque index, and caries experience by the DMFT and DMFS indices. The combined use of these indices in a single investigation may be inappropriate because of the transient nature of plaque deposits. Plaque indices refer strictly to the standard of oral cleanliness at the moment of the examination whilst caries indices give the total caries experience accumulated from the time of tooth eruption. Thus an investigation into the permanent dentitions of 12-year-olds assumes that the standard of oral cleanliness has remained the same for roughly 6 years. This assumption may be more valid when only the children with extreme standards of oral cleanliness are selected for comparison.

The reported studies appear to have been conducted almost exclusively on children between the ages of 3 and 15 years, and mainly with older children. Where mean DMFT or DMFS values may be identified the results of the studies are summarized in Table 4.1.

Trubman (1963) studied 397 children from Jackson, Missouri, aged between 12 and 14 years, and found a weak negative and statistically insignificant correlation between caries experience and oral cleanliness. The children with the cleanest oral hygiene scores had a mean of 15.0 DMF surfaces compared with 14.2 in the worst group.

McHugh et al. (1964) found no significant correlation between oral hygiene scores and the mean numbers of DMF teeth in 2905 children aged 13 years from Dundee, Scotland. Similar results have been reported from Finland and Canada. Parviainen et al. (1977) studied 365 13- to 15-year-olds from three Finnish communities with varying amounts of fluoride in the drinking water. In none of the communities was a correlation found between visible plaque index scores and DMF caries scores. Richardson et al. (1977) found no significant

Table 4.1. Prevalence studies of caries and oral cleanliness

Reference	Age of subjects	Index of oral cleanliness	No. of subjects	Mean caries experience	% increase	Significance
McCauley and Frazier (1957)	6–10	Oral hygiene score				
		(good) 4,0	983	2.4 DMFT		Not given
		3.0–3.9	1238	2.9	21	
		2.0–2.9	247	3.5	46	
		(poor) 1.0–1.9	30	4.4	83	
Mansbridge (1960)	12–14	Good	146	9.6 DMFT		
		Fair	162	10.2	6	$p < 0.05$
		Neglected	118	11.5	20	$p < 0.01$
Trubman (1963)	12–14	Oral hygiene index				
		(good) 0.0–0.4	99	15.0 DMFS		$r = -0.07$
		0.5–0.9	142	15.9	6	$p > 0.05$
		1.0–1.4	80	14.6	–3	
		1.5–1.9	37	11.1	–26	
		(poor) 2.0 +	39	14.2	–5	
McHugh *et al.* (1964)	13	Oral hygiene index				
		(good) Under 5	341	9.6 DMFT		n.s.
		6–7	730	9.7	1	
		8–9	869	10.3	7	
		(poor) 10–12	965	9.9	3	
Sutcliffe (1977)	3–4	Simplified debris				
		(good) 0.0–0.5	259	1.6 dmft		$p < 0.001$
		(poor) 1.5 +	236	3.6 dmft	125	
Bjertness *et al.* (1986)	35 (1973)	OHI-S 0.00–0.99	35	81.7 DMFS		
		1.00–1.99	54	86.1	11	
		2.00+	27	95.6	17	$0.5 > p > 0.01$
	35	OHI-S 0.00–0.99	47	80.3 DMFS		
		1.00–1.99	62	89.8	12	
		2.00+	35	82.9	3	$0.05 > p > 0.01$

correlation between oral hygiene indices and caries when they examined a total of 457 7- and 13-year-old Canadian children. In this study of first- and seventh-grade children, refined and total carbohydrate consumption was also measured. It was found that the children with high caries indices did not have the poorest oral hygiene nor consume the most carbohydrates. The children with low caries indices did not have the cleanest teeth nor consume lesser amounts of carbohydrates.

The authors commented that the lack of correlation between caries and carbohydrate consumption may have been due to the limitations of self-recorded diet surveys and to the problem of correlating indices with different time bases. However, in a study of the dental health of 1015 school-children, aged 11 to 12 years, living in South Wales, Addy *et al.* (1986) reported highly statistically significant but low Pearson correlation coefficients between plaque scores and DMFT ($r = 0.14$) or DMFS ($r = 0.09$).

In an earlier and broadly similar study of 12- to 14-year-olds from Miami the diet and oral cleanliness of 46 caries-free children was contrasted with data from 40 caries-active children. Diet scores, based upon the frequency and quality of sugar eating, were found to be significantly associated with caries experience. However a negligible inverse relationship between caries and oral cleanliness was found that may have occurred because many children who normally did not brush

their teeth did so because they expected the dental examination (Duany *et al.* 1972).

Bay and Ainamo (1974) adopted a slightly different approach: 293 7-year-old Copenhagen children were ranked according to caries experience, and the PLG plaque index scores were compared between 89 low caries-risk children (4 or fewer affected tooth surfaces) and 56 high caries-risk children (22 or more affected tooth surfaces). The first group had a mean plaque score of 1.9 and the second group 2.2. Although this difference was significant ($p < 0.05$), the authors commented that it was of no clinical importance. Additional analysis did reveal that most of the heavy plaque scores were in the high caries group.

In a comparison of the dental caries experience and oral cleanliness of Asian and white Caucasian children aged 5 and 6 years attending multiracial schools in Greater Glasgow and Greater Manchester it was found that caries experience and oral cleanliness varied between the white children and sub-groups of the Asian children divided according to religion and the English-speaking ability of the mother. Oral cleanliness scores were found to follow a similar pattern to dental caries experience although no coefficients of correlation are given (Bedi and Elton 1991).

The relative importance of associations between caries occurrence and exposure to sugar, fluoride, medication with drugs affecting saliva secretion and the standard of oral cleanliness was assessed in 125 mentally disadvantaged and 79 healthy 9- to 10-year-old Finnish children. The evaluation of the relative importance of the associations was based on logistic regression analyses. For mentally disadvantaged children the most important determinant of caries risk was their poor standard of oral hygiene (Palin-Palokas *et al.* 1987).

In two studies of random samples of 35-year-old Oslo citizens carried out in 1973 and 1984 the participants were grouped together according to their simplified oral hygiene index scores (Bjertness *et al.* 1986). The mean numbers of DMFS surfaces were then compared between each of the three oral hygiene groups. In each survey a statistically significant increase in caries experience was found with increase in the OHI-S score. In the 1973 survey there was a 17 per cent increase in DMF surfaces between the low and high oral-hygiene score groups: in 1984 the increase was 3 per cent. These average differences amounted to 13.9 and 2.6 DMF surfaces respectively.

McCauley and Frazier (1957), Mansbridge (1960), and Sutcliffe (1977) found that poorer standards of oral cleanliness in children were accompanied by an increase in the total caries experience. When the results of the three studies are taken together and only the 'best' and 'worst' children are compared then it can be seen that the greatest increase was found in the youngest children (3- and 4-year-olds), and the smallest increase in the oldest subjects (12- to 14-year-olds).

Kleemola-Kujala (1978) examined the relationship between the amount of plaque that had accumulated on groups of teeth and caries experience in a total of 806 5-, 9-, and 13-year-old Finnish children. The results showed an increase in caries experience of all tooth types with increasing plaque at all ages, although only slight increases were found in permanent molar teeth. Mansbridge (1960) came to a similar conclusion when he compared the 12- to 14-year-olds with 'good' and 'neglected' oral hygiene. He found that the differences in the caries experience were greatest in the premolar and incisor teeth, and smallest in molars. Similarly a greater response to poor oral cleanliness was found in deciduous incisor and canine teeth, rather than molar teeth, in 4-year-olds (Sutcliffe 1977).

In a review of oral hygiene and caries, Bellini *et al.* (1981) commented: 'The association between plaque and caries was most apparent in front teeth and in free smooth surfaces. Since these areas are most easily reached by self applied brushing, the findings support the opinion of a direct effect of oral hygiene on caries'.

In a further report on Finnish children in low fluoride areas the relative contribution of increased plaque accumulation and sugar consumption to the total load of caries was assessed (Kleemola-Kujala and Rasanen 1982). A total of 543 children, aged 5–9 and 13 years, took part in the study. They were divided into three groups of plaque level according to their plaque indices, and into three groups of sugar consumption assessed by a 24-hour recall method. Caries experience was expressed as the proportion of tooth surfaces examined which were found carious or filled.

The results suggest that when oral hygiene is poor, even a relatively low total sugar consumption can promote decay in caries-susceptible primary and young permanent teeth. The association between the amount of plaque and dental caries was statistically significant at all levels of sugar consumption. With increasing total sugar consumption the risk of caries increased significantly only when oral hygiene was simultaneously poor.

RETROSPECTIVE LONGITUDINAL STUDIES (Table 4.2)

Data collected during clinical trials have been used to look back upon the relationship between successive estimations of oral cleanliness and the increase in caries that has occurred over the same period. This approach goes some way towards avoiding the combined use of indices with different time bases, but children recruited to take part in clinical trials are selected for their qualities of cooperation and motivation, and may not be typical of all children.

In a 3-year study with adolescents, Holloway and Teagle (1976) compared mean caries increments in 63 subjects with good oral cleanliness at annual examinations with the increment measured in 52 subjects with poor oral cleanliness

Table 4.2. Retrospective longitudinal studies of caries increments and oral cleanliness

Reference	Initial age of subjects	Duration of study	Index of oral cleanliness	Number of subjects		Mean caries increments	% increase	Significance
Sutcliffe (1973)	11–12	3 years	Good	Boys	8	3.00 DMFT		n.s.
			Fair		131	3.17	6	
			Poor		78	3.47	16	
			Good	Girls	34	4.21 DMFT		n.s.
			Fair		118	3.97	−6	
			Poor		29	4.52	7	
Tucker *et al.* (1976)	11	3 years	Good		184	4.25 DMFT		*p* < 0.05
			Poor		192	4.96	17	
			Good		184	8.35 DMFS		n.s.
			Poor		192	9.27	11	
Beal *et al.* (1979)	11–12	3 years	Clean		59	7.59 DMFS	36	*p* < 0.05
			Not clean		101	10.29		

throughout. Although lower increments were found in those with good oral cleanliness the difference, which amounted to only one attacked tooth surface in 3 years, did not attain statistical significance.

In a similar 3-year study, Sutcliffe (1973) compared the caries increments between 42 children who had good oral cleanliness at annual examinations and 107 children with poor oral cleanliness. The children were initially aged between 11 and 12 years. Those children with clean teeth at each examination had the smallest mean increment, but the difference was rather less than 0.5 DMFT and was not statistically significant.

The dry weight of plaque collected from one side of the mouth at intervals of one, two, and three years after baseline examinations had been completed was compared with the 3-year increment in DF surfaces in 51 boys, aged between 11 and 14 years. All of the coefficients of correlation showed a weak, positive association but only the correlation for first-year plaque was significant (Ashley and Wilson 1977). The correlation between the 3-year DF surface increment and the mean dry weight of plaque from the three samples was also weak and positive and was again not statistically significant.

Tucker *et al.* (1976) examined the relationship between the 3-year increment in caries experience in 184 children with 'good' and 192 with 'poor' oral cleanliness measured at three annual intervals. Initially the children were between 11 and 12 years old. Children with good oral cleanliness had mean increments of 4.3 DMFT or 8.4 DMFS, the mean values in children with 'poor' oral cleanliness were greater by 0.7 DMFT or 0.9 DMFS respectively. Only the difference between DMF teeth was statistically significant ($p < 0.05$). The results were more clear-cut for teeth which had erupted during the trial. The mean caries increment in teeth which were unerupted at the baseline examination was 1.3 DMFT or 1.6 DMFS in those with good oral cleanliness, and 1.9 DMFT or 2.5 DMFS in those with poor oral cleanliness. These differences were highly statistically significant ($p < 0.001$).

Beal *et al.* (1979) also contrasted the 3-year increment in caries experience in children initially aged 11 to 12 years whose dental status was consistently clean or not clean. There were 59 children with consistently clean mouths with

a mean increment of 7.59 DMFS compared with a mean of 10.29 DMFS in 101 children with consistently unclean mouths—the difference was statistically significant ($p < 0.05$).

In a prospective 2-year study involving 405 English children, initially aged 11.5 years, the results of 3-day diet records, collected on five occasions, were compared with the increments in caries experience (Rugg-Gunn *et al.* 1984). Correlations between caries increment and dietary factors were low due to the low caries increments observed and the large error associated with dietary data where analyses attempt to discriminate between individuals. The highest correlation was between caries increment and weight of daily intake of sugars (+0.143, $p < 0.01$). At each annual examination the level of gingival inflammation was used as a measure of plaque accumulation for each child. Of the non-dietary variables studied (sex, social class, gingival index, and tooth-brushing frequency) only gingival index significantly increased the correlation between weight of sugars and caries increment. This interesting result parallels the finding by Kleemola-Kujala and Rasanan (1982) of an interaction between increased plaque accumulation and sugar consumption.

A similar finding was reported by Sundin *et al.* (1992) in a study of the 3-year incidence of proximal surface caries in molars and premolars in 69 children initially aged 15 years. A number of variables were studied, including oral cleanliness as indicated by gingival health. It was concluded that sweet eating was particularly harmful when oral hygiene was poor and consumption of other sugary products was high.

THE FREQUENCY OF TOOTH-BRUSHING AND DENTAL CARIES (Table 4.3)

The reported frequency of tooth-brushing has also been used to investigate the relationship between oral cleanliness and dental caries. This indirect method has considerable limitations because those who frequently brush their teeth are probably those who are most likely to carry out other procedures to improve their dental health such as restricting sugar eating and seeking regular dental check-ups. An addi-

Table 4.3. Studies of caries and frequency of tooth-brushing

Reference	Age of subjects	Daily brushing frequency	Number of subjects	Mean caries experience	% increase	Significance
Smith and Stiffler (1963)	18–44	Twice or more yesterday	1043	9.51 DMFT		n.s.
		Once yesterday	752	7.57	−20	
		Did not brush yesterday	171	5.73	−40	
Dale (1969)	17–29	Three times	31	17.19 DMFT		n.s.
		Twice	188	19.11	11	
		Once	327	19.47	13	
		Less than once	67	18.67	9	
Miller and Hobson (1961)	12	Regular	115	5.8 DMFT		$p < 0.05$
Miller (1961)		Irregular	264	5.0	−14	
		None	357	5.0	−14	
				3 year increment		
Tucker *et al.* (1976)	11–14	Twice or more	187	4.29 DMFT		$p < 0.05$
		Less than twice	189	4.94	15	

tional complication is that dental attenders have been found to have higher mean numbers of DMF teeth than irregular attenders (Todd 1975; Todd and Walker 1980). Regular adult tooth-brushers have also been found to have a lower mean number of decayed, that is untreated teeth, than irregular brushers (Dale 1969; Ainamo 1971). This may be seen as evidence of the relationship between regular brushing and other tooth-preserving habits. Finally a direct relationship between tooth-brushing and oral hygiene status has not always been found (Tucker *et al.* 1976). Frequent tooth-brushing need not necessarily lead to freedom from plaque if the brushing is inefficient. An exaggerated claim for frequent brushing may be checked by an oral examination (Miller and Hobson 1961).

In a study of 555 children, aged between 1 and 5 years, from Camden in London, parents were asked whether or not they brushed their child's teeth each day. A total of 295 children (53 per cent of the total study population) were reported to have daily tooth-brushing: 84 per cent of these children were caries-free compared with 89 per cent among those who did not clean daily. This small difference was not statistically significant (Holt *et al.* 1982).

In the study of Danish 7-year-olds already referred to, Bay and Ainamo (1974) found no difference in frequency of tooth-brushing between the low- and high-caries risk groups. A correlation was not found between the frequency of tooth-brushing and DFS scores in 13- to 15-year-old Finnish children (Ainamo and Parviainen 1979).

A total of 115 12-year-old English children who brushed once a day and who were also found to have clean teeth had a mean of 5.8 DMF teeth, which was significantly greater ($p < 0.05$) than the mean of 5.0 found in 621 children who brushed less than once a day (Miller 1961; Miller and Hobson 1961).

In their 3-year retrospective study, Tucker *et al.* (1976) reported that the increment in caries experience was 4.3 DMF teeth in those who brushed their teeth as least twice daily compared with a mean of 4.9 DMF teeth in those who brushed less frequently. The difference was significant ($p < 0.05$).

This type of investigation has also been carried out on adults. The reported frequency of tooth-brushing was not found to be related to the mean DMFT in 1976 adults aged 18 to 44 years from New Mexico (Smith and Striffler 1963). No relationship was found between tooth-brushing frequency and DMFT in 613 regular servicemen aged between 17 and 29 years from Sydney, Australia (Dale 1969).

In an interesting study Rajala *et al.* (1980) tried to disentangle the influence of behaviours associated with tooth-brushing upon caries experience. Information was obtained from 212 male employees at a Finnish paper mill. Potential risk indicators other than tooth-brushing were controlled by stratification using a multivariate confounder summarizing score. The variates included in the model were number of teeth, education, sucrose consumption, previous fluoride exposure, income, and use of dental services. In general it was found that caries experience was consistently higher for sporadic tooth-brushers. The authors also commented that their results indicated that the positive association between reported daily tooth-brushing and low caries experience may be more pronounced in groups with higher overall risk status, for example, in the strata where education and income was low, frequency of dental visits irregular, number of teeth small, use of sucrose high, and fluoride exposure low. This finding suggests that in situations where the 'baseline prevention' is weak, tooth-brushing may be useful in caries prevention, or vice versa, the true effect of tooth-brushing may be hidden by other, perhaps more powerful, means of caries prevention.

PROSPECTIVE STUDIES (Table 4.4)

The most satisfactory method of examining the relationship between oral cleanliness and caries is by means of controlled prospective studies in which randomly assigned test subjects experience an improved standard of oral cleanliness. The improvement may be achieved by either encouraging the participants to thoroughly clean their teeth under supervision or by cleaning the teeth professionally.

SELF-CLEANING STUDIES

Fosdick compared the 2-year caries increment in 423 students who continued with their customary oral hygiene habits, with the increment in 523 test subjects who undertook to brush their teeth thoroughly within 10 minutes after eating food or sweets or, when brushing was impossible, to rinse the mouth thoroughly with water. A significantly smaller increment was recorded in the test group but deficiencies in the design of this early study complicate an overall assessment of the result (Fosdick 1950; Smith and Striffler 1963).

Alice M. Horowitz and her colleagues studied the effect of an intensive school-based plaque-removal programme on children initially aged from 10 to 13 years. A fluoride-free dentifrice was used. Children from the same school were randomly placed in the test or control group. For 32 months the subjects in the treatment group carried out tooth-brushing and flossing each school day. Of the 481 children initially examined, 295 remained in the study for 32 months. Of these, 279 were present at all of the six examinations, 111 in the treatment group and 168 in the control group. Data were reported for these children only. Most of the children found the system of cleaning boring, the school staff became increasingly less co-operative, and the supervising personnel commented that the programme was very demanding. After 32 months only the test-group girls showed a significant reduction in plaque score ($p < 0.01$) although the boys showed some improvement. Both boys and girls showed a significant improvement in gingival health ($p < 0.01$). Losses of subjects during the trial resulted in an imbalance on the initial mean caries experience of the children seen at every examination and adjusted mean incremental DMFS scores are presented in the results. The adjusted mean increment in the treatment group was 4.3 DMF surfaces and 4.9 DMF surfaces in the control group. This 1.3 per cent reduction was not significant. The biggest reduction of 26 per cent or 0.7 DMF surfaces was seen in proximal sites but this was not statistically significant (Horowitz *et al.* 1980).

Table 4.4. Prospective studies of caries increments and improved oral cleanliness

Reference	Age of subjects	Duration of study	Group	Number of subjects		Mean caries increment	% decrease	Significance
Horowitz *et al.* (1980)	10–13	32 months	Self-cleaning		111	4.27 DMFS	13	n.s.
			Control		168	4.89		
Silverstein *et al.* (1977)	12	29 months	Montera					
			Self-cleaning		42	4.17 DMFS	–157	n.s.
			Control		45	1.62		
			Lowell					
			Self-cleaning		76	6.51 DMFS	7	n.s.
			Control		73	7.00		
Ashley and Sainsbury (1981)	11	3 years	Professional cleaning		119	4.83 DFS	–11	n.s.
			Control		102	4.34		
						New proximal lesions		
Wright *et al.* (1979)	5.8	20 months	Professionally flossed surfaces	Group 1.	44	13	55	$p = 0.004$
			Control		44	29		
			Professionally flossed surfaces	Group 2.	44	12	52	$p = 0.014$
			Control		44	25		

Another study from the United States produced broadly similar results (Silverstein *et al.* 1977, and personal communication). At each of two junior high schools in Oaklands, California, 393 12-year-olds were randomly allocated to control and test groups. The treatment groups brushed without a dentifrice and flossed every school day under supervision. At the fifth and final examination after 29 months, 227 children remained in the study. In one school significant reductions in plaque and gingivitis scores were measured in the test children but in the other school only a reduction in gingivitis scores was recorded. Caries examinations at both schools showed no significant differences in DMFS increments. In this study the control group experienced only slightly smaller improvements in gingivitis and plaque deposits than those in the test group, perhaps as a result of peer pressure from the test-group children.

The value of limited self-flossing under supervision in schools has also been investigated. The aim was to test a very simple style of flossing, which was achieved by pulling the waxed floss once up and down through each contact point. A half-mouth technique was adopted for the evaluation and 140 Swedish children aged between 12 and 13 years flossed the right or the left lateral region once every school day for 2 years. The children were stratified according to their dietary and oral hygiene habits. After 2 years no statistically significant differences were found in caries increments between the flossed and unflossed surfaces. The authors commented that this was probably due to the inadequate flossing technique (Granath *et al.* 1979).

PROFESSIONAL TOOTH-CLEANING

In order to investigate the value of more thorough flossing against proximal caries, Wright and his co-workers carried out two successive short studies each of 20 months duration. The combined results from the two studies are referred to here. The first-grade Canadian children had an initial mean age of 5.8 years. A half-mouth technique was used in which quadrants were assigned randomly to test and control groups. Initially 118 children took part in the study yielding 528 pairs of contralateral surfaces. To qualify for inclusion the pairs of surfaces had to be initially caries-free and in contact with the adjacent tooth. Six surfaces were studied, from the distal of the deciduous canine tooth to the mesial of the first permanent molar. Caries assessments depended upon a combination of mirror and probe examinations supplemented by radiographic data. Drop outs and losses at individual examinations reduced the number of participants to 88. Research assistants flossed the test surfaces each school day and no other oral hygiene procedure or instruction was provided. The 20-month study period included a 4-month summer vacation when flossing was discontinued. The study yielded 374 test and 374 control surfaces. After 20 months, 25 of the test surfaces had developed caries compared with 54 control surfaces. The difference in the incidence of new proximal lesions was significant ($p = 0.014$).

The authors concluded that professionally applied flossing reduces proximal caries but also added that the results were produced under strictly controlled circumstances that could not necessarily be found in an individual or community flossing programme (Wright *et al.* 1979). It is also appropriate to comment that a clinical trial of 20 months' duration is rather short. It is impossible to set out precise guidelines but a test period of 2 years for teeth erupting during a trial has been recommended (Horowitz 1968).

The effect of a 3-year school-based plaque-control programme with English girls initially aged 11 years has been reported (Ashley and Sainsbury 1981). Initially 261 children agreed to take part in the study and 221 were seen at the final examination, 119 in the experimental group and 102 in the control group. The children all attended the same school but the classes were randomly assigned to experimental or control groups. Girls in the experimental group visited a dental hygienist, based at the school, every 2 weeks during term time and, following disclosing, brushing, and oral hygiene reinforcement, received a professional prophylaxis using a fluoride-free polishing paste. Girls in the control group received oral hygiene instruction during the first term of the baseline year only. All participants received a new toothbrush each term and were encouraged to use a fluoride-containing toothpaste at home. Caries was assessed clinically supplemented by bitewing radiographs of posterior teeth. Mean dry weights of plaque are given for the first 2 years of the study.

The baseline mean number of DF surfaces in the 119 experimental group of children was 6.8 compared with 7.0 in the 102 control group girls. The 3-year mean increments in DF surfaces were 4.8 and 4.3 respectively; the difference was not statistically significant. The authors commented that a 'spill-over effect' from the experimental group regime to the control group may have influenced the results; there is some evidence of this from the changes in gingival health in both groups of participants. At the end of the first and second years the experimental group of girls had fewer inflamed gingival sites but by the end of the third year there was only a slight difference in favour of the experimental group which did not reach statistical significance. A second factor may have been the effect of selecting girls for the study since they have a higher dental awareness than boys. Even the most unkempt girls may not have accumulated sufficient quantities of plaque to permit an evaluation on the initiation of caries. However, at the end of the first and second years the experimental group had a significantly smaller mean dry weight of plaque. Home use of fluoride dentifrice in both groups may have obscured benefits arising from the professional cleaning. Twelve months after the end of the study 109 children from the experimental group and 93 from the control group were re-examined. The experimental group still had significantly less plaque than the control group. However, no significant differences were observed in caries increments between the groups, indicating that the programme had no delayed effect on caries experience (Ashley and Sainsbury 1982).

A number of Scandinavian studies have shown remarkable reductions in caries increments in children who have received regular professional prophylaxis combined with some form of fluoride therapy (Lindhe et al. 1975; Badersten et al. 1975; Hamp et al. 1978). The individual contributions of the effects of the prophylaxis and of fluoride to the reductions in caries increments remains speculative. The result of a cross-over study has been published, which was designed to measure the relative effects of fluoride and plaque control. Initially 164 13- to 14-year-old Swedish children were randomly assigned to one of four groups. The value of chlorhexidine gel, mechanical tooth-cleaning with and without fluoride, rinsing with fluoride solution or distilled water, and the use of fluoride or placebo dentifrices were all evaluated over a 2-year period with changes in the regimes after 1 year. The authors found that the results of the trial revealed the overall importance of regularly repeated inter-proximal plaque

elimination in the prevention of proximal surface caries in children (Axelsson et al. 1976). However, 1 year is probably too short a time to judge the effect of a regime on mean caries increment

In an interesting 3-year Danish study of 56 test children and 58 control children initially aged 6–8 years a significant reduction in occlusal caries of erupting first permanent molars was achieved by intensive patient education and professional tooth-cleaning including the use of 2 per cent sodium fluoride solution and a fluoridated dentifrice (0.1 per cent F). The approach was found to require less clinical time than the more conventional approach of applying fissure sealants (Carvalho et al. 1992).

In their review of oral hygiene and caries, Bellini and co-workers (1981) concluded that the results of clinical trials show that self-performed oral hygiene can lead to reductions in caries increments but that professional tooth-cleaning programmes demonstrate more clearly that efficient oral hygiene is a caries-preventive measure.

In a review of 22 studies of the effectiveness of frequent professional prophylaxis, Ripa (1985) commented that although this technique can apparently significantly reduce dental caries incidence in both children and adults, a wide range of preventive techniques had been employed in the investigations. He observed that in the studies that did not employ a fluoride-containing prophylaxis paste or in which the children were not making use of fluoride, statistically significant differences in the caries increments between control and treatment groups were not achieved.

DISCUSSION

As a starting point three ways of investigating the relationship between caries and oral cleanliness have been described. About half of the prevalence studies reviewed earlier have shown a positive association between plaque and caries (McCauley and Frazier 1957; Mansbridge 1960; Bay and Ainamo 1974; Sutcliffe 1977; Kleemola-Kujala 1978; Bjertness et al. 1986). The remaining studies revealed no relationship (McHugh et al. 1964; Nordling and Ainamo 1977; Richardson et al. 1977) or a weak negative relationship (Trubman 1963; Duany et al. 1972). The list of prevalence studies is not exhaustive but those selected are sufficient to show the pattern of results. All of the retrospective studies showed a positive trend with an increase in caries experience associated with poorer standards of oral cleanliness although the results seldom reached significance (Sutcliffe 1973; Holloway and Teagle 1976; Tucker et al. 1976; Ashley and Wilson 1977; Beal et al. 1979).

Studies of the relationship between brushing frequency and caries represent the least satisfactory approach because of the indirectness of the method and most of the results showed no relationship (Smith and Striffler 1963; Dale 1969; Bay and Ainamo 1974; Ainamo and Parviainen 1979; Holt et al. 1982). One study showed a significant negative relationship (Miller 1961). Two studies showed a positive relationship (Tucker et al. 1976; Rajala et al. 1980).

The consensus of the results of the more preferable prevalence and retrospective studies point towards the presence of a weak positive association between plaque and caries. As possessing clean teeth may be associated with other caries-preventing behaviours it is important to establish if oral cleanliness alone has a direct relationship with caries. This is best achieved by clinical trials of a least two, and preferably three years' duration, in which caries-susceptible subjects are randomly assigned to control and test groups that are initially well balanced. Because the presence of plaque, as measured in epidemiological studies, is likely to have only a weak influence on caries increments, other powerful preventive agents such as fluoride should preferably be absent. A treatment-controlled study is also preferable since a high level of restorative care provided outside the control of the investigators may obscure a preventive effect (Jackson and Sutcliffe 1967). None of the prospective studies that has been described completely fulfil these criteria. This in itself is an indication of the difficulty of conducting such studies.

Unfortunately the well-designed study by Horowitz and her co-workers suffered losses that upset the initial balance of the groups, and the final caries increment data was adjusted to accommodate the influence of the losses. The effect of this adjustment on the final overall conclusion of a positive but statistically insignificant relationship between plaque and caries is not clear.

In the similar study conducted by Silverstein and his colleagues the control group experienced marked reductions in gingivitis and plaque as the trial continued, possibly as a result of peer pressure. It is a fundamental requirement in self-cleansing studies that the experimental group should have measurably less plaque after the baseline examinations and the absence of this difference, particularly at one of the schools, makes it difficult to interpret the final result of no significant differences in caries increments between the control and experimental groups.

The problem of ensuring that the participants maintain high levels of oral cleanliness is eliminated if teeth are cleaned professionally. The clearest indication that daily interproximal cleaning reduces the incidence of proximal surface caries in the deciduous dentition comes from a study conducted by Wright *et al.* (1979). It is tantalizing that the study continued for only 20 months.

Both the control and experimental groups of girls in the school-based plaque-control programme described by Ashley and Sainsbury (1981) were encouraged to use a fluoride-containing toothpaste at home and it is possible that this was sufficient to mask the effect of the fortnightly disclosing, brushing, and fluoride-free professional prophylaxis.

Thus there is no unequivocal evidence that good oral cleanliness reduces caries experience, nor is there sufficient evidence to condemn the value of good oral cleanliness as a caries-preventive measure. When the effects of a number of variables upon caries experience were studied the results indicated that poor standards of oral cleanliness enhance the cariogenicity of sucrose in the diet (Kleemola-Kujala and Rasanen 1982; Rugg-Gunn *et al.* 1984). Fortunately there is no conjecture about the advice that may be given to patients. Fluoride toothpastes are capable of reducing the incidence of caries and their regular and frequent use is recommended.

FLUORIDE DENTIFRICES AND TOOTH-BRUSHING HABITS

In 1973, in a low fluoride area in Finland, no association was found between brushing frequency and mean DFS scores in 13- to 15-year-olds. When similarly aged children from the same area were re-examined in 1982, dental health had significantly improved and high brushing frequency was found to be associated with low mean DFS scores. During the time between the two examinations the average amount of fluoride toothpaste used in Finland per inhabitant per year had almost doubled, from 80 to 150 ml, and the proportions of children brushing their teeth at least once a day had increased from 56 to 75 per cent. The authors concluded that the decrease in mean DFS scores between 1973 and 1982, was at least in part to be associated with the increased frequency of brushing the teeth with fluoride dentifrice (Ainamo and Parviainen 1989). Similarly, in a study of reported daily tooth-brushing frequency and caries experience in 12- to 15-year-old children from a fluoride-deficient community in New York State it was found that more frequent brushing was associated with less caries activity. Since 90 per cent of the children were found to be using brands of dentifrice that contained fluoride, it was concluded that the inverse relationship between brushing frequency and caries activity may have been related to the more frequent fluoride contact when the children brushed (Leske *et al.* 1976).

Thorough rinsing after using a fluoride dentifrice may be expected to reduce the subsequent salivary fluoride levels; in a trial involving eight subjects, the salivary fluoride concentration which was measured 5 minutes after dentifrice application, decreased significantly with increasing rinse volume, rinse duration, and rinse frequency. The investigators concluded that rinsing habits may play an important role in the oral retention of fluoride from dentifrices which may, in turn, affect their clinical efficacy (Duckworth *et al.* 1991).

Data on tooth-brushing habits were collected during a 3-year caries clinical trial of sodium monofluorophosphate toothpastes in Lanarkshire, Scotland, involving 3005 schoolchildren of mean age 12.5 years at baseline (Chesters *et al.* 1992). Differences in oral habits were observed between the sexes, with 42 per cent of girls and 52 per cent of boys being non-beaker rinsers and 73 per cent of girls but only 44 per cent of boys, brushing their teeth at least twice per day. Twice a day brushers had a consistently lower caries increment than less frequent brushers. This was also seen in the baseline caries experience data, but did not account for all incremental differences noted. The proportion of the children who stated that they brushed once a day or more, increased during the trial. Over the 3-year interval of the trial, 403 children stated that they brushed once a day or less at each of the four annual examinations and 856 consistently stated that they brushed twice per day or more. The mean DMFS values at baseline were 10.57 in the once a day or less brushers and 8.96 in the twice a day or more brushers. The mean three year increments in DMFS were 6.95 in the least frequent brushers and 5.38 in the most frequent brushers. These differences were statistically significant ($p < 0.001$).

Half of the children in the Lanarkshire study used beakers for rinsing after tooth-brushing and had consistently higher increments in caries experience than non-beaker rinsers. Again this difference could not be explained by variation in baseline caries experience. Differences in the caries increment were also observed between boys and girls, these appearing to be linked both to the cumulative effect of variations in brushing and rinsing habits between males and females in addition to a difference in the baseline caries experience. The mean baseline DMFS of the 1066 non-beaker users was 9.25 compared with 10.98 in the 1213 beaker users. The mean 3-year increments in DMFS were 5.77 in the non-beaker users and 6.87 in the beaker users. These differences were statistically significant ($p < 0.001$).

Several aetiological variables were assessed over a 2-year period in 431 adolescents residing in non-fluoridated Clwyd, in Wales, and in 93 adolescents living in economically deprived areas of Cork, Ireland, which is fluoridated (Kavanagh 1994). In the non-fluoridated community brushing frequency with a fluoride toothpaste was observed to be a valuable predictor of final caries experience in males, but not in females. It was also found that the male subjects who used a cup to rinse toothpaste from their mouths after brushing, increased their risk of developing caries. Once again, this correlation was not observed within the female group. Brushing frequency and rinsing method were not useful predictors of caries experience in the fluoridated area, although in the case of brushing frequency this may have been due to unavoidable limitations in the study design. The author concluded that brushing frequency (with a fluoride toothpaste) and rinse methods after brushing were important predictors of caries risk within a non-fluoridated community.

SUMMARY

- Although tooth cleaning with unmedicated agents may be expected to reduce caries experience, the lack of consistent epidemiological corroboration of the relationship has led to a questioning of the value of oral hygiene practices against caries.

- Of the investigations quoted, about half of the prevalence studies showed a positive association between plaque and caries. All of the retrospective studies showed a positive trend with an increase in caries experience associated with poorer standards of oral cleanliness, although the results seldom reached statistical significance. The majority of the studies of brushing frequency (with a non-fluoride dentifrice) showed no relationship with caries.

- The most satisfactory method of investigating oral hygiene practices is by means of controlled prospective studies of improved oral cleanliness and increments in caries experience. Relatively few such studies have been undertaken and the results point towards a weak positive association between plaque and caries. Professional cleaning appears to be more effective than self-cleaning.

- Tooth-brushing with fluoridated dentifrices has been shown to be an effective caries preventive measure. The effectiveness of fluoride toothpastes has been shown to improve with increased brushing frequency and if the minimum amount of water is used to rinse after brushing.

REFERENCES

Addy, M., Dummer, P.M.H., Griffiths, G., Hicks, R., Kingdom, A., and Shaw, W.C. (1986). Prevalence of plaque, gingivitis and caries in 11–12 year old children in South Wales. *Commun. Dent. oral Epidemiol.* **14**, 115–18.

Ainamo, J. (1971). The effect of habitual toothcleansing on the occurrence of periodontal disease and dental caries. *Proc. Finn. dent. Soc.* **67**, 63–70.

Ainamo, J. and Parviainen, K. (1979). Occurrence of plaque, gingivitis and caries related to self reported frequency of toothbrushing in fluoride areas in Finland. *Commun. Dent. oral Epidemiol.* **7**, 142–6.

Ainamo, J. and Parviainen, K. (1989). Influence of increased toothbrushing frequency on dental health in low, optimal, and high fluoride areas in Finland. *Commun. Dent. oral Epidemiol.* **17**, 296–9.

Ashley, F.P. and Sainsbury, R.H. (1981). The effect of a school based plaque control programme on caries and gingivitis. *Br. dent. J.* **150**, 41–5.

Ashley, F.P. and Sainsbury, R.H. (1982). Post study effects of a school based plaque control programme. *Br. dent. J.* **153**, 337–8.

Ashley, F.P. and Wilson, R.F. (1977). Dental plaque and caries, a three year longitudinal study in children. *Br. dent. J.* **142**, 85–91.

Axelsson, P., Lindhe, J., and Waseby, J. (1976). The effect of various plaque control measures on gingivitis and caries in schoolchildren. *Commun. Dent. oral Epidemiol.* **4**, 232–9.

Badersten, A., Egelberg, J., and Koch, G. (1975). Effect of monthly prophylaxis on caries and gingivitis in schoolchildren. *Commun. Dent. oral Epidemiol.* **3**, 1–4.

Bay, I. and Ainamo, J. (1974). Caries experience among children in Copenhagen. *Commun. Dent. oral Epidemiol.* **2**, 75–9.

Beal, J.F., James, P.M.C., Bradrock, G., and Anderson, R.J. (1979). The relationship between dental cleanliness, dental caries incidence and gingival health. *Br. dent. J.* **146**, 111–14.

Bedi, R. and Elton, R.A. (1991). Dental caries experience and oral cleanliness of Asian and white Caucasian children aged 5 and 6 years attending primary schools in Glasgow and Trafford, UK. *Commun. dent. Health*, **8**, 17–23.

Bellini, H.T., Arneberg, P., and von der Fehr, F.R. (1981). Oral hygiene and caries. A review. *Acta odont. Scand.* **39**, 257–65.

Bibby, B.G. (1966). Do we tell the truth about preventing caries? *J. dent. Child.* **33**, 269-79.

Bjertness, E., Eriksen. H.M., Hansen, B.F. (1986). Caries prevalence of 35 year old Oslo citizens in 1973 and 1984. *Commun. Dent. oral Epidemiol.* **14**, 277-82.

Carvalho, J.C., Thylstrup, A., and Ekstrand, K.R. (1992). Results after 3 years of non-operative occlusal caries treatment of erupting permanent first molars. *Commun. Dent. oral Epidemiol.* **20**,187–92.

Chesters, R.K, Huntington, E., Burchell, C.K., and Stephen, K.W. (1992). Effect of oral care habits on caries in adolescents. *Caries Res.* **26**, 299–304.

Dale, J.W. (1969). Toothbrushing frequency and its relationship to dental caries and periodontal disease. *Australian. dent. J.* **14**, 120–3.

Duany, L.F., Zinner, D.D., and Jablon, J.M. (1972). Epidemiologic studies of caries free and caries active students: II. Diet, dental plaque, and oral hygiene. *J. dent. Res.* **51**, 727–33.

Duckworth, R.M., Knoop, D.T.M., and Stephen, K.W.(1991). Effect of mouthrinsing after toothbrushing with a fluoride dentifrice on human salivary fluoride levels. *Caries Res.* **25**, 287–91.

Fisher, F.J. (1968). A field survey of dental caries, periodontal disease and enamel defects in Tristan da Cunha. *Br. dent. J.* **125**, 398–401; 447–53.

Fosdick, L.S. (1950). The reduction of the incidence of dental caries I. Immediate toothbrushing with a neutral dentifrice. *J. Am. dent. Ass.* **40**, 133–43.

Gillham, J. and Lennon, D. (1958). The biology of the children of Hopewood House. Bowral, N.S.W. II. Observations extending over five years (1952–1956 inclusive). 4. Dietary survey. *Australian dent. J.* **3**, 378–82.

Granath, L.E., Martinsson, T., Matsson, L., Nilsson, G., Schröder, U., and Söderholm, B. (1979). Intraindividual effect of daily supervised flossing on caries in schoolchildren. *Commun. Dent. oral Epidemiol.* **7**, 147–50.

Hamp, S.E., Lindhe, J., Fornell, J., Johansson, L.A., and Karlsson, R. (1978). Effect of a field programme based on systematic plaque control on caries and gingivitis in schoolchildren after 3 years. *Commun. Dent. oral Epidemiol.* **6**, 17–23.

Holloway, P.J. and Teagle, F. (1976). The relationship between oral cleanliness and caries increment. *J. dent. Res.* 55 (special issue. D), Abstr. No. 1.

Holloway, P.J., James, P.M.C., and Slack, G.L. (1963). Dental disease in Tristan da Cunha. *Br. dent. J.* **115**, 19–25.

Holt, R.D., Joels, D., and Winter, G.B. (1982). Caries in pre-school children, the Camden study. *Br. dent. J.* **153**, 107–9.

Horowitz, A.M. Suomi, J.D., Peterson, J.K., Mathews, B.L., Voglesong, R.H., and Lyman, B.A. (1980). Effects of supervised daily dental plaque removal by children after 3 years. *Commun. Dent. oral Epidemiol.* **8**, 171–6.

Horowitz, H.S. (1968). In *Art and science on dental caries research.* (ed. R.S. Harris), p. 179. Academic Press, New York.

Jackson, D. and Sutcliffe, P. (1967). Clinical testing of a stannous fluoride-calcium pyrophosphate dentifrice in Yorkshire schoolchildren. *Br. dent. J.* **123**, 40–8.

Kavanagh, D.A. (1994). The relationship between measurements on saliva in children and dental caries. D. Phil. thesis. University College Cork, Ireland.

Kleemola-Kujala, E. (1978). Oral hygiene and its relationship to caries prevalence in Finnish rural children. *Proc. Finn. dent. Soc.* **74**, 76–85.

Kleemola-Kujala, E. and Rasanan, L. (1982). Relationship of oral hygiene and sugar consumption to risk of caries in children. *Commun. Dent. oral Epidemiol.* **10**, 224–33.

Leske, G.S., Ripa, L.W., and Barenie, J.T. (1976). Comparisons of caries prevalence of children with different daily toothbrushing frequencies. *Commun. Dent. oral Epidemiol.* **4**, 102–5.

Lindhe, J., Axelsson, P., and Tollskog, G. (1975). Effect of proper oral hygiene on gingivitis and dental caries in Swedish schoolchildren. *Commun. Dent. oral Epidemiol.* **3**, 150–5.

McCauley, H.B. and Frazier, T.M. (1957). Dental caries and dental care needs in Baltimore school children (1955). *J. dent. Res.* **36**, 546–51.

McHugh, W.D., McEwen, J.D., and Hitchin, A.D. (1964). Dental disease and related factors in 13-year-old children in Dundee. *Br. dent. J.* **117**, 246–53.

Mansbridge, J.N. (1960). The effects of oral hygiene and sweet consumption on the prevalence of dental caries. *Br. dent. J.* **109**, 343–8.

Miller, J. (1961). Relationship of occlusion and oral cleanliness with caries rates. *Archs. oral Biol.* (special suppl.) **6**, 70–9.

Miller. J. and Hobson, P. (1961). The relationship between malocclusion, oral cleanliness, gingival conditions and dental caries in school children. *Br. dent. J.* **111**, 43–52.

Palin-Palokas, T., Hausen, H., and Heinonen, O.P. (1987). Relative importance of caries risk factors in Finnish mentally retarded children. *Commun. Dent. oral Epidemiol.* **15**, 19–23.

Parviainen, K., Nordling, H., and Ainamo, J. (1977). Occurrence of dental caries and gingivitis in low, medium and high fluoride areas in Finland. *Commun. Dent. oral Epidemiol.* **5**, 287–91.

Rajala, M., Selkainaho, K., and Paunio, I. (1980). Relationship between reported toothbrushing and dental caries in adults. *Commun. Dent. oral Epidemiol.* **8**, 128–31.

Richardson, A.S., Boyd, M.A., and Conry, R.F. (1977). A correlation study of diet, oral hygiene and dental caries in 457 Canadian children. *Commun. Dent. oral Epidemiol.* **5**, 227–30.

Ripa, L.W. (1985). The roles of prophylaxes and dental prophylaxis pastes in caries prevention. In *Clinical uses of fluorides,* (ed. S.H.Y. Wei). Lea and Febiger; Philadelphia.

Rugg-Gunn, A.J., Hackett, A.F., Appleton, D.R., Jenkins, G.N., and Eastoe, J.E. (1984). Relationship between dietary habits and caries increment assessed over two years in 405 English adolescent school children. *Archs. oral Biol.* **29**, 983–92.

Schou, L., Currie, C., and McQueen, D. (1990). Using a 'lifestyle' perspective to understand toothbrushing behaviour in Scottish schoolchildren. *Commun. Dent. oral Epidemiol.* **18**, 230–4.

Silverstein, S., Gold. D., Heilbron, D., Nelms, D., and Wycoff, S. (1977). Effect of supervised deplaquing on dental caries, gingivitis and plaque. *J. dent. Res.* 56 (special iss. A) A85. Abstr. 169.

Smith, A.J. and Striffler, D.F. (1963). Reported frequency of toothbrushing as related to the prevalence of dental caries in New Mexico. *Publ. Hlth. Dent.* **23**, 159–75.

Sullivan, H.R. and Harris, R. (1958). The biology of children of Hopewood House, Bowral, N.S.W.2. Observations on oral conditions. *Australian dent. J.* **3**, 311–17.

Sundin, B., Granath, L., and Birkhed, D.(1992). Variation of posterior approximal caries incidence with consumption of sweets with regard to other caries-related factors in 15–18-year-olds. *Commun. Dent. oral Epidemiol.* **20**, 76–80.

Sutcliffe, P. (1973). A longitudinal clinical study of oral cleanliness and dental caries in school children. *Archs. oral Biol.* **18**, 765–70.

Sutcliffe, P. (1977). Caries experience and oral cleanliness of 3 and 4 year old children from deprived and non-deprived areas in Edinburgh, Scotland. *Commun. Dent. oral Epidemiol.* **5**, 213–19.

Todd, J.E. (1975). *Children's dental health in England and Wales,* 1973. HMSO, London.

Todd, J.E. and Walker, A.M. (1980). *Adult dental health.* Vol. 1. *England and Wales 1968–1978.* HMSO, London.

Trubman, A. (1963). Oral hygiene: its association with periodontal disease and dental caries in children. *J. Am. dent. Ass.* **67**, 349–51.

Tucker, G.J., Andlaw, R.J., and Birchell, C.K. (1976). The relationship between oral hygiene and dental caries incidence in 11-year-old children. *Br. dent. J.* **141**, 75–9.

Wright, G.Z., Banting, D.W., and Feasby, W.H. (1979). The Dorchester dental flossing study: final report. *Clin. prevent. Dent.* **1**, 23–6.

5. Fissure sealants

P.H. GORDON and J.H. NUNN

INTRODUCTION

Fissure sealants are materials which are designed to prevent pit and fissure caries. They are applied mainly to the occlusal surfaces of molar teeth in order to obliterate the occlusal fissures, and remove the sheltered environment in which caries may thrive.

Fissure sealing is a very conservative way of tackling the problem of occlusal caries, involving a minimum of treatment which most children have no difficulty in accepting. Fissure sealants are so effective and the reaction of the patients and parents is so favourable, that it is difficult to understand why these materials have not gained widespread acceptance, and why they are not in general use. A look at the history of fissure sealing, and dental practitioners' views on these materials will help to explain how this situation has arisen.

EARLY MATERIALS

There was a surge of interest in fissure sealing in the early 1970s, and a casual observer could be forgiven for assuming that fissure sealing was a new and exciting development. In fact, there had been a longstanding interest in sealing as a method of preventing occlusal caries, ever since the early part of the century, when a number of workers had attempted to prevent the onset of decay by applying silver nitrate (W.D. Miller 1905; Miller 1950), nitrocellulose (Gore 1939), and zinc chloride (Ast et al. 1950). Miller's paper (1905) was not the result of a scientific study, but rather a report that he had used silver nitrate to prevent the onset of occlusal caries and had found it useful. The other studies did not demonstrate any detectable benefit from using the materials that were being tested.

Silver nitrate, and the other materials mentioned above, would not work by physical occlusion of the fissure. They would exert their effect, if they worked at all, by altering the composition of the enamel in the depths of the fissure, to make it more resistant to bacterial action. The work was carried out at a time when the proteolytic theory of the initiation of caries was in fashion, and it was hoped that by precipitating inorganic material on to the tooth surface, it would be possible to block organic pathways into the tooth.

A different approach had been tried by other researchers (Hyatt 1923; Miller 1950). They attempted to fill the occlusal fissure with a sealant material which, by blocking the fissure, would prevent bacteria and their substrate from coming into contact with that part of the tooth. Clearly, if successfully retained on the tooth, this would have a good chance of preventing caries of the underlying enamel. The difficulty was to ensure the retention of the sealing material.

Hyatt recommended that the occlusal fissure of the erupting tooth should be sealed with zinc phosphate cement, as soon as possible, and that when the tooth was sufficiently erupted a minimal Class I cavity should be prepared, and the tooth filled with amalgam before it became carious. There was considerable resistance to his proposals from the dental profession, which objected to cutting cavities in caries-free teeth. One might also expect a certain amount of 'consumer resistance' to the idea of having a tooth filled, before it had a cavity in it. From the patient's point of view it was as well to wait until caries developed, because the operative procedures were the same. Hyatt's argument was that it was almost inevitable that the first permanent molar would develop occlusal caries. One should fill the tooth before progression of this caries made restoration difficult, and there was no time like the present. Hyatt's concept, sometimes called 'prophylactic odontotomy', never gained wide acceptance, probably because the procedure involved drilling the child's teeth.

Miller (1950) tested the preventive action of black copper cement when used as a fissure sealant. The copper cement was compared with silver nitrate, and neither material was found to be effective in preventing caries when contrasted with a group of control teeth, which received no treatment. The copper cement was not retained on the occlusal surfaces.

ACID-ETCH RETAINED MATERIALS

While investigating different methods of improving the edge-seal of acrylic resin filling materials, Buonocore decided to test the effect of etching the tooth surface with an acid solution before applying the filling material (Buonocore 1955). This alteration in technique had a dramatic effect on the adhesion of the resin to the tooth, and acid-etch techniques were soon introduced into the field of fissure sealing. When the cyanoacrylate resins became available a number of research workers reported on the use of these materials as fissure sealants, and most used an acid-etch technique as part of the application procedure (Takeuchi et al. 1966, 1971; Cueto and Buonocore 1967; Ripa and Cole 1970). In these studies, a respectable number of teeth retained the sealant resin on the occlusal surface. They were essentially short-term studies, and as such were not designed to detect a reduction in the incidence of caries. The promising results from these studies encouraged other research workers to take an interest in cyano-acrylate resins as fissure sealing materials (Parkhouse and Winter 1971), but the outcome of the subsequent trial did not inspire confidence in the material.

Rock (1974) reported on the use of two polyurethane materials as fissure sealants; one was retained by an acid-etch, the other was applied directly to the enamel with no etch to prepare the surface. Neither material was retained on the tooth, and it appeared that any effect on caries was minimal, despite the incorporation of a fluoride compound in the resins, in the hope that this would have some local effect as an anti-caries agent.

Following the introduction of the bis-(glycidyl-methacrylate) (GMA) resins, several studies were carried out in quick succession, testing the suitability of the new resins for use as fissure sealants (Buonocore 1970, 1971; Rock 1972, 1973; Ibsen 1973; McCune *et al.* 1973). The results from these studies show very satisfactory retention rates from the materials they were using. These results reawakened interest in fissure sealing, and more trials were undertaken, but once again it soon became apparent that there were considerable differences in the results obtained by different workers. The promising results reported in the early trials were not always repeated in subsequent studies, with very variable retention figures in the follow-up studies (Table 5.1).

RESULTS OF CLINICAL TRIALS

There are several possible explanations for this variation: for example, the different workers may have used slightly different materials, they may have sealed different teeth (premolars as opposed to molars), possibly they were working under different conditions, and they were certainly working on different groups of children. In addition, there may have been variations in the application technique. To what extent are these different factors responsible for the varying results obtained in clinical trials?

The first obvious possibility is that the different studies may have been testing different materials. Modern sealant studies have been conducted on a variety of materials, the cyano-acrylates, the polyurethanes, the GMA resins, and the glass ionomer cements forming the main groups. The GMA resins and the glass ionomer cements have produced the most consistent results, with retention figures generally better than the cyano-acrylates and polyurethanes. Although differences between materials may account for some of the variation in the results of clinical trials, there must be other factors involved.

Variation in application technique may account for some of the differences found between the studies. The majority of studies do not give a detailed account of the application technique, simply stating that the material was applied according to the manufacturer's instructions. There is seldom any mention of the degree of difficulty experienced by the operators in complying with these instructions. In particular, only a very few reports indicate whether or not children were discarded from the trial if the operator found it difficult to maintain a dry working field when applying the resin to the child's teeth. This very important aspect of the protocol under

which the trials were conducted is hardly ever mentioned directly, though there are oblique references to difficulties that have been encountered (Ibsen 1973): '... the clinical studies of fissure sealants are, in reality, a study of the proficiency of the operators ... best results are achieved when the sealants are applied under conditions approaching the ideal of private practice, and (the resins) are less effective when applied under conditions of mass prophylaxis'. Good results, as in other areas of paediatric dentistry, require the co-operation of the child, and although this is relatively easy to obtain when using fissure sealants, there will always be a number of children who find it difficult to co-operate sufficiently to allow the successful placement of a sealant.

APPLICATION TECHNIQUE

It is apparent from the literature that application technique is very important to the success of a fissure sealant, but it is difficult, using clinical data, to decide which aspects of the application technique are most important. Most of the research work carried out on the strength of the bond between resin and tooth, and the effect of changing various aspects of the application technique, has been done in the laboratory, where it is easier to test the effect of changing one factor in isolation.

The application procedure is similar for all the modern materials, which depend on acid-etching for their retention. The manufacturer will usually recommend that the tooth concerned is first polished, then isolated and etched with the material provided (usually phosphoric acid), for a specific time. The acid is then rinsed off the tooth, keeping the tooth isolated from contact with saliva, and the tooth dried, using compressed air. The sealing material is placed on the occlusal surface, which must be kept isolated until the material has polymerized.

The whole area of prophylaxis before placing a sealant has been controversial. Indeed, one recent article maintained that intensive professional tooth-cleaning on its own obviated the need for fissure sealants and backed up the statement with data from a clinical trial (Carvalho *et al.* 1992). There has been a shift away from cleaning surfaces to be sealed after the publication of results indicating that sealant retention was unaffected by the procedure (Donnan and Ball 1988). However, other studies indicate that air polishing, both *in vitro* and *in vivo*, not only aids in the cleaning of the fissure but enhances the penetration of resin into the enamel and should be considered before etching (Brocklehurst *et al.* 1992; Kuba *et al.* 1992). Brockmann *et al.* (1989) comparing different surface preparation prior to sealing noted that although the combination of air-polishing and etching gave the best bond strengths, they were not significantly greater than the rubber cup with pumice and etch combination.

Recent years have seen the advent of etchant in a gel as well as liquid form. Whilst Rock *et al.* (1990) showed that gel etchant was as effective as the liquid form the clinical disadvantage lies in the doubling of the rinsing time required with the gel form.

Variation in the concentration of the etching material appears to have little effect: provided that the concentration of

Table 5.1. Clinical trials of fissure sealants applied to first permanent molars

Length of trial	Per cent of teeth retaining sealant	Age of children (yrs)
6 months		
Burt *et al.* (1975)	36	5–17
Charbeneau *et al.* (1977)	91	5–8
Cueto and Buonocore (1967)	75	5–17
Dorignac (1987)	98	6–8
Eidelman *et al.* (1984)	99	5.5–6.5
Ferguson (1980)	78	3–16
	62	3–16
Harris *et al.* (1976)	81	6–14
Helle (1975)	100	5–7
Higson (1976)	64	6–8
Hinding and Buonocore (1974)	100	10.2
Leake and Martinello (1976)	84	6–8
Li *et al.* (1981)	94	5–16
	88	5–16
Luoma *et al.* (1973)	100	7 mean
Raadal (1978)	95	5–7
Ripa and Cole (1970)	72	5–10
Rock *et al.* (1978)	51	6–7
	80	6–7
Rock and Evans (1982)	81	7–8
	84	7–8
Sheykholeslam and Houpt (1978)	97	6–10
Stephen *et al.* (1978)	97	6–10
Stephen *et al.* (1981*a*)	100	6–7
	99	6–7
Stephen *et al.* (1981*b*)	90	6–11
	98	6–11
Stephen *et al.* (1985)	100	5–8
	94	5–8
Vrbic (1986)	93	6.8 mean
12 months		
Alvesalo *et al.* (1977)	74	6–7
Bojanini *et al.* (1976)	91	6–8
Brooks *et al.* (1976)	95	6–8
Brooks *et al.* (1976)	83	6–8
Charbeneau *et al.* (1977)	79	5–8
Collins *et al.* (1985)	71	> 9
	79	5–8
Cueto and Buonocore (1967)	63	5–17
Dorignac (1987)	96	6–8
Eidelman *et al.* (1984)	99	5.5–6.5
Ferguson (1980)	72	3–16
Foreman and Matis (1991)	91	Various
	60	3–16
Fuks *et al.* (1982)	28	6–10
Going *et al.* (1976)	78	10–14
Harris *et al.* (1976)	72	6–14
Helle (1975)	96	5–7
Higson (1976)	32	6–8
Hinding and Buonocore (1974)	92	10.2 mean
Leake and Martinello (1976)	65	6–8
Leske *et al.* (1976)	77	6–8
Li *et al.* (1981)	91	5–16
	73	5–16

Table 5.1. *continued*

Length of trial	Per cent of teeth retaining sealant	Age of children (yrs)
McCune *et al.* (1973)	72	5–14
McCune *et al.* (1979)	92	6–8
Poulsen *et al.* (1979)	82	Kindergarten
Raadal (1978)	90	5–7
	88	5–7
Richardson *et al.* (1978)	80	7–8
Ripa and Cole (1970)	36	5–10
Risager and Poulsen (1974)	69	6–8
Rock *et al.* (1978)	41	6–7
	75	6–7
Rock and Evans (1982)	76	7–8
	75	7–8
Sheykholeslam and Houpt (1978)	92	6–10
Stephen *et al.* (1976)	2	6
Stephen *et al.* (1978)	93	6–10
Stephen *et al.* (1981*a*)	100	6–7
	99	6–7
Stephen *et al.* (1981*b*)	86	6–11
	93	6–11
Stephen *et al.* (1985)	100	5–8
	95	5–8
18 months		
Charbeneau *et al.* (1977)	74	5–18
Collins *et al.* (1985)	66	5–8
	68	> 9
Dorignac (1987)	96	6–8
Harris *et al.* (1976)	60	6–14
Helle (1975)	91	5–7
Higson (1976)	16	6–8
Leake and Martinello (1976)	54	6–8
Li *et al.* (1981)	88	5–16
	65	5–16
Meurman *et al.* (1975)	98	7 mean
Poulsen *et al.* (1979)	78	Kindergarten
Raadal (1978)	85	5–7
	85	5–7
Stephen *et al.* (1981*b*)	71	6–11
	84	6–11
Stephen *et al.* (1985)	92	5–8
	93	5–8
24 months		
Alvesalo *et al.* (1977)	40	6–7
Ball (1981)	91	Various
Barrie *et al.* (1990)	71	5–6
	53	5–6
	81	5–6
	88	5–6
Brooks *et al.* (1979*a*)	84	< 8
	58	< 8
Brooks *et al.* (1988)	79	5–14
	86	5–14
	92	5–14

Table 5.1. *continued*

Length of trial	Per cent of teeth retaining sealant	Age of children (yrs)
Burt (1977)	20	5–12
Burt *et al.* (1977)	19	5–17
Charbeneau *et al.* (1979)	71	5–8
Collins *et al.* (1985)	48	5–8
	54	> 9
Dorignac (1987)	92	6–8
Feigal *et al.* (1993)	92	6–15
	86	6–15
Gandini *et al.* (1991)	93	6–11
	66	6–11
	84	6–11
Going *et al.* (1976)	58	10–14
Harris *et al.* (1976)	50	6–14
Higson (1976)	3	6–8
Hinding and Buonocore (1974)	89	10.2 mean
Horowitz *et al.* (1974)	48	5–14
Leake and Martinello (1976)	43	6–8
Leske *et al.* (1976)	50	6–8
Li *et al.* (1981)	88	5–16
	69	5–16
McCune *et al.* (1979)	89	6–8
Poulsen *et al.* (1979)	58	Kindergarten
Raadal (1978)	82	5–7
	84	5–7
Raadal *et al.* (1991)	97	6–14
	96	6–14
Richardson *et al.* (1978)	86	7–8
Richardson *et al.* (1977)	51	6–20
Sheykholeslam and Houpt (1978)	85	6–10
Simonsen (1980*a*)	59	3–15
Stephen *et al.* (1981*b*)	70	6–11
	81	6–11
Stephen *et al.* (1985)	91	5–8
	92	5–8
Thylstrup and Poulsen (1978)	60	7
Ulvestad (1976)	98	6–9
Vrbic (1986)	86	6.8 mean
Williams *et al.* (1978)	98	6–8
	50	6–8
	62	6–8
Williams *et al.* (1986)	16	7.5 mean
	77	7.5 mean
	80	7.5 mean
30 months		
Le Bell and Forsten (1980)	93	7–8
	88	7–8
Dorignac (1987)	81	6–8
Harris *et al.* (1976)	48	6–14
Raadal (1978)	84	5–7
	75	5–7
36 months		
Bagramian *et al.* (1979)	11	6–7
	29	14
Brooks *et al.* (1979*b*)	80	< 8
	60	< 8

Table 5.1. *continued*

Length of trial	Per cent of teeth retaining sealant	Age of children (yrs)
Charbeneau and Dennison (1979)	61	5–8
Harris *et al.* (1976)	42	6–14
Houpt and Shey (1983)	83	6–10
Ismail *et al.* (1989)	79	5–7
Leake and Martinello (1976)	29	6–8
Leske *et al.* (1976)	33	6–8
McCune *et al.* (1979)	88	6–8
Meurman and Helminen (1976)	92	7 mean
Richardson *et al.* (1980*a*)	75	7–8
Rock and Evans (1983)	43	7–8
	56	7–8
Simonsen (1980*b*)	71	6–8
	97	6–8
	99	6–8
Vrbic (1986)	67	6.8 mean
48 months		
Charbeneau and Dennison (1979)	52	5–8
Going *et al.* (1977)	34	10–14
Horowitz *et al.* (1976)	13	5–8
	8	10–14
Houpt and Shey (1983)	73	6–10
Leake and Martinello (1976)	20	6–8
Richardson *et al.* (1980*b*)	69	7–8
Vrbic (1986)	61	6.8 mean
Williams and Winter (1981)	64	6–8
	31	6–8
	13	6–8
60 months		
Gibson *et al.* (1982)	67	7–8
Horrowitz *et al.* (1977)	7	5–8
	1	10–14
Houpt and Shey (1983)	67	6–10
Meurman *et al.* (1978)	73	7 mean
Richardson *et al.* (1981)	9	6–20
Shapira *et al.* (1990)	59	6–8
	48	6–8
Simonsen (1987)	82	5–15
Vrbic (1986)	52	6.8 mean
72 months		
Houpt and Shey (1983)	58	6–10
84 months		
Heidmann *et al.* (1990)	40	12
Mertz-Fairhurst *et al.* (1984)	31	< 8
	66	< 8
120 months		
Romcke *et al.* (1990)	85	3–16
Simonsen (1987)	57	5–15
180 months		
Simonsen (1991)	28	5–15

ortho-phosphoric acid (which is the most widely used etching material) lies between 30 and 50 per cent by weight, small variations in the concentration do not appear to affect the quality of the etched surface (Silverstone 1974).Variation in the time during which the tooth enamel is exposed to etching solution is more important, but provided the enamel is exposed to the etching material for 20 seconds, there will be sufficient demineralization to allow adequate retention of the sealant (Eidelman *et al.* 1984). Even in areas where there is an optimal level of fluoride in the water supply, it appears there is little to be gained by increasing the etching time (Beech and Jalaly 1980; McCabe and Storer 1980; Barkmeier *et al.* 1985). Laboratory studies indicate it may be more difficult to gain adequate retention by etching the enamel of primary teeth, but clinical studies (Simonsen 1979) suggest it may not, in fact, be necessary to increase the etching time when sealing primary molars since perfectly adequate retention figures are obtained using the same sort of etching times as are recommended for permanent teeth. McConnachie (1992) disagrees with this view suggests that the etching time for primary molars should be double that for permanent teeth due, they say, to the differences in surface enamel formation. Relatively small variations in the time for which the etched enamel is rinsed have a more marked effect on the strength of the bond between resin and enamel (Williams and von Fraunhofer 1977), and the operator applying sealant resins should take particular care over the rinsing and drying of the tooth surface, before applying the resin. It would appear that the enamel should be rinsed for a full 20 to 25 seconds before being dried.

It has always been maintained that the most critical parts of the application procedure are the rinsing of the etched enamel, drying the tooth surface, and maintaining the isolation of the teeth until the sealant material has polymerized. Rubber dam has been advocated for isolation during sealant application but since it is desirable to place sealants on newly erupted teeth that have not achieved their full clinical crown height, this is often impractical (Williams 1990); neither does it seem to be necessary since equally good retention rates can be achieved using cotton wool rolls and a saliva ejector, alone or in combination (Wood *et al.* 1989) as an alternative means of isolation (Eidelman *et al.* 1983; Straffon *et al.* 1985).

Some investigators have set out to determine whether it is possible to improve the bond between sealant and an enamel surface that has been contaminated by saliva. Recent studies have thrown doubt on the absolute need to maintain a perfectly dry tooth surface for good retention; in a 2-year trial of sealed teeth which were intentionally contaminated with saliva, results showed that sealant retention was possible provided a bonding agent was interspersed between enamel and sealant, but the number of children in this study was small (Feigal *et al.* 1993). Other authors have shown that bonding agents have no influence on retention rates, albeit in a trial that was not looking at the issue of contamination of the etched surface (Boksman *et al.* 1993). The outcome from this limited number of studies is equivocal and it is probably wise to adhere to the existing protocol of ensuring, where possible, a dry field for the application of sealants until more conclusive evidence emerges. The tooth having been adequately prepared the operator has only to choose between types of

materials: a filled or unfilled resin and clear or tinted/opaque. Surprisingly, filled and unfilled resins wear at the same rate but the greater viscosity of the former means that a larger volume will be applied to the tooth surface, which will vary from operator to operator, and so some occlusal adjustment may be required (Jensen *et al.* 1981; Stach *et al.* 1992). Reported differences in retention rates of filled versus unfilled resins may relate more to differences in diagnosis in that it is easier to detect opaque, filled sealants (Rock *et al.* 1990). This study also confirmed that there was no difference in retention rates between materials that had been light cured or chemically cured, but reported, as have other authors (Strang *et al.* 1984), that longer curing times were needed than were generally recommended by the manufacturers Interestingly, Chosack and Eidelman (1988) reported that sealant penetration into etched enamel was less when the time between sealant application and the exposure to the light source was reduced. The longest tag length was achieved when the time lapse between placement of the sealant and the subsequent light polymerization was 20 seconds. This was significantly better than with the shorter intervals but still not as good as the tag length achieved by the use of auto-polymerizing resins. It may not be practical, however, to delay polymerization of light cured resins because of the likely contamination of the unset resin by saliva. The authors conclude that clinical trials are required to investigate the minimum tag length required, as a function of time between application and curing, for optimal retention.

As a final comment on the difficulties of assessing the effectiveness of application technique, it is ironic to note that in a trial in which the operators graded the ease with which the resin was applied, there was no relationship between the retention of the resin and the operator's assessment of the level of the child's co-operation (Rock and Evans 1982).

FURTHER CLINICAL TRIALS

After the early studies that have already been mentioned, there has been a flood of reports of clinical trials of fissure sealants. For reasons that are discussed later, attention should be focused on the first permanent molars; Table 5.1 shows the results of some of the clinical trials that have considered the extent to which fissure sealants are retained on these teeth. The first permanent molar, shortly after eruption, is a severe testing ground for any fissure sealant. The children are young, the teeth are only partly erupted, right at the back of the mouth, and if the resin will stay on this tooth, it has done all that can reasonably be expected.

The mass of results in Table 5.1 shows that the sealant resins do indeed stay on the great majority of these teeth, and for a considerable length of time. Resin material is progressively lost from the tooth surface as time goes by. The loss of resin is most marked in the first six months, but there is a further progressive loss of about 10 per cent per annum (Horowitz *et al.* 1977). More recent trials generally report better retention rates than earlier studies, perhaps reflecting an increasing familiarity on the part of the operators with the use of acid-etch retained materials.

USE OF FISSURE SEALANTS

It is entirely proper that any new material should be examined critically before being accepted into general use, and this principle applies especially in cases where a whole new technique being introduced, rather than a new material. Arguments have been put forward that fissure sealants will be ineffective in general use, due to failure of retention, or that the operator will inadvertently damage the tooth by sealing in caries, or that the teeth may be more liable to caries following loss of the sealant resin, since the enamel surface has been damaged by etching. These arguments cannot simply be ignored, and we should now consider to what extent these reservations are justified.

As to whether or not fissure sealants will be effective in general use, it is worth noting that the most frequently used design of clinical trial does not test the material in the way in which it would, in fact, be used. The usual procedure adopted in sealant studies has been to apply the material to the occlusal surfaces of a number of teeth, and then observe the children over a period of time in order to determine how many teeth retain the resin, and for how long. If a sealant was being used as part of a programme to prevent dental caries, and it was noticed at a recall appointment that the sealant had been lost from any particular surface, then the resin would be re-applied and the tooth would not be left without its protective covering. When this approach has been adopted, the results have been very encouraging (Bagramian *et al.* 1978; Rantala 1979; Isler *et al.* 1980).

Concern has been expressed about the likelihood of sealing a tooth that already had a carious lesion. This is an obvious possibility and is still a real concern for dental practitioners (Hicks *et al.* 1989); the accurate diagnosis of early occlusal caries is very difficult, and there are bound to be occasions where the operator has difficulty in deciding whether or not a tooth has already been attacked. A number of studies have highlighted the discrepancies between the clinical appearance of the occlusal surface and its radiographic appearance and it is likely, no matter what method of diagnosis is employed, that on occasions sealant will be applied to teeth with early occlusal caries (Kidd *et al.* 1992; Weerheijm *et al.* 1992a). Another study by one of these authors highlights the fact that in a longitudinal study of teenagers and young adults there was evidence of occlusal caries below fissure sealants on bitewing radiographs (Weerheijm *et al.* 1992b). This the authors attribute to the difficulty of diagnosing occlusal caries at a time when these sealants were placed (in the 20-year-olds). Fortunately, clinical research indicates that if a tooth with early occlusal caries, or even more advanced dentinal caries, is treated with a fissure sealant, then one might reasonably hope for a favourable outcome (Handelman 1991; Swift 1988). These studies show that there is a decrease in the number of viable organisms in the affected dentine, and that the metabolic activity of the remaining bacteria is reduced. It appears that, providing the sealant layer remains intact, the cavity will not progress to any significant extent. Although, other authors are more cautious and maintain that continuing microbial activity and softened, carious dentine in these situations indicate that such hidden lesions are not totally inactive (Weerheijm *et al.* 1993). The evidence in

favour of sealing over clinically intact enamel, where there is no doubt over the integrity of the occlusal surface, is now so persuasive that the conscientious practitioner should be encouraged to adopt the maxim 'when in doubt, seal', rather than the alternative 'when in doubt, fill'.

Some of the clinical trials quoted in Table 5.1 and in the References give figures for caries reductions obtained by the use of sealants. These data should be interpreted with caution, particularly in the case of the shorter 1- or 2-year trials, since the diagnosis of early occlusal caries is very liable to error. Some sealant studies, however, have run for several years, and these studies indicate that teeth which lose the sealant resin are not more likely to become carious than the control teeth which were never sealed. It appears that the acid-etch applied to the enamel in the process of sealing the tooth does not make the tooth more susceptible to decay.

In an era of declining caries prevalence one might question the need for fissure sealants. However, two recent papers have highlighted the continuing susceptibility of occlusal surfaces to caries attack. At the end of a clinical trial in the Isle of Wight, Kidd *et al.* (1992) noted that approximately 50 per cent of subjects had at least one molar tooth affected by caries. In the Netherlands a similar comparison of the clinical and radiographic state of permanent molars indicated that 15 per cent of occlusal surfaces diagnosed as sound did in fact have caries into dentine evident on radiographs. The authors went on to conclude that fissure sealing, soon after eruption, of teeth that appear sound both radiographically and clinically, is justified (Weerheijm *et al.* 1992a, b). Indeed, in a study by Vehkalahti *et al.* (1991) first permanent molars sealed at 7 years of age developed less caries than teeth that had been unsealed or filled at the baseline examination. Stephen *et al.* (1990) writing about a 6-year trial of preventive dentistry concluded that the differences between different preventive regimes could be ascribed solely to the effectiveness of sealant presence.

In the USA, the National Institute of Dental Research published the results of their nation-wide survey in 1986–7. The results of that survey (Brunelle 1989) showed that only 8 per cent of children had at least one tooth fissure sealed. This should be viewed in the light of the fact that 95 per cent of all caries in American children is pit and fissure caries. The routine use of sealants could virtually eliminate caries. In the UK, the picture is similar, with generally poor uptake of this preventive measure. Even in the trial of a capitation scheme, which was supposed to foster a preventive approach, very few fissure sealants were placed (Lennon *et al.* 1990). In Denmark, there is a marked contrast in the use of sealants between the publically funded services as opposed to the private practitioners (Ekstrand *et al.* 1991). A similar difference in targeting between private and public dental practitioners was highlighted by Riordan *et al.* (1993) in their review from Australia. Interestingly, in the Danish study, there was no difference in socio-economic status or caries prevalence to account for the difference between the two services in their provision of sealants, whereas there was a difference in caries susceptibility between groups in the Australian study.

Questionniare surveys on the use of fissure sealants have often concluded that education programmes are what is needed to increase the use of sealants (Nakata *et al.* 1989; Bowen and Fitzgerald 1990; Cohen and Sheiham 1990). Although some of these authors were able to demonstrate large increases in the application rates of fissure sealants, others are less positive about the effects of education programmes, maintaining that education programmes have an impact on dentists' knowledge but little effect on their attitudes (Lang *et al.* 1991).

Many reasons have been put forward for the low utilization of dental sealants by dental practitioners. They tend to centre around the belief that sealants do not work or that they fall off, or that decay may develop beneath a sealant. Simonsen (1989) maintains that, certainly in the USA where sealants are not covered in all third-party insurance plans, the real reason is economic. This may well be the case in the UK since the change in the system of paying dentists in the general dental services. Even in areas where sealants are used, albeit minimally, they are often placed on teeth at times well removed from their eruption dates and thus their period of higher risk (Corbin *et al.* 1990). Because of such uncertainties, the British Society of Paediatric Dentistry produced a policy document on the use of fissure sealants which was updated in 1993 and which addressed the doubts and uncertainties raised by many practitioners (British Society of Paediatric Dentistry 1993).

Overall, the pattern of usage of fissure sealants as reported in the literature is governed by many factors but there are a number of characteristics that emerge as positive indicators of increased sealant use: Gonzales *et al.* (1991), in their survey of dentists, reported that sealants were more likely to be used if dental hygienists were employed, if there were more sources of information, where there were higher knowledge scores, and also by dentists who had more favourable opinions about sealants.

COST-EFFECTIVENESS OF SEALANTS

There are a number of factors to take into account when considering the cost-effectiveness of a procedure. As this relates to fissure sealants an important consideration nowadays is the community's caries incidence; the lower the incidence of dental caries, the less cost-effective fissure sealing becomes (Weintraub *et al.* 1993). Another consideration, and a more fundamental one, is the very nature of the comparisons. There is a major philosophical issue at stake when making comparisons, for cost-effectiveness purposes, between a procedure which prevents caries (fissure sealing) and a measure to treat caries (amalgam restorations). However, comparisons with other preventive measures, which are less labour-intensive, put fissure sealants in a less favourable light. The alternative is to view sealants as a treatment for incipient lesions and a measure aimed at protecting tooth tissue. Then comparisons with restorations become valid (Burt 1989; Lewis and Morgan 1994).

It is difficult to be dogmatic about whether or not fissure sealants are 'cost-effective' (Houpt and Shey 1980). This is a difficult question to answer in a straightforward way since the answer depends on the value, in money terms, that is placed on intangible benefits such as the prevention of pain and suffering, the adoption of a reversible, non-traumatic procedure for the treatment of 'sticky fissures', and a change in attitude on the part of the public at large (Mitchell and Murray 1987).

Sealing every tooth that has an occlusal surface, would mean that fissure sealing would become more expensive than the alternative approach, which is the restoration of carious teeth with amalgam (Horowitz 1980; Eklund 1986). The process of applying the resin is not particularly time consuming, and the resin itself is not expensive; the difficulty lies in the fact that if every premolar and molar tooth is sealed, then a lot of teeth are sealed unnecessarily, because they are not going to decay in the first place. Far fewer teeth are treated if treatment is confined to the teeth which do develop caries, but who can say in advance which teeth are going to decay, and which are not? It is the treatment of all these extra teeth that increases the cost. Over a 6- to 7-year review period, Heidmann *et al.* (1990) showed that for girls, five occlusal surfaces in first permanent molars had to be sealed in order to save one filling, compared with eight surfaces for boys. To avoid this potential cost, treatment should be confined to the particular teeth which are most likely to decay at any given time. It is known which teeth are liable to decay, and at what age, because this information is available from epidemiological studies, and it is evident that the first permanent molar, shortly after eruption, emerges as the prime target for fissure sealants (Walter 1982). Simonsen (1982) carried out a clinical trial of over 5 years of a white sealant. The benefit–cost ratio for caries-inactive subjects amounted to only 0.3, while for the caries active group it was 1.0. It was concluded that for the caries-prone, sealing was beneficial and alternative preventive measures would have enhanced this difference.

If fissure sealants are used on the first permanent molars, shortly after the eruption of these teeth, the procedure soon becomes 'cost-effective', even though it is known that in a proportion of cases the resin will have to be re-applied. There is no doubt that it can be very difficult to keep the teeth isolated when using the resin on young children, and the retention of the resin does depend very much on this particular aspect of the technique, but as with most other skills, one can expect some improvement with practice. In one study (Rantala 1979), fissure sealants were applied to the first permanent molars, as part of an overall programme of caries prevention. After about 2 years, sealing all the first molars had become cheaper, simply in terms of money, than filling those teeth that would have become carious. There were, of course, all the additional benefits arising from the use of a procedure that was very acceptable to the children involved.

Naturally, the amount of money saved as a result of the sealing depends on the number of teeth that would otherwise have become carious. According to a number of recent studies, as much as 90 per cent of carious lesions occur in the pits and fissures of molars and premolars (Rock *et al.* 1981*a*; Dummer *et al.* 1988; Mertz-Fairhurst *et al.* 1992). Indeed, because of the extension of the period of susceptibility, due to a slowing in the rate of the caries process, the caveat that teeth should be sealed within two years of eruption needs to be withdrawn (Ripa 1990). There is no doubt that the first permanent molar is still liable to suffer occlusal caries in the first few years after its eruption. The diagram reproduced here as Fig. 5.1 was published in a study reported in 1981 (Rock

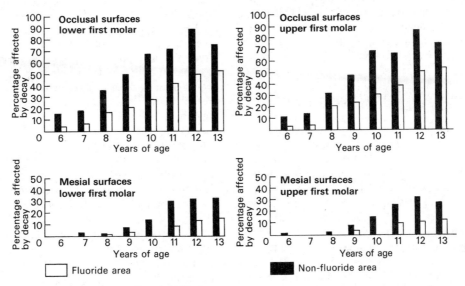

Fig. 5.1. Caries in first permanent molars. (After Rock *et al.* 1981*a*.)

et al. 1981*a*), and it gives indication of the rate at which first molars are affected by caries, in fluoride and non-fluoride areas. In the non-fluoride area approximately half the first molars were decayed by the age of 9, while in the fluoride area the children had reached the age of 12 before half the teeth were affected. Virtually all the affected teeth suffered from occlusal caries.

With regard to the onset of approximal caries, at the age of 13, 30 per cent of first permanent molars in the non-fluoride area had mesial cavities or restorations, while only 10 per cent of mesial surfaces of the first molars in the fluoride area were similarly affected. The effectiveness of fissure sealing is reduced unless some measures are taken to reduce the incidence of approximal caries. Both fissure sealing and some form of fluoride supplement should be employed in any programme designed to prevent caries. The use of either measure in isolation will provide only partial benefit.

Improvements in the cost-effectiveness of fissure sealants can be obtained if the technique is employed in the care of particular target groups, for example: children with medical conditions which make the prevention of dental caries particularly important, or children whose previous dental history indicates they are susceptible to caries. Ancillary staff may be trained to apply fissure sealants, and can achieve retention rates similar to those obtained by dentists (Calderone and Mueller 1983; Leske *et al.* 1976; Stephen *et al.* 1978). Clearly the choice of staff employed to apply the resin will have an impact on the cost-effectiveness of the procedure.

COMPARISONS WITH AMALGAM

When considering the cost-effectiveness of fissure sealing, the durability of sealants should not be considered in isolation; whatever the methodological arguments used against comparisons with restorative procedures, currently this is the argument which the clinician perceives as relevant. As with

sealants, the durability of amalgam restorations has been shown to improve as the age of the patient increases (Walls *et al.* 1985). Fissure sealants are best used in newly erupted first permanent molars, and therefore a comparison should be made with amalgam restorations in young children, at the age at which first permanent molars develop occlusal caries.

There have been relatively few studies which have considered the life-expectancy of amalgam restorations in this age group. Walls *et al.* (1985) found a median survival time of 26 months for amalgam restorations in children aged 5 to 7 years when the restoration was provided. This means that half the restorations had failed after 26 months. The median survival time for amalgam restorations placed in 7- to 9-year-old children was 33 months. If a local anaesthetic had not been used, these survival times were reduced by 23 per cent. Similar figures are quoted by Hunter (1985) who found a median survival time of 26 months for amalgam restorations placed in a group of children aged 8 years or younger. The only published study to directly compare amalgam restorations against fissure sealants in the same mouth was carried out over 7 years (Straffon and Dennison 1988). These authors not only found that fissure sealed teeth had a lower caries experience compared with teeth restored with amalgam, but that they also required half the time investment, including topping up, over the 7-year follow-up period.

Mitchell and Murray (1987) used a type of analysis similar to that employed by Walls *et al.* (1985) and examined data from a similar group of children. They found a median survival time of 27 months for fissure sealants used on first permanent molars in a group of 5- to 8-year-old children.

These figures suggest that there is no great difference between the survival of fissure sealants and amalgams in this age group, provided that a local anaesthetic is employed when a cavity is prepared for amalgam. The type of analysis used (median survival times from life-table analysis) is likely, however, to be operating to the disadvantage of the sealant group. The children in the amalgam studies were followed-up for 12 years (Walls *et al.* 1985) and 20 years (Hunter 1985). The sealant group was followed-up for 5.5 years. This means that no sealant had the opportunity to last longer than 5.5 years, while some of the amalgam restorations were given the opportunity to last for 12 or 20 years.

PREVENTIVE RESIN RESTORATION

There is no doubt that the only remaining controversy which exists in relation to fissure sealants is the caries status of the tooth (Ripa and Wolff 1992) and thus the subsequent management of the occlusal surface. The evidence that sealing over incipient lesions does not lead to gross coronal destruction has encouraged some to advocate sealing over early caries lesions (Elderton 1985). One 6-year clinical trial has reported on cariostasis achieved by the application of sealed amalgam restorations over radiographically detectable caries into dentine (Mertz-Fairhurst *et al.* 1992). Other authors are more circumspect about endorsing the sealing over of hidden or 'occult' caries noting that such teeth still have viable cariogenic microorganisms and softened dentine on later inspection (Weerheijm *et al.* 1992*a*).

An alternative approach that has been employed to deal with the problem of early fissure caries is to use a procedure which employs a minimal composite restoration (Ripa and Wolff 1992). The technique involves making a very small, local cavity preparation in the immediate area of the fissure system at which the presence of caries is suspected. No attempt is made to extend the cavity beyond the immediate area affected by caries. Exposed dentine is protected with a calcium hydroxide lining material and the occlusal surface of the tooth etched in the conventional way. The defect in the occlusal surface is restored, usually with a bonded composite resin filling material. Following this, the entire occlusal surface of the tooth is sealed, the sealant being applied over the top of any composite resin filling material as well as the etched fissure system. The advantage of this approach is that the absolute minimum of tooth substance is removed. Welbury *et al.* (1990) reported that the occlusal amalgam restorations in their study occupied, on average, 25 per cent of the occlusal surface of the tooth, compared with 5 per cent for the minimal composite restoration. In addition, the procedure avoids the unfortunate consequences of an error in diagnosis. If a healthy tooth is investigated, little harm is done, since it quickly becomes evident that there is no caries present and the resulting defect, if contained within enamel, is readily filled with a fissure sealant. If the caries is more extensive than was originally supposed, this will become apparent during the procedure and a conventional amalgam restoration can be placed.

The results of clinical trials which have included this type of restoration would suggest that the durability of preventive resin restorations is similar to the durability of fissure sealants, whether the operator be a dentist, ancilliary, or student (Granath *et al.* 1992; Roth and Conry 1992). The longest reported trial of preventive resin restorations is 9 years (Houpt *et al.* 1994). After 9 years, 43 restorations had survived totally intact; 24 per cent of the teeth which had lost some sealant had experienced caries attack and in addition, 16 teeth had proximal caries unrelated to the occlusal

restoration. None of the restorations were topped up during the 9-year review period.

The composite restorations are small and are positioned at the bottom of a pit or fissure. These factors, taken together, minimize any potential problems arising from wear of the composite filling material. New or recurrent caries has not been shown to be a significant problem with this type of restoration but where it occurs is correlated with loss of the sealant from the composite surface (Houpt *et al.* 1994; Roth and Conry 1992), which in some series has been topped up at intervals to maintain the integrity of the restoration (Straffon and Dennison 1988).

Preventive resin restorations were first included in the National Health Service fee scale for the UK general dental services in 1987. A postal/telephone survey of dental practitioners working in one of the Scottish Health Boards a year later showed that a high proportion (81 per cent) of them were using this type of restoration, but that an even higher proportion would welcome more facts about their use (Paterson *et al.* 1990). In response to this request a distance learning package was designed and distributed. A follow-up survey a year later indicated that more dentists were using preventive resin restorations and that a number had modified their clinical practice as a result of reading the programme (Paterson *et al.* 1991).

A variant of the preventive resin restoration, namely a glass ionomer sealant restoration, also appeared as an item on the fee scale at the same time, and was endorsed by a joint working party of the British Dental Association and the Department of Health (British Dental Association 1986), despite the fact that there were no published clinical trials to substantiate its use. Advocates of the technique published details of the procedure but gave no clinical results (Henry and Jessel 1989). The only clinical trial comparing the longevity of glass ionomer sealant restorations with preventive resin restorations has recently been reported; this study was carried out over 27 months and involved 66 pairs of restorations. Over the period of the trial four restorations failed, 3 (4.5 per cent) of the glass ionomer sealant restorations and 1 (1.5 per cent) of the resin restorations. Glass ionomer sealant restorations required topping up with sealant more frequently than did the preventive resin restorations but none of the restorations had recurrent caries (Kilpatrick 1993). Reports of newer materials combining the advantages of both the glass ionomer cements and the composite resins are now beginning to appear, but as yet these materials are in their infancy (Croll 1992*a*, *b*).

In summary, it is the view of the British Society of Paediatric Dentistry (1993) that if early dentine caries is suspected in a tooth surface, either from clinical examination alone or in combination with evidence from radiographs, then the surface should be investgated. If minimal caries is discovered a composite restoration should be placed and the surface should be sealed.

NEW DEVELOPMENTS

Fissure sealants are marketed in a variety of formats; they can be filled, unfilled, tinted, clear or opaque and they may be polymerized in a variety of ways. The first generation fissure sealants were ultraviolet light cured, the second generation chemically cured (auto-polymerized), and the third generation were visible light cured. The fourth generation fissure sealants are those containing fluoride.

Fluoride is incorporated into resins in one of two ways; the first utilizes a soluble fluoride salt which after application dissolves releasing fluoride ions, possibly compromising the integrity of the resin. The other system uses an organic fluoride compound chemically bound to the resin. The fluoride is subsequently released by an exchange with other ions in the system (Ripa 1993). Fluoride containing fissure sealants have been tested some time ago (Rock 1974), but were not found to reduce caries incidence perhaps because they were poorly retained on the tooth surface. More recent studies, both *in vivo* and *in vitro*, show promising results (Cooley *et al.* 1990; Jensen *et al.* 1990a, b). Fluoride release from the sealant is rapid and it is unlikely therefore that the potential benefits to be gained from such a material can be long-lasting. In particular, as sealants are known not to penetrate the depths of the fissure, it is difficult to see how fluoride releasing sealants can exert their optimal effect (Atwan and Sullivan 1987). The other drawbacks with these studies as yet are that the trials have only reported results after one year, and little is known about the effect on the integrity of the sealant after the fluoride is released (Forsten 1990; Zimmerman *et al.* 1984). By comparison with other fluoride-releasing materials this type of sealant shows enhanced caries inhibition on smooth surfaces.

Other materials incorporating fluoride which have been advocated for use as fissure sealants are the glass ionomer cements. The early results of trials using glass ionomer cements as fissure sealants were disappointing, with early loss of the material reported almost universally (Shimokobe *et al.* 1986; Williams and Winter 1976). Later studies have given more encouraging results with either conventional glass ionomer or silver cermet cements. Retention rates vary: 93 per cent full retention at 6 months (McKenna and Grundy 1987), 85 per cent complete retention at 12 months (Widmer and Jayasekara 1989), and 83 per cent complete retention of silver cermet cement at 24 months (Mills and Ball 1993). These results compare at least as favourably if not better than conventional resin retention rates. All studies reported that no caries was observed with the glass ionomer based materials at recall. Authors do make the point, however, that although the bulk of the material is lost some remains within the fissure system and that, combined with fluoride release from the glass ionomer, may account for the low incidence of caries observed when these materials are used (Mejare and Mjor 1990; Ovrebo and Raadal 1990).

McLean (1988) maintains that with meticulous attention to technique, glass ionomer cements can be well retained, provided fissure widening techniques are employed, the enamel surface is pre-conditioned with polyacrylic acid, and the finished sealant is protected with a coating of light cured bonding resin. Certainly, the results quoted by McLean and Wilson (1984) lend credibility to this approach with loss of glass ionomer sealant reported in only 10 per cent of cases in the first year and 4 per cent in the second year. Adequate preparation of the fissure system is emphasized by another advocate of glass ionomer sealants, this time for newly erupted molars vulnerable to caries attack. Kubo *et al.* (1992) attributes the success of their technique (retention rates of 96 per cent after 12 months) to elaborate prophylaxis of the surface to be treated. This included a combination of mechanical and chemical means, the former either ultrasonic or low frequency and the latter using chemical solvents known to soften carious dentine. Croll (1992b) reports favourably on 4-year results using light cured glass ionomer cements, but only reports on their use as a restorative material in small pit and fissure restorations.

CONCLUSIONS

There is little doubt that the need for fissure sealants still exists despite the recent decline in dental caries prevalence, with upward of 90 per cent of carious lesions occurring in pits and fissures (Mertz-Fairhurst *et al.* 1992), together with the evidence that caries in pits and fissures of teeth increases with age (Ripa 1990; Walter 1982). A more preventively orientated approach to these lesions is indicated, particularly in the light of the traditional restorative approach to occlusal caries with inconsistent treatment decisions, poor durability of restorations, and unfortunate consequences of the replacement of those restorations (Eccles 1989). Since the demise of the early ultraviolet light polymerized sealants the more recent auto-polymerized sealants have come into their own and have reported 15-year results. Clinical results over 5 years of the visible-light cured materials are encouraging, but their greater sensitivity to operator technique means that longer-term studies are indicated. Fluoride-releasing cements are in their infancy, but are showing promise (Ripa 1993). The utilization of glass ionomers as fissure sealant materials is beginning to produce good results in terms of retention of material and there have been encouraging results on caries inhibition. New materials combining glass ionomers and resins may have a role in the treatment of the early carious lesion in the future, combining the desirable qualities of both materials. New techniques of tooth-cleaning and tooth preparation may yield even better results for many of the materials currently in use (Brocklehurst *et al.* 1992; De Craene *et al.* 1989, 1992; Kuba *et al.* 1992; McLean 1988).

Other factors to be considered because of their impact on outcome are: the effectiveness of sealants decreases with time and therefore the sealants should be topped up; there appears to be a positive interaction between fluoride in the drinking water and fissure sealants in preventing dental caries (Weintraub 1989). In addition, more studies are needed to determine if effectiveness is influenced by the operator (Llodra *et al.* 1993).

In the USA, less than 8 per cent of children have one or more molar teeth sealed and from a questionnaire survey to general dental practitioners in the UK, use of sealants was reported for just under 14 per cent of child patients (Brunelle 1989; Cohen and Sheiham 1990). What is essential for a more effective uptake in the use of fissure sealants is better targeting of both susceptible children and susceptible teeth (Kuthy *et al.* 1990). The British Society of Paediatric Dentistry in its policy document underlined the need for fissure sealants beyond the age which has been accepted as the normal 'window of vulnerability' of caries attack on the occlusal surfaces of permanent molar teeth (Dummer et al. 1990; Walter 1982). The document produces guidelines for patient selection: children with special needs and children with extensive caries in the primary dentition, and tooth selection: pits and fissures of permanent molar teeth when there is evidence of caries involving one or more molar teeth. The policy document stresses the need for constant monitoring, including radiographic review at appropriate intervals (British Society of Paediatric Dentistry 1993; Riordan et al. 1993; Williams 1990). The need for education programmes to the dental profession and the public cannot be underestimated in furthering the use of this preventive measure (Cohen 1990; Nakata et al. 1989).

SUMMARY

- 90% of carious lesions occur in pits and fissures.

- Caries in pits and fissures increases with age.

- A preventively oriented approach to these lesions is indicated.

- Fifteen-year results are now available for fissure sealants in clinical use.

- Light-curing and auto-polymerizing sealants are equally effective.

- Fissure sealants should be employed on clinical grounds based on a thorough clinical examination, supported by radiographs where necessary.

- Fissure sealants are indicated for patients with special needs, a history of extensive caries in the primary dentition or caries involving one or more molars.

- Sealed teeth should be reviewed at regular intervals and sealant resin applied as necessary.

REFERENCES

Alvesalo, L., Brummer, R., and Le Bell, Y. (1977). On the use of fissure sealants in caries prevention. A clinical study. *Acta odont. Scand.* **35**, 155–9.

Ast, D.B., Bushel, A., and Chase, H.C. (1950). A clinical study of caries prophylaxis with zinc chloride and potassium ferrocyanide. *J. Am. dent. Ass.* **41**, 427–42.

Atwan, S.M.A. and Sullivan, R.E. (1987). In vitro investigation of the tensile bond strengths of chemically initiated and a visible light initiated sealants with SEM observations. *Ped. Dent.* **9**, 147–51.

Bagramian, R.A., Graves, R.C., and Srivastava, S. (1978). A combined approach to preventing dental caries in schoolchildren: caries reductions after 3 years. *Commun. Dent. oral Epidemiol.* **6**, 166–71.

Bagramian, R.A., Srivastava, S., and Graves, R.C. (1979). Pattern of sealant retention in children receiving a combination of caries-preventive measures: Three-year results. *J. Am. dent. Ass.* **98**, 46–50.

Ball, I.A. (1981). Pit and fissure sealing with Concise Enamel Bond. *Br. dent. J.* **151**, 220–2.

Barkmeir, W.M., Gwinnett, A.J., and Shaffer, S.E. (1985). Effect of enamel etching time on bond strength and morphology. *J. clin. Orthod.* **19**, 36–8.

Barrie, A.M., Stephen, K.W., and Kay, E.J. (1990). Fissure sealant retention: a comparison of three sealant types under field conditions. *Commun. dent. Health*, **7**, 273–7.

Beech, J.L. and Jalaly, T. (1980). Bonding of polymers to enamel: influence of deposits formed buring etching, etching time and period of water immersion. *J. dent. Res.* **59**, 1156–62.

Bojajini, J., Garces, H., McCune, R.J., and Pineda, A. (1976). Effectiveness of pit and fissure sealants in the prevention of caries. *J. prev. Dent.* **3**, 31–4.

Boksman, L., McConnell, R.J., Carson, B., and McCutcheon-Jones, E.F. (1993). A 2-year clinical evaluation of two pit and fissure sealants placed with and without the use of a bonding agent. *Quintess. Int.* **24**, 131–3.

Bowen, P.A. and Fitzgerald, C.M. (1990). Utah dentists' sealant usage survey. *J. dent. Child.* **57**, 134–8.

British Dental Association (1986). Fissure Sealants. Report of the joint BDA/DHSS Working Party. *Br. dent. J.* **161**, 343.

British Society of Paediatric Dentistry (1993). A policy document on fissure sealants. *Int. J. paed. Dent.* **3**, 99–100.

Brockmann, S.L., Scott, R.L., and Eick, J.D. (1989). The effect of an air-polishing device on tensile bond strength of a dental sealant. *Quintess. Int.* **20**, 211–7.

Brocklehurst, P.R., Joshi, R.I., and Northeast (1992). The effect of air-polishing occlusal surfaces on the penetration of fissures by a sealant. *Int. J. paed. Dent.* **2**, 157–62.

Brooks, J.D., et al. (1976). A comparative study of the retention of two pit and fissure sealants: one-year results. *J. prev. Dent.* **3**, 43–6.

Brooks, J.D., Pruhs, J.J., Azhadari, S., and Ashrafi, M.H. (1988). A pilot study of three tinted unfilled pit and fissure sealants: 23-month results in Milwaukee, Wisconsin. *Clin. prev. Dent.* **10** 18–22.

Brooks, J.D., et al. (1979a). A comparative study of two pit and fissure sealants: two-year results in Augusta, GA. *J. Am. dent. Ass.* **98**, 722–5.

Brooks, J.D., et al. (1979b). A comparative study of two pit and fissure sealants: three-year results in Augusta, GA. *J. Am. dent. Ass.* **99**, 42–6.

Brunelle, J. (1989). Prevalence of dental sealants in U.S. schoolchildren (abstract). *J. dent. Res.* **68** (Special issue), 183.

Buonocore, M.G. (1955). A simple method of increasing the adhesion of acrylic filling materials to enamel surfaces. *J. dent. Res.* **34**, 849–53.

Buonocore, M.G. (1970). Adhesive sealing of pits and fissures for caries prevention, with use of ultra-violet light. *J. Am. dent. Ass.* **80**, 324–8.

Buonocore, M.G. (1971). Caries prevention in pits and fissures sealed with an adhesive resin polymerised by ultra-violet light: a two-year study of a single adhesive application. *J. Am. dent. Ass.* **82**, 1090–3.

Burt, B.A. (1977). Tentative analysis of the efficiency of fissure sealants in a public program in London. *Commun. Dent. oral Epidemiol.* **5**, 73–7.

Burt, B.A. (1989). Cost-effectiveness of sealants (letter; comment). *Commun. Dent. oral Epidemiol.* **17**, 220.

Burt, B.A., Berman, D.S., Gelbier, S., and Silverstone, L.M. (1975). Retention of a fissure sealant six months after application. *Br. dent. J.* **138**, 98–100.

Burt, B.A., Berman, D.S., and Silverstone, L.M. (1977). Caries retention and effects on occlusal caries after 2 years in a public program. *Commun. Dent. oral Epidemiol.* **5**, 15–21.

Calderone, J.J. and Mueller, L.A. (1983). The cost of sealant application in a state dental disease prevention programme. *J. publ. hlth Dent.* **43**, 249–54.

Carvalho, J.C., Thylstrup, A., and Ekstrand, K.R. (1992). Results after 3 years of non-operative occlusal caries treatment of erupting permanent first molars. *Commun. Dent. oral Epidemiol.* **20**, 187–92.

Charbeneau, G.T. and Dennison, J.B. (1979). Clinical success and potential failure after a single application of a pit and fissure sealant: a four-year report. *J. Am. dent. Ass.* **98**, 559–64.

Charbeneau, G.T., Dennison, J.B., and Ryge, G. (1977). A filled pit and fissure sealant: 18 month results. *J. Am. dent. Ass.* **95**, 299–306.

Chosack, A. and Eidelman, E. (1988). Effect of the time from application until exposure to light on the tag lengths of a visible light-polymerised sealant. *Dent. Mater.* **4**, 302–6.

Cohen, L. and Sheiham, A. (1990). Influence of dental school experience on sealant use by British dentists. *Int. dent. J.* **40**, 249–52.

Cohen, L.D. (1990). Pit and fissure sealants. An under utilized preventive technology. *Int. J. tech. assess. Hlth Care*, **6**, 378–91.

Collins, W.J.N., *et al.* (1985). Experience with a mobile fissure sealing unit in the greater Glasgow area: results after three years. *Commun. dent. Health*, **2**, 195–202.

Cooley, R.L., McCourt, J.W., Huddleston, A.M., and Casmedes, H.P. (1990). Evaluation of a fluoride-containing sealant by SEM, microleakage, and fluoride release. *Ped. Dent.* **12**, 38–42.

Corbin, S.B., Clark, N.L., McClendon, B.J., and Snodgrass, N.K. (1990). Patterns of sealant delivery under variable third party requirements. *J. publ. Hlth Dent.* **50**, 311–8.

Croll, T.P. (1992a). Glass ionomers and esthetic dentistry. *J. Am. dent. Ass.* **123**, 51–4.

Croll, T.P. (1992b). Glass ionomer/resin preventive restorations. *J. dent. Child.* **59**, 269–72.

Cueto, E.I. and Buonocore, M.G. (1967). Sealing of pits and fissures with an adhesive resin: its use in caries prevention. *J. Am. dent. Ass.* **75**, 121–8.

De Craene, L.G.P.., Martens, L.C., Dermant, L.R., and Surmount, P.A.S. (1989). A clinical evaluation of a light cured fissure sealant (Helioseal). *J. dent. Child.* **56**, 97–101.

Dorignac, G.F. (1987). Efficacy of highly filled composites in the caries prevention of pits and fissures: two and one half years of clinical results. *J. pedod.* **11**, 139–45.

Donnan, M.F. and Ball, I.A. (1988). A double blind clinical trial to determine the importance of pumice prophylaxis on fissure sealant retention. *Br. dent. J.* **165**, 283–6.

Doyle, W.A. and Brose, J.A. (1978). A five-year study of the longevity of fissure sealants. *J. dent. Child.* **45**, 127–9.

Dummer, P.M.H., Addy, M., Oliver, S.J., and Shaw, W.C. (1988). Changes in the distribution of decayed and filled tooth surfaces and the progression of approximal caries in children between the ages of 11–12 years and 15–16 years. *Br. dent. J.* **164**, 277–82.

Dummer, P.M.H., *et al.* (1990). Factors influencing the initiation of carious lesions in specific tooth surfaces over a 4-year period in children between the ages of 11–12 years and 15–16 years. *J. dent. Res.* **18**, 190–7.

Eccles, M.F. (1989). The problem of occlusal caries and its current management. A review. *New Zealand dent. J.* **85**, 50–5.

Eidelman, E., Fuks, A.B., and Chosak, A. (1983). The retention of fissure sealant, rubber dam or cotton rolls in a private practice. *J. dent. Child.* **50**, 259–61.

Eidelman, E., Shapira, J., and Houpt, M. (1984). The retention of fissure sealants using twenty-second etching time. *J. dent. Child.* **51**, 422–4.

Eklund, S.A. (1986). Factors affecting the loss of fissure sealants: a dental insurers perspective. *J. publ. Hlth Dent.* **46**, 133–40.

Ekstrand, K., Neilsen, L.A., Westergaard, D., Reinert, M., and Thylstrup, A. (1991). Indications and use of fissure sealants in public dental health care in Denmark. A questionnaire-investigation. *Tandlaegebladet*, **95**, 741–7.

Elderton, R.J. (1983). Longditudinal study of dental treatment in the general dental service in Scotland. *Br. dent. J.* **155**, 91–6.

Elderton, R.J. (1985). Management of early dental caries in fissures with fissure sealant. *Br. dent. J.* **158**, 254–8.

Feigal, R.J., Hitt, J., and Splieth, E. (1993). Retaining sealant on salivary contaminated enamel. *J. Am. dent. Ass.* **124**, 88–97.

Ferguson, F.S. (1980). Retention of two sealant systems applied by inexperienced operators: results after 6 months and 12 months. *J. prev. Dent.* **7**, 355–8.

Foreman, F.J. and Matis, B.A. (1991). Retention of sealants placed by dental technicians without assistance. *Ped. Dent.* **13**, 59–61.

Forsten, L. (1990). Short and long term fluoride intake from glass ionomers and other fluoride containing filling materials in vitro. *Scand. J. dent. Res.* **98**, 179–85.

Fuks A.B., *et al.* (1982). A comparison of the retentive properties of two filled resins used as fissure sealants. *J. dent. Child.* **49**, 127–30.

Gandini M., Vertuan V., and Davis J.M. (1991). A comparative study between visible-light-activated and autopolymerizing sealants in relation to retention. *J. dent. Child.* **58**, 297–9.

Gibson, G.B., Richardson, A.S., and Waldman, R. (1982). The effectiveness of a chemically polymerized sealant in preventing occlusal caries: five-year results. *Ped. Dent.* **4**, 309–10.

Going R.E., *et al.* (1976). Two-year clinical evaluation of a pit and fissure sealant Part 1: Retention and loss of substance. *J. Am. dent. Ass.* **92**, 388–97.

Going, R.E., *et al.* (1977). Four-year clinical evaluation of a pit and fissure sealant. *J. Am. dent. Ass.* **95**, 972–81.

Gonzalez C.D., Frazier P.J., and Messer L.B. (1991). Sealant use by general practitioners: a Minnesota survey. *J. dent. Child.* **58**, 38–45.

Gore J.T. (1939). Etiology of dental caries. Enamel immunization experiments. *J. Am. dent. Ass.* **26**, 958–9.

Granath, L., Schroder, U., and Sundin, B. (1992). Clinical evaluation of preventive and Class I composite resin restorations. *Acta odont. Scand.* **50**, 359–64.

Handelman, S.L. (1991). Therapeutic use of sealants for incipient or early carious lesions in children and young adults. A review. *Proc. Finn. dent. Soc.* **87**, 463–75.

Harris, N.O., *et al* (1976). Adhesive sealant clinical trial: effectiveness in school population of the U.S. Virgin Islands. *J. prev. Dent.* **71**, 91–5.

Heidmann, J., Poulsen, S., and Mathiassen, F. (1990). Evaluation of a fissure sealing programme in a Danish Public Child Dental Service. *Commun. dent. Health*, **7**, 379–88.

Helle, A. (1975). Two fissure sealants tested for retention and caries reduction in Finnish children. *Proc. Finn. dent. Soc.* **71**, 91–5.

Henry, R.J. and Jessell, R.G. (1989). The glass ionomer, rest-a-seal. *J. dent. Child.* **56**, 283–7.

Higson, J.F. (1976). Caries prevention in first permanent molars by fissure sealing: a 2-year study in 6–8 year old children. *J. Dent.* **4**, 218–22.

Hinding J.H. and Buonocore M.G. (1974). The effects of varying the application protocol on the retention of pit and fissure sealant: a two-year clinical study. *J. Am. dent. Ass.* **89**, 127–31.

Horowitz, H.S. (1980). Pit and fissure sealants in private practice and public health programmes: analysis of cost-effectiveness. *Int. dent. J.* **30**, 117–26.

Horowitz, H.S., Heifetz, S.B., and McCune R.J. (1974). The effectiveness of an adhesive sealant in preventing occlusal caries: findings after two years in Kalispell, Montana. *J. Am. dent. Ass.* **89**, 885–90.

Horowitz, H.S., Heifetz, S.B., and Poulsen, S. (1976). Adhesive sealant clinical trial: an overview of results after four years in Kalispell, Montana. *J. prev. Dent.* **3**, 38–49.

Horowitz, H.S., Heifetz, S.B., and Poulsen, S. (1977). Retention and effectiveness of a single application of an adhesive sealant in preventing dental caries: final report after five years of a study in Kalispell, Montana. *J. Am. dent. Ass.* **95**, 1133–9.

Houpt, M.I. and Shey, Z. (1980). Cost-effectiveness of fissure sealant placement. *J. prev. Dent.* **6**, 7–10.

Houpt, M. and Shey, Z. (1983). The effectiveness of a fissure sealant after six years. *Ped. Dent.* **5**, 104–6.

Houpt, M.I., Fuks, A., and Eidelmann, E. (1994). The preventive resin (composite resin/sealant) restoration: Nine-year results. *Quintess. Int.* **25**, 155–9.

Hunter, B. (1985). Survival of dental restorations in young patients. *Commun. Dent. oral Epidemiol.* **13**, 285–7.

Hyatt T.P. (1923) Prophylactic odontotomy. The cutting into the tooth for the prevention of disease. *Dent. Cosmos,* **65**, 234–41.

Ibsen, R.L. (1973). Use of a filled diacrylate as a fissure sealant: one-year clinical study. *J. Am. Soc. Prev. Dent.* **3**, 60–5.

Isler S.L. and Doline S.L. (1981). Practical application of pit and fissure sealants. A seven year retrospective study. *Clin. Prev. Dent.* **3**, 18–20.

Isler, S.L., Malecz, R., and Ruff, J. (1980). A pedodontic preventive dentistry practice. Part 1. Pit and fissure sealants: 5-year clinical evaluation. *J. prev. Dent.* **6**, 201–14.

Ismail, A.I., King, W., and Clark, D.C. (1989). An evaluation of the Saskatchewan pit and fissure sealant program: a longitudinal follow-up. *J. publ. Hlth Dent.* **49**, 206 and 11.

Jensen, O.E., Handleman, S.L., and Pameijer, L.T. (1981). Clinical assessment of wear of the pit and fissure sealants. *J. prosthet Dent.* **46**, 639–41.

Jensen, M.E., Wefel, J.S., Triolo, P.T., and Hammesfahr, P.D. (1990*a*). Effects of a fluoride-releasing fissure sealant on artificial enamel caries. *Am. J. Dent.* **3** 75–8.

Jensen, M.E., Billinghas, R.J., and Featherstone, J.D. (1990*b*). Clinical evaluation of Fluroshield pit and fissure sealant. *Clin. prev. Dent.* **12**, 24–7.

Kidd, E.A.M., Naylor, M.N., and Wilson, R.F. (1992). Presence of clinically undetected and untreated molar occlusal caries in adolescents on the Isle of Wight. *Caries Res.* **26**, 397–40.

Kilpatrick, N.M. (1993). Glass ionomer cements. Factors influencing their durability. D. Phil. thesis. University of Newcastle-upon-Tyne, UK.

Kuba Y., Miyazaki K., Ichiki K., Kawazoe H., and Motokawa W. (1992). Clinical application of visible light-cured fluoride-releasing sealant to non-etched enamel surface of partially erupted permanent molars. *J. Clin. ped. Dent..* **17**, 3–9.

Kuthy, R.A., Branch, L.G., and and Clive, J.M. (1990). First permanent molar restoration. Differences between those with and without dental sealants. *J. dent. Educ.* **54**, 653–60.

Lang, W.P., Faghaly, M.M., Woolfolk, M.W., Ziemiecki, T.L., and Fuja, B.W. (1991). Educating dentists about fissure sealants: effects on knowledge, attitudes and use. *J. publ. Hlth Dent.* **51**, 164–9.

Le Bell, Y. and Forsten, L. (1980). Sealing of preventively enlarged fissures. *Acta odont. Scand.* **38**, 101–4.

Leake, J.L. and Martinello, B.P. (1976). A four-year evaluation of a fissure sealant in a public health setting. *Can. dent. Ass. J.,* **42**, 409–15.

Lennon, M.A., Worthington, H.V., Coventry, P., Mellor, A.C., and Holloway, P.J. (1990). The Capitation Study. 2. Does capitation encourage more prevention?. *Br. dent. J.* **168**, 213–5.

Leske, G.S., Pollard, S., and Cons, N. (1976). The effectiveness of dental hygienist teams in applying a pit and fissure sealant. *J. prev. Dent.* **3**, 33–6.

Lewis J.M. and Morgan, M.V. (1994). A critical review of the methods for the economic evaluation of fissure sealants. *Commun. dent. Health,* **11**, 79–82.

Li S.H., *et al.* (1981). Evaluation of the retention of two types of pit and fissure sealants. *Commun. Dent. oral Epidemiol,* **9**, 151–8.

Llodra, J.C., Biano, M., Delgado-Rodriguez, M., Baca, P., and Galvez, R. (1993). Factors influencing the effectiveness of sealants—a meta analysis. *Commun. Dent. oral Epidemiol.* **41**, 261–8.

Luoma H., *et al.* (1973). Retention of a fissure sealant with caries reduction in Finnish children after six months. *Scand. J. dent. Res.* **81**, 510–12.

McCabe, J. and Storer, R. (1980). Adaptation of resin restorative materials to etched enamel and the interfacial work of fracture. *Br. dent. J.* **148**, 155–8.

McClean, J.W. (1988). Glass ionomer cements. *Br. Dent. J.* **164**, 293–9.

McConnachie, I. (1992). The preventive resin restoration: a conservative alternative. *Can. dent. Ass. J.* **58**, 197–200.

McCune R.J., *et al.* (1973). Pit and fissure sealants: one-year results from a study in Kalispell, Montana. *J. Am. dent. Ass.* **87**, 1177–80.

McCune, R.J., Bojanini, J., and Abodeely, R.A. (1979). Effectiveness of a pit and fissure sealant in the prevention of dental caries: three-year clinical results. *J. Am. dent. Ass.* **99**, 619–23.

McKenna, E.F. and Grundy, G.E. (1987). Glass ionomer cement fissure sealants applied by operative dental auxiliaries—retention rate after one year. *Australian dent. J.* **32**, 200–3.

McLean, J.W. and Wilson, A.D. (1994). Fissure sealing and filling with an adhesive glass ionomer cement. *Br. dent. J.* **136**, 269–76.

Mejar, I. and Mjor, I.A. (1990). Glass ionomer and resin-based fissure sealants: a clinical study. *Scand. J. dent. Res.* **98**, 345–50.

Mertz-Fairhurst, E.J., Fairhurst, C.W., Williams, J.E., Della-Giustina, V.E., and Brooks, J.D. (1984). A comparative clinical study of two pit and fissure sealants: 7- year results. *J. Am. dent. Ass.* **109**, 252–5.

Mertz-Fairhurst, E.J., *et al.* (1992). Cariostatic and ultra-conservative sealed restorations: six year results. *Quintess. Int.* **23**, 827–38.

Meurman, J.H. and Helminen, S.K.J. (1976). Effectiveness of fissure sealant 3 years after application. *Scand. J. dent. Res.* **84**, 218–23.

Meurman, J.H., Helminen, S.K.J., and Luoma, H. (1978). Caries reduction over five years from a single application of a fissure sealant. *Scand. J. dent. Res.* **86**, 153–6.

Meurman, J.H. *et al.* (1975). Caries reduction 1.5 years after application of a fissure sealant as related to dietary habits. *Scand. J. dent. Res.* **83**, 1–6.

Miller J. (1950). A clinical investigation in preventive dentistry. *Dent. Practit.* **1**, 66–75.

Miller, W.D. (1905). The preventive treatment of teeth with special reference to nitrate of silver. *Dent. Cosmos*, **47**, 913–22.

Mills, R.W. and Ball, I.A. (1993). A clinical trial to evaluate the intention of a solvent cement-ionomer cement used as a fissure sealant. *Oper. Dent.* **18**, 148–54.

Mitchell, L. and Murray, J.J. (1987). The durability of fissure sealants placed in children attending a dental hospital. *Br. dent. J.* **163**, 353–6.

Nakata, M., Kuriyama, S., Mitsuyasu, K., Morimoto, M., and Tomioka, K. (1989). Transfer of innovation for advancement in dentistry: a case study on pit and fissure sealants' use in Japan. *Int. dent. J.* **39**, 263–8.

National Institutes of Health (1984). Consensus development conference statement on dental sealants in the prevention of tooth decay. *J. Am. dent. Ass.* **108**, 233–6.

Ovrebo, R.L. and Raadal, M. (1990). Microleakage in fissures sealed with resin or glass ionomer cement. *Scand. J. dent. Res.* **98**, 66–9.

Parkhouse R.C. and Winter G.B. (1971). A fissure sealant containing methyl-2-cyanoacrylate as a caries preventive agent. *Br. dent. J.* **130**, 16–19.

Paterson, R.C., Blinkhorn, A.S., and Paterson, F.M. (1990). Reported use of sealant restorations in a group of general practitioners in the west of Scotland. *Br. dent. J.* **169**, 18–22.

Paterson, F.M., Paterson, R.C., and Blinkhorn, A.S. (1991). General practitioner's perceptions of the effects of a distance learning programme. *Br. dent. J.* **171**, 21–5.

Poulsen S., *et al.* (1979). Evaluation of a pit-and-fissure sealing program in a public dental health service after 2 years. *Commun. Dent. oral Epidemiol.* **7**, 154–7.

Raadal, M. (1978). Follow-up study of sealing and filling with composite resins in the prevention of occlusal caries *Commun. Dent. oral Epidemiol.* **6**, 176–80.

Raadal, M., Utkilen, A.B., and Nilsen, O.L. (1991). A wo-year clinical trial comparing the retention of two fissure sealants. *Int. J. paed. Dent.* **1**, 77–81.

Rantala, E.V. (1979). Caries incidence in 7–9-year-old children after fissure sealing and topical fluoride therapy in Finland. *Commun. Dent. oral Epidemiol.* **7**, 213–17.

Richardson, A.S., Waldman, R., and Gibson, G.B. (1978). The effectiveness of a chemically polymerised sealant preventing occlusal caries: 2 year results. *Can. dent. Ass. J.* **44**, 269–72.

Richardson, A.S., Gibson, G.B., and Waldman, R. (1980*a*). Chemically polymerised sealant in preventing occlusal caries. *Can. dent. Ass. J.* **46**, 259–60.

Richardson, A.S., Gibson, G.B., and Waldman, R. (1980*b*). The effectiveness of a chemically polymerised sealant: four-year results. *Ped. Dent.* **2**, 24–6.

Richardson, B.A., Smith D.C., and Hargreaves, J.A. (1977). Study of a fissure sealant in mentally retarded Canadian children. *Commun. Dent. oral Epidemiol.* **5**, 220–6.

Richardson, B.A., Smith, D.C., and Hargreaves, J.A. (1981). A five-year clinical evaluation of the effectiveness of a fissure sealant in mentally retarded Canadian children. *Commun. Dent. oral Epidemiol.* **9**, 170–4.

Riordan, P.J., Dalton-Ecker, L., and Edwards, T.S. (1993). Dental status of 12-year-olds treated in private practice and a school dental service. *Commun. Dent. oral Epidemiol.* **21**, 198–202.

Ripa, L.W. (1990). Has the decline in caries prevalence reduced the need for fissure sealants in the U.K? *J. paed. Dent.* **6**, 79–84.

Ripa, L.W. (1993). Sealants revisted: an update of the effectiveness of pit and fissure sealants. A review. *Caries Res.* **27** (suppl. 1), 77–82.

Ripa L.W. and Cole W.W. (1970). Occlusal sealing and caries prevention: results 12 months after a single application of adhesive resin. *J. dent. Res.* **49**, 171–3.

Ripa, L.W. and Wolff, M.S. (1992). PRR: Indications, techniques and success. *Quintess. Int.* **23**, 307–15.

Risager, J. and Poulsen, S. (1974). Fissure sealing with Nuva-Seal in a public health program for Danish schoolchildren after 12 months observation. *Scand. J. dent. Res.* **82**, 570–3.

Rock W.P. (1972). Fissure sealants. Results obtained with two different sealants after one year. *Br. dent. J.* **133**, 146–51.

Rock W.P. (1973). Fissure sealants. Results obtained with two different bis-GMA type sealants after one year. *Br. dent. J.* **134**, 193–6.

Rock, W.P. (1974). Fissure sealants. Further results of clinical trials. *Br. dent. J.* **136**, 317–21.

Rock W.P. (1977). Fissure sealants. REsults of a 3-year clinical trial using an ultra-violet sensitive resin. *Br. dent. J.* **142**, 16–18.

Rock W.P. and Evans, R.I.W. (1982). A comparative study between a chemically polymerised fissure sealant resin and a light cured resin. *Br. dent. J.* **152**, 232–4.

Rock, W.P. and Evans, R.I.W. (1983). A comparative study between a chemically polymerised fissure sealant resin and a light-cured resin: three-year results. *Br. dent. J.* **155**, 344–6.

Rock W.P., Gordon P.H., and Bradnock G. (1978). The effect of operator variability and patient age on the retention of fissure sealant resin. *Br. dent. J.* **145**, 72–5.

Rock W.P., Gordon P.H., and Bradnock G. (1981*a*). Dental caries experience in Birmingham and Wolverhampton school children following the fluoridation of Birmingham water in 1964. *Br. dent. J.* **150**, 61–6.

Rock W.P., Gordon P.H., and Bradnock G. (1981*b*). Caries experience of West Midland school children following fluoridation of Birmingham water in 1964: caries of first permanent molars. *Br. dent. J.* **150**, 269–73.

Rock W.P., Weatherill S., and Anderson R.J. (1990). Retention of three fissure sealant resins. The effects of etching agent and curing method. Results over 3 years. *Br. dent. J.* **168**, 323–5.

Romcke, R.G., Lewis, D.W., Maze, B.D., and Vickerson, R.A. (1990). Retention and maintenance of fissure sealants over 10 years. *Can. dent. Ass. J.* **56**, 235–7.

Roth, A.G. and Conry, J.P. (1992). A restrospective cohort evaluation of preventive resin restorations. *Can. dent. Ass. J.* **58**, 223–6.

Shapira, J., Fuks, A., Chosack, A., Houpt, M., and Eidelman, E. (1990). Comparative clinical study of autopolymerized and light-polymerized fissure sealants: five-year results. *Ped. dent.* **12**, 168–9.

Sheykholeslam, Z. and Houpt, M. (1978). Clinical effectiveness of an auto-polymerised fissure sealant after 2 years. *Commun. Dent. oral Epidemiol.* **6**, 181–4.

Shimokobe H., Komatsu H., Kawakanui S., and Hirota K. (1986). Clinical evaluation of glass ionomer cement need for sealants (abstract). *J. dent. Res.* **65**, 780.

Silverstone, L.M. (1974). Fissure sealants, laboratory studies. *Caries Res.* **8**, 2–26.

Simonsen, R.J. (1979). Fissure sealants in primary molars: retention of coloured sealants with variable etch times at 12 months. *J. dent. Child.* **46**, 382–4.

Simonsen, R.J. (1980*a*). The clinical effectiveness of a colored pit and fissure sealant at 24 months. *Ped. Dent.* **2**, 10–16.

Simonsen, R.J. (1980*b*). Preventive resin restorations: three-year results. *J. Am. dent. Ass.* **100**, 535–9.

Simonsen, R.J. (1982). Five year results of sealant effects on caries prevalence and treatment cost (abstract). *J. dent Res.* **61**, 330.

Simonsen, R.J. (1987). Retention and effectiveness of a single application of white sealant after 10 years. *J. Am. dent. Ass.* **115**, 31–6.

Simonsen, R.J. (1989). Editorial. Why not prevention? *Quintess. Int.* **20**, 785.

Simonsen, R.J. (1991). Retention and effectiveness of dental sealant after 15 years. *J. Am. dent. Ass.* **122**, 34–42.

Stach, D.J., Hatch, R.A., and Tilliss, T.S. (1992). Change in occlusal height resulting from placement of pit and fissure sealants. *J. prosthet. Dent.* **68**, 750–3.

Stephen, K.W., Sutherland, D.A., and Trainer, J. (1976). Fissure sealing by practitioners. First year retention data in Scottish 6-year-old children. *Br. Dent. J.* **140**, 45–51.

Stephen K.W., *et al.* (1978). Fissure sealing of first permanent molars. An improved technique applied by a dental auxilliary. *Br. dent. J.* **144**, 7–10.

Stephen K.W., *et al.* (1981*a*). A clinical comparison of two filled fissure sealants after one year. *Br. dent. J.* **150**, 282–4.

Stephen, K.W., Kirkwood, M., Campbell, D., Young, K.C., Gillespie, F.C., and Boyle, P. (1981*b*). Fissure sealing with Nuva-seal and Alpha-seal: two-year data. *J. Dent.* **9**, 53–7.

Stephen, K.W., Campbell, D., Kirkwood, M., and Strang R. (1985). A two-year visible light/UV light filled sealant study. *Br. dent. J.* **159**, 404–5.

Stephen, K.W., Kay, E.J., and Tullis J.I. (1990). Combined fluoride therapies. A 6-year double-blind school-based preventive dentistry study in Inverness, Scotland. *Commun. Dent. oral Epidemiol.* **18**, 244–8.

Straffon L.H., Dennison J.B., and More F.G. (1985). Three year evaluation of sealant: effect of isolation on efficacy. *J. Am. dent. Ass.* **110**, 714–17.

Straffon L.H. and Dennison J.B. (1988). Clinical evaluation comparing sealant and amalgam after 7 years: Final report. *J. Am. dent. Ass.* **117**, 755–7.

Strang, R., Cummings A., and Stephen, K.W. (1984). Laboratory examination of new fissure sealants: Microhardeners and setting times. *Caries Res.* **18**, 179–80.

Swift, E.J. (1988). The effect of sealants on dental caries: a review. *J. Am. dent. Ass.* **116**, 700–4.

Takeuchi M., *et al.* (1966). Sealing of the pit and fissure with resin adhesive II. Results of nine months' field work, and investigation of electrical conductivity of teeth. *Bull. Tokyo Dent. Coll.* **7**, 50–9.

Takeuchi M., *et al.* (1971). Sealing of the pit and fissure with resin adhesive IV. Results of 5 year field work and a method of evaluation of field work for caries prevention. *Bull. Tokyo Dent. Coll.* **12**, 295–320.

Thylstrup, A. and Poulsen, S. (1978). Retention and effectiveness of a chemically polymerised pit and fissure sealant after two years. *Scand. J. dent. Res.* **86**, 21–4.

Ulvestad, H. (1976). A 24-month evaluation of fissure sealing with a diluted composite material. *Scand. J. dent. Res.* **84**, 51–5.

Vehkalahti, A.M., Solvaara, L., and Rytomaa, I. (1991). An eight-year follow-up of the occlusal surfaces of first permanent molars. *J. dent. Res.* **70**, 1064–7.

Vrbic, V. (1986). Five-year experience with fissure sealing. *Quintess. Int.* **17**, 371–2.

Walls A.W.G., Wallwork M.A., Holland I.S., and Murray J.J (1985). The longevity of occlusal amalgam restorations in first permanent molars of child patients. *Br. dent. J.* **158**, 133–6.

Walter, R.G. (1982). A longitudinal study of caries development in initially caries free naval recruits. *J. dent. Res.* **61**, 1405–7.

Welbury, R.R., Walls, A.W.G., Murray, J.J., and McCabe, J.F. (1990). The management of occlusal caries in permanent molars. A 5 year clinical trial comparing a minimal composite with an amalgam restoration. *Br. dent. J.* **169**, 361–6.

Weerheijm, K.L., Groen, H.J., Bast, A.J.T., Kuft, I.A., Eijkman, M.A.J., and Van Amerongen M.E. (1992*a*). Clinically undetected occlusal dentine caries: a radiographic comparison. *Caries Res.* **26**, 305–9.

Weerheijm, K.L., Gruythuysen, R.J., and Van Amergongen W.E. (1992*b*). Prevalence of hidden caries. *J. dent. Child.* **59**, 408–12.

Weerheijm, K.L., De Soet, J.J., Van Amerongen, W.E., and De Graff, J. (1993). Hidden caries under sealants. *ORCA 39th Congress Abstract*, No. 94.

Weintraub, J.A. (1989). The effectiveness of pit and fissure sealants. *J. publ. Hlth Dent.* **49**, 317–27.

Weintraub, J.A., Stearns, S.C., Burt, B.A., Beltran, E., and Eklund, S.A. (1993). A retrospective analysis of the cost-effectiveness of dental sealants in a children's health centre. *Soc. Sci. Med..* **36**, 1483–93.

Widmer, R.P. and Jayasekara, T.R. (1989). Fissure sealing with a glass ionomer cement: 2 year results (abstract). *J. dent. Res.* **68**.

Williams, B. (1990).Fissure sealant: a review. *J. Int. Ass. dent. Child.* **20**, 35–41.

Williams B. and von Frauenhofer J.A. (1977). The influence of the time of etching and washing on the bond strength of fissure sealants applied to enamel. *J. oral Rehabil.* **4**, 139–43

Williams, B. and Winter, G.B. (1976). Fissure sealants: a 2 year clinical trial. *Br. dent. J*, **141**, 15–18.

Williams, B. and Winter, G.B. (1981). Fissure sealants. Further results at 4 years. *Br. dent. J.* **150**, 183–7.

Williams, B., Price, R., and Winter, G.B. (1978). Fissure sealants. A 2-year clinical trial. *Br. dent. J.* **145**, 359–64.

Williams, B., Ward R., and Winter, G.B. (1986). A two-year clinical trial comparing different resin systems used as fissure sealants. *Br. dent. J.* **161**, 367–70.

Wood A.J. *et al.* (1989). Cotton roll isolation versus Vac-Ejector isolation. *J. dent. Child.* **56**, 438–41.

Zimmerman, B.F., Rauis, H.R., and Bassett, R.G. Jr. (1984). Fluoride release and physical properties of experimental resin-filled sealant. *J. dent. Res.* **63**, 11–16.

PLATES

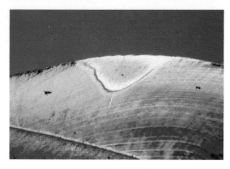

Plate 6.1 Longitudinal ground section through a small lesion of enamel caries examined in quinoline with polarized light. The translucent zone is clearly differentiated from sound enamel and the dark zone shows positive birefringence. The striae of Retzius are well marked within the body of the legion. × 50.

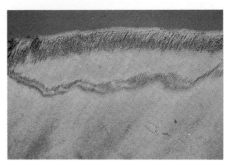

Plate 6.4 Longitudinal ground section of a small lesion examined in quinoline with polarized light before exposure to a calcifying fluid. The advancing front of the lesion shows a translucent zone and a positively birefringent dark zone. × 50. (From Silverstone (1977), by courtesy of *Caries Research*).

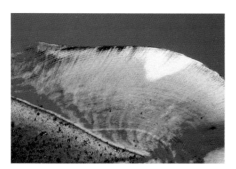

Plate 6.2 Longitudinal ground section through a small lesion of enamel caries examined in quinoline with polarized light. The body of the lesion is seen as a translucent area. No dark zone is present in this specimen. × 50.

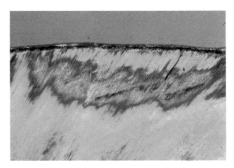

Plate 6.5 The same section as in Plate 6.4 after exposure to a synthetic calcifying fluid. The section is again examined in quinoline. The dark zone appears much broader than prior to the experiment. Whilst its deep border is approximately at the original position, its superficial boundary has extended towards the enamel surface into the region previously identified as the body of the lesion. This legion of 'new' dark zone has a pore volume of between 2 and 4 per cent and shows a negative birefringence in water. This region previously had been demineralized to a stage exhibiting a pore volume of between 5 and 20 per cent. × 50. (From Silverstone (1977), by courtesy of *Caries Research*).

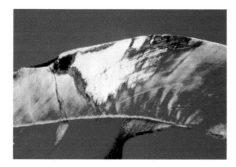

Plate 6.3 Longitudinal ground section of a natural carious lesion in a tooth extracted from a patient aged 70 years, examined in quinoline with polarized light. Wide, well-developed dark zones are obvious at the advancing front of the lesion, within the body of the lesion, and at the surface of the lesion. × 50.

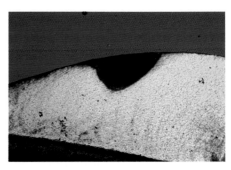

Plate 6.6 The same section as in Plate 6.1 now examined in water with polarized light. The body of the lesion shows as an area of positive birefringence. × 50.

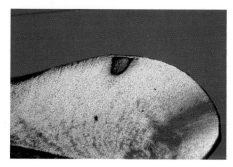

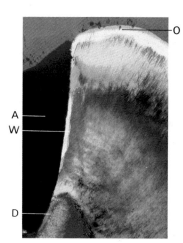

Plate 6.11 Longitudinal ground section of a natural secondary carious lesion. The gound section is in quinoline and viewed with polarized light. An amalgam restoration is present (A). The wall lesion is seen as a translucent zone (W). Dentine involvement is obvious (D). An outer lesion, caused by primary attack on the enamel surface, is also present (O). × 50. (By courtesy of *Dental Update*.)

Plate 6.7 The same section as in Plate 6.2 now examined in water with polarized light. The body of the lesion, positioned in the subsurface enamel, shows positive birefringence. The surface overlying the lesion exhibits a negative birefringence. × 50.

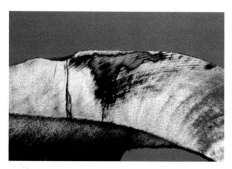

Plate 6.8 The same section as in Plate 6.3 now examined in water with polarized light. Well-mineralized laminations are obvious within the body of the lesion, particularly on its occlusal aspect. × 50.

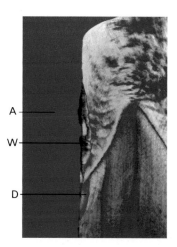

Plate 6.12 Longitudinal ground section of a natural secondary carious lesion. The ground section is in quinoline and viewed with polarized light. An amalgam restoration was present but lost during section preparation (A). The wall lesion is seen as a dark zone (W) Dentine involvement is obvious (D). × 50. (By courtesy of *Dental Update*).

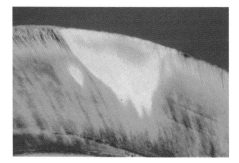

Plate 6.9 Longitudinal ground section through a deciduous molar tooth examined in quinoline with polarized light. The lesion is seen as a translucent area, there being no evidence of a dark zone in this specimen. × 50.

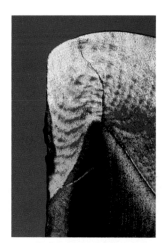

Plate 6.13 The same section as in Plate 6.12 now viewed in water with polarized light. The wall lesion is now seen as an area of positive birefringence indicating a demineralization in excess of 5 per cent. × 50.

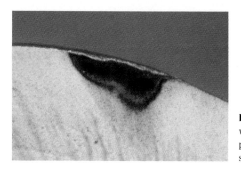

Plate 6.10 The same section as in Plate 6.9 now examined in water with polarized light. The body of the lesion shows as an area of positive birefringence beneath an intact, negatively birefringent, surface zone. × 50.

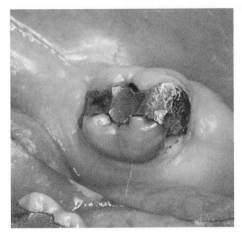

Plate 6.14 A cavitated lesion adjacent to a restoration.

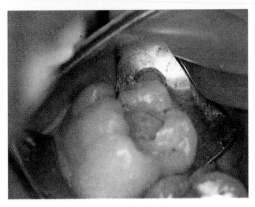

Plate 6.17 The same cavity as in Plate 6.16 after use of the caries detector dye. Note areas of red stain at the enamel-dentine junction.

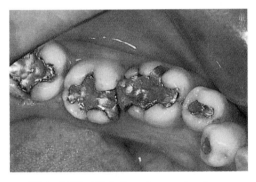

Plate 6.15 Ditched amalgam restorations.

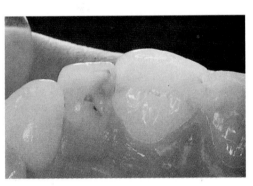

Plate 6.18 Caries is present beneath the restoration on the mesial aspect of the lateral incisor.

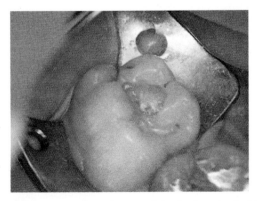

Plate 6.16 A cavity where the enamel-dentine junction had been judged to be clinically caries-free.

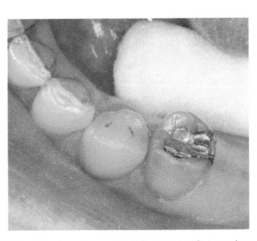

Plate 6.19 Discolouration around the margin of an amalgam restoration. Is this caries or corrosion products?

6. The carious lesion in enamel

E.A.M. KIDD

NEARLY a hundred years ago a remarkable American dentist, Dr G.V. Black, was studying the problem of dental caries. He wrote extensively on the pathology of the disease (Black 1908) and based on his observations he laid the foundations for the operative management of the disease. He wrote, 'The complete divorcement of dental practice from studies of the pathology of dental caries, that existed in the past, is an anomaly in science that should not continue. It has the apparent tendency plainly to make dentists mechanics only.'

In the intervening years a mass of information has been gathered. It is now appreciated that the carious process is not a simple process of demineralization but is characterized by alternating periods of destruction and arrest or even repair. When the destructive forces pre-dominate demineralization will progress. Conversely, preventive measures, such as dietary control, effective plaque removal, and judicious use of fluoride, can arrest the process.

Part of this chapter will describe the pathology of enamel caries as this is the scientific basis on which the management strategies rest. In addition, the clinical detection of enamel carious lesions will be discussed, for without accurate diagnosis it is not possible to formulate a sensible approach to the management of the disease.

MACROSCOPIC FEATURES OF THE EARLY ENAMEL LESION

The earliest macroscopic evidence of enamel caries is known as the 'white spot lesion'. The lesions form in areas of plaque stagnation, such as enamel pits and fissures in the occlusal surface of molars and premolars, approximal enamel smooth surfaces just cervical to the contact point (Fig. 6.1), and the enamel of the cervical margin just coronal to the gingival margin. The lesion is best seen on dried teeth where the opaque, white appearance distinguishes it from the adjacent sound enamel. At this stage the enamel is still hard and shiny. Sometimes the lesion may appear brown in colour, the so-called 'brown spot lesion'. Eventually, if the lesion progresses, the intact surface breaks down (cavitation) and a hole is formed (a cavity).

Although the white spot lesion is the earliest visual sign of the disease it has been preceded by destructive processes which are not discernible macroscopically. Research workers have used the scanning electron microscope to observe the early enamel reaction to acids produced by bacteria in the dental plaque. At this ultrastructural level direct dissolution of

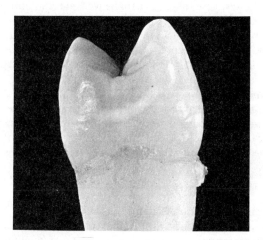

Fig. 6.1. Premolar showing a white spot lesion on the approximal tooth surface.

the outer enamel surface can be seen (Thylstrup and Fejerskov 1986). This involves partial dissolution of the crystal peripheries leading to an enlargement of inter-crystalline spaces. In addition, the tissue immediately beneath the outer microsurface appears more porous than the micro-surface itself. Eventually these changes, involving an increase in porosity of the tissue, become macroscopically visible after air-drying.

It is perhaps worth considering why air-drying makes these changes easier to see. The explanation concerns the refractive indices of hydroxyapatite (1.62), water (1.33), and air (1.0). When the tissue is dried, air will replace the water in the intercrystalline spaces. The difference between the refractive index of hydroxyapatite and air is now so large that the porous tissue loses its translucency and appears opaque. Lesions which appear opaque without air-drying are more demineralized than those which are only apparent on a dry surface. Thus to pick up early demineralization visually, teeth must be both clean and dry.

MICROSCOPIC FEATURES OF THE EARLY ENAMEL LESION

To examine carious enamel in the light microscope, ground sections are required. On a smooth surface the lesion is usually triangular in shape, the apex of the triangle pointing towards the enamel–dentine junction (Plate 6.1). The small lesion has been divided into zones based upon its histological appearance when longitudinal ground sections are examined with the light microscope. Four zones may be distinguished. There is a translucent zone at the inner advancing front of the lesion, while a dark zone may be found just superficial to this. The body of the lesion is the third zone, lying between the dark zone and the apparently undamaged surface enamel. This is the zone that makes up the major part of the lesion and shows the most marked demineralization. The relatively unaffected surface zone, superficial to the lesion, is the fourth zone.

While each of these zones may be seen in plain transmitted light, the lesion is particularly clear when examined with polarized light.

When ground sections are examined in polarized light, it is usual to place the section in a liquid; this liquid is called an 'imbibition medium'. Two imbibition media will be referred to in the description that follows—water and quinoline.

Enamel has a refractive index of 1.62. Water, however, has a different refractive index of 1.33. Quinoline, on the other hand, has a refractive index of 1.62, the same as enamel. The appearance of each of the four zones of enamel caries in polarized light will now be described.

Zone 1: the translucent zone

The translucent zone of enamel caries lies at the advancing front of the lesion and is the first recognizable zone of alteration from normal. This zone is only seen when a longitudinal ground section is examined in a clearing agent, such as quinoline, having the same refractive index (1.62) as that of enamel. The translucent zone appears structureless, the tranlucency being demarcated from normal enamel on its deep aspect and the dark zone on its superficial aspect (Plate 6.1).

The translucent zone is a more porous region than sound enamel, the pores having been created by the demineralization process. Sound enamel has a pore volume of about 0.1 per cent. The translucent zone, however, has a pore volume of approximately 1 per cent. The pores are probably located at junctional sites such as prism borders, cross-striations, and striae of Retzius (Silverstone 1966). Once these areas are imbibed with quinoline these structural markings are lost, due to the penetration of a medium having an identical refractive index to that of enamel apatite.

A translucent zone is not present in all lesions and may sometimes only be observed on the lateral aspects of a lesion, close to the enamel surface.

Zone 2: the dark zone

If a translucent zone is present at the advancing front of a lesion when examined in quinoline, the dark zone is the second zone of alteration from normal and lies just superficial to the translucent zone. The zone appears dark or positively birefringent after imbibition with quinoline (Plate 6.1). The dark zone may show considerable variation in its width and is not present in all lesions (Plate 6.2).

The dark zone is more porous than the translucent zone, having a pore volume of 2–4 per cent. The explanation of why the dark zone appears dark, or positively birefringent, is

an intriguing one. It would seem that in this zone the pores are of varying sizes, large and small. Quinoline is a large molecule and cannot enter the small pores, which remain filled with air (Darling *et al.* 1961). Because the refractive index of air is remote from that of enamel, positive-form birefringence is produced. Thus, some of the pores of the dark zone act as a 'molecular sieve', excluding large molecules such as quinoline.

There are two theoretical ways in which these small pores may have formed. They may have been created by demineralization, that is by an opening up of sites not previously attacked. Alternatively, the small pores could represent areas of healing where mineral has been redeposited. There is now considerable evidence to support the view that the dark zone can represent an area of remineralization. If arrested lesions that have been present clinically for many years (Fig. 6.2) are examined histologically (Kidd 1983), they show wide, well-developed dark zones at the front of the lesion, within the body of the lesion, and on the surface of the lesion (Plate 6.3).

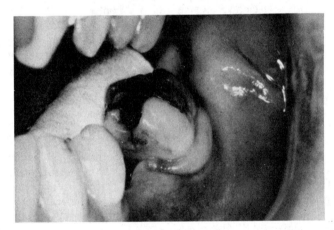

Fig. 6.2.   Arrested caries on the mesial surface of the lower second molar.

Attempts have been made to remineralize enamel lesions in the laboratory using human saliva and calcifying fluids prepared from synthetic hydroxyapatite with added fluoride (Silverstone 1973). After such exposure there were changes in the histological appearance of the lesions including significant broadening of the dark zones (Plates 6.4 and 6.5).

Zone 3: the body of the lesion

The body is the largest proportion of carious enamel in the small lesion. It lies superficial to the dark zone and deep to the relatively unaffected surface layer. When a longitudinal ground section is examined in quinoline in polarized light, the area appears translucent, negatively birefringent, and the striae of Retzius may be well marked (Plates 6.1 and 6.2).

The body of the lesion is particularly clearly seen if the ground section is examined after imbibition with water. The body now shows as an area of positive birefringence in contrast to the negative birefringence of sound enamel and the rest of the lesion (Plates 6.6 and 6.7). The region has a minimum pore volume of 5 per cent at its periphery, increasing to 25 per cent or greater in the centre. After imbibition with water the striae of Retzius are often particularly clear.

Several workers have described natural enamel lesions that show bands of well-mineralized tissue passing through the body of the lesion (Kostlan 1962; Crabb 1966; Silverstone 1970). Histologically this appearance may be found in 'old' or 'chronic' lesions (Plate 6.8). This feature may represent a lesion which has developed very slowly with alternating periods of de- and re-mineralization, or a lesion which having developed has arrested and partially healed.

Zone 4: the surface zone

One of the important characteristics of enamel caries is that the greatest degree of demineralization occurs at a subsurface level. The small lesion remains covered by a surface layer which appears relatively unaffected by the attack. When such a lesion is examined in polarized light after imbibition with water, the porous subsurface region is positively birefringent while the surface zone retains a negative birefringence (Plate 6.7).

This relatively unaffected surface zone is usually some 30 μm in depth and has a pore volume of approximately 1 per cent. If the lesion progresses, this surface layer is eventually destroyed and a cavity forms.

The subsurface demineralization that characterizes the enamel lesion has intrigued research workers for many years. Some have suggested that the formation of this relatively unaffected surface layer is associated with the special properties of surface enamel, which shows a high degree of mineralization, a higher fluoride content, and possibly a greater amount of insoluble protein than subsurface enamel. However, in the laboratory, artificial caries-like lesions can be produced in enamel when the original surface has been ground away. Consequently the existence of surface enamel with 'special' characteristics cannot be entirely responsible.

Another explanation for the relative protection of this outermost enamel, which is next to the pellicle and plaque, must be the dynamic processes taking place at this interface. The surface zone may, in part, be a manifestation of remineralization.

FISSURE CARIES

Occlusal fissures and buccal pits are obvious stagnation areas where plaque can form and mature, anatomically protected from the toothbrush bristle by the dimensions of the fissure.

The histological features of fissure caries are similar to those already described for smooth surfaces. The lesion forms on either side of the fissure walls, giving the appearance of two small, smooth surface lesions (Fig. 6.3) (Mortimer 1964). Eventually the lesions increase in size, coalescing at the base of the fissure. The enamel lesion broadens as it approaches the underlying dentine, guided by prism direction. With lateral spread at the enamel–dentine junction, the area of involved dentine is larger than with smooth surface lesions.

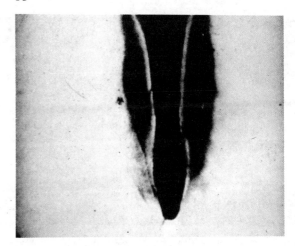

Fig. 6.3. Microradiograph of fissure caries showing lesion formation on either side of the fissure walls. × 30. (From Mortimer (1964), by courtesy of *Caries Research*.)

THE EARLY LESION IN DECIDUOUS TEETH

The histological features of enamel caries in deciduous teeth are essentially similar to those already described in permanent enamel (Plates 6.9 and 6.10). All of the four zones described for the classical lesion of caries in permanent enamel may be present in the lesion of primary enamel (Silverstone 1970). However, the enamel in deciduous teeth is much thinner than in permanent teeth and the pulps are relatively large. Thus, early diagnosis of the incipient lesion in primary enamel is of particular importance.

MICRORADIOGRAPHY

In the laboratory, it is possible to take a radiograph of a ground section. This is called a microradiograph and may be examined in the light microscope.

Microradiography is sufficiently sensitive to demonstrate demineralization in excess of 5 per cent as a radiolucent area whose size corresponds almost exactly with the body of the lesion as seen in polarized light after imbibition with water (Fig. 6.4). The striae of Retzius and prism structure are often well marked. Superficially the radiolucent region is limited by the presence of a well-mineralized radiopaque layer at the surface of the lesion, which may or may not coincide with the presence of a surface zone.

ELECTRON MICROSCOPY

The *scanning electron microscope* has been used to examine the surface of white spot lesions (Thylstrup and Fejerskov 1981). On approximal surfaces the contact facet has a smooth appearance without perikymata. In the active lesion the opaque surface of the enamel cervical to the facet shows numerous irregular holes which represent deepened and more irregular Tomes' processes pits and an increased number of eroded focal holes. These areas may merge together to form larger areas of irregular cracks or microcavities. Thus, although polarized light shows that the early lesion is principally a subsurface demineralization, the scanning elec-

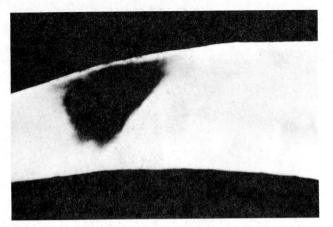

Fig. 6.4. Microradiograph of an early carious lesion in a deciduous molar tooth. The body of the lesion, in the subsurface enamel, shows marked radiolucency in contrast to the surface of the tooth, which remains well mineralized. × 70.

tron microscope shows a distinct disintegration of the very surface.

The first evidence of a change from sound enamel that can be recognized with the *transmission electron microscope* appears to coincide with the body of the lesion as seen in the light microscope. Demineralization of enamel is diffuse, affecting both intra- and inter-prismatic enamel. Prism junctions would appear to be sites of preferential dissolution, with narrow channels occurring between prisms (Fig. 6.5) (Johnson 1967*a*, *b*). In these areas, crystallites larger than those in sound enamel may be seen, which probably represent areas of recrystalization. Carious destruction of individual crystals results in loss of crystal centres and in surface damage.

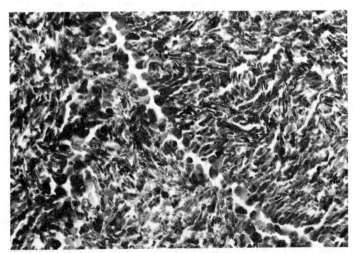

Fig. 6.5. Electronmicrograph showing parts of two transversely sectioned prisms from carious enamel. Inter-crystallite space containing embedding material can be differentiated from artefact. A double row of enlarged, polyhedral cells is present at the prism junction lining a channel which is largely artefact, but which does contain Araldite. This is seen where it forms a halo to the crystals. The majority of crystals are irregular flattened hexagons with central deficiencies. × 42 500. (By courtesy of Professor N.W. Johnson.)

DENTAL CARIES AND THE ORGANIC MATRIX OF ENAMEL

As enamel mineralizes much of its organic contents disappear so that the mature tissue contains relatively little organic material.

For many years there has been argument as to whether the initial lesion of enamel caries was caused by demineralization or by alteration of the organic matrix. Microdissection techniques have been developed which allow the various histological zones of enamel caries, as seen with the light microscope, to be dissected out and analysed chemically. Such experiments have shown that mineral is lost from the translucent zone with no evidence of change in the organic matrix (Hallsworth *et al.* 1972). Thus, it is now thought that demineralization precedes organic destruction.

However, the role of the organic matrix in the initiation and progress of caries is not fully known. It has been shown by microchemical studies that the composition of interior enamel is variable with pockets of high and low mineral content (Robinson *et al.* 1971). Mineral content has been found to correlate inversely with protein distribution. It might be thought that areas of comparatively low mineralization and increased protein would be more susceptible to acid attack. However, enamel protein could be protective by preventing the spread of the small ions responsible for dissolving mineral. It is known that fluorosed enamel, which is relatively poorly mineralized, is remarkably resistant to acid attack (Kidd *et al.* 1978). This could be related to its high protein content. Alternatively, the high level of fluoride in the tissue may be the important factor.

It is thought that the organic content of carious enamel is greater than that of sound tissue. The organic material is of exogenous origin, bacterial or salivary, but little is known of the effect this has on the carious process.

ARRESTED LESIONS

It is important to realize that enamel lesions do not automatically progress and the clinician will frequently see arrested carious lesions. These are particularly common on proximal surfaces where the adjacent tooth is missing (Fig. 6.2). Such lesions commonly are heavily stained and it has been suggested that extraction of the adjacent tooth changes the environment so that the lesion becomes more cleansable and accessible to saliva.

Another situation where arrested lesions are commonly seen is cervically where bands of demineralized enamel, which formed during tooth eruption, are left 'high and dry' as passive eruption occurs. This arrest of the carious process may allow some redeposition of mineral (remineralization) within the lesion, which probably explains why these chronic lesions in old teeth appear quite different histologically from acute lesions. Sometimes a white spot lesion can actually disappear. A well-known example of this is found in the work of Backer-Dirks (1966), who studied 184 buccal surfaces of maxillary first molars in the same children at age 8 and again at age 15. Of 72 surfaces with white spots at age 8, 37 appeared sound at age 15. Alternatively, a white spot lesion may lose the matt surface indicative of active disease and become shiny. Clean, dry teeth, viewed with magnification, are required to detect these clinically relevant visual changes.

EVIDENCE OF REMINERALIZATION FROM EXPERIMENTAL CARIES IN MAN

The concept of arrest and partial remineralization of the carious lesion has attracted a great deal of research interest, and several experiments have been carried out *in vivo*.

When blocks of enamel, covered with Teflon gauze to facilitate bacterial colonization, were mounted in removable bridges in the mouths of human subjects, the enamel blocks showed surface softening as detected by micro-hardness testing. When the gauze was removed, to expose the enamel to the saliva *in vivo*, an increase in hardness occurred in the test blocks. This increase in hardness was thought to be due to remineralization (Koulourides 1966).

In subsequent work with the same method (Koulourides *et al.* 1980), fluoride solutions were used to encourage remineralization. Subsequently the 'healed' lesions were again covered with gauze to create a cariogenic environment. The enamel which had remineralized was now found to be more resistant to dental caries than an adjacent area of sound enamel which had not previously been exposed. It thus seems possible that a remineralized white spot lesion may be more resistant to carious attack than sound enamel.

Other experiments have been carried out on teeth destined for extraction. Plates or bands were placed on the teeth to induce plaque accumulation and thus produce a cariogenic environment. Once lesions had formed, the plates or bands were removed to expose the enamel to the oral fluids. Remineralization occurred and the lesions either disappeared or remained as hard, discoloured areas (Von der Fehr 1965; Holmen *et al.* 1987).

Experimental caries has also been induced with sucrose mouth rinses in human subjects over a 23-day period. After this time, oral hygiene procedures were recommenced and the subjects used daily mouth rinses with 0.2 per cent sodium fluoride solutions for 1 month. Caries scores showed regression or 'healing' of the experimental lesions during the fluoride mouth-rinsing regime (Von der Fehr *et al.* 1970).

THE CLINICAL RELEVANCE OF ARREST AND REMINERALIZATION

As caries progression is not inevitable an important role for the dentist is the early diagnosis of caries. The dentist can then show the patient how to arrest the disease by dietary control, judicious use of fluorides, and effective plaque removal. These diagnostic and preventive efforts are just as much *treatment* of the disease as is operative dentistry, and should be recognized and rewarded as such.

It is important to realize that once cavitation occurs, remineralization will not 'fill up the hole'. Indeed the cavity will favour progression rather than arrest if it hinders effective plaque removal. This does not mean, however, that cavitated lesions will automatically progress, because if they are cleansable and if the diet is modified, the disease can still be arrested.

CLINICAL DETECTION OF THE ENAMEL LESION

The diagnosis of caries requires good lighting and dry, clean teeth. If heavy deposits of plaque or calculus are present the mouth should be cleaned before attempting accurate diagnosis.

FREE SMOOTH SURFACES

Enamel lesions are easily seen on free, smooth surfaces and can be diagnosed at the stage of the white or brown spot lesion, before cavitation has occurred, provided the teeth are clean, dry and well lit (Fig. 6.6). Traditionally, sharp probes have also been used to detect the 'tacky' feel of early cavitation. However, this approach should *not* be used because the sharp probe can physically damage an incipient carious lesion.

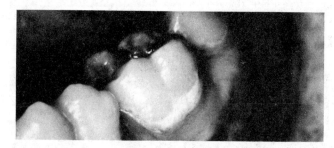

Fig. 6.6. White spot lesions on the buccal aspect of first and second molars.

PITS AND FISSURES

While caries on free smooth surfaces is easy to see, caries in pits and fissures is difficult to diagnose at this early stage because, histologically, the white spot lesion forms on the walls of the fissure. Thus, the fissure which looks clinically caries-free may histologically show signs of an early lesion. In addition, the fissure that is sticky to a sharp probe may not be carious histologically. The stickiness may relate to the fissure shape or the pressure exerted rather than caries, and indeed a sharp probe can actually damage an incipient carious lesion. The probe should be used to remove any plaque from the fissure to allow sharp eyes to pick up discoloration, cavitation, and the grey appearance of enamel undermined by caries in the dentine beneath. Despite all this care, however, occlusal lesions penetrating into dentine are frequently missed (Kidd *et al.* 1993). It is important to remember that clinical cavitation may represent a relatively late presentation of the carious process particularly since the widespread use of fluoride toothpastes. In addition, the concept of dental caries being exclusively a disease of young, newly erupted teeth is no longer tenable. Fluoride delays lesion progression thus the carious process may present at the cavitation level in young adults as well as in children.

Today bitewing radiographs are essential in the diagnosis of occlusal caries although by the time a lesion can be seen on radiograph it is well into dentine. It must be appreciated that large dentine lesions may be present in teeth which appear clinically sound. This phenomenon has been called occult or hidden caries. (Weerheijm *et al.* 1992).

Thus the early diagnosis of caries in pits and fissures is difficult and is giving rise to considerable concern among practitioners. However, help may be on the way in the form of an electronic caries detector (Rock and Kidd 1988). The principle behind this machine is that the spaces in the porous tissue fill with fluid and therefore the electrical conductivity increases with increasing demineralization. A machine was produced commercially (Vanguard Electronic Caries Detector) where a battery-generated current was applied to the fissure through a probe (Fig. 6.7). The probe was placed co-axially in an air tube which dries the tooth surface, and the machine gave a digital read-out varying from 0 to 9, representing increasing degrees of demineralization. The possibility may well exist for monitoring progression or arrest of early enamel fissure lesions in this way. Unfortunately, this machine is no longer commercially available but there is now a resurgence of interest in the technique and a Dutch physicist is developing a new machine for use by practitioners (Ricketts *et al.* 1993).

contact point. A carious lesion has a lowered index of light transmission and therefore appears as a dark shadow that follows the outline of the decay through the dentine. This technique has been used for many years in the diagnosis of approximal lesions in anterior teeth. Light is reflected through the teeth using the dental mirror and the carious lesions are seen readily in the mirror. In posterior teeth a stronger light source is required and fibre-optic lights, with the beam reduced to 0.5 mm in diameter, have been used (Mitropoulus 1985). However, the technique is unreliable in the diagnosis of the enamel lesion although once the caries is in dentine, reliability improves.

The bitewing radiograph is still the most important diagnostic tool for approximal caries but the technique is relatively insensitive and is not able to detect early subsurface demineralization. The earliest radiographic sign of approximal caries is seen on a bitewing radiograph as a small, triangular radiolucent area just cervical to the contact point (Fig. 6.8). Although the lesion appears confined the outer enamel, histological examination shows that it penetrates into the underlying dentine.

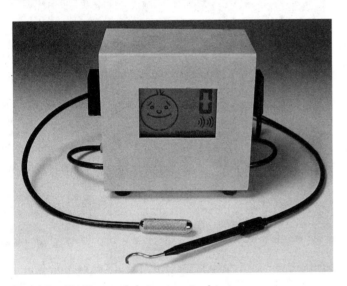

Fig. 6.7. The Vanguard electronic caries detector.

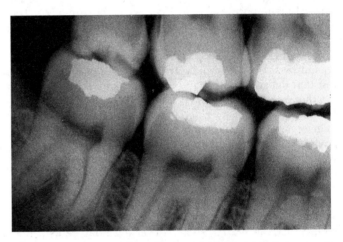

Fig. 6.8. A bitewing radiograph showing early carious lesions on the distal surface (46) and the mesial surface (47).

APPROXIMAL SURFACES

As with the fissure, it will be difficult to see the enamel lesion on an approximal surface. Vision is obscured by the adjacent tooth. The lesion is discovered visually at a relatively late stage when it has already progressed into dentine and is seen as a pinkish grey area shining up through the marginal ridge.

It is, however, possible to insert circles of elastic between teeth to separate them. This technique is extensively used in orthodontic treatment when bands are to be placed on teeth. An interdental gap of 0.5–1.0 mm is readily produced in 48 hours. The method is non-destructive, reversible, and inexpensive, and may be a useful aid in the diagnosis and management of some lesions (Pitts 1987).

Visual diagnosis can be aided by the use of transmitted light. The technique consists of shining light through the

Unfortunately, in spite of rigorous attempts to standardize all aspects of the radiographic method and viewing techniques, visual estimates of lesion size remain subjective and liable to considerable error. Beam aiming and film holding devices, which automatically aim the central ray at the centre of the film, should be used in practice to ensure that reproducible radiographs are taken (Pitts and Kidd 1992). Only then may such radiographs be used to monitor lesion progression or arrest.

THE RELEVANCE OF THE DIAGNOSTIC INFORMATION TO THE MANAGEMENT OF THE DISEASE

The preceding section has discussed the clinical methods available for the detection of the enamel lesion. How should this information be used clinically? First of all it is important to remember that clinical and radiographic diagnoses may be inaccurate. No one can be sure of recording the same caries diagnosis on different occasions on one patient and even the trained epidemiologist in only 70 to 80 per cent reliable.

Once lesions have been recognized, consideration should be given to what these appearances mean in the particular mouth being examined. In a young child or young adult this appearance may be indicative of active and progressive disease. Unless preventive measures are instituted, cavitation will occur as the disease progresses. A similar appearance in the mouth of an older person might indicate a period of active disease some years earlier. Alternatively, this same picture could indicate a recent change in diet, such as sweets substituted for cigarettes, and active disease which will progress unless prevented.

As with all clinical problems, a careful history from the patient is of obvious importance. In addition, knowledge of the mouth as it was months and years previously is invaluable.

The frequency of radiographic examination depends on a caries risk assessment and such assessment is fundamental to contemporary practice so that preventive efforts may be sensibly targeted (Pitts and Kidd 1992). Unfortunately, caries risk assessment is difficult and no one method, or combination of methods, has yet been developed that can be used reliably to predict future caries activity in individuals. However, clinical observation of signs or symptoms of past disease experience still seems to be the most significant predictor. Thus, a thorough clinical examination showing multiple primary and/or recurrent carious lesions (whether these are small sub-surface lesions or open cavities), a heavily restored dentition with missing teeth and multiple endodontic treatments may be taken to indicate a high-risk individual. The pattern of caries attack is also relevant. Individuals developing lesions on smooth surfaces, or anterior teeth, or on exposed root surfaces, are high risk. In some high-risk individuals many sites will be involved, in others the caries attack may be focused more towards one type of site; for example, pits and fissures or approximal surfaces. Similarly, a history of extractions for caries and multiple new restorations for new decay should alert the practitioner.

To this picture can be added factors which in themselves have so far been shown to be less reliable but, taken with the above, may be relevant. Such factors include social deprivation, irregular attendance, poor oral hygiene, an unfavourable diet or fluoride history and, for a child, the condition of the mother's teeth. Medical problems which cause reduced salivary flow, such as radiotherapy in the region of the salivary glands for a head and neck malignancy, and Sjögren's syndrome, are also highly relevant, and medication known to induce xerostomia may be important.

If the clinician detects multiple white spot lesions and decides that these represent active disease, the correct treatment is to institute prevention and observe the lesions rather than to attack them immediately with the dental drill. Plaque control and dietary advice are of obvious importance. As the fluoride ion appears to be so important in remineralization, some form of topical fluoride therapy should be begun. It would appear that the remineralization effect requires the presence of the fluoride ion in the fluid environment of the tooth surface. For this reason, frequent, low-dose, topical applications such as fluoridated water, toothpastes, mouth rinses, and tablets, would seem particularly useful. On occlusal surfaces a fissure sealant is a sensible additional preventive measure.

SECONDARY CARIES

Dentists spend a considerable amount of their time and derive a substantial part of their income from replacing restorations in teeth. One in three restorations present at any time is unsatisfactory and has failed to meet the clinical criteria commonly used to define success (Elderton 1976). Secondary caries is often the single most important factor given by dentists for the replacement of restorations and yet dentists vary widely in their treatment planning decisions (Elderton and Nuttall 1983). This must call into question the ability of dentists to diagnose caries within restored teeth.

HISTOLOGICAL FEATURES OF THE EARLY LESION

When a filling is placed, the adjacent enamel may be considered in two planes: the surface enamel and the enamel of the cavity wall. For this reason, a secondary carious lesion has been described as occurring in two parts; an 'outer lesion' formed on the surface of the tooth as a result of primary attack and cavity 'wall lesion', which will only be seen if hydrogen ions can pass between the restoration and the cavity wall.

The early secondary carious lesion in enamel is most clearly seen in polarized light when ground sections are imbibed with quinoline. In this medium, the wall lesion appears as either a translucent zone or a dark zone extending along the cavity wall. If the lesion reaches the enamel-dentine junction, it spreads laterally to involve the dentine on a wider front (Plates 6.11 and 6.12). An outer lesion may also be present (Plate 6.11). Examination of sections after imbibition with water will reveal areas of enamel demineralization in excess of 5 per cent as positively birefringent (Plate 6.13).

THE PREVENTION OF SECONDARY CARIES

It appears that the interface between a restoration and the dental tissue is susceptible to demineralization whenever leakage of bacteria, fluids, molecules, or ions can occur between a cavity wall and the restorative material applied to it. This clinically undetectable leakage around restorations has come to be referred to as 'microleakage' and has been extensively investigated over the last 30 years (see review by Kidd 1976).

Many techniques have been devised to test the cavity sealing properties of restorations both *in vitro* and *in vivo*. These include the use of dyes, radioactive isotopes, air pressure, bacteria, neutron activation analysis, scanning electron microscopy, and artificial caries. The salient point in all this work is that all filling materials leak and therefore, in a caries-prone mouth, all restorations may potentially fail because of recurrent caries. Thus, restorations cannot be regarded as a treatment for dental caries. Fillings merely replace missing tissue with a poor substitute for unblemished enamel and dentine. The management of dental caries, be it primary or secondary, rests with assessing risk and reducing the rate of caries progression by dietary control, judicious use of fluorides, and plaque control.

However, there are measures the clinician can take during the restoration of teeth which make secondary caries less likely (Elderton 1987) and these measures will now be discussed.

Plaque Control and Restorative Technique

It is well known that caries forms in areas of plaque stagnation. The junction between a restoration and a tooth is a potential plaque trap and it is important that this area can be cleaned easily. For many years it was held that cavity margins be finished in 'self-cleansing' areas but it is now known that 'self-cleansing' is an unreliable method of plaque control. Thus, cavity margins should normally allow access for tooth-brush filaments, dental floss, or interdental wood points. This implies that on occlusal surfaces, cavity margins should not be finished in deep fissures where plaque would tend to collect unless these fissures are sealed, as in the sealant (preventive resin) restoration (Simonsen 1978).

Approximally, the bucco-axial and linguo-axial margins of the Class II cavity should not be finished at the contact point but brought into the embrasure so that they may be cleaned with a toothbrush. It could, of course, be argued that if patients were routinely to use dental floss this would not be necessary. However, finishing these margins in a cleansable area has the added advantage that the dentist is able to see the margin to check it at subsequent visits. Cavity margins should also be placed coronal to gingival margin wherever possible, because subgingival margins encourage plaque accumulation and therefore recurrent caries and periodontal disease.

Ditching is a particular problem with amalgam restorations (Plate 6.15). As early as 1895, G.V. Black noted this appearance and attributed it to deformation under the stress of mastication. Recent research has confirmed this observation as it has been shown that those amalgams with the lowest creep rate display the least incidence of marginal breakdown. The high copper-content alloys show a significant reduction in creep rate in comparison with conventional alloys and in addition are more resistant to corrosion. Jorgensen (1965) has suggested that the mechanism of marginal fracture is related to corrosion, so these newer alloys are likely to show improved marginal adaptation and clinical trials have confirmed this (Duperon *et al.* 1971).

In addition, ditching may be reduced by attention to detail in cavity preparation. As amalgam is a brittle material the amalgam-margin angle must exceed 70° as angles less than this are prone to fracture (Elderton 1984).

Although ditched margins may predispose to plaque accumulation and therefore caries, restorations with ditched margins should not automatically be replaced. Histological examination of extracted teeth with occlusal restorations with both ditched and unditched margins showed a low prevalence of carious lesions in the outer enamel and wall lesions in 54 per cent of specimens irrespective of whether the margin was defective or sound (Kidd and O'Hara 1990). In addition, research has shown that replacement restorations frequently contain the same in-built errors as their predecessors (Elderton 1977). Thus, where a margin is severely ditched, it may be more logical to repair that part of the restoration, concentrating efforts on improving it. Alternatively, ditched restorations may be accepted and put under review so that they may serve a little longer. This approach would seem particularly applicable in mouths which are not caries-prone.

Ditching is not the only discrepancy of fit than can hinder plaque control. Overhanging margins, which are particularly likely to occur gingivally, are very difficult to clean, encouraging both caries and periodontal diseases.

Every effort should be made to achieve a smooth junction between restoration and tooth by careful use of matrix bands and wedges, and by meticulous carving as soon as the band is removed. Despite all this care, ledges may still occur and may be obvious on bitewing radiographs. Such ledges should be removed by grinding with abrasive strips or with specially designed reciprocating handpieces and diamond-coated points or rotary instruments. Alternatively the restoration should be replaced.

Choice of Restorative Material in Posterior Teeth

Amalgam alloy is the material most commonly used in the restoration of posterior teeth. The freshly packed amalgam restoration has been shown to leak but cavity seal is improved when restorations have been in the mouth for some time (Nelson *et al.* 1952). This phenomenon has been attributed to the formation of corrosion products at the amalgam/dental tissue interface. Thus, corrosion of the alloy, a property long deplored by clinicians, may be responsible for its success in giving long clinical service (for review see Kidd 1976).

Many studies have shown that the initial leakage around an amalgam restoration may be minimized by applying a thin layer of cavity varnish to the walls and floor of the cavity before packing the amalgam. Little information is available on the duration of this beneficial effect, but it may prevent leakage around the freshly packed filling until corrosion products form and block the microspace between restoration and cavity wall. It would seem wise, therefore, to use a cavity varnish routinely in the caries-prone mouth.

Cast gold inlays are an alternative to amalgam for the restoration of posterior teeth. In any cast restoration the gap between restoration and tooth is filled by cement. It is thus obvious that the cavity sealing ability of a gold inlay is dependent on the seal of the cement lute. Unfortunately, very little research work has been done on the cavity sealing ability of such cemented restorations, either in the laboratory or in the mouth. However, a limited comparison of zinc phosphate and glass ionomer cement using an *in vitro* artificial-caries system has shown that secondary caries-like lesions were formed adjacent to both materials. In addition, it is known that the commonly used luting agents are to some extent soluble in the oral fluids. For these reasons, current teaching is that cemented restorations are positively contraindicated in the caries-prone mouth.

When composite resin materials first appeared on the market, it was hoped that their physical properties would make them suitable for posterior teeth. However, clinical trials showed that abrasion of the material led to a loss of anatomical form over the years. As far as recurrent caries was concerned, clinical trials carried out in dental hospitals were reassuring (for review see Barnes and Kidd 1980) but many practitioners reported a high incidence of recurrent caries around these restorations. It is interesting to speculate why clinical trials and general practitioner experience differed. It is possible that caries-susceptible patients were not used in the clinical trials. In addition, there may have been differences in the way the two groups handled the materials.

With the advent of newer, more highly filled, composite materials, designed specifically for use in posterior teeth, the subject has come under discussion again. It appears that the wear resistance of the new materials is greatly improved but resistance to recurrent caries at the cervical margin of the Class II cavity may be poor, despite the fact that composites are bonded to enamel via the acid-etch technique and to dentine via bonding resins.

The problem is that these materials shrink as they set (Kidd 1985) and any adhesive material that shrinks in this way will move towards the stronger bond as it polymerizes. As the bond with the thick enamel of the axial wall is stronger than the bond with the thin enamel or dentine at the cervical margin, a gap is likely to form in this area. The fact that the materials are light cured could exacerbate the problem because the surface nearest the light sets first and the material then shrinks towards the light, that is away from the cervical margin. To help to solve this problem light-reflectant wedges have been produced, and the polymerizing light is then applied buccally and reflected into the cervical area.

A novel concept in treatment of approximal caries has been to use an occlusal approach to the carious lesion which preserves the marginal ridge. This is called the internal cavity preparation (McLean and Gasser 1985). The cavity is restored with a glass ionomer cement or silver cermet, which are injected through the occlusal access cavity. This is an ingenious idea because it preserves as much sound tooth as possible while restoring the lesion with a fluoride-releasing material. The material adheres to enamel and dentine and may thus support and strengthen the tissues. The results of clinical trials are awaited with interest.

Choice of Restorative Material in Anterior Teeth

When restoring intracoronal cavities in anterior teeth the clinician may choose to use composite resin, glass ionomer cement, or a combination of the two. With the composite materials acid-etching of the enamel, possibly combined with bevelling of the cavity wall, should improve marginal seal.

Glass ionomer cement contains available fluoride which will exert a cariostatic effect (Kidd 1978). This makes it the material of choice in a caries-prone mouth. The material also has the advantage of being chemically adhesive to enamel and dentine. Thus, where cavities are bounded by both enamel and dentine, it is possible to use glass ionomer cement to replace the missing dentine, then etch this material and the adjacent enamel before adding composite resin to complete the restoration (McLean *et al.* 1985).

Patient Education and Review

The responsibility for patient care neither begins nor ends with the placement of a restoration. Unless patients are educated and motivated to prevent disease, time and money will be wasted. The experienced clinician will have learnt this by hard experience as, unless myopic or peripatetic, he will have seen his work fail over the years.

Having completed the restorative part of a treatment plan, every attempt must be made to ensure that the patient is able to clean perfectly around the restorations. This is particularly important where Class II restorations, crowns, or bridges are present. Interdental cleaning is obligatory (see Chapter 8, p. 126). Attempts should be made to find out whether the advice given on diet is being followed (see Chapter 2). Consideration must also be given to whether some form of topical fluoride therapy, such as mouth rinses should be continued. Finally, the dentist must decide when the patient should be seen again. The timing of the recall appointment will be based on the state of the mouth when the patient originally presented and the patient's response to preventive measures during treatment.

PROBLEMS IN DIAGNOSIS OF CARIES IN RESTORED TEETH

One of the tasks of the dentist at the recall visit is to inspect restorations for any sign of new disease. This is so much a part of the everyday practice that the reader may consider the process is straightforward. However, the problems are enormous and a search for their solution is probably one of the most pressing problems in preventive dentistry today.

One problem is the filling with a defective margin, particularly the ditched amalgam restoration (Plate 6.15). There is a widely held view that recurrent caries is largely the result of marginal failure of restorations (Goldberg *et al.* 1981) and it has become common dental practice and teaching to replace defective restorations as a preventive procedure. The laboratory study of Jorgensen and Wakumoto (1968) is often quoted to support this approach. In this study, caries was not found in gaps smaller than 35–50 µm but the larger the marginal defect, the more likely it was to develop secondary caries. However, this latter correlation was only found at fissure sites and it is possible that primary caries was being diagnosed rather than recurrent disease. Recent laboratory studies have shown a poor correlation between caries prevalence and marginal defects (Soderholm *et al.* 1989; Kidd and O'Hara 1990; Kidd *et al.* 1994).

Another problem to be considered in the diagnosis of caries in restored teeth is whether the dentist can distinguish new, recurrent caries around a restoration from residual caries that the dentist left during cavity preparation.

Two studies (Anderson and Charbeneau 1985; Kidd *et al.* 1989 have shown how commonly dentists leave residual caries in cavities. These investigations used caries detector dyes (Fusayama and Terachima 1972) in cavities passed as clinically satisfactory by teachers at a dental school. It is claimed that this red dye enhances the visual recognition of dentinal caries by staining the infected demineralized dentine which should be removed during cavity preparation (Plates 6.16, 6.17) but leaving unstained dentine which is only mildly demineralized, not infected, and capable of remineralization.

These studies showed that parts of the enamel–dentine junction were stained red by the dyes in over 50 per cent of teeth where cavities had been passed as clinically satisfactory using ordinary visual and tactile criteria. However, this is the very area where it is currently taught that the cavity should be made clinically caries-free because it is argued that residual caries in this area may flourish beneath a leaking restoration. It is thought-provoking that dentists cannot even diagnose caries within cavities when they can look directly at it and use probes! Fortunately, subsequent microbiological sampling of dye-stained and dye-unstained sites resulted in the recovery of low levels of bacteria and revealed no difference in the level of infection of the two sites (Kidd *et al.* 1993).

Thus, to judge by these studies the incidence of residual demineralization is very high indeed. Will this residual demineralization progress? Logic suggests that the relevant factor is what happens in the plaque at the tooth surface because recurrent caries may be inevitable if a cariogenic plaque with a suitable dietary substrate remains.

One further problem in the diagnosis of caries within restored teeth is distinguishing active caries, which is likely to progress, from chronic, static lesions that are already arrested. Currently, there are no clinical criteria on which to base this judgement.

CLINICAL METHODS TO DIAGNOSE RECURRENT CARIES IN RESTORED TEETH

As in the diagnosis of primary caries, the clinician needs good lighting, dry clean teeth, sharp eyes but 'blunt' probes, and good bitewing radiographs. Recurrent disease occurs more frequently at cervical and approximal margins so particular care must be taken in these areas (Mjor 1985).

A freshly cavitated lesion adjacent to a restoration will be obvious clinically (Plate 6.14) but sharp eyes may also pick up the pink, grey, or brown appearance of enamel undermined by caries (Plate 6.18).

Marginal staining of composite restorations produces considerable difficulty in diagnosis. Such staining represents marginal deterioration, but is this necessarily synonomous with caries?

The colour of corrosion products around amalgam restorations can also cause diagnostic problems as this grey or blue discoloration may also indicate caries (Plate 6.19).

Once again it is relevant to consider whether the discoloured area is new caries or residual disease. It has been suggested that arrested or slowly progressing dentine lesions are darkly staining (Miller and Massler 1962); such stain is probably picked up from exogenous dietary sources. If recurrent lesions pick up stain in a similar way it is possible that those lesions which are most obvious clinically because of their colour, may be the ones that are inactive, arrested, or slowly progressing! The interpretation of the relevance of stain around a restoration where the margin is clinically intact is a major problem to which there is no obvious answer at present (Kidd *et al.* 1994).

Sharp probes should be used with as much care in the diagnosis of caries around restorations as in the diagnosis of primary disease. The probe may catch in a marginal discrepancy which is not carious or it may cause damage to the cavity margin or the filling. Despite these reservations, a curved probe is helpful cervically where evidence from bitewing radiographs is difficult to interpret. However, the probe should be used with a light touch not a heavy hand.

Bitewing radiographs are very important in the diagnosis of caries within restored teeth although they usually reveal the caries once it is in dentine rather than showing the early lesion. Provided that the restorative material is radiopaque, the bitewing can be of value in detecting caries both proximally and occlusally.

THE CONSEQUENCES OF DIAGNOSTIC DIFFICULTIES

An experiment has been conducted where nine dentists were asked to examine in the laboratory specific areas of 228 extracted and filled teeth and indicate whether caries was present and the treatment that was required (Merrett and Elderton 1984). They found that caries was clearly considered to be a good reason for treatment in that these dentists proposed to treat 95 per cent of the teeth in which they diagnosed it. The teeth were then sectioned and the presence or absence of caries determined. Unfortunately, there was a considerable lack of correspondence between the teeth in which caries was identified as present in the laboratory after sectioning and those in which it was assessed as present in the simulated clinical examinations.

One consequence of this depressing finding is that clinicians, and those who fund them, must currently accept that fillings may be done unnecessarily, or that caries may be missed and therefore the appropriate preventive and operative measures not taken. It is also currently inevitable that dentists will not agree in their diagnoses. This creates enormous problems for the practitioner who must continue to provide care in an uncertain situation. The academic is privileged to be paid to address these problems and teachers should discuss them with students.

SUMMARY

- The carious process is characterized by alternating periods of destruction and arrest.

- Primary and secondary carious lesions form in areas of plaque stagnation.

- Since caries progression is not inevitable, an important role for the dentist is the early diagnosis of caries.

- Caries diagnosis requires good lighting, dry clean teeth and good bitewing radiographs.

- Enamel caries can be arrested by effective plaque control, dietary control and judicious use of fluoride. This is preventive treatment.

- Cavitation favours lesion progression because it hinders plaque removal. Operative treatment may now be required.

REFERENCES

Anderson. M.H. and Charbeneau, G.T. (1985). A comparison of digital and optical criteria for detecting carious dentine. *J. prosthet. Dent.* **53**, 643–6.

Anderson, M.H., Loesch, W.J., and Charbeneau, G.T. (1985). Bacteriologic study of a basic fuchsin caries-disclosing dye. *J. prosthet. Dent.* **54**, 51–5.

Backer-Dirks, O. (1966). Post-eruptive changes in dental enamel. *J. dent. Res.* **45**, 503–11.

Barnes, I.E. and Kidd, E.A.M. (1980). Composite resin restorative materials—a review, *Dent Update*, **7**, 273–83.

Black, G.V. (1895). An investigation of the physical characters of the human teeth in relation to their disease, and to practical dental operations, together with the physical characters of filling materials. *Dent. Cosmos*, **37**, 553–71.

Black, G.V. (1908). *A work on operative dentistry*, Vol. I. *The pathology of the hard tissues of the teeth.* Medico-Dental Publishing Company, Chicago.

Crabb, H.S.M. (1966). Enamel caries. Observations on the histology and patterns of progress of the approximal lesion. *Br. dent. J.* **121**, 115–29.

Darling, A.I., Mortimer, K.V., Poole, D.F.G., and Ollis, W.D. (1961). Molecular sieve behaviour of normal and carious human dental enamel. *Archs. oral Biol.* **5**, 251–73.

Duperon, D.F., Neville, M.D., and Kasloff, Z. (1971). Clinical evaluation of corrosion resistance of conventional alloy, spherical-particle alloy and dispersion-phase alloys. *J. prosthet. Dent.* **25**, 650–6.

Elderton, R.J. (1976). The prevalence of failure of restorations: a literature review. *J. Dent.* **4**, 207–10.

Elderton, R.J. (1977). The quality of amalgam restorations. In *Assessment of the quality of dental care*, (ed. H. Allred), pp. 45–81. London Hospital Medical College.

Elderton, R.J. and Nuttall, N.M. (1983). Variation among dentists in planning treatment. *Br. dent. J.* **154**, 201–6.

Elderton, R.J. (1984). Cavo-surface angles, amalgam-margin angles and occlusal cavity preparations. *Br. dent. J.* **156**, 319–24.

Elderton, R.J. (1987). Preventively-orientated restorations and restorative procedures. In *Positive dental prevention*, pp. 82–92. Heinemann, London.

Fusayama, T. and Terachima, S. (1972). Differentiation of two layers of carious dentine by staining. *J. dent. Res.* **51**, 866.

Goldberg. J., Tanzer, J., Munster, E., Amara, J., Thal, F., and Birkhead, D. (1981). Cross sectional clinical evaluation of recurrent enamel caries, restoration of marginal integrity and oral hygiene status. *J. Am. dent. Ass.* **102**, 635–41.

Hallsworth, A.S., Robinson, C., and Weatherell. J.A. (1972). Mineral and magnesium distribution within the approximal carious lesion of dental enamel. *Caries Res.* **6**, 156–68.

Holmen, L., Thylstrup, A., and Artun, J. (1987). Clinical and histological features observed during arrestment of active enamel carious lesions *in vivo*. *Caries Res.* **21**, 546–54.

Johnson, N.W. (1967a). Transmission electron microscopy of early carious enamel. *Caries Res.* **1**, 356–69.

Johnson, N.W. (1967b). Some aspects of the ultrastructure of early human enamel caries seen with the electron microscope. *Archs. oral Biol.* **12**, 1505–21.

Jorgensen, K.D. (1965). The mechanism of marginal fracture of amalgam fillings. *Acta odont. Scand.* **23**, 347–89.

Jorgensen, K.D. and Wakumoto, S. (1968). Occlusal amalgam fillings: marginal defects and secondary caries. *Odont. Tids.* **76**, 43–53.

Kidd, E.A.M. (1976). Microleakage: a review. *J. Dent.* **4**, 199–206.

Kidd, E.A.M. (1978). Cavity sealing ability of composite and glass ionomer restorations. An assessment *in vitro*. *Br. dent. J.* **144**, 139–42.

Kidd, E.A.M. (1983). The histopathology of enamel caries in young and old permanent teeth. *Br. dent. J.* **155**, 196–8.

Kidd, E.A.M. (1985). Microleakage and shrinkage. In *Posterior composite resin dental materials*, (ed. G. Vanherle and D. Smith) pp. 263–8. 3M Co.

Kidd, E.A.M., Thylstrup, A., Fejerskov, O., and Silverstone, L.M. (1978). Histopathology of caries-like lesions created *in vitro* in fluorosed and sound enamel. *Caries Res.* **12**, 268–74.

Kidd, E.A.M., Joyston-Bechal, S., Smith, M.M., Allan, R., Howe, L., and Smith, S.R. (1989). The use of a caries detector dye in cavity preparation. *Br. dent. J.* **167**, 132–4.

Kidd, E.A.M., and O' Hara, J.W. (1990). The caries status of occlusal amalgam restorations with marginal defects. *J. dent. Res.* **69**, 1275–7.

Kidd, E.A.M., Toffenetti F., and Mjör, I.A. (1992). Secondary caries. *Int. dent. J.* **42**, 127–38.

Kidd, E.A.M., Joyston-Bechal, S., and Beighton, D. (1993). The use of a caries detector dye during cavity preparation: a microbiological assessment. *Br. dent. J.* **174**, 245–8.

Kidd, E.A.M., Ricketts, D.N.J., and Pitts, N.B. (1993). Occlusal caries diagnosis: a changing challenge for clinicians and epidemiologists. *J. Dent.* **21**, 323–31.

Kidd, E.A.M., Joyston-Bechal, S., and Beighton, D. (1994). Diagnosis of secondary caries: a laboratory study. *Br. dent. J.* **176**, 135–9.

Kostlan, J. (1962). Translucent zones in the central part of the carious lesion of enamel. *Br. dent. J.* **113**, 244–8.

Koulourides, T. (1966). Dynamics of tooth surface—oral fluid equilibrium. *Adv. oral Biol.* **2**, 149–71.

Koulourides, T., Keller, S.E., Manson-Hing, L., and Lilley, V. (1980). Enhancement of fluoride effectiveness by experimental cariogenic priming of human enamel. *Caries Res.* **14**, 32–9.

McLean, J.W. and Gasser, O. (1985). Glass-cermet cements. *Quintess. Int.* **16**, 333–43.

McLean, J.W., Prosser, H.J., and Wilson, A.D. (1985). The use of glass-ionomer cements in bonding composite resins to dentine. *Br. dent. J.* **158**, 410–14.

Merrett, M.C.W. and Elderton, R.J. (1984). An *in vitro* study of restorative dental treatment decisions and dental caries. *Br. dent. J.* **157**, 128–33.

Mjor, I.A. (1985). Frequency of secondary caries at various anatomical locations. *Oper. Dent.* **10**, 88–92.

Miller, W.A. and Massler, M. (1962). Permeability and staining of active and arrested lesions in dentine. *Br. dent. J.* **112**, 187–97.

Mitropoulos, C.M. (1985). A comparison of fibreoptic trans-illumination with bitewing radiographs. *Br. dent. J.* **159**, 21–3.

Mortimer, K.V. (1964). Some histological features of fissure caries in enamel. *Eur. Org. caries Res.* **2**, 85–94.

Nelson, R.J., Wolcott, R.B., and Paffenbarger, G.C. (1952). Fluid exchange at the margins of dental restorations. *J. Am. dent. Ass.* **44**, 288–95.

Pitts, N.B. (1987). Temporary tooth separation with special reference to the diagnosis and management of equivocal approximal carious lesions. *Quintess. Int.* **18**, 563–73.

Pitts, N.B. and Kidd, E.A.M. (1992). Some of the factors to be considered in the prescription and timing of bitewing radiography in the diagnosis and management of dental caries. *J. Dent.* **20**, 74–84.

Pitts, N.B. and Kidd, E.A.M. (1992). The prescription and timing of bitewing radiography in the diagnosis and management of dental caries: contemporary recommendations. *Br. dent.* **172**, 225–7.

Ricketts, D.N.J., Kidd, E.A.M., Liepins, P., and Wilson, R.F. (1993). Evaluation of electrical impedance changes in the detection of fissure caries *in vivo*. *Caries Res.* **27**, 207.

Robinson, C., Weatherell, J.A., and Hallsworth, A.S. (1971). Variation in composition of dental enamel within thin ground sections. *Caries Res.* **5**, 44–57.

Rock, W.P. and Kidd, E.A.M. (1988). The electronic detection of demineralization in occlusal fissures. *Br. dent. J.* **164**, 243–7.

Silverstone, L.M. (1966). The primary translucent zone of enamel caries and of artificial caries-like lesions. *Br. dent. J.* **120**, 461–71.

Silverstone, L.M., (1968). The surface zone in caries and in caries-like lesions produced *in vitro*. *Br. dent. J.* **125**, 145–57.

Silverstone, L.M. (1970). The histopathology of early enamel caries in the enamel of primary teeth. *J. Dent. Child.* **37**, 17–27.

Silverstone, L.M. (1973). The structure of carious enamel, including the early lesion. In *Oral sciences reviews*, No. 4. *Dental enamel*, (ed. A.H. Melcher and G. Zarb) pp. 100–60. Munksgaard, Copenhagen.

Simonsen, R.J. (1978). *Clinical applications of the acid-etch technique.* Quintessence, Chicago.

Söderholm, K.J., Antonson, D.E., and Pischlschweiger, W. (1989). Correlation between marginal discrepancies at the amalgam-tooth interface and recurrent caries. In *Quality evaluation of dental restorations*, (ed. K.J. Anusavice), pp. 95–110. Quintessence, Chicago.

Thylstrup, A., and Fejerskov, O. (1981). Surface features of early carious enamel at various stages of activity. In *Proceedings of a workshop on tooth surface interactions and preventive dentistry*, (ed. G. Rolla, T. Sonju, and G. Embery), pp. 193–205. IRL Press, London.

Thylstrup, A. and Fejerskov, O. (1986). *Textbook of cariology*, pp. 204–34. Munksgaard, Copenhagen.

Von der Fehr, F.R. (1965). Maturation and remineralization of enamel. *Adv. Fluor. Res.* **3**, 83–95.

Von der Fehr, F.R., Loe, H., and Theilade, E. (1970). Experimental caries in man. *Caries Res.* **4**, 131–48.

Weerheijm, K.L., Gruythuysen, R.J.M., and van Amerongen W.E., (1992). Prevalence of hidden caries. *J. Dent. Child.* **59**, 408–12.

7. Prevention of caries: immunology and vaccination

W.M. EDGAR

INTRODUCTION

Mobilization or augmentation of the defence systems of the body is perhaps the most attractive approach to the prevention of infectious disease, as it involves working with natural functions, rather than cutting across them. The idea that caries might by prevented by such methods has a long history, but in the last two decades has stimulated increasing interest. There now exists a large body of research into the defence mechanisms of the mouth, and the possibility of preventing caries by stimulating these mechanisms.

The defences of the body are of two types, non-specific and specific. In the mouth, properties of saliva, such as its buffering power, its calcium and phosphate levels, and its lubricating and cleansing functions, may be thought of as non-specific defence mechanisms, but the term is normally reserved for antibacterial systems of saliva such as lysozyme, lactoperoxidase, and lactoferrin, which are active against many species of bacteria. However, no more will be said here of these non-specific antibacterial mechanisms as although they may be important in host resistance, ways of increasing their effectiveness are for the most part unknown.

Specificity of antibacterial action is the hallmark of the immune systems of the body. These systems have been exploited since the time of Jenner in controlling disease that result from infection by a single, pathogenic strain or species of micro-organism, by vaccination. This process involves exposing the host to killed or attenuated forms of the organism (or to characteristic components or products) in order to instruct the host's immunological memory to mount an effective antibacterial response when the fully virulent organism is encountered.

To achieve the aim of mobilizing these specific immunological defences to prevent caries, we therefore need to understand the microbial aetiology of caries, the mechanisms involved in recognition of the aetiological agents by the immune system, and the ways in which the system might interfere with the pathological process leading to caries. With this knowledge, we can then sift the evidence relating caries and immunological responses in human populations and in animal experiments, with a view to arriving at a prognosis for successful and safe vaccination against caries in man.

MICROBIAL SPECIFICITY IN CARIES

The search for a single organism as the cause of caries began shortly after the recognition of the role of bacteria in the aeti-

ology of the disease. Clarke, in 1924, isolated an organism which he named *Streptococcus mutans* (because of its variable appearance on different culture media) in large numbers from human carious teeth, but the subsequent description of increased levels of lactobacilli in saliva from subjects with active caries led for many years to the widespread incrimination of that group of organisms as the major cause of caries.

EVIDENCE FROM ANIMAL CARIES

It was not until the development of techniques whereby experimental animals could be bred and reared under germ-free conditions that the bacterial aetiology of caries could be proved. In the absence of bacteria, no caries developed in the teeth of susceptible animals fed a high-sugar, caries-conducive diet (Orland *et al.* 1955). When individual species were allowed to infect the mouths of these otherwise germ-free animals, variable levels of caries occurred depending upon the species introduced. Re-isolated from these animals, the organisms could be transferred to other germ-free animals who then also developed caries. Caries was induced in animals not normally susceptible by infecting them with faeces from animals having caries. All these observations indicated that (in animal experiments at least) caries was an infectious, transmissible disease (Fitzgerald and Keyes 1960).

Of the organisms studied (mostly isolated from human mouths) the evidence rapidly became overwhelming that one species, subsequently identified as the *Strep. mutans* of Clarke, was pre-eminent in causing caries in rats and hamsters both when introduced into germ-free animals (gnotobiotic experiments) and when inoculated in high numbers (superinfected) into the mouths of animals with their normal bacterial flora (Table 7.1). A few other species were also capable of producing caries, but usually less extensive and rapid, and not involving the smooth surface of the teeth.

This pre-eminence has led some workers to believe that *Strep. mutans* is specifically involved in caries in man. However, certain strains of other species (for example, lactobacilli and *Strep. milleri*) may give rise to almost as much caries under controlled test conditions as *Strep. mutans*. Furthermore, with most animal caries experiments, diets containing high levels of sugar (40–60 per cent) are usually administered in order to elicit rapid development of caries, and it has been argued that *Strep. mutans* is among the few organisms which can tolerate such high levels of sugar— much higher than in the mixed human diet. Experiments using a less severe dietary challenge have tended to suggest

Table 7.1. Cariogenicity of various microbial groups in rats with gnotobiotic and conventional floras. (Modified after Gibbons and van Houte 1975.)

Organism	Caries		
	Smooth surfaces	Fissures	Root caries
Streptococci			
Strep. mutans	+++	+++	+
Strep. salivarius	–	–	–/++
Strep. sanguis	–	–/+	–
Strep. milleri	–/+	+/++	–
Strep. mitis	–	–/+	–
Enterococci	–	–/+	–
Lactobacilli	–	+/++	–
Filaments	–	–/+	+++

References: Drucker and Green (1978); Fitzgerald (1968); Fitzgerald *et al.* (1960, 1980); Frank *et al.* (1972); Gibbons and van Houte (1975); Guggenheim (1968); Jordan and Hammond (1972); Keyes (1962, 1968); Krasse and Carlsson (1970); Orland *et al.* (1955); Rosen *et al.* (1968); Socransky (1970).

that animals whose oral flora included *Strep. mutans* were not markedly more caries-prone than those in which the organism was absent. In one experiment for example, with a group of rats fed a cariogenic diet for 21 days with a naturally acquired flora, only 67 out of 214 (31 per cent) of fissures with caries harboured the organisms, while in five out of 29 (17 per cent) of non-carious fissures the organism was nevertheless present (Huxley 1978). Thus caries could occur without detectable infection by *Strep. mutans*, and vice versa.

VIRULENCE FACTORS AND *STREP. MUTANS*

The properties of an organism responsible for its pathogenicity are called virulence factors. With *Strep. mutans*, the most prominent features are its ability to form acid rapidly from dietary carbohydrates (in practice, mainly sucrose), its ability to tolerate acid conditions, and its ability to synthesize from sucrose an insoluble extracellular polysaccharide which is believed to help the organism to become attached to the teeth. This polysaccharide, a polymer of glucose (glucan) linked by $1 \rightarrow 3$ and $1 \rightarrow 6$ bonds, has been called 'mutan' to distinguish it from glucans synthesized by other species in which the $1 \rightarrow 6$ bond predominates.

The importance of these properties has been investigated by studying the amount of caries produced when a mutant form of the organism deficient in one of the properties is used to infect gnotobiotic animals. If, for example, mutan synthesis is an important virulence factor, than a mutant lacking this property should produce less caries than the parent strain. This was in fact the case (Tanzer and Freedman 1978; Mao and Rosen 1980), but only for caries of smooth surfaces and not for the pits and fissures. Conversely, a mutant synthesizing excessive mutan produces more rapid and extensive caries than the parent strain (Michalek *et al.* 1975). However, other organisms capable of producing extensive caries in animals do not synthesize mutan (Drucker and Greene 1978; Fitzgerald *et al.* 1980).

Mutants forming less acid than the parent strain gave greatly reduced caries, while those lacking the property of acid tolerance failed to become established on the animals teeth and did not produce any caries. Acid production from sugars by *Strep. mutans* has been found to be more rapid than other organisms from the mouth in test-tube experiments (e.g. Ranke and Ranke 1970; Minah and Loesche 1977), especially when the pH of the medium is low (Komiyama and Kleinberg 1974; Iwami and Yamada 1980). These properties are therefore probably the most important features of *Strep. mutans* giving rise to its virulence in animal experiments.

It is increasingly accepted that strains formerly designated as serotypes belonging to a single *Strep. mutans* species should more correctly be classified into five separate species on the basis of DNA homology and other studies. The two species predominant in man are *Strep. mutans* (formerly serotypes c, e, and f) and, less important, *Strep. sobrinus* (formerly serotypes d and g). *Strep. cricetus* (serotype a), *Strep. ferus* (serotype c), and *Strep. macacae* (serotype c) strains are rarely, if ever, isolated from the human mouth.

As defined above, *Strep. mutans* has been shown to produce more acid from sucrose and glucose than other members of the group and, in particular, to show enhanced acid production at pH 5 compared with pH 6.5. *Strep. mutans* and *Strep. sobrinus* are attached to pellicle by different receptors. Species differences such as these may contribute to variations in prevalence and virulence, such as these may contribute to variations in prevalence and virulence, although the relative cariogenicity of the various species is not well established.

Genetic fingerprinting techniques (e.g. ribotyping and RNA gene analysis) are now defining the clonal nature of *Strep. mutans* populations, and thus the acquisition and spread of oral bacteria in human populations and the variation in cariogenic properties between clonal lines. Genetic engineering techniques have also allowed the development of isogenic mutants of *Strep. mutans* for testing in animal models. Isogenic mutants are identical in genetic make-up to the wild type, with the exception of a single inactivated gene.

Cariogenicity testing of isogenic mutants with specific genes inactivated can thus give specific information on the importance of virulence factors associated with the genes in question. For example, inactivation of a gene (*gtf*A), known to include a stretch of chromosome containing other *Strep. mutans* genes involved in sugar transport, had no effect on cariogenicity in rats. Other non-essential genes were; a gene for fructanase, and *spa*P—a gene encoding for a wall protein formerly known as Antigen B or antigen I/II (see below). On the other hand, defective genes for fructosyltransferase or for intracellular polysaccharide storage led to loss of cariogenicity of the mutants.

STREP. MUTANS AND CARIES IN MAN

Numerous analyses of the microbial make-up of plaque in subjects of different caries experience have revealed a correlation between the presence of *Strep. mutans* and caries. Typically, subjects with high levels of caries harbour many *Strep. mutans*, but only occasionally caries is found in the absence of detectable numbers of *Strep. mutans*, and the organism may be found in the absence of disease.

Simple correlations of this kind do not of course prove that the organism causes the disease—it is equally possible that the acid conditions in a carious lesion favour the growth of the organism. To demonstrate a cause-and-effect relationship, it is necessary to carry out longitudinal studies observing microbial populations in plaque over a period of years during which caries develops in the underlying enamel. As such studies are laborious and expensive, only a few have been reported. In one, proportions of *Strep. mutans* (and *lactobacilli* rose *after* caries was diagnosed, suggesting that the carious lesion acted as a preferred ecological niche for these acid-tolerant organisms (Hardie *et al.* 1977). Another study found a significant rise in levels of *Strep. mutans* in the fissures of some children at the same time as caries was diagnosed, but not before diagnosis. In a minority of subjects, the appearance of caries was accompanied by an increase in lactobacilli, but not of *Strep. mutans* (Loesche and Straffon 1979). However, a further study by this group found that the proportion of *Strep. mutans* in molar fissures in caries-active children rose 6–24 months before diagnosis of caries in the fissures. Plaque in fissures in the same subjects which did not become carious, or in caries-inactive subjects, did not show the same rise in pro-portions of *Strep. mutans* (Loesche *et al.* 1984). Kristofferson *et al.* (1985) found that 83 per cent of approximal surfaces which never harboured *Strep. mutans* in 13-year-olds remained intact over 2 years, compared with only 35 per cent of surfaces from which the organism was regularly recovered. Caries incidence over 2 years was significantly associated with *Strep. mutans* counts in pre-school children (Alaluusua and Renkonen, 1983; Aaltonen *et al.* 1987). Overall, these studies show that *Strep. mutans* is an important factor in caries, but that it can not be regarded as the specific cause of the disease in man, as caries can occur in the absence of the organism.

Further evidence is given by studies of naturally occurring antibodies to oral organisms in subjects with varying levels of caries. Antibodies specific for *Strep. mutans* are present in higher concentrations in the sera of subjects with low levels of the disease, suggesting that they are exerting a protective effect. A similar relationship is not shown with antibodies to other species of organism, implying that they are not causally related to caries (Challacombe 1980). However, as we shall see later, the evidence relating naturally occurring antibodies and caries is confused, and as evidence for the specific role of *Strep. mutans* these findings must be viewed with caution.

IMMUNOLOGY OF THE ORAL CAVITY

ANTIGENS OF ORAL BACTERIA

The study of natural immune responses to a caries-producing organism, and the development of a vaccine, depend upon knowledge of the antigenic properties of the organism. The cell surface of *Strep. mutans* possesses very many antigens. The cell-wall enzyme glucosyltransferase (GTF) responsible for synthesis of insoluble extracellular mutan, has been extens-ively studied, as has the serotype-specific polysaccharide con-taining glucose, rhamnose, and sometimes galactose and galactosamine. In addition, the cell wall contains lipoteichoic acid, a polymer of glycerol and phosphate covalently linked to a glycolipid, which is found in virtually all Gram-positive organisms. This antigen may be responsible for some immunological cross-reactions between bacterial species, but specificity may be imparted by carbohydrate groups on the glycerol phosphate backbone. Glucans may be antigenic, but some reactions with glucans may have arisen from contamination with lipoteichoic acid or GTF.

A highly immunogenic antigen tightly bound to the cell wall of *Strep. mutans* gives antibodies in rabbits (Van de Rijn and Zabriski 1976) which cross-react with human heart tissue. Purification of antigens from cells of *Strep. mutans* has revealed at least two highly immunogenic proteins (Russell 1979). One, designated 'antigen A', is of low molecular weight (29 000 daltons) and the other, 'antigen B' (molecular weight 185 000 daltons) is similar to a protein having two antigenic determinants and called 'antigen 1/11' (Russell *et al.* 1980). It has been suggested that antigen B (and possibly 1/11) is responsible for cross-reactivity with heart tissue (Hughes *et al.* 1980; Russell 1979; Forester *et al.* 1983), although no evidence of heart damage has been reported in monkeys vaccinated for caries protection. Antigen 1/11 is present in all strains of *Strep. mutans* and *Strep. sobrinus*. Genetic techniques have shown that Antigen B (Antigen I/II) is a product of a gene given the symbol *spa*P. The gene product is an adhesin, involved in experimental adhesion to saliva-coated hydroxyapatite particles. Its importance in adhesion was confirmed by inactivating the gene.

Most studies of natural immune responses in man and vaccination experiments in animals have used as the antigen whole bacterial cells, usually killed by heat or with formalin, but GTF preparations and ribosomal proteins have been employed as a vaccine in rats and monkeys, and purified cell-wall associated antigens (A, B, 1/11) have been used to vaccinate monkeys.

ANTIBODIES IN THE MOUTH

Bacteria on the surface of the teeth may be affected by anti-bodies of two types—the secretory (salivary) antibodies of the isotype called s-IgA (Tomasi *et al.* 1965), and the serum anti-bodies (IgG, IgM, and IgA), which enter the mouth mainly via the gingival crevice (Challacombe *et al.* 1978).

s-IgA is present in external secretions such as tears, milk, sweat, and the products of glands of the respiratory and gastrointestinal tracts, including saliva. In this secretory form it is dimeric, comprising two molecules of IgA united by a polypeptide 'secretory component' together with a shorter junctional peptide known as the 'J-chain'. Synthesis of monomeric IgA in response to antigenic stimulation occurs in the lumphoid tissue associated with the gastrointestinal tract, both locally and in collections of lymphoid tissue such as the tonsils, mesenteric lymph nodes, and Peyers patches; addition of the secretory piece and dimer formation occurs during passage of the molecule through the epithelium of the gland. There is evidence that s-IgA antibodies formed by minor buccal and labial salivary glands may be elicited by penetration of antigen into the glands via the ducts (Krasse *et al.* 1978).

The functions of s-IgA are to bind with and aggregate foreign bodies and to inactivate antigens and toxins to prevent them adhering to surfaces and penetrating the epithelium. Formation of a s-IgA-antigen complex does not activate the complement mechanism, and s-IgA does not 'opsonize' bacteria to promote phagocytosis by polymorphonuclear leukocytes (PMNLs). IgA occurs in two subclasses; IgA1, which is susceptible to a proteolytic enzyme produced by certain oral bacteria including *Strep. sanguis*, and IgA2, which is more prevalent in secretions and is not cleaved by bacterial protease because it lacks a 13-peptide sequence where enzymic cleavage occurs.

Serum IgG is the major isotype in serum and is responsible for the humoral immune response, particularly the secondary or anamnaestic response where memory of a prior encounter with an antigen carried by primed lymphocytes leads to a brisk and sustained synthesis of antibody. The antigen is probably first bound and concentrated by macrophages and then 'presented' to the lymphocytes for more effective triggering of the cells to proliferate to antibody-secreting plasma cells. The B-lymphocytes involved in this humoral response are assisted in their function through the co-operative action of T-helper lymphocytes.

The principal functions of IgG are activation of complement, opsonization, and inhibition of antigens with biological activity, e.g. enzymes. In the activation of complement, antigen–antibody complexes stimulate a cascade-like sequence of changes in a group of nine serum factors ending up with release of a chemotactic factor which attracts phagocytic PMNLs, histamine release, and lysis of susceptible bacteria. Opsonization—coating of foreign particles such as bacteria with IgG molecules—results in increased phagocytosis by PMNLs, which have a binding site on their surfaces specific for parts of the bound IgG. Inhibition of GTF from *Strep. mutans* and of cell adhesion to surfaces may occur with sera from immunized animals (Ciardi *et al.* 1978; Hamada *et al.* 1979).

Cellular Immune Responses

Besides their helper function mentioned above, the principal function of T-lymphocytes is in the cell-mediated immune response. Antigens in the tissues, perhaps on the surface of a macrophage, are detected by specific receptors (not antibodies) on the surfaces of the T-cells, which are then stimulated to blastic transformation and proliferation. The blast cells form two populations, one of which (the killer T-cells) is cytotoxic to virally infected host cells or to cells bearing foreign histocompatability antigens—i.e. graft cells; the other subpopulation is responsible for release of soluble factors—the lymphokines—which have a large range of functions including chemotaxis and activation of macrophages, vascular permeability, and both stimulation and inhibition of other lymphocytes, perhaps related to T-cell helper and suppressor functions.

Cellular immune responses may be elicited in animals vaccinated with *Strep. mutans*, but it is unlikely that they play a direct part in the immunology of caries. However, they may modify a humoral immune response through (i) helper and suppressor actions of T-cells, and (ii) inflammation of the gingiva with accompanying increase in gingival fluid flow and hence access of IgG and PMNLs to the mouth.

Immunological Microenvironments in the Mouth

The plaque in the cervical region of the tooth and on root surfaces in older subjects is thus subjected to the influence both of salivary s-IgA and of serum immunoglobulins, complement factors, and PMNLs from the gingival crevice. IgA, IgG, IgM and the third component of complement can be detected in plaque extracts, and in the free aqueous phase of plaque (plaque fluid) separated from the solid phase by centrifugation, but in view of the proteolytic activity of many plaque bacteria (including IgA protease) the proportion of these components present as functional antibodies is unknown.

Plaque in the fissures and more coronal parts of the smooth surfaces of the teeth is probably influenced only by salivary antibodies. PMNLs survive only for a very short time in human saliva, although in monkeys their survival may be more prolonged and in the gingival crevice they may persist for long periods.

IMMUNOLOGY AND CARIES

Naturally Induced Immune Responses to Caries in Man

Antibodies or oral bacteria including *Strep. mutans* can be detected in human serum and saliva. In order to see whether or not these antibodies might play a part in natural caries immunity, numerous comparisons of caries experience and levels of immunoglobulin or specific antibody have been carried out, but consistency in the results of such experiments is not apparent (Table 7.2). For example, IgA levels in saliva have been found to be higher, lower, or unchanged in subjects with little or no caries compared with subjects with high caries experience. Raised levels of serum antibodies to cariogenic bacteria have been found in caries-free or -inactive subjects and in those with active caries. Serum antibody against *Strep. mutans* fell in a group of subjects with high caries experience and active caries, during a 9-month period when their active lesions were treated, suggesting that a protective antibody response was no longer stimulated by the presence of antigen; in contrast salivary agglutinating activity rose during the same period. No similar changes in salivary or serum antibodies against *Strep. mutans* were observed. However, in view of the many conflicting reports noted above, the general applicability of such evidence remains in doubt.

Another approach has been to examine the caries experience of patients suffering from selective deficiencies in immunoglobulins of various classes. Such patients are rare, and numbers available for study have been small, but a trend emerges towards increased caries in patients with disturbances of salivary IgA secretion. However, these patients have often received antibiotic therapy for long periods, and caution is needed in making comparisons with normal age-matched controls.

Given these weak and uncertain correlations between antibody responses and caries, the apparent failure of naturally acquired immune mechanisms to prevent caries in the vast majority of people living in developed countries is not

Table 7.2. Immunoglobulins (Igs) and antibodies (abs) to *Strep. mutans* in serum and saliva related to caries experience in man

Reference	Saliva	Serum	Caries status
Geller and Rovelstad (1959)	high Igs	–	low
Kraus and Sinsinha (1962)	no corr Igs[1]	–	–
Toto *et al.* (1960)	no corr Igs	–	(Lactobacillus count)
Lehner *et al.* (1967)	low IgA, IgG	high IgG	low
Zengo *et al.* (1971)	high IgA[2]	–	caries free
Sims (1972)	no corr Igs	–	–
Serre *et al.* (1972)	no corr Igs	–	–
Everhart *et al.* (1972)	high IgA[3]	–	low
Örstavik and Brandtzaeg (1975)	high IgA, parotid[4]	–	low
Stuchel and Mandel (1978)	high IgA[5]	–	caries free
Arnold *et al.* (1978)	low s-IgA ± IgM[6]	–	increased caries
Cole *et al.* (1978)	high IgS, IgG[7]	–	low caries
Kennedy *et al.* (1968)	–	high abs	caries free
Challacombe *et al.* (1973)	low abs[8]	high abs	low, treated
Lehner *et al.* (1978a)	no corr IgA, abs	low IgG:IgA, IgG:IgM abs	high (deciduous)
Huis in't Veld *et al.* (1978)	no corr IgA, abs	low IgG abs	caries free
McGhee *et al.* (1978)	rise in IgA abs	no abs elicited	oral vaccine
Gahnberg and Krasse (1983)	no rise IgA abs	–	oral vaccine
Cole *et al.* (1984)	no rise IgA abs	–	oral vaccine
Challacombe (1980)	rise in IgA abs	fall in IgG abs	treatment of caries
Weinmann (1936)	no cor PMNLs	–	–
Wright and Jenkins (1953)	no corr PMNLs	–	–
Friedman and Tonzetich (1968)	no corr PMNLs	–	–
Shklair *et al.* (1969)	high PMNLs	–	caries free
Lehner *et al.* (1976)	–	low SI[9]	high, treated
Ivanyi and Lehner (1978)	–	high SI[9] mothers, neonates	active (mothers)
Aaltonen *et al.* (1985)	–	high IgG abs[10]	low (deciduous)
Aaltonen *et al.* (1987)	–	low IgG abs	high 2 yr increment (deciduous)

[1] No correlation between Ig levels and caries.
[2] In submandibular saliva.
[3] 20–29 year age group only.
[4] Output/min, SIg negative correlation, SIgA vs DMF
[5] Output/min
[6] Subjects with deficiences in various Ig classes.
[7] Subjects from communities with contrasting caries levels.
[8] abs to GTF.
[9] Stimulation index; lymphoproliferative response to *Strep. mutans*.
[10] Related to maternal transmission of *Strep. mutans* in saliva.

surprising. It seems likely that in communities where the dietary factors lead to weak cariogenic challenge, natural immune mechanisms might be effective in controlling caries, but that they fail in the face of the overwhelming challenge presented by the modern Western diet.

The aim of those attempting to develop a vaccine for human use is to stimulate an enhanced, prolonged response to cope with this increased dietary challenge. In other diseases effectively controlled by vaccination such as smallpox, diphtheria, etc., natural immunity occurs, preventing re-infection or limiting the disease process, and the purpose of vaccination is to provide the lymphocytes with information allowing them to function optimally. Vaccination to prevent caries in man may therefore be more difficult to achieve as its purpose is to stimulate a response greater than that observed naturally.

Caries Vaccines in Animals

Vaccination of rats and hamsters fed a cariogenic diet has given variable levels of protection using a range of antigens and routes of immunization (Table 7.3). In the past, the most

popular type of vaccine was prepared from whole cells of *Strep. mutans*, usually killed by heat or by treatment with formalin, but increasingly, antigen preparations of varying purity derived from *Strep. mutans* are used as vaccines. Reductions in caries have usually been accompanied by a demonstrable antibody response in serum, saliva, or both.

Subcutaneous inoculation with formalin-killed cells of *Strep. mutans* in Freund's adjuvant in the vicinity of the salivary glands of rats whose mouths were subsequently infected with the same strain resulted in protection, but inoculation with similar antigens in sites remote from the salivary glands were less consistently successful. Both serum and salivary antibody responses were elicited by these subcutaneous injections close to the salivary glands. Injection of GTF preparations both from the same strain used for infection, and from different strains, have usually been effective, but in some cases increased levels of caries have been observed.

Oral vaccination elicits a s-IgA response in saliva and milk without detectable serum antibodies, and such vaccines have given protection. Passive immunization via antibodies in the milk of immunized dams has conferred protection in their pups, and rats fed with dried milk from cows immunized with

Table 7.3.　Vaccination with *Strep. mutans* against caries in rats and hamsters

Reference	C or G[1]	Vaccine	Route	Antibodies		Protection against caries (%)
				Saliva	Serum	
Guggenheim *et al.* (1970)	C	live whole cells	i.v.	NR[2]	yes	−25 to−40
	G	live whole cells	i.v.	NR	yes	6 to 16
	C	GTF	i.v.	NR	yes	−15 to−27
	G	GTF	i.v.	NR	yes	−9 to 19
Hayashi *et al.* (1972)	C	GTF	i.p.	NR	yes	59
		GH[3]				28
Tanzer *et al.* (1973)	C	fk[4] whole cells	s.c.	yes?	yes	0 to 69
Taubman and Smith (1974)	C	fk whole cells	s.c. (SGV)[5]	yes	yes	15 to 58
McGhee *et al.* (1975)	G	fk whole cells	s.c. (SGV)	yes	yes	64
Gaffar (1976)	C[6]	fk whole cells	i.p.	NR	NR	−40
	C[6]	GTF	i.p.	yes	yes	−11 to 37
Taubman and Smith (1977)	C	crude GTF	s.c. (SGV)	yes	yes	34
	G	pure GTF	s.c. (SGV)	yes	yes	58
	C[6]	pure GTF	s.c. (SGV)	yes	yes	65
Michalek and McGhee (1977)	G	hk whole cells[7]	dams milk	yes	yes	45 (in pup)
	G	fk whole cells[8]	dams milk	yes, in milk		51 (in pup)
Smith *et al.* (1978)	C[6]	GTF, various[9]	s.c. (SGV)	yes	yes	36 to 69
Michalek *et al.* (1978)	G	fk whole cells	oral	yes	NR	21 to 68
	G	fk whole cells	cows' milk	NR	NR	56 to 88[10]
Schöller *et al.* (1978)	G	GTF[11]	s.c. (SGV)	yes	yes	95[12]
Hughes *et al.* (1983)	C	antigen A	s.c. (SGV)	NR	NR	72[12]
Gregory *et al.* (1984)	G	ribosomes	s.c. (SGV)	IgA	IgG	18–94

[1] Conventional flora or gnotobiotic.

[2] Not recorded.

[3] Glycosidic hydrolases injected directly into the submandibular glands.

[4] Formalin-killed

[5] In the vicinity of the salivary glands.

[6] Hamsters.

[7] Heat killed cells injected i.v. elicited ab in milk.

[8] Injected s.c. in mammary gland region or orally via drinking water.

[9] GTF from one strain protective against caries on infecting with same or different strain.

[10] Milk from immunized cows fed to non-immunized rats.

[11] From *Strep. sanguis.*

[12] Smooth-surface lesions only.

Strep. mutans developed less caries than controls receiving conventional dried milk.

The evidence in rats and hamsters thus demonstrates the possibility of protection against caries, and that this protection may be afforded by s-IgA. The effect of the antibody seems to be to interfere with attachment of *Strep. mutans* to the tooth, either by inhibiting GTF activity, or blocking cell surface sites of attachment, or both. However, rodent teeth and saliva composition are very different from those of man, and experimental caries in rodents is known to differ in some respects from human caries, notably in the fact that only short-term experiments are possible owing to the animals' brief life-span. The immune response may last long enough to prevent caries over weeks or months, but not persist to confer protection over a number of years.

Caries in monkeys more closely resembles that in man, and their teeth, saliva, and immune systems are similar to the human pattern. For these reasons, vaccination experiments in monkeys can be expected to give more applicable findings. Reports of such experiments are fewer than with rodents owing to the expense of acquiring and maintaining the monkeys. However, protection against caries has been achieved by inoculation subcutaneously or submucosally with broken cells, cell walls, or heat-killed whole cells of *Strep.*

mutans and by intravenous injection of live cells (Table 7.4). Vaccination with enzymes including GTF has given variable results; in some experiments protection was observed but in the experiments of Bowen *et al.* (1975) increased caries occurred in animals vaccinated with GTF. It is likely that some of the GTF preparations have been contaminated with other antigens. Vaccination with purified protein antigens from *Strep. mutans* have been successful in protecting against caries. It has been suggested that antigen A gives the most reliable protection, and that antigen B (perhaps the same as antigen 1/11) is less effective and may be responsible for cross-reactivity with heart tissue. Antigen A can be purified from the supernatants of cultures of *Strep. mutans* by passing the fluid through an immunosorbent affinity column prepared with monoclonal anti-antigen A antibody, followed by elution of the bound pure antigen.

The nature of the protective antibody response to vaccination in these experiments is not certain, but the present evidence suggests that IgG may play a more important part in monkeys than in rodents. Salivary IgA antibodies were elicited in monkeys using an oral vaccine (Challacombe and Lehner 1979), but the response was of short duration (Lehner *et al.* 1980*b*; Walker 1981). Protection against caries has been linked with increased phagocytosis (Scully and Lehner

Table 7.4. Vaccination with *Strep. mutans* against caries in monkeys

Reference	Vaccine	Route	Antibodies		N[1]	Protection against caries (%)
			Saliva	Serum		
Bowen (1969)	live cells	i.v.	NR	yes	3	80
Lehner *et al.* (1975)	hk[2] whole cells	s.c.	yes	yes	6	65[3]
	hk[2] whole cells	s.m.[4]	yes	yes	6	51[3]
Bowen *et al.* (1975)	live cells	i.v.	NR	yes	5	53
	broken cells	s.m.	NR	yes	4	100
	GTF	s.m.	yes	yes	11	increased caries
Evans *et al.* (1975)	fk[5] whole cells and GTF	s.c. (SGV)[6]	no	yes		
		SGD[7]	yes	yes	4	NR[8]
Lehner *et al.* (1977)	hk or fk cells	s.c.	?yes	yes	6	69[9]
Bahn *et al.* (1977)	GH[10]	s.m.	NR	yes	10	23[11]
	GTF	s.m.	NR	yes	5	69
	FTF[12]	s.m.	NR	yes	5	62
	GH	s.m.	NR	yes	5	57
Schick *et al.* (1978)	cell walls[13]	s.m.	no	yes	6	33–50
	GTF	s.m.	no	yes	3	70
Lehner *et al.* (1978*b*)	passive[14]	–	no	yes	3	80
Cohen *et al.* (1979)	fk whole cells	s.c.	NR	NR	8	55
	fk whole cells	s.m.	NR	NR	8	28[15]
Lehner *et al.* (1980*a*)	antigen 1/11	s.c.	yes	yes	3	70
	fk whole cells	s.c.	yes	yes	3	73
Lehner *et al.* (1980*b*)	live cells	oral	?yes	no	6	34 (NS)
Russell *et al.* (1982)	antigen A	s.c.	NR	yes	10	yes
	antigen B	s.c.	NR	yes	9	variable
Russell and Colman (1981)	GTF	s.c.	NR	yes	4	0
Lehner *et al.* (1985)	3800D fragment	s.c.	?yes	yes	6	100

[1] Number of animals per group.
[2] Heat killed.
[3] Fissures only, two years.
[4] Submucosal injection.
[5] Formalin killed.
[6] Salivary gland vicinity.
[7] Instilled via salivary gland duct.
[8] Reduced infection with *Strep. mutans*

[9] First permanent molars only.
[10] Glycoside hydrolase enzyme.
[11] Short-term experiment.
[12] Fructosyl transferase enzyme.
[13] Two strains.
[14] Immune plasma injected; protection associated with IgG fraction.
[15] Estimated from graph.

1979), and passive immunization by injection of IgG (but not IgA) fractions separated from immune monkey plasma prevented caries in the recipients of the plasma, but no salivary antibodies were found in the animals receiving injections of the IgA fraction. It is possible that in monkeys, both serum and salivary antibodies are necessary to obtain maximum protection, with the former being more important in protecting the approximal and free smooth surfaces, and the latter having more effect in occlusal pits and fissures.

TOWARDS A HUMAN CARIES VACCINE

The protection against caries achieved in the animal experiments just described has generated hopes for developing an effective vaccine for use in man. However, a number of major problems remain. First, in most of the experiments the caries in the control animals has been induced by infection with *Strep. mutans*, usually of the same strain as that used for vaccination. In gnotobiotic experiments, the plaque consists of a pure culture of the organism, while in animals with conventional flora, superinfection with *Strep. mutans* has been employed because of the need to achieve rapid caries in view of the prolonged vaccination period, after weaning and before administering the cariogenic diet. With monkeys, superinfection has also been employed. Thus the successful results of vaccination against caries associated with *Strep. mutans* may underestimate the difficulty of achieving success in man, where the association between the organism and caries is less clear, as discussed earlier.

Even if a vaccine were successful in giving a response which eliminated the target organism, other organisms might step in to fill the gap. A vaccine against the most prevalent of the serotypes of *Strep. mutans* (serotype c) that acted specifically to eliminate this serotype might simply lead to a shift towards other members of the *Strep. mutans* group without reducing the level of cariogenic challenge. A less specific vaccine giving rise to antibodies reacting with *Strep. sobrinus* as well as *Strep. mutans* would avoid this problem. This type of cross-protection has been observed when caries resulting from infection with one strain of *Strep. mutans* was prevented by immunizing with GTF from a different strain (Table 7.3). However, elimination of all strains of *Strep. mutans* may not necessarily lead to reduced caries, as other species may take over the role of the target species.

The evidence at present does not allow us to decide confidently the nature of the antibody action or actions which is likely to confer maximum protection. Inhibition of bacterial attachment, perhaps including inhibition of GTF activity, may be important in the action of salivary IgA antibodies, while the action of IgG antibodies derived from the serum may involve opsonization and subsequent phagocytosis by crevicular PMNLs as well as complement-mediated lysis. We have seen that the two classes of antibody may be involved in protecting different tooth surfaces, but IgA may also inhibit the functions of IgG and so the proportion of the two isotypes elicited by vaccination, as well as their concentrations, may be important.

Recent work using purified cell wall protein antigens for *Strep. mutans* as vaccines has established their effectiveness, and after more extensive investigation of their relationship with the cell-wall antigen responsible for reaction with human heart tissue the development of a vaccine for human testing is under way. However, the immunization schedules used must be readily acceptable for human use, and further elucidation of the mechanisms involved in conferring protection might reveal more acceptable antigens, adjuvants, and routes.

GTF preparations are attractive possible vaccines, as they may constitute an important target of the antibacterial mechanism of the immune response, have the advantage of not eliciting heart-reactive antibodies, and have been shown in rats to offer cross-protection between different strains of *Strep. mutans*. However, these antigens have been less successful in conferring protection both in rats and monkeys.

In some animal studies, oral vaccination with whole-cell or cell-wall vaccines elicited a secretary immune response, without eliciting serum antibodies (including a possible heart-reactive antibody). If it can be shown that salivary s-IgA confers protection, the secretory immune route offers hope of a safe and acceptable method (Ciardi *et al.* 1992). Genetic engineering techniques may assist in generating more effective vaccines against specific targets while excluding possible harmful responses.

Passive immunization with antibodies from the yolks of immunized hens or from colostrum from immunized cows can prevent caries in rats, but has so far been unpromising in man. Such a method would by-pass the need for active immunization of children, and could prove acceptable if effective.

A programme of vaccination against caries could probably be easily implemented alongside other vaccination procedures in childhood. It is uncertain however if it would be widely accepted in the present climate of public opinion which is cautious about vaccination against disease that are not life-threatening. With falling levels of caries in children in most developed countries, it may be that vaccination would be most valuable for high-risk groups, or perhaps for developing countries where other caries control methods are less applicable.

It should be clear from the foregoing that formidable obstacles must be overcome before safety and effectiveness could be guaranteed. Furthermore, in view of the complex bacterial aetiology of caries in man, it seems likely that even the most effective vaccination programme targeted against a single cariogenic species could only provide partial protection. The potential benefits of vaccination (alongside other preventive measures including treatments and diet control) in the elimination of caries from the community may, if they can be achieved, prove sufficient to warrant the effort and expense of development. However even if the effort is successful, vaccination will not remove the need for continued fluoride therapy, or allow young patients to consume limitless cariogenic foods with impunity.

SUMMARY

- Defence mechanisms against caries are non-specific and specific; exploitation of specific mechanisms by vaccination implies a degree of bacterial specificity in aetiology.

- Strains of the Mutans group of streptococci are among the most cariogenic in animal caries experiments, principally because they are acidogenic and aciduric, but also because of their ability to synthesize extracellular and intracellular polysaccharides.

- Mutans streptococcal infection tends to be associated with caries incidence and prevalence in man, but this association is not invariable—caries can occur without detectable levels of these organisms.

- Cariogenic bacteria possess many antigens which may elicit antibody formation when whole cells are injected in vaccination experiments. Important antigens which may be virulence factors include glucosyl transferase enzyme (responsible for insoluble extracellular polysaccharide formation), and Antigen B, a cell-wall protein involved in adhesion of mutans streptococci to saliva-coated hydroxyapatite.

- Immune responses in the mouth may be of the humoral type, involving antibodies of the class S-IgA in saliva or Ig G in serum (entering the mouth via the gingival crevicular fluid); or cellular immune responses which may modify the humoral response and increase gingival crevicular fluid flow.

- Evidence of natural immunity to caries in man is weak and contradictory, but vaccination experiments in rodents and in monkeys have given promising levels of protection against caries.

- Development of human caries vaccines may be assisted by molecular genetic techniques providing more active and specific antigenic components of cariogenic organisms. However, uncertainty as to the route by which immunity is to be achieved, the level of protection which can be expected, and the acceptability of vaccination against a background of falling disease prevalence has removed much of the impetus for further research.

RECOMMENDED READING

Roit, I.M. and Lehner, T. (1980). *Immunology of oral diseases.* Blackwell, Oxford.

Hamada, S. and Slade, H.D. (1980). Biology, immunology and cariogenicity of *Streptococcus mutans*. *Microbiol. Rev.* **44**, 331–44.

Hamada, S., Michalek, S.M., Kiyona, H., Menaker, L., and McGhee, J.R. (1986) (ed.). *Molecular microbiology and immunobiology of Streptococcus mutans*. Elsevier, Amsterdam.

McGhee, J.R. and Michalek, S.M. (1981). Immunobiology of dental caries. *Ann. Rev. Microbiol.* **35**, 595–638.

Russell, R.R.B. and Johnson, N.W. (1987). The prospects for vaccination against dental caries. *Br. dent. J.* **162**, 29–34.

Krasse, B., Emilson, C-G., and Gahnberg, L. (1987). An anticaries vaccine: report on the status of research. *Caries Res.* **21**, 225–76.

Russell, R.R.B. (1994). Control of specific plaque bacteria. *Adv. dent. Res.*, 285–90.

REFERENCES

Aaltonen, A.S., Tenovuo, J., Lehtonen, O-P., Saksala, R., and Meurman, O. (1985). Serum antibodies against oral *Streptococcus mutans* in young children in relation to dental caries and maternal close-contacts. *Archs. oral Biol.* **30**, 331–35.

Aaltonen, A.S., Tenovuo, H., and Lehtonen, O-P (1987). Increased dental caries activity in preschool children with low baseline levels of serum IgG antibodies against the bacterial species *Streptococcus mutans*. *Archs. oral Biol.* **32**, 55–60.

Alaluusua, S. and Renkonen, O-V. (1983). *Streptococcus mutans* establishment and dental caries experience in children from 2 to 4 years old. *Scand. J. dent. Res.* **91**, 453–7.

Arnold, R.R., Prince, S.J., Mestecky, J., Lynch, D., Lynch, M., and McGhee, J.R. (1978). Secretory immunity and immunodeficiency. In *Secretory immunity and infection*, (ed. J.R. McGhee, J. Mestecky, and J.L. Babb). pp. 401–10. Plenum Press, New York.

Bahn, A.N., Shklair, I.L., and Hayashi, J.A. (1977). Immunization with dextransucrases, Levansucrases and glysocidic hydrolases from oral streptococci. *J. dent. Res.* **56**, 1586–98.

Bowen, W.H. (1969). A vaccine against dental caries. A pilot experiment in monkeys (*Macaca irus*). *Br. dent. J.* **126**, 159–60.

Bowen, W.H., Cohen, B., Cole, M.F., and Colman, G. (1975. Immunization against dental caries. *Br. dent. J.* **139**, 45–58.

Challacombe, S.J. (1980). Serum and salivary antibodies to *Streptococcus mutans* relation to the development and treatment of human dental caries. *Archs. oral Biol.* **25**, 495–502.

Challacombe, S.J. and Lehner, T. (1979). Salivary antibody responses in Rhesus monkeys immunized with *Streptococcus mutans* by the oral, submucosal or subcutaneous routes. *Archs. oral Biol.* **24**, 917–25.

Challacombe, S.J., Guggenheim, B., and Lehner, T. (1973). Antibodies to an extract of *Streptococcus mutans*, containing glycosyltransferase activity, related to dental caries in man. *Archs. oral Biol.* **18**, 657–68.

Challacombe, S.J., Russell, M.W., Hawkes, J.E., Bergmeier, L., and Lehner. T. (1978). Passage of immunoglobulins from plasma to the oral cavity in Rhesus monkeys. *Immunology*, **35**, 923–31.

Ciardi, J.E., Bowen, W.H., Reilly, T.A., Hsu, S.D., Gomez, I., Kuzmiak-Jones, H., and Cole, M.F. (1978). Antigens of *Streptococcus mutans* implicated in virulence-production of antibodies. In *Secretory immunity and infection*, (ed. J.R. McGhee,

J. Mestecky, and J.L. Babb), pp. 281–92. Plenum Press, New York.

Ciardi, J.E., McGhee, J.R., and Keith, J.M. (1992) (ed.). Genetically engineered vaccines. In *Advances in experimental medicine and biology*, Vol. 327. Plenum Press, New York.

Clarke, J.K. (1924). On the bacterial factor in aetiology of dental caries. *J. exp. Pathol.* **5**, 141–7.

Cohen, B., Colman, G., and Russell, R.R.B. (1979). Immunization against dental caries: further studies. *Br. dent. J.* **147**, 9–14.

Cole, M.F. *et al.* (1978). Immunoglobulins and antibodies in plaque fluid and saliva in two populations with contrasting levels of caries. In *Secretory immunity and infection*, (ed. J.R. McGhee, J. Mestecky, and J.L. Babb), pp. 383–92. Plenum Press, New York.

Cole, M.F., Emilson, C-G., Hsu, S.D., Li, S-H., and Bowen, W.H. (1984). Effects of peroral immunization of humans with *Streptococcus mutans* on induction of salivary and serum antibodies and inhibition of experimental infection. *Infec. Immunity* **46**, 703–9.

Drucker, D.B. and Green, R.M. (1978) The relative cariogenicities of *Streptococcus milleri* and other viridans group streptococci in gnotobiotic hooded rats. *Archs. oral Biol.* **23**, 183–7.

Evans, R.T., Emmings, F.G., and Genco, R.J. (1975). Prevention of *Streptococcus mutans* infection of tooth surfaces by salivary antibodies in Irus monkeys (*Macaca fascicularis*). *Infec. Immunity* **12**, 293–302.

Everhart, D.L., Grisby, W.R., and Carter, W.H. (1972). Evaluation of dental caries experience and salivary immunoglobulins in whole saliva. *J. dent. Res.* **51**, 1487–91.

Fitzgerald, R.J. (1968). Dental caries research in gnotobiotic animals. *Caries Res.* **2**, 139–46.

Fitzgerald, R.J. and Keys, P.H. (1960). Demonstration of the etiologic role of streptococci in experimental caries in the hamster. *J. A.m dent. Ass.* **61**, 9–19.

Fitzgerald, R.J., Jordan, H.V., and Stanley, H.R. (1960). Experimental caries and gingival pathologic changes in the gnotobiotic rat. *J. dent. Res.* **39**, 923–35.

Fitzgerald, R.J., Fitzgerald, D.B., Adams, B.O., and Duany, L.F. (1980). Cariogenicity of human oral lactobacilli in hamsters. *J. dent. Res.* **59**, 832–7.

Forester, H., Hunter, N., and Knox, K.W. (1983). Characteristics of a high molecular weight extracellular protein of *Streptococcus mutans*. *J. gen. Microbiol.* **129**, 2779–88.

Frank, R.M., Guillo, B., and Llory H. (1972). Caries dentaires chez le rat gnotobiote inoculé avec *Actinomyces viscosus et Actinomyces naeslundii*. *Archs. oral Biol.* **17**, 1249–53.

Friedman, S.D. and Tonzetich, J. (1968). A study of human oral leucocytes in relation to caries incidence. *Archs. oral Biol.* **13**, 647–59.

Gaffar, A. (1976). Effects of specific immunization on dental caries in hamsters. *J. dent. Res.* **55**, C221–3.

Gahnberg, L. and Krasse, B. (1983). Salivary immunoglobulin A antibodies and recovery from challenge of *Streptococcus mutans* after oral administration of *Streptococcus mutans* vaccine in humans. *Infec. Immunity*, **39**, 514–19.

Geller, J.H. and Rovelstad, G.H. (1959). Electrophoresis of saliva: relationship of protein components to dental caries. *J. dent. Res.* **38**, 1060–5.

Gibbons, R.J. and van Houte, J. (1975). Dental caries. *Ann. Rev. Med.* **26**, 121–36.

Gregory, R.L., Michalek, S.M., Schechmeister, I.L., and McGhee, J.R. (1984). Effective immunity to dental caries: protection of gnotobiotic rats by a local immunisation with a ribosomal preparation from *Streptococcus mutans. Microbiol. Immunol.* **27**, 787–800.

Guggenheim, B. (1968). Streptococci of dental plaque. *Caries Res.* **2**, 147–64.

Guggenheim, B., Mühlemann, H.R., Regolati, B., and Schmid, R. (1970). The effect of immunization against streptococci or glucosyltransferases on plaque formation and dental caries in rats. In *Dental plaque*, (ed. W.D. McHugh), pp. 287–96. Churchill Livingstone, Edinburgh.

Hamada, S., Tai, S., and Slade, H.D. (1979). Serotype-dependent inhibition of glucan synthesis and cell adherence of *Streptococcus mutans* by antibody against glucosyltransferase of serotype e *S. mutans. Microbiol. Immunol.* **23**, 61–70.

Hardie, J.M. *et al.* (1977). A longitudinal epidemiological study on dental plaque and the development of dental caries—interim results after two years. *J. dent. Res.* **56**, C90–8.

Hayashi, J.A., Shlair, I.L., and Bain, A.N. (1972). Immunization with dextransucrases and glycosidic hydrolases. *J. dent. Res.* **51**, 436–42.

Huis in't Veld, J., Bannet, D., van Palenstein Helderman, W., Sampaio Camargo, P., and Backer Dirks. O. (1978). Antibodies against *Streptococcus mutans* and glucosyltransferases in caries-free and caries-activity military recruits. In *Secretory immunity and infection*, (ed. J.R. McGhee, J. Mestecky, and J.L. Babb). Plenum Press, New York.

Hughes, M., MacHardy, S.M., Sheppard, A.J., and Woods, N.C. (1980). Evidence for an immunological relationship between *Streptococcus mutans* and human cardiac tissue. *Infec. Immunity,* **27**, 576–88.

Hughes, M., MacHardy, S.M., and Sheppard, A.J. (1983). Manufacture and control of a dental caries vaccine for parenteral administration to man. In *Glycosyltransferases, glucans, sucrose and dental caries*, (ed. R.J. Doyle and J.E. Ciardi), pp. 259–68. I.R.L. Press, Washington, D.C.

Huxley, H.G. (1978). *Streptococcus mutans* and dental caries in Long-Evans rats with a naturally-acquired oral flora. *Archs. oral Biol.* **23**, 703–7.

Iwami, Y. and Yamada, T. (1980). Rate-limiting steps of the glycolytic pathway in the oral bacteria *Streptococcus mutans* and *Strep. sanguis* and the influence of acidic pH on the glucose metabolism. *Archs. oral Biol.* **25**, 163–9.

Ivanyi, L. and Lehner, T. (1978). The relationship between caries index and stimulation of lymphocytes by *Strep. mutans* in mothers and their neonates. *Archs. oral Biol.* **23**, 851–6.

Jordan, H.V. and Hammond, B.F. (1972). Filamentous bacteria isolated from human root surface caries. *Archs. oral Biol.* **17**, 1333–42.

Kennedy, A.E., Shklair, I.L., Hayashi, J.A., and Bahn, A.N. (1968). Antibodies to cariogenic streptococci in humans. *Archs. oral Biol.* **13**, 1275–9.

Keyes, P.H. (1962). Recent advances in dental caries research. Bacteriology. *Int. dent. J.* **12**, 443–64.

Keyes, P.H. (1968). Research in dental caries. *J. Am. dent. Ass.* **76**, 1357–73.

Komiyama, K. and Kleinberg, I. (1974). Comparison of glucose utilization and acid formation by *Strep. mutans* and *Strep. sanguis* at different pH. *J. dent. Res* **53** (special issue), 241.

Krasse, B. and Carlsson, J. (1970). various types of streptococci and experimental caries in hamsters. *Archs. oral Biol.* **15**, 25–32.

Krasse, B., Gahnberg, L., and Bratthall, D. (1978). Antibodies reacting with *Strep. mutans* in secretions from minor salivary

glands in humans. In *Secretory immunity and infection.* (ed. J.R. McGhee, J. Mestecky, and J.L. Babb), pp. 349–54. Plenum Press, New York.

Krause, F.W. and Sirisinha, S. (1961). Gamma-globulin in saliva. *Archs. oral Biol.* **7**, 221–33.

Kristoffersson, K., Grondahl, H-G., and Bratthall, D. (1985). The more *Streptococcus mutans*, the more caries on approximal surfaces. *J. dent. Res.* **64**, 58–61.

Lehner, T., Caldwell, J., and Clarry, E.D. (1967). Immunoglobulins in saliva and serum in dental caries. *Lancet,* **I**, 1294–6.

Lehner, T., Challacombe, S.J., and Caldwell. J. (1975). An immunological investigation into the prevention of caries in deciduous teeth of Rhesus monkeys. *Archs. oral Biol.* **20**, 305–10.

Lehner, T., Challacombe, S.J., Wilton. J.M.A., and Ivanyi, L. (1976). Immunopotentiation by dental microbial plaque and its relationship to oral disease in man. *Archs. oral Biol.* **21**, 749–53.

Lehner, T., Caldwell, J. and Challacombe, S.J. (1977). Effects of immunization on dental caries in the first permanent molars in Rhesus monkeys. *Archs. oral Biol.* **22**, 393–7.

Lehner, T., Murray, J.J., Winter, G.B., and Caldwell, J. (1978a). Antibodies to *Strep. mutans* and immunoglobulin levels in children with dental caries. *Archs. oral Biol.* **23**, 1061–7.

Lehner, T., Russell, M.W., Wilton, M.M.A., Challacombe, S.J., Scully, C.M., and Hawkes, J.E. (1978b). Passive immunization with antisera to *Streptococcus mutans* in the prevention of caries in Rhesus monkeys. In *Secretory immunity and infection*, (ed. J.R. McGhee, J. Mestecky, and J.L. Babb), pp. 303–16. Plenum Press, New York.

Lehner, T., Russell, M.W., and Caldwell, J. (1980a). Immunization with a purified protein from *Streptococcus mutans* against dental caries in rhesus monkeys; *Lancet,* **I**, 995–6.

Lehner, T., Challacombe, S.J., and Caldwell, J. (1980b). Oral immunization with *Streptococcus mutans* in rhesus monkeys and the development of immune responses and dental caries. *Immunology,* **41**, 857–64.

Lehner, T., Caldwell, J., and Giasuddin, A.S.M. (1985). Comparative immunogenicity and protective effect against dental caries of a low (3800) and high (18 000) molecular weight protein in rhesus monkeys (*Macaca mulatta*). *Archs. oral Biol.* **30**, 207–12.

Loesche, W.J. and Straffon, L.H. (1979). Longitudinal investigation of the role of *Streptococcus mutans* in human fissure decay. *Infec. Immunity,* **26**, 498–507.

Loesche, W.J., Eklund, S., Earnest, R., and Burt, B. (1984). Longitudinal investigation of bacteriology of human fissure decay: epidemiological studies in molars shortly after eruption. *Infec. Immunity,* **46**, 765–72.

McGhee, J.R., Michalek, S.M., Webb., J., Navia, J.M., Rahman, A.F.R., and Legler, D.W. (1975). Effective immunity to dental caries: protection of gnotobiotic rats by local immunization with *Streptococcus mutans. J. Immunol.* **114**, 300–5.

McGhee, J.R., Mestecky, J., Arnold, R.R., Michalek, S.M., Prince, S.J., and Babb, J.L. (1978). Induction of secretory antibodies in humans following ingestion of *Streptococcus mutans*. In *Secretory immunity and infection*, (ed. J.R. McGhee, J. Mestecky, and J.L. Babb), pp. 177–84. Plenum Press, New York.

Mao. M.W.H. and Rosen, S. (1980). Cariogenicity of mutants of *Strep. mutans. J. dent. Res.* **59**, 1620–6.

Michalek, S.M. and McGhee J.R. (1977). Effective immunity to dental caries: passive transfer to rats of antibodies to *Strep. mutans* elicits protection. *Infec. Immunity* **17**, 644.

Michalek, S.M., Shiota, T., Ikeda, T., Navia, J.M., and McGhee, J.R. (1975). Virulence of *Streptococcus mutans*: biochemical and pathogenic characteristics of mutant isolates. *Proc. Soc. exp. Biol. Med.* **150**, 498–502.

Michalek, S.M., McGhee, J.R., Arnold, R.R., and Mestecky, J. (1978). Effective immunity to dental caries: selective induction of secretory immunity by oral administration of *Streptococcus mutans* in rodents. In *Secretory immunity and infection.* (ed. J.R. McGhee, J. Mestecky, and J.L. Babb), pp. 261–70. Plenum Press, New York.

Minah, G.E. and Loesche, W.J. (1977). Sucrose metabolism by prominent members of the flora isolated from cariogenic and non-cariogenic dental plaque. *Infec. Immunity,* **17**, 55–61.

Orland, F.J., Blayney, J.R., Harrison, R.W., Reyniers, J.A., Trexler, P.C., Ervin, R.F., Gordon, H.A., and Wagner, M. (1955). Experimental caries in germfree rats inoculated with enterococci. *J. Am. dent. Ass.* **50**, 259–72.

Örstavik, D. and Brandtzaeg, P. (1975). Secretion of parotid IgA in relation to gingival inflammation and dental caries experience in man. *Archs. oral Biol.* **20**, 701–4.

Ranke, E. and Ranke, B. (1970). Zur Bedeutung verschiedener Plaque-Streptokokken für die Karies. *Deut. zahnartl. Z.* **25**, 270–3.

Rosen, S. Lenny, W.S., and O'Malley, J.E. (1968). Dental caries in gnotobiotic rats inoculated with *Lactobacillus casei. J. dent. Res.* **47**, 358–63.

Russell, M.W., Bergmeier, L.A., Zanders, E.D., and Lehner, T. (1982). Protein antigens of *Streptococcus mutans*: purification and properties of a double antigen and its protease-resistant component. *Infec. Immunity,* **28**, 486–93.

Russell, R.R.B. (1979). Wall-associated protein antigens of *Streptococcus mutans. J. gen. Microbiol.* **114**, 109–15.

Russell, R.R.B., Beighton, D., and Cohen, B. (1980). Immunizatin of monkeys (*Macaca fascicularis*) with antigens purified from *Streptococcus mutans. Br. dent. J.* **152**, 81–4.

Russell, R.R.B. and Colman, G. (1981). Immunization of monkeys. (*Macaca fascicularis*) with purified *Streptococcus mutans* glucosyltransferase. *Archs. oral Biol.* **26**, 23–6.

Schick, H.J., Klimek, F.J., Weimann, E., and Zwisler, O. (1978). Preliminary results in the immunization of Irus monkeys against dental caries. In *Secretory immunity and infection.* (ed. J.R. McGhee, J. Mestecky, and J.L. Babb), pp. 703–12. Plenum Press, New York.

Schöller, M., Klein, J.P., and Frank, R.M. (1978). Dental caries in gnotobiotic rats immunized with purified glycosyltransferase from *Strep. sanguis. Archs. oral Biol.* **23**, 501–4.

Scully, C.M. and Lehner, T. (1979). Opsonization, phagocytosis and killing of *Strep. mutans* by polymorphonuclear leucocytes, in relation to dental caries in the Rhesus monkey (*Macaca mulatta*). *Archs. oral Biol.* **24**, 307–12.

Serre. A., Benfredi, G., and Levey, D. (1972). Les immunoglobulines A salivaires. Étude des corrélations avec les indices de carie et de quelques facteurs de variabilité de resultats. *Revue Immunol., Paris,* **36**, 47–54.

Shklair, I.L., Rovelstad, G.H., and Lamberts, B.L. (1969). Study of some factors influencinig phagocytosis of cariogenic streptococci by caries-free and caries-active individuals. *J. dent. Res.* **48**, 842–5.

Sims, W. (1972). The concept of immunity in dental caries. II. Specific responses. *Oral Surg.* **34**, 69–86.

Smith, D.J., Taubman, M.A., and Ebersole, J.L. (1978). Effects of local immunization with glucosyltransferase fractions from *Streptococcus mutans* on dental caries in hamsters caused by homologous and heterologous serotypes of *Streptococcus mutans. Infec. Immunity.* **21**, 843–51.

Socransky, S.S. (1970). Relationship of bacteria to the etiology of periodontal disease. *J. dent. Res.* **49**, 203–22..

Stuchel. R.N. and Mandel, I.D. (1978). Studies of secretory IgA in caries-resistant and caries-susceptible adults. In *Secretory immunity and infection,* (ed. J.R. McGhee, J. Mestecky, and J.L. Babb), pp. 341–8. plenum Press, New York.

Tanzer, J.M. and Freedman, M.L. (1978). Genetic alteration of *Streptococcus mutans* virulence. In *Secretory immunity and infection,* (ed. J.R. McGhee, J. Mestecky, and J.L. Babb), pp. 661–72. Plenum Press, New York.

Tanzer, J.M., Hageage, G.L., and Larson, R.H. (1973). Variable experiences in immunization of rats against *Streptococcus mutans*–associated dental caries. *Archs. oral Biol.* **18**, 1425–40.

Taubman, M.A. and Smith, D.J. (1974). Effects of local immunization with *Streptococcus mutans* on induction of salivary immunoglobulun A antibody and experimental dental caries in rats. *Infec. Immunity* **9**, 1079–91.

Taubman, M.A. and Smith, D.J. (1977). Effect of local immunization with glucosyltransferase fractions from *Streptococcus mutans* in dental caries in rats and hamsters. *J. Immunol.* **118**, 710–20.

Tomasi, T.B., Tan, E.M., Solomon, A., and Prendergast, R.A. (1965). Characteristics of an immune system common to certain external secretions. *J. exp. Med.* **121**, 101–24.

Toto, P.D., Grisamore, T., Rapp, G.W., Delow, R., and Hammond, H. (1960. The correlation of *Lactobacillus* count and gamma globulin level of human saliva. *J. dent. Res.* **39**, 285–8.

Van de Rijn, I. and Zabriskie, J.B. (1976). Immunological relationship between *Streptococcus mutans* and human myocardium. In *Immunological aspects of dental caries,* (ed. W.H. Bowen, R.J. Genco, and T.C. O'Brien), pp. 187–94. Information Retrieval Inc., Washington, D.C.

Walker, J. (1981). Antibody responses of monkeys to oral and local immunization with *Streptococcus mutans. infec. Immunity,* **31**, 61–70.

Weinmann, J. (1936). Role of leukocytes in saliva. *J. dent. Res.* **15**, 360.

Wright, D.E. and Jenkins, G.N. (1953). Leukocytes in the saliva of caries-free and caries-active subjects. *J. dent. Res.* **32**, 511–23.

Zengo, A.N., Mandel, I.D., Goldman, R., and Khurana, H.J. (1971). Salivary studies in human caries resistance, *Archs. oral Biol.* **16**, 557–60.

8. The prevention and control of chronic periodontal disease

W.M.M. Jenkins

THE PATHOGENESIS OF PERIODONTAL DISEASE

The appearance of normal healthy periodontium is illustrated diagrammatically in Fig. 8.1a. The oral epithelium is keratinized but the crevicular (sulcular) epithelium and the junc-

tional epithelium are not. The junctional epithelium is attached to the enamel surface and underlying connective tissue by a basal lamina and hemi-desmosomes, and its free surface (from which desquamation takes place) lines the bottom of the histological crevice. The depth of the histological crevice—the distance from the crest of the free gingiva to the coronal extent of the junctional epithelium—measures only 0.5 mm. Clinically, however, the crevice depth is considered to be the distance to which a blunt probe will penetrate and, because it will readily produce a tear in the fragile junctional epithelium, the clinical crevice depth is more in the order of 2 mm. If gingival recession occurs, the junctional epithelium will form an attachment to cementum.

When plaque is allowed to accumulate freely there is an acute exudative inflammatory response within 2–4 days in the connective tissue underlying the coronal portion of junctional epithelium. This occurs without any change in clinical appearance. After 10–21 days of persistent plaque accumulation, collagen destruction in this zone is marked and a dense infiltrate of chronic inflammatory cells is found. The clinical changes of chronic gingivitis can now be detected: redness, swelling, reduced resistance to probing, and an increased tendency of the gingiva to bleed on probing or when the teeth are brushed.

Bacterial deposits do not extend below the gingival margin in the subclinical stages of developing gingivitis. Gingival enlargement, however, helps to create a subgingival flora as supragingival deposits become located within the gingival pocket. Apical advancement of subgingival plaque occurs at a later stage (Fig. 8.1b) as the junctional epithelium separates from the tooth surface and becomes 'pocket epithelium', characterized by the formation and lateral extension of rete pegs, and by areas of micro-ulceration.

After the development of chronic gingivitis, an equilibrium is usually established between the increased mass of bacteria and the host defences, maintaining a state of chronic gingivitis indefinitely. If and when periodontitis does supervene, it is thought to be precipitated either by a proportional increase in pathogenic micro-organisms within the subgingival bacterial flora, by impaired host resistance, or by both factors in combination.

As soon as the destructive process extends apically to affect the alveolar bone and fibre attachment of the root surface, periodontitis is said to have developed (Fig. 8.1c). Thus, periodontitis is characterized by loss of (connective tissue)

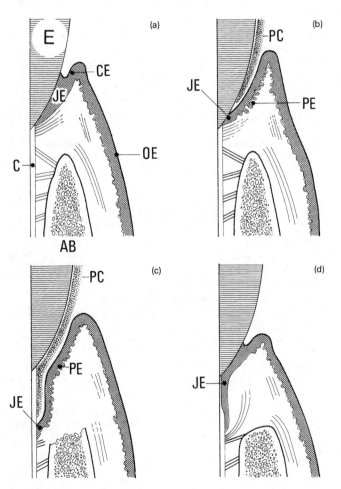

Key: AB, alveolar bone; C, cementum; CE, crevicular epithelium; E, enamel; JE, junctional epithelium; OE, oral epithelium; PC, plaque/calculus; PE, pocket epithelium

Fig. 8.1. (a) Periodontal health, (b) chronic gingivitis (late phase), (c) chronic periodontitis, (d) repair following debridement.

attachment. Junctional epithelium proliferates apically to maintain an epithelial barrier at the base of the deepening pocket, and the denuded cementum becomes contaminated by microorganisms and their products. Periodontitis is detected most readily with a probe, a blood-stained or purulent exudate being elicited by probing to the base of the pocket beyond the amelocemental junction.

Chronic gingivitis is a condition which can be largely reversed by plaque control. On the other hand, the loss of fibre attachment, which is the principal feature of periodontitis, is virtually irreversible. Periodontitis is treated by removal of plaque and calculus, together with pathologically altered cementum, and by establishing daily plaque control. Following treatment of periodontitis, repair processes take place in which the junctional epithelium is re-established by involution of pocket epithelium, and supported by new gingival connective tissue, consisting of functionally orientated (but not tooth-attached) collagen fibres (Fig. 8.1d). More advanced lesions may not respond to treatment without surgical intervention.

IMPLICATIONS FOR PREVENTION

As gingivitis is caused by supragingival plaque accumulation and as gingivitis is a prerequisite for the development of periodontitis, both diseases can be prevented by an adequate standard of plaque control.

Although there is great variation in individual susceptibility, there are, at present, no predictive tests which would single out, for priority preventive care, individuals at high risk of developing the more aggressive forms of periodontitis. Regular and frequent dental visits are, therefore, indicated to establish and maintain good oral hygiene and to identify inflammatory changes at an early and reversible stage.

EPIDEMIOLOGY

Unlike caries, periodontal disease has existed since ancient times.

FACTORS AFFECTING THE PREVALENCE AND SEVERITY OF PERIODONTAL DISEASES

Evaluation of large populations invariably reveals that older people have more attachment loss. This is thought to reflect, not the ageing process itself, but the duration of exposure to aetiological agents.

Studies of large populations also show that periodontal conditions are worse in males, lower socioeconomic groups, and infrequent dental attenders (Oliver *et al.* 1991), presumably because these groups demonstrate poorer standards of preventive health behaviour.

It is established beyond doubt that plaque is the primary aetiological factor both in gingivitis and in periodontitis. Not surprisingly, therefore, differences between large populations with respect to the prevalence and severity of gingivitis and periodontitis are largely explained by differences in oral hygiene when comparison is limited to similar age groups. While this may be universally true of gingivitis, some populations are peculiarly susceptible to periodontitis and may experience more attachment loss than others with comparable levels of oral hygiene (Baelum *et al.* 1991).

In comparisons between individuals, the association of periodontal diseases with plaque is much weaker, and variations in disease levels cannot be explained solely by the amount of plaque present. This is because of secondary aetiological factors such as pregnancy, smoking, inherited characteristics, immune function, etc., which are peculiar to individuals and which determine their levels of susceptibility. In obtaining population mean severity scores, these variations in susceptibility between individuals are 'smoothed' so that oral hygiene emerges as the overwhelming risk factor. The variation in periodontal disease experience among different individuals of the same age and standard of oral hygiene has important implications; preventive measures, applied randomly to a large group, may not be appropriate for all individuals in that group.

PREVALENCE AND SEVERITY OF GINGIVITIS

The epidemiology of gingivitis has been reviewed by Stamm (1986). From the deciduous dentition stage, gingivitis increases in prevalence and severity with increasing age, to reach a peak prevalence of 90–100 per cent at puberty. A slight decline in prevalence and severity during adolescence is then followed by a gradual rise throughout adult life. The hormonal changes associated with puberty may be responsible for the peak which is recognized in this age group (Sutcliffe 1972). Alternatively, the rising prevalence before puberty may be attributed to an increase in gingival sites at risk as the permanent dentition develops (Murray 1974). Furthermore, the temporary decline in prevalence and severity after puberty may reflect an increased social awareness and resulting improved oral hygiene (Greene 1963).

PREVALENCE AND SEVERITY OF PERIODONTITIS

The absolute diagnostic criterion of periodontitis is the demonstration of inflammation apical to the amelo-cemental junction by the occurrence of bleeding on probing. Such painstaking examination, however, is inappropriate for large epidemiological surveys. Instead, rough estimates of the damage caused by periodontitis are obtained clinically by measuring loss of attachment, or radiographically by measuring loss of marginal bone. Neither of these methods gives a precise diagnosis. Loss of attachment and reduction in alveolar bone height are evidence of previous destruction, not of existing disease. Furthermore, attachment loss with gingival recession may occur due to trauma from oral hygiene devices rather than inflammatory processes, making attachment loss on facial surfaces difficult to interpret. Radiographs, on the other hand, can reveal the destructive effect of periodontitis only on proximal surfaces. For all these reasons, the data which follow must be interpreted with caution.

Periodontitis may be found even in the deciduous dentition of young children. In a bitewing radiographic study, Sjödin and Matsson (1994) detected marginal bone loss (amelocemental junction to bone crest distance > 2 mm) in 4.5 per cent of a sample of 2017 9-year-old Swedish children. By contrast, the detection rate among 4-year-olds from a mainly Hispanic community in the USA was 7.6 per cent (Bimstein *et al.* 1988): probably a reflection of the different socio-economic backgrounds of the two samples.

The true prevalence of periodontitis in teenage populations is much disputed, and to a large extent this is due to lack of uniformity in the stringency of diagnostic criteria which are applied. There is wide agreement that large amounts of periodontal destruction are unusual, but minor amounts may be quite common. In a 5-year longitudinal study of 167 British adolescents, initially 14 years of age, from a low socio-economic area, Clerehugh *et al.* (1990) determined the prevalence of attachment loss by examining the mesial surfaces of first molars, first premolars, and central incisors for evidence of a reduction in attachment level of 1 mm or more. The prevalence increased from 3 per cent at 14 years, through 37 per cent at 16 years, to 77 per cent at 19 years. Attachment loss greater than 1 mm was found only at 19 years when it affected 14 per cent of the group, and did not exceed 2 mm. The proportion of *sites* with loss of attachment increased from less than 1 per cent at 14 years, through 7 per cent at 16 years, to 31 per cent at 19 years.

According to Brown *et al.* (1990), by 18–24 years of age, virtually 100 per cent of the US population of employed adults were affected by attachment loss of 1 mm or more (Table 8.1). Of course, prevalence estimates of periodontitis are a function of the criteria used for diagnosis, and rates of almost 100 per cent are frequently obtained when assignment of a diagnosis of periodontitis depends on attachment loss or marginal bone height reductions of only 1 mm. By selecting higher disease thresholds, as shown in Table 8.1, the following is apparent:

1. Both the prevalence and extent of clinically significant disease is low in early adulthood and increases with age.

2. Only a minority of teeth, affected by periodontitis, progress eventually to an advanced stage of the disease.

The figures quoted in Table 8.1 should not be regarded as definitive since these data were obtained by a partial recording system which is likely to have underestimated both the proportion of subjects and the number of sites affected by

Table 8.1. Prevalence, severity, and extent of loss of attachment in employed adults in the United States (After Brown *et al.* 1990)

	Loss of attachment (mm)					
Age (yrs)	Prevalence (% subjects)			Extent (no. of sites*)		
	≥ 1	≥ 3	≥ 5	≥ 1	≥ 3	≥ 5
10–24	99	16	2	33	0.7	< 0.1
35–44	100	49	14	35	4	1
55–64	100	77	35	34	8	2

*Maximum number of affected sites in a 28-tooth dentition = 56.
Reprinted by permission of ADA Publishing Co., Inc.

severe attachment loss. By contrast, a detailed full mouth survey in a Japanese population revealed that the prevalence of attachment loss >5 mm affected 6 per cent of 20- to 29-year-olds, 35 per cent of 40- to 49-year-olds, and 68 per cent of 60- to 69-year-olds (Okamoto *et al.* 1988). These latter figures are consistent with the findings of radiographic surveys of dentate adults in Sweden (Papapanou *et al.* 1988) and Scotland (Jenkins and Kinane 1989). Like the US data in Table 8.1, these three full-mouth surveys show that the more severe levels of periodontal destruction follow a skewed distribution in the general population.

Although, in older age groups, there may be a high frequency of individuals with advanced attachment loss affecting at least one tooth surface, the proportion of individuals with severe *generalized* periodontitis is smaller. Hugoson *et al.* (1992), for example, reported that *generalized* marginal bone loss, exceeding one-third of root length, affected only 13 per cent of a population of 550 randomly selected dentate adults aged 20–70 years. Nevertheless, although generalized bone loss of this magnitude was uncommon at 40 years, it was detected in 32 per cent of 60-year-olds and 42 per cent of 70-year-olds.

Cross-sectional data such as those depicted in Table 8.1, or as obtained in the other studies mentioned above, must be interpreted with caution. It cannot be assumed that the younger cohorts, as they grow older, will exhibit the same periodontal conditions as the older ones, and, therefore, the rate of progression of periodontal disease with age cannot be firmly extrapolated from these data.

AGE OF ONSET OF PERIODONTITIS

As noted above, minor amounts of attachment loss occur frequently in children and adolescents, although in most cases the disease progresses slowly and is unlikely to become clinically significant until the fourth decade. This form of periodontitis is often termed *adult periodontitis*. It is the most common form of periodontitis and is responsible for the majority of cases of advanced destructive disease in middle-aged and elderly individuals.

Those forms of the disease which are characterized by advanced destruction in early childhood, adolescence or early adulthood are described respectively as *pre-pubertal*, *juvenile* or *'rapidly progressive'* periodontitis. These early-onset types of periodontitis have been linked to specific subgingival microfloras, to impairment of immune and inflammatory mechanisms, and to familial distributions.

Generalized pre-pubertal periodontitis is very rare and is invariably associated with underlying systemic disease, such as neutropenia, hypophosphatasia, etc. Juvenile periodontitis affects approximately 0.1 per cent of adolescent Caucasians while, in ethnic negroid races, prevalence rates are 1–3 per cent. 'Rapidly progressive periodontitis' is a term used to describe severe generalized periodontitis affecting young adults between 20 and 35 years of age. There are no reliable epidemiological data on its occurrence but a prevalence rate of 1–2 per cent for Caucasians has been suggested.

On the whole, with the exception of localized juvenile periodontitis, the various forms of chronic periodontitis are poorly characterized. There is considerable overlap and a precise diagnosis is frequently impossible: the time lapse between onset and diagnosis may be unknown; different diagnoses may be appropriate for different teeth in one mouth; and the influence of concurrent systemic disease may be difficult to assess.

PERIODONTAL TREATMENT NEEDS

The epidemiological data summarized above yield important information on the prevalence and severity of periodontal disease at different ages and in various populations. However, they cannot easily be converted to give a reliable estimate of treatment needs or, therefore, to plan and develop preventive or curative services. This deficiency has been addressed by introduction of the Community Periodontal Index of Treatment Needs (CPITN), devised by the World Health Organization and the International Dental Federation (Ainamo *et al.* 1982).

Examination is carried out with a specially designed probe; colour-coded for pocket depth measurement and with a ball tip for calculus detection. A score is given to each sextant according to the worst finding in all teeth of that sextant as follows:

Pocket of 6 mm depth or more	Code 4
Pocket of 4 or 5 mm depth	Code 3
Supra- or subgingival calculus	Code 2
Bleeding on probing	Code 1
No disease	Code 0

Using the CPITN, Cushing and Sheiham (1985) examined a random sample of 448 dentate individuals, aged 20 to 60 years, in the north-west of England, and assessed their treatment needs. Only 2 per cent (Code 0) did not require any treatment. Seven per cent (Code 1) required oral hygiene instruction only. Eighty-four per cent (Codes 2 and 3) required oral hygiene instruction and scaling, while 7 per cent (Code 4) required complex treatment. By combining these data with the number of sextants requiring treatment, the manpower resource requirements were estimated at 1 week of work for a dental surgeon and 6 months of work for a dental hygienist. These estimates did not include time taken for initial examination, treatment planning, and monitoring and maintenance care, which would increase the dentist-time required.

It is worth noting that extensive loss of attachment on proximal as well as facial and lingual surfaces is often associated with gingival recession, and, therefore with shallow pockets (Wilson *et al.* 1988). Thus, CPITN surveys, while providing valid data on pocket depths, and therefore on type of treatment required, are certain, by ignoring gingival recession, to underestimate the degree of periodontal breakdown.

INTRA-ORAL DISTRIBUTION OF PERIODONTAL DISEASE

The tooth surfaces most often coated in plaque and affected by gingivitis or periodontitis are the proximal surfaces (Hugoson and Koch 1979). The teeth most severely affected by gingivitis are the molars and lower anteriors (Suomi and Barbano 1968). The first teeth to be affected by periodontitis are usually the first molars (Hugoson and Rylander 1982). The rate of attachment loss, on average, is greater in the maxilla than in the mandible, and slowest at the canines, mandibular first premolars, and maxillary central incisors (Wennström *et al.* 1990).

Although studies of large populations suggest that certain teeth are preferentially affected by periodontitis, this pattern is frequently not detectable in single subjects where attachment loss may appear to follow a random distribution throughout the dentition. At present, there is no satisfactory explanation for differences in susceptibility to periodontitis between teeth or individual tooth surfaces.

TOOTH MORTALITY

There is great variation in tooth mortality statistics in different parts of the world depending on oral hygiene, caries susceptibility, and the availability and effectiveness of dental services. The dentist's and patient's attitude, together with technical difficulties associated with provision of treatment, may also be significant factors determining the timing of extractions which obscure the significance of caries and periodontal disease. This must be borne in mind when interpreting tooth mortality statistics.

Several recent studies, reviewed by Oliver and Brown (1993), show that caries greatly exceeds periodontal disease as a cause of tooth loss. While caries was responsible for 43–63 per cent of all extractions, periodontitis accounted for 21–36 per cent. Furthermore, while periodontal disease, with increasing age, assumes greater importance as a cause of tooth loss, it remains, according to some studies, a less frequent cause of extraction than caries, even in older age groups.

THE RATE OF PERIODONTAL DESTRUCTION

Recent introduction of the automated pressure-sensitive probe has permitted relatively small increments of attachment loss to be detected, allowing the progress of single lesions to be monitored (Jeffcoat and Reddy 1991). It is, thereby, apparent that progression may be linear, proceeding very slowly, consistent with tooth survival, or progressing more quickly, leading eventually to tooth loss. Attachment loss may also occur at a continuous, but exponential rate. Alternatively, progression may be episodic, acute episodes being interspersed with periods of remission or repair. Different patterns of progression may affect the same site at different times, and prolonged remission may not be uncommon.

The difference in rate of progress between individuals has been highlighted by Löe *et al.* (1986), who reported on a 15-year longitudinal study of Sri Lankan tea labourers, aged initially 14–31 years. All displayed gross accumulation of plaque and calculus, and widespread gingivitis. Nevertheless, three distinct subpopulations were identified, based on proximal surface loss of attachment and tooth mortality rates. Eight per cent of the total population exhibited rapid loss of attachment and had a peak annual rate of proximal surface attachment loss of 1 mm per year. Eighty-one per cent exhibited moderate progression with a peak annual rate of destruction of 0.5 mm per year. Eleven per cent exhibited essentially no progression beyond gingivitis.

Thus, the rate of periodontal destruction may vary at different stages of the disease, between single tooth surfaces and between individuals.

PERIODONTAL DISEASE TRENDS

Evidence has accumulated of an improvement in gingivitis in children and adults during the last 30 years. This evidence has been obtained by repeating cross-sectional studies of the same age range after an interval of several years using the same survey criteria. Thus, Anderson (1981) reported a decline in gingivitis and improvement in dental cleanliness over a 15-year period among 12-year-old English children from two schools. Cutress (1986) reported a decline in gingivitis prevalence over a 6-year period in the 15–19 year age group in New Zealand, from 98 per cent of subjects and 51 per cent of teeth to 79 per cent of subjects and 34 per cent of teeth.

Improvements in gingivitis and oral hygiene among adults as well as children have been reported in the USA over a 12-year period (Douglass *et al.* 1985), and in Sweden over a 10-year period (Hugoson *et al.* 1986). In the Swedish study, the improvement in gingivitis and plaque control was most noticeable on buccal and lingual surfaces and was less marked interproximally (Hugoson *et al.* 1986).

Evidence to suggest that *periodontitis* is declining is harder to obtain because of changing attitudes to tooth extraction. Thus, Hugoson *et al.* (1992), in comparing periodontal conditions of 20-to-70-year-olds between 1973 and 1983, found a substantial *increase* in the proportion of individuals with generalized bone loss within the range of one-third to two-thirds of normal bone height. This was particularly marked among 60-year-olds (affecting 3 per cent of the dentate population in 1973, but rising to 26 per cent in 1983) and 70-year-olds (6 per cent in 1973 rising to 38 per cent in 1983). There was, however, a considerable *reduction* in tooth loss at these age levels over the 10-year period, suggesting that, in 1983, periodontal disease *per se* was no longer sufficient reason for extraction.

AETIOLOGY OF PERIODONTAL DISEASE

It is well established that periodontal disease is initiated by bacterial plaque. It is, however, recognized that other aetiological factors exist—those which predispose to plaque accumulation and those which modify the inflammatory response.

PLAQUE AND OTHER ACQUIRED TOOTH DEPOSITS

'*Plaque* is the soft, non-mineralized, bacterial deposits which form on teeth that are not adequately cleaned' (Löe 1969). It accumulates on tooth surfaces not exposed to friction from cheeks, lips, tongue, and food, and its composition varies according to its location.

The earliest deposit to form on a cleaned tooth surface is the 'acquired pellicle'. It is a structureless film of salivary glycoproteins selectively adsorbed to the surface of hydroxy-apatite crystals, and is visible within minutes following a polish with pumice. The formation of pellicle is accompanied by bacterial colonization as micro-organisms in saliva adsorb to the pellicle. After three or four hours a thin layer of plaque, composed mainly of Gram-positive cocci (principally streptococci) will be established. These remain the predominant micro-organisms for approximately seven days, although, during this time, there is a proportional increase in Gram-positive rods and in Gram-negative cocci and rods, and, after seven days, filaments, fusobacteria, and spirilla are found in greater numbers. As the plaque matures further, spirochaetes and vibrios appear, and filamentous bacteria, especially *Actinomyces*, may become predominant.

There appear to be many mechanisms for bacterial adherence: *Streptococcus sanguis* is adapted for adherence to hydroxyapatite and is among the pioneer bacteria to be found in the deepest layers of plaque; some organisms interact with salivary constituents which serve as the binding material; and the occurrence in plaque of *Streptococcus mutans* is dependent on sucrose from which it synthesizes extracellular polysaccharides to mediate its attachment. The synthesis of surface polymers may also account for the ability of bacteria of one species to bind to one another or to bacteria of a different species. 'Corn-cob' structures, i.e. filamentous bacteria coated with cocci, represent one example of such interspecies binding. In addition to extracellular polysaccharides, plaque contains intracellular polysaccharides in the form of storage granules synthesized from dietary sugars.

Microorganisms constitute at least 70 per cent of the bulk of plaque and the intermicrobial matrix comprises a protein and carbohydrate substrate derived partly from endogenous sources, namely, saliva, epithelial cells, and crevicular exudate, and partly from the diet. The exact structural, bacteriological, and biochemical composition of plaque is subject to great variation depending on: the concentration of bacteria in saliva; the site and duration of plaque formation; the nature of competitive resident flora; oxygen and nutrient availability; the composition of the diet; and the presence of periodontal disease.

Bacteriological studies of plaque during development of gingivitis suggest that there are more than 200 different species in mature plaque. Gingivitis is believed to result from quantitative changes in plaque rather than the overgrowth of specific micro-organisms.

Periodontitis is caused by subgingival downgrowth of those bacteria best able to evade host defences and survive in a low oxygen environment. Thus, the composition of subgingival plaque differs from plaque on the adjacent visible tooth surface. For example, in subgingival plaque, Gram-positive bacteria are found in lower proportions and Gram-negative bacteria in higher proportions than in supragingival plaque. The subgingival flora comprise a layer of tooth-attached plaque as well as a loosely adherent component in direct association with the pocket epithelium. The tooth-attached plaque consists mainly of Gram-positive rods and cocci, while the unattached plaque consists predominantly of Gram-negative organisms including motile forms. Many different bacterial species are thought to be of aetiological significance in periodontitis.

The mechanisms by which bacteria may provoke an inflammatory and immune response and cause tissue destrution are complex. Bacterial invasion of the tissues, if it occurs at all, is thought to be relatively unimportant. Instead, tissue damage is sustained mainly by penetration of the tissues by various soluble substances produced by plaque bacteria. These 'toxins' have wide-ranging effects: in addition to toxic effects on host cells and enzymic degradation of tissue, chemotactic and antigenic effects occur, as well as activaiton or suppression of inflammatory and immune mechanisms, and stimulation of bone resorption.

Mineralization within plaque results in calculus formation. Its inorganic content (70–90 per cent) is mostly crystalline and amorphous calcium phosphate. The organic component includes protein, carbohydrates, lipid, and various non-vital microorganisms, predominantly filamentous ones. The rate of calculus formation between individuals is very variable, and children form less calculus than adults. Calcification may commence in 1-day-old plaque but the mechanism for calculus formation is not known. In supragingival locations, however, it is thought to result from interactions between saliva, tooth surfaces, and plaque, while, in subgingival locations, inflammatory exudate within pockets is the fluid medium involved. Subgingival calculus forms more slowly and is usually more difficult to remove by virtue of the intimate relationship which it forms with the rougher root surface. Calculus is always covered by soft plaque and retains toxic bacterial products.

Stains are caused by food substances such as tea and coffee, by tobacco, by the products of chromogenic bacteria, or by metallic particles. These pigments become absorbed by plaque or pellicle.

FACTORS PREDISPOSING TO PLAQUE ACCUMULATION

Tooth malalignment

It is well recognized that gingivitis is more common and more severe around malaligned teeth because they are harder to clean (Silness and Røynstrand 1985).

Restorations

Bacteria accumulate more readily on restoration surfaces (Glantz 1969), with the possible exception of porcelain (Newcomb 1974), than on tooth enamel. Furthermore, the surface finish of a restorative material may influence the degree of plaque accumulation. A highly polished surface should be more amenable to cleansing procedures than a rough surface.

Restorations with overhanging or otherwise defective cervical margins form retention sites for plaque and may have a profound effect on periodontal health (for review see Brunsvold and Lane 1990). Subgingival restoration margins produce more plaque accumulation and result in poorer gingival health than margins which are level with the gingival crest or in a supragingival position (Silness 1980). Excessive axial crown contours tend to enhance plaque accumulation and gingival inflammation (Yuodelis *et at.* 1973).

Removable partial dentures

It has been observed that patients provided with partial dentures accumulate more plaque on abutment teeth (Addy and Bates 1979). The fitting surfaces of the dentures themselves become coated with plaque, and plaque accumulation both on abutment teeth and denture is increased by day and night wear. These factors help to account for the common observation of gingivitis around abutment teeth. Moreover, El Ghamrawy (1979) has shown that the microbial composition of plaque in denture subjects changes more rapidly, resembling the 4-to 9-day-old plaque of non-denture wearers as early as the second day.

Calculus

The surface texture of calculus promotes plaque accumulation and retention of irritant bacterial deposits. There is no evidence, however, that calculus itself is capable of initiating periodontal disease.

FACTORS MODIFYING THE INFLAMMATORY RESPONSE

Host defence mechanisms appear to be both protective and destructive, and in most cases the tissue damage sustained is minor relative to the protection provided. An intact and normal functioning host response would appear to be compatible with, at worst, slowly progressive periodontal disease. However, subtle changes in the capacity of various components of the host response to deal with the bacterial challenge may cause an increased susceptibility to periodontal disease. In addition, a number of identifiable systemic factors are thought to affect the host response to local irritants, increasing the severity of periodontal disease. These factors include diabetes mellitus, smoking, stress, blood dyscrasias, certain genetic disorders, and alteration in the levels of circulating sex hormones during puberty, pregnancy or medication with oral contraceptives.

RATIONALE FOR PREVENTION AND MANAGEMENT OF PERIODONTAL DISEASE

PROFESSIONAL CARE

Dental health education

The objective of oral hygiene education is to produce a change in behaviour which will result in a reduction of plaque accumulation sufficient, if possible, to prevent the initiation and progression of dental caries and periodontal disease, and to make the patient as independent as possible of professional support. A successful outcome will depend not only on mastery of plaque control techniques but also on a change of behaviour and compliance with the suggested plaque control regime. Kegeles (1963) has suggested various steps which must be taken before a recommended health action is adopted:

1. belief in susceptibility to the disease;
2. belief that the disease is undesirable;
3. belief that prevention is possible;
4. belief that prevention is desirable.

Clearly, therefore, the clinician must use an educative approach aimed at changing the patient's attitude to periodontal disease and dental care (Blinkhorn *et al.* 1983). Furthermore, plaque control skills must be taught using proper educational principles such as step-size advancement, self-pacing, repeated feedback, and reinforcement, as well as active participation by the patient.

Dental health education and instruction in oral hygiene is traditionally carried out by dental personnel at the chairside, but this process is labour-intensive and, with repetition, is likely to affect the mood of the instructor and, thereby, the effect of the instruction. In recent years, however, the need for oral hygiene instruction to be given at the chairside has been questioned. Glavind *et al.* (1985) have shown that a self-educational programme, comprising self-examination and instruction manuals, was as effective as chairside instruction by dental personnel in changing oral hygiene habits.

The dental surgery has frightening overtones for many people, who then find it difficult to concentrate on advice being given (Blinkhorn *et al.* 1983). This fact alone might explain the success of self-education manuals—the freedom to assimilate information in a less hostile environment compensating for the lack of personal contact.

Regardless of the means employed, it is well known that oral hygiene instruction usually has no long-term effect unless periodically reinforced. Gjermo (1967), for example, found that the initial improvement observed 1 month after individual instruction of schoolchildren was not maintained at the second examination 7 months later. Thus, initial incentives for behavioural change appear to fade after the target behaviour has been achieved. According to the Committee on Oral Health Care for the Prevention and Control of Periodontal Disease (Committee Report 1966): 'Probably the most important and difficult problem that remains to be solved before much progress can be made in the prevention of periodontal disease is how to motivate the individual to follow a prescribed effective oral health-care programme throughout his life'. This remains as true today as it was 30 years ago.

Improved oral hygiene alone has little effect on gingival condition, pocket depth, or subgingival flora of deep periodontal lesions (Corbet and Davies 1993). In patients with existing periodontal disease, therefore, dental health education must be supported by attention to the subgingival environment.

Scaling and root planing

Scaling alone is sufficient to remove plaque and calculus from enamel completely leaving a smooth clean surface. Root surfaces, however, whether supra- or subgingival, may have deposits of calculus embedded in cemental irregularities. A portion of cementum must, therefore, be removed to eliminate these deposits. Furthermore, plaque accumulation results in contamination of cementum by toxic substances, notably endotoxins. Some evidence suggests that this cementum may be biologically unacceptable to adjacent gingival tissue and should be removed by root planing, a procedure which may result in exposure of dentine. While this is not the aim of treatment, it may be unavoidable. There is little evidence that the degree of root smoothing *per se* is of biological importance although it gives the best clinical indication that calculus and altered cementum have been completely removed.

Subgingival débridement should result in a sufficiently plaque-free environment to allow renewal of junctional epithelium and the epithelial attachment. The degree of subgingival root surface cleansing necessary to achieve this is likely to vary from patient to patient and from site to site. Although it is well established that non-surgical instrumentation often fails to achieve complete removal of plaque and calculus, incomplete débridement may still be compatible with clinical periodontal health in many cases. In other cases, failure to achieve complete plaque removal will allow recolonization of the root surface to take place, and inflammation to persist or recur.

Following subgingival instrumentation, good supragingival plaque control is a prerequisite for pocket healing. At sites of persistent supragingival plaque accumulation, pocket débridement has no effect on gingivitis (Sbordone *et al.* 1990), an initial, small reduction in probing depth is reversed within 8 weeks (Sbordone *et al.* 1990), and the main periodontal pathogens are re-established within 4–8 weeks in the proportions observed prior to débridement (Magnusson *et al.* 1984; Sbordone *et al.* 1990).

Polishing

Polishing enamel may result in reorientation of surface crystals to create a smoother surface (Boyde 1971). However, although early experimental studies have shown that polishing to a high gloss inhibits formation of pellicle (Muhler *et al.* 1964), plaque (Swartz and Philips 1957), and calculus (Barnes *et al.* 1971), there is no documented evidence of periodontal health benefits from this practice. Removal of extrinsic tooth stains for cosmetic reasons, and the psychological effect of having clean teeth after a dental appointment may be the principal benefits of polishing, while removal of fluoride from superficial layers of the enamel could be a significant drawback (Billier *et al.* 1980). Clearly, tooth polishing cannot be supported on scientific grounds as a routine procedure, but may be indicated in special instances where plaque removal is obviously inhibited by surface roughness.

Surgical pocket therapy

There is no certain magnitude of initial probing depth beyond which non-surgical instrumentation is ineffective, provided sufficient skill and perseverance are applied (Badersten *et al.* 1984). Non-surgical scaling and root planing, however, as a definitive procedure in deep pockets, is very time-consuming, and surgical intervention may be required to provide the operator with better access to the plaque-infected root surface for pockets of more than approximately 5 mm depth (Lövdal 1961).

HOME CARE

The manual tooth-brush

Design characteristics

Design variations include dimensions of the head, the length, diameter, and modulus of elasticity of the filaments and their number, distribution, and angulation. Operating efficiency may further depend on moisture content, temperature of the water used, and brushing technique. These variables confound comparison of the many investigations carried out to determine optimum tooth-brush characteristics. Although current opinion favours a soft-textured nylon multi-tufted brush with a short head, there is no clear-cut evidence that one particular type of tooth-brush is superior to others with respect to plaque removal and prevention of gingivitis (Bergenholtz 1972). Frequent use of a hard-textured brush has been linked to gingival recession (Khocht *et al.* 1993).

Tooth-brushing methods

Greene (1966) grouped tooth-brushing methods into the following categories based on the direction of the brushing stroke: (i) vertical; (ii) horizontal; (iii) roll technique; (iv) vibrating techniques (Charters, Stillman, Bass); (v) circular technique; (vi) physiological technique; (vii) scrub brush method. Comparative studies of these different methods have yielded conflicting results and each technique has its own protagonists. In a sample of 800 individuals, Wade (1971) showed that more than one-third used no definite brushing stroke but, of those who employed an identifiable stroke, almost half used the roll method. This, however, may be one of the least efficient methods according to the Health Education Council (1979). Current opinion now favours the Bass method (Gibson and Wade 1977) or a modification of it.

The electric tooth-brush

Electric tooth-brushes have long been advocated for physically or mentally handicapped individuals (Smith and Blankenship 1964), and for those responsible for assisting others with tooth-cleaning. Well-informed individuals with reasonable digital skill, however, use the manual brush just as effectively as the traditional electric tooth-brush (McKendrick *et al.* 1968). In recent years, *rotational* electric tooth-brushes have been marketed, and evidence is accumulating to suggest that these are more efficient than both the manual and traditional electric tooth-brushes, especially at proximal surface plaque removal, when used either by students or by periodontal patients with normal manual dexterity (Van der Weijden *et al.* 1993; Yukna and Shaklee 1993; Stoltze and Bay 1994). Use of the wrong power setting may cause gingival abrasions (Yukna and Shaklee 1993).

Interdental cleaning

It is well established that periodontal conditions are worst in interdental areas where standard tooth-brushes are ineffective at removing proximal surface plaque. Furthermore, bacterial deposits remaining after brushing will promote the regrowth of fresh plaque (De La Rosa *et al.* 1979). The importance of total plaque removal is emphasized by Brecx *et al.* (1980) in a study of early plaque formation. Using light and electron microscopy, they concluded that the establishment of a complex and presumably pathogenic flora on cleaned tooth surfaces may be accelerated when plaque remains on other tooth surfaces.

The need for effective interdental cleaning has led to the manufacture of various devices. They should be recommended in accordance with individual dexterity and interdental anatomy.

Woodpoints (toothpicks)

The woodpoint is effective only where sufficient interdental space is available to accommodate it. Bergenholtz *et al.* (1974), in a study of open interdental spaces, demonstrated that triangular woodpoints are superior to round or rectangular ones, which are ineffective on lingual aspects of proximal surfaces. Triangular woodpoints in this study were more effective overall than dental floss. In a more recent study, testing various characteristics both *in vitro* and *in vivo*, Bergenholtz *et al.* (1980) concluded that triangular woodpoints with low surface hardness and high strength values are preferable. Axelsson (1993) advocates that, to clean posterior teeth, which normally have wider lingual than buccal embrasures, woodpoints should be fixed in a handle and inserted from the lingual side.

Dental floss

Although flossing requires more digital skill and is almost twice as time-consuming as the use of woodpoints (Gjermo and Flötra 1970), there appears to be no alternative method of cleaning proximal surfaces when a normal papilla fills the interdental space. Bergenholtz *et al.* (1974) and Kiger *et al.* (1991) showed that, when tooth-brushing was accompanied by flossing, more plaque was removed from the proximal surfaces than by tooth-brushing alone. Graves *et al.* (1989), in a 2-week supervised clinical trial of patients with gingivitis, showed that interdental bleeding was reduced by about 67 per cent by flossing and brushing compared to a 35 per cent reduction achieved by tooth-brushing alone. There is little apparent difference in the cleaning ability of waxed and unwaxed floss (Gjermo and Flötra 1970; Bergenholtz and Brithon 1980), nor is there any difference between dental tape and waxed or unwaxed dental floss with regard to their effectiveness at reducing interdental gingival bleeding (Graves *et al.* 1989). Gjermo and Flötra (1970) and Bergenholtz and Brithon (1980) demonstrated that floss was superior to woodpoints especially in removing plaque from the lingual aspect of proximal surfaces.

Interspace brush (single-tufted tooth-brush)

This device was introduced to improve access to tipped, rotated or displaced teeth and teeth affected by gingival recession. Gjermo and Flötra (1970) demonstrated that the combined use of the interspace brush and woodpoints compensated for the lack of effectiveness of woodpoints alone within lingual embrasures. The interspace brush is of limited value on its own at cleaning proximal surfaces except for surfaces adjacent to an extraction space.

The interdental brush (bottle brush)

Open interdental spaces are cleaned most thoroughly by the interdental brush (Gjermo and Flötra 1970), which is manufactured in different sizes. The larger type is held by its wire handle while smaller versions are attachable to a metal or plastic handle. Studies comparing the interdental brush with dental floss (Bergenholtz and Olsson 1984; Kiger *et al.* 1991) have shown it to be superior in cleaning large interdental spaces. Waerhaug (1976) showed that individuals who used the interdental brush habitually were able not only to maintain supragingival proximal surfaces free of plaque, but also to remove subgingival plaque to a depth of 2–2.5 mm below the gingival margin.

In patients with gingivitis, swollen papillae may initially limit the choice of interdental aid to dental floss. If, however, any proximal attachment loss has occurred, the gingival recession, which will inevitably occur with treatment, should, in due course, allow interdental brushes to be used instead.

Irrigation devices

These provide a steady or pulsating stream of water escaping through a nozzle under pressure. Oral irrigators should not be used as a substitute for tooth-brushing and are time-consuming and messy to use. There is also a risk that patients using irrigation devices may believe them to be more effective than proved, and reduce their efforts in manual plaque control. Only surface layers of soft plaque are removed and the findings reported from numerous clinical trials are conflicting with regard to an effect on gingivitis. Nevertheless, Rethman and Greenstein (1994), reviewing the literature, conclude that supragingival irrigation has a small adjunctive effect on plaque removal and gingivitis, particularly in areas of the dentition not readily accessed by conventional mechanical means. In special cases, irrigation devices may have a role in the delivery of chemical agents to the oral cavity (Cumming and Löe 1973*a*; Lang and Ramseier-Grossman 1981)—see the section on chemical plaque control, p. 131.

Toothpaste

It was established many years ago that brushing with a conventional fluoride toothpaste was a more effective means of plaque control than brushing with water alone. One study demonstrated that, during the 24-hour period after brushing, the rate of plaque regrowth in the group using toothpaste was 27 per cent lower than in the group brushing without toothpaste (De La Rosa *et al.* 1979). This effect may be attributed to detergents, abrasives or the antimicrobial effect of fluoride. Nowadays, many toothpastes are formulated with more effective antimicrobial agents which make significant contributions to plaque removal and reduction of gingivitis (Van der Ouderaa 1992) (see also p. 133). Although the degree of abrasivity may not influence the amount of plaque removal achieved, the abrasive property of toothpaste keeps the pellicle layer thin and prevents the accumulation of surface stains (Bergenholtz 1972). Paste with a high dentine abrasion value may cause destructive lesions in the cervical tooth region, but the optimum degree of abrasivity which will reduce surface pellicle without damaging tooth structure has

not been determined. Some toothpastes are now formulated with crystallization inhibitors such as soluble pyrophosphates, zinc citrate or a polymer system (Gantrez), which have been shown to reduce supragingival calculus formation (for review see White 1992).

Frequency of tooth-cleaning

Plaque forms continuously and tooth surfaces cannot be maintained in a plaque-free state by conventional mechanical means. The object of plaque control in prevention of periodontal disease is, therefore, the periodic removal of accumulated plaque at intervals which are sufficiently frequent to prevent pathological effects arising from recurrent plaque formation. Accordingly, individuals with healthy gingivae and no history of periodontal disease can prevent gingivitis by *complete* mechanical plaque removal every 48 hours (Lang *et al.* 1973). On the other hand, if inflammation is already present, colonization of the cleaned tooth surface occurs much sooner (Saxton 1973), plaque grows more rapidly (Lang *et al.* 1973; Ramberg *et al.* 1994), and matures faster (Brecx *et al.* 1980). This may be attributable to the presence of bacterial growth factors in gingival fluid which is secreted in larger amounts by inflamed gingival tissues. Dental plaque accumulation may also increase adjacent to swollen gingival tissues due to impaired natural cleansing by the tongue, cheeks, and lips (Ramberg *et al.* 1994). To control gingivitis, rather than prevent its onset, therefore, more frequent plaque removal may be necessary.

Individual susceptibility to gingivitis and periodontitis (Van der Velden *et al.* 1985) may be another important factor to consider in selecting a suitable frequency of tooth-cleaning. In their experimental gingivitis model, Löe *et al.* (1965) showed that, following the first clinical signs of inflammatory change, the introduction of oral hygiene measures, twice daily, achieved resolution of gingivitis within a few days. This was true even of the more susceptible individuals who had developed gingivitis at an early stage of plaque accumulation. Accordingly, to achieve gingival health, the interval between tooth-cleaning sessions need be no less than 12 hours and no greater than 48 hours, depending on prevailing gingival conditions and individual susceptibility to periodontal disease.

Duration and technique of tooth-cleaning

Questionnaire surveys in Scandinavian countries (e.g. Frandsen 1985) have revealed that, although the reported use of floss was negligible, tooth-brushing was practised once or twice daily by a majority of individuals. When gingivitis occurs, therefore, it is important not to jump to the convenient, but probably erroneous conclusion that tooth-brushing has been too infrequent. Cumming and Löe (1973*b*) have shown that, among individuals who brush at least twice daily, the same surfaces consistently remain cleaned or not cleaned at each tooth-cleaning session. Thoroughness of technique, therefore, is an important factor in prevention of gingivitis. Furthermore, in a study to analyse the effect of habitual tooth-brushing in 13-year-old children, the duration of brushing was found to have a greater influence on plaque removal than either its frequency or pattern (Honkala *et al.*

1986). Studies of tooth-brushing duration in uninstructed children (MacGregor *et al.* 1986) and uninstructed adults (MacGregor and Rugg-Gunn 1985) revealed brushing times of only 51 and 33 seconds, respectively.

Diet and natural cleansing

It has been shown by tube-feeding experiments in dogs (Egelberg 1965) and monkeys (Bowen 1974) that plaque formation is not dependent on the presence of food in the mouth.

The effect of diet on plaque accumulation is reviewed by E. Theilade and J. Theilade (1976). They conclude that the effect of dietary sugars on plaque quantity in man is generally far less pronounced than could be anticipated from theoretical considerations. They further state that there is great individual variation in the amount of plaque formation and its response to different dietary regimes. Although diet may influence the quantitative proportions of plaque micro-organisms, the clinical significance of such changes with respect to the initiation and progress of periodontal disease is not known.

It has been shown conclusively in a number of studies that the traditional concept of natural cleansing by detersive foodstuffs is not valid. This concept is cited by the Health Education Council (1979) as an example of a dental health message, popular in the past, which has little or no evidence to support it. Cervical tooth regions are not subject to much physical stress from food particles during mastication (Wilcox and Everett 1963) and excessive chewing of raw vegetables and fruit has a limited effect on the quantity of plaque accumulating there (Bergenholtz *et al.* 1967; Lindhe and Wicén 1969).

It is clear, therefore, that dietary advice, although important in caries prevention, is not beneficial with respect to periodontal disease.

PROLONGED PREVENTIVE PROGRAMMES BASED ON PLAQUE CONTROL

The components of an effective preventive programme based on plaque control are dental health education, oral hygiene instruction, and professional tooth-cleaning. The relative importance of each component has been assessed in a number of studies. These have measured various parameters of oral cleanliness and periodontal health, namely, plaque and calculus accumulation, gingival inflammation, gingival bleeding, pocket depths, attachment levels, and bone resorption. This work has been carried out both in children and adults. The discussion which follows concerns non-surgical methods of periodontal care which have been standardized for testing on large groups of individuals. The participants were 'ordinary' members of the public rather than periodontal patients *per se*, and the various procedures were tested both for their effects on pre-existing periodontal disease and for their ability to prevent new or recurrent disease. Because of the 'treatment' element, these programmes cannot be solely regarded as primary prevention.

PREVENTIVE PROGRAMMES IN CHILDREN

It is generally assumed that good oral hygiene practices are best acquired in childhood when they may be integrated with other developing health habits. Preventive programmes in schools provide continual opportunities for peer influence and the stimulating effect of daily personal interaction.

Evidence for the effectiveness of dental health education programmes in schools is equivocal (for review see Flanders 1987). Although there may be significant improvements in knowledge and attitudes, changes in behaviour, as measured by reduction in plaque and gingivitis, are usually short-lived. Craft (1984) reported the effect of the 'Natural Nashers' health education programme in the UK. This was a large trial involving 6700 13- to 14-year-olds who received a teacher–mediated dental health education programme comprising three 70–80 minute sessions, at weekly intervals. The programme employed active learning principles and included a slide presentation, experimental work, and use of work sheets. Improvement in plaque and gingivitis levels, while statistically significant, was small and faded considerably between the 5- and 28-week observation periods. Nevertheless, the exposure to such a dental health programme might conceivably improve the uptake of subsequent practice-based preventive care.

Supervised tooth-brushing in schools is an alternative approach which has been evaluated in several studies. Lindhe and Koch (1966), for example, in a study of 12- to 13-year-old schoolchildren, showed that a 3-year supervised daily brushing regimen in the last year of the study *reduced* gingivitis in 56 per cent of all tooth areas examined, whereas the control group showed a 75 per cent *increase* in gingivitis, typical of this stage of childhood.

Although supervised tooth-brushing may produce an overall improvement in gingival health, the reduction of gingivitis is unevenly distributed within the dentition. Lindhe *et al.* (1966) found that their test group had 80 per cent less gingivitis than controls in the upper anterior region but only 13 per cent less in the lower molar regions. Furthermore, Lindhe and Koch (1966) noted that gingivitis scores were somewhat higher for proximal surfaces than for buccal and lingual surfaces. Another major criticism of this type of preventive programme is the lack of any prolonged effect after it is withdrawn. Lindhe and Koch (1967) showed a substantial increase in gingivitis one year after the end of their 3-year supervised tooth-brushing programme in children who at follow-up were 16–17 years of age. Likewise, Horowitz *et al.* (1977), observing the effect of a 2-year supervised daily brushing and flossing regime in schoolchildren, initially 10–13 years old, noted that the benefits virtually disappeared during the summer vacation. These limitations, inherent in a tooth-brushing regimen, have to some extent been overcome in later studies in which dental personnel have introduced various other preventive strategies to children on an individual basis.

In 1974, Axelsson and Lindhe reported the effect of a rigorous preventive programme in schoolchildren aged initially 7–14 years. The test groups received fortnightly professional tooth-cleaning, oral hygiene instruction, and topical fluoride applications. Parental involvement was obtained at the beginning of the study and after 1 year. The experimental group after 2 years demonstrated low plaque scores and negligible signs of gingivitis. The control group children, on the other hand, had much higher plaque and gingivitis scores. In the test groups there were no significant differences between gingivitis scores of proximal and buccal/lingual areas. Thus it appears that careful fortnightly interproximal cleaning with floss or polishing tips prevents gingivitis in those areas in children. Furthermore the plaque control programme was equally effective for molars and incisors.

This study was continued for two further years. During the third year, the interval between prophylactic sessions was prolonged to 4 weeks in the younger age groups and to 8 weeks in the oldest age group (Lindhe *et al.* 1975). During the fourth year, all children were recalled every 8 weeks (Axelsson and Lindhe 1977). The excellent standard of oral hygiene was maintained during the third and fourth years and there was no significant change in gingival condition. Significant differences, however, were once again observed between test and control groups. This introductory 2-year programme of fortnightly prophylactic and oral hygiene sessions, followed by recall at intervals of one or two months during the third and fourth years, practically eliminated all signs of gingivitis in schoolchildren.

A further trial with a similar design was carried out by Hamp *et al.* (1978) primarily to assess the effect of preventive measures in a large group (1100) of schoolchildren between the ages of 7 and 17 years. Specially trained dental nurses administered oral hygiene instruction and professional tooth-cleaning, and applied topical fluoride every third week. Over the 3-year trial period, the frequency of plaque-infected surfaces in the experimental group fell from 64.1 per cent to 29.2 per cent, and the frequency of inflamed gingival units from 41.1 per cent to 18.8 per cent. Differences between test and control groups were highly significant at re-examination.

Further studies were designed to ascertain the separate effect of each component of the prophylactic regimen.

Poulsen *et al.* (1976) attempted to determine the benefits that might be obtained by professional tooth-cleaning alone in 78 7-year-old children. Thus the experimental group received thorough mechanical cleaning every 2 weeks while a control group were given no professional tooth cleaning. Both groups received fortnightly supervised fluoride rinsing. Throughout the study, home-care standards were not intentionally influenced. After 1 year, there was a statistically significant difference in plaque accumulation between the groups and an improvement in gingivitis in the test group. This study was continued for one further year during which the interval between professional tooth-cleaning sessions was increased to 3 weeks. Results were reported by Agerbaek *et al.* (1978). Plaque and gingivitis scores increased in the experimental group but remained significantly lower than in the control group where there was no appreciable change in oral cleanliness or gingival health. These studies demonstrate that the frequency of professional tooth-cleaning is of major importance when it is the only plaque control measure used, although it is difficult to assess the value of tooth-cleaning *per se* because the involvement of the children itself may have motivated them to practise better home-care.

That the benefits of fortnightly professional tooth-cleaning cannot be attributed entirely to the repeated removal of 2-week old plaque has also been demonstrated in a study by Axelsson and Lindhe (1981) involving 13- to 14-year-old children who received fortnightly professional tooth-cleaning in a split-mouth design. The children were divided into two groups only one of which received oral hygiene instruction at 2-week intervals. There was an equal reduction in plaque and gingivitis in the untreated quadrants of both groups of children suggesting that the subjective impression of tooth cleanliness, as identified in the cleaned jaw quadrants of the group not receiving oral hygiene instruction, was sufficient to motivate the children towards a standard of home-care which was equal to that achieved by the group which did receive oral hygiene instruction.

The fortnightly programme of Axelsson and Lindhe (1974), which has produced the most impressive reductions not only of gingivitis but also of caries, required about 160 min/child per year (Lindhe and Axelsson 1973). Traditional dental treatment, for children not participating in the trial, required about 140 min/child per year and cost over twice as much as the preventive programme. Furthermore, the trial participants achieved a much better standard of dental health—gingivitis was negligible and practically no caries developed. Attempts by others to match these results have, however, been unsuccessful. Although other trials (Ashley and Sainsbury 1981) have achieved similar reductions in plaque and gingivitis, their effect on caries has not been sufficiently large to make such programmes cost-effective.

PREVENTIVE PROGRAMMES IN ADULTS

From a practical standpoint, it is more important to prevent the progression of periodontitis, which is widespread in adults, than to abolish gingivitis. However, as gingivitis either precedes or accompanies destructive periodontal disease and plaque is the common aetiological agent, those measures which effect a reduction of gingivitis in children are pertinent also for adults. On the other hand, in adults, subgingival as well as supragingival deposits of plaque and calculus are common so that professional tooth cleaning may include an element of subgingival instrumentation to treat early destructive lesions (Fig. 8.1 d).

The success of a preventive regimen depends largely on the extent to which it will preserve attachment levels. In children, attachment loss occurs infrequently, and the consequences of plaque accumulation can be measured only by its effect on the gingivae. Preventive regimens in adults, however, may be assessed by comparing changes in attachment level with untreated control values.

The fundamental importance of oral hygiene instruction in preventing periodontitis was demonstrated by Suomi *et al.* (1973*b*) who found that when scaling and polishing was carried out, unsupported by oral hygiene instruction, the 17- to 22-year-old participants showed progressive gingivitis and attachment loss regardless of whether the procedure was repeated annually, 6-monthly or 3-monthly.

The need for scaling will clearly depend to a large extent on the rate of calculus formation and the presence of pathological pockets which harbour subgingival deposits of plaque and calculus. When pockets are less than 3 mm deep, therefore, gingivitis may be substantially reduced by oral hygiene instruction alone even when abundant supragingival calculus is present (Gaare *et al.* 1990). Pockets of 4–5 mm, on the other hand, will not respond to oral hygiene instruction until subgingival débridement has been performed (Cercek *et al.* 1983), and, once pocket depths exceed 5 mm, adequate non-surgical treatment becomes much less predictable. This was established by the earlier work of Lövdal *et al.* (1961), who carried out the first long-term study to evaluate the combined effect of oral hygiene instruction and scaling on the incidence of gingivitis. Their study group, originally comprising 1428 men and women, was followed for a period of 5 years, during which time prophylactic visits were arranged at 3- or 6-month intervals according to the severity of individual cases. After 5 years, there was a reduction in gingivitis of between one-eighth and one-half, depending on whether the participants started the study with good or poor oral hygiene respectively. The improvement was limited, however, to those areas where pocket depths did not exceed 5 mm and which, therefore, were reasonably accessible to scaling instruments.

The effect of such a prophylactic regimen, not only on gingival health but also on attachment levels, was later observed by Suomi *et al.* (1971*a*), who carried out a 3-year study in which they subjected their test group to dental health education, oral hygiene instruction, and professional tooth-cleaning at 2–4 month intervals. They showed that a matched control group, who were not recruited to the preventive programme, had substantially greater plaque scores, more gingivitis, and their rate of attachment loss, at 0.1 mm/year, was more than $3\frac{1}{2}$ times greater than their experimental counterparts. Furthermore, Suomi *et al.* (1971*b*) showed that, during the 3-year trial period, the experimental group showed almost no radiographic evidence of bone loss in the region studied—the lower right posterior segment—whereas the controls exhibited 0.19 mm of marginal bone destruction. Two and a half years after the experiment had been discontinued and the preventive regimen disbanded, Suomi *et al.* (1973*a*) showed that the former experimental group continued to demonstrate cleaner teeth and better periodontal health than the former control group. Nevertheless, the difference between groups with respect to oral hygiene and gingivitis had diminished.

A similar 3-year study was carried out by Axelsson and Lindhe (1978) to include an investigation on caries increment. Their experimental group of 375 adults received oral hygiene instruction and thorough scaling and root planing at the beginning of the study. These measures were repeated as necessary at 2-month intervals for the first 2 years and at 3-month intervals during the third year. A total of 180 matched controls received only traditional dental care at yearly intervals and, during this period, demonstrated persistent gingivitis and progressive loss of periodontal attachment. The experimental group, on the other hand, showed negligible signs of gingivitis and no loss of periodontal support.

This maintenance schedule was discontinued after 6 years. Then, during the following 9 years, the recall programme was designed to be needs-related. Thus, 65 per cent of the subjects were recalled once per year, 30 per cent twice per year, and 5 per cent (those with a recent history of progressive attachment loss) were recalled 3–6 times per year, and the low incidence of periodontal disease and caries was maintained (Axelsson *et al.* 1991). This study showed that, by tailoring supportive measures to individual requirements, it was possible to reduce greatly the overall professional input to a standardized preventive programme without detriment to dental or periodontal health. Furthermore, this type of study serves as a model for periodontal care: initial treatment to achieve optimum periodontal conditions, followed by a standard programme of maintenance care during which stability is assessed, ending with needs-related preventive maintenance.

Söderholm (1979) described a longitudinal study of 454 Swedish shipyard workers who, for 9 years between 1965 and 1974, received traditional dental care. Then, for 4 years between 1974 and 1978, they were enrolled instead on a treatment programme with a strong preventive emphasis which included scaling and oral hygiene instruction at 3-monthly intervals. The preventive programme reduced the proportion of tooth surfaces coated in plaque from 60 per cent to approximately 20 per cent, and the rate of periodontal bone loss from about 0.1 mm per year to zero; the rate of tooth loss was halved, at 0.1 teeth per individual per year. A cost-benefit analysis was reported by Björn (1982). Thus, traditional care was estimated at 2 hours of 'dentist time' and 16 minutes of 'dental auxiliary time' per year, while the preventive programme required 54 minutes of 'dentist time' and 1 hour 54 minutes of 'dental auxiliary time' per year. Although the participants spent 32 minutes more per year in the dental chair during the preventive programme, their dental care cost 10–20 per cent less, because the greater proportion of dental care was performed by a dental auxiliary. Furthermore, during the 4 years of prevention the participants enjoyed a much better standard of periodontal health and an improved periodontal prognosis.

CHEMICAL PLAQUE CONTROL

Plaque control by mechanical débridement is highly labour-intensive, whether professionally administered or practised personally. Satisfactory home-care further demands a measure of manual dexterity and a high degree of motivation which many individuals do not possess. Not surprisingly, therefore, a large number of chemical agents have been tested for their ability to reduce plaque accumulation. Some chemicals act by preventing colonization of the enamel or by removing attached organisms but, on the whole, these have shown less promise than antimicrobial agents.

This review will be limited to a consideration of those antimicrobials which have been tested as preventive agents for their effects on *supragingival* plaque accumulation. Therapeutic agents directed against *subgingival* plaque lie outwith the scope of this discussion.

Chemical antiplaque agents are assessed in several different ways: *in vitro* studies may be employed to evaluate antimicrobial action; short-term studies of a few days can assess the ability of the chemical agent to inhibit plaque formation *in vivo*; however, studies of 2–3 weeks are necessary to establish an inhibitory or therapeutic effect on gingivitis; and long-term studies of unsupervised use for several months are required to assess fully the adjunctive value of the agent when used in conjunction with tooth-brushing.

In spite of the wide range of antimicrobial substances of proven effectiveness in the treatment of many different infections, the nature of dental plaque infection limits the usefulness of chemical agents. Of major significance are the apparent non-specific nature of chronic gingivitis and the proliferative capacity of oral bacteria. Therefore, while various antiseptic mouthwashes can achieve a temporary reduction in the number of bacteria in plaque (Strålfors 1962), only those agents that remain active in the mouth, to exert a prolonged effect after administration, are capable of significant plaque inhibition. Thus, Gjermo et al. (1970) demonstrated that the cationic bisbiguanide, chlorhexidine, was a much more effective plaque-inhibitor *in vivo* than other antiseptics with equal or better *in vitro* activity. Indeed, it is well established that the antiplaque and antigingivitis effects of chlorhexidine are unsurpassed by all other chemical agents. Phenolic agents (Listerine) are moderately effective, and triclosan formulations hold some promise, but have not been fully evaluated. Quaternary ammonium compounds, metal salts, fluorides, sanguinarine, oxygenating agents, hexetidine, and enzymes are of little value. This literature has been reviewed by Ciancio (1992), Cummins and Creeth (1992), and Addy et al. (1994).

CHLORHEXIDINE

Chlorhexidine may be administered as a mouth rinse, as a toothpaste or gel, in an oral irrigator, or as a spray. Inconvenient local side-effects make it unsuitable for long-term use.

Mode of action

Chlorhexidine has a broad spectrum of bactericidal activity against Gram-positive and Gram-negative organisms. It was marketed by ICI (Macclesfield, England) in 1953 as a general disinfectant for skin and mucous membranes. It is used principally in the form of chlorhexidine digluconate.

The positively charged chlorhexidine binds to bacterial cell walls and to various oral surfaces including the hydroxyapatite of tooth enamel, the organic pellicle covering the tooth surface, mucous membrane, and salivary protein. Besides acting immediately on oral bacteria it is retained on the tooth surface to exert a prolonged bactericidal effect, and subsequently, as its concentration falls, a bacteriostatic effect for several hours. It interacts with bacteria, damaging permeability barriers and precipitating cytoplasm. The pharmacodynamics of chlorhexidine in the mouth indicate that the frequency of application should not be less than twice daily. A 0.2 per cent aqueous mouth rinse in 10 ml doses for 1 minute twice daily, has been shown to reduce the salivary bacterial count by 85–95 per cent over a 22-day period (Schiött et al. 1970), and essentially to prevent plaque accumulation and gingivitis development in subjects whose habitual mechanical cleaning is suspended (Löe and Schiött 1970a). Suppression of the salivary flora, however, does not appear to play a major part in dental plaque inhibition, which is primarily a result of the local antibacterial activity of chlorhexidine that has become bound to tooth-surface components (Davies et al. 1970).

Mouthwash

The antiplaque effects of chlorhexidine are dose-, not concentration-related. Thus, optimum plaque control is achieved with a divided daily dose of 18–20 mg; for example 10 ml of 0.2 per cent chlorhexidine twice daily (Löe and Schiött 1970a), or 15 ml of 0.12 per cent chlorhexidine twice daily (Grossman et al. 1986; Segreto et al. 1986; Siegrist et al. 1986). Significant, although suboptimal effects may be obtained with reduced dosage and frequency of use, namely 15 ml of 0.2 per cent chlorhexidine once daily (Lang et al. 1982); 10 ml of 0.1 per cent chlorhexidine twice daily (Flötra et al. 1972; Axelsson and Lindhe 1987); and 15 ml of 0.1 per cent chlorhexidine once daily (Lang et al. 1982). In theory, those side-effects, such as taste disturbance, which are concentration-dependent, should be less when using reduced concentrations of the drug, thereby leading to better compliance for long-term usage.

It must be stressed that antimicrobial agents, chlorhexidine included, have little or no effect on *established* plaque in doses intended for inhibition of *new* plaque formation. To resolve a superficial gingivitis, produced by 17 days of uninterrupted plaque accumulation, a more intensive programme of mouth rinsing was required (Löe and Schiött 1970b). This regimen comprised six 1 minute rinses with 10 ml of 0.2 per cent chlorhexidine in the space of 1 hour followed by twice daily rinsing with the same solution. After 6 days the teeth were virtually plaque-free.

It was further shown by Flötra et al. (1972) that twice daily 0.2 per cent chlorhexidine mouthwashes, accompanied by customary personal oral hygiene regimens, although producing a large reduction in supragingival plaque, had a less dramatic effect on established gingivitis where subgingival plaque had formed. Following subgingival scaling, the experimental group receiving chlorhexidine showed substantial improvement in gingival health in those areas where pocket depths did not exceed 3 mm. However, even after subgingival scaling, the continued use of chlorhexidine had no therepeutic effect where pocket depths exceeded 3 mm. This suggested, therefore, that chlorhexidine mouthwash is unable to eliminate subgingival plaque or to prevent recolonization of deep pathological pockets from subgingival deposits of bacteria not removed by scaling.

Oral irrigation

Taste disturbance can be reduced by reducing the concentration of chlorhexidine, and to achieve an effective dose, an oral irrigator can be used to deliver a larger volume. Indeed, by improving the distribution of chlorhexidine to the more inaccessible areas of the dentition, this use of an oral irrigator may achieve better plaque control than a 0.2 per cent mouthwash (Cumming and Löe 1973a). In a more recent study on the use of chlorhexidine with an oral irrigator, Lang and Ramseier-Grossman (1981) established that 400 ml of a 0.02 per cent solution of chlorhexidine once daily was the lowest concentration and dose to achieve complete plaque inhibition. Reducing the concentration further did not achieve complete plaque control even when the dose was increased.

Toothpaste

Many toothpaste ingredients, notably anionic detergents, will interact with, and inactivate chlorhexidine. As a result, attempts to formulate an active chlorhexidine-containing toothpaste have, on the whole, met with little success. Yates *et al.* (1993), however, have recently evaluated two experimental 1 per cent chlorhexidine toothpastes, one with fluoride. Anionic detergents were omitted from the formulations and both pastes achieved modest reductions in plaque and gingivitis throughout the 6-month period of the study. Staining and calculus were significantly increased in the experimental groups compared with the control group.

Tooth gel

Aqueous gels containing 1 per cent chlorhexidine have been commercially available for many years. Most studies have demonstrated modest reductions in plaque (Hansen *et al.* 1975; Hoyos *et al.* 1977; Bain and Strahan 1978) or in plaque and gingivitis (Bassiouny and Grant 1975; Joyston-Bechal *et al.* 1979) among participants who brushed with the gel. However, the necessary absence of detergents and abrasives from gel formulations of chlorhexidine, reduces patient acceptance since there is then nothing in the product to counteract stain formation.

Although chlorhexidine gel is of little adjunctive value in individuals with moderate or good oral hygiene, it may have a greater therapeutic effect among those with high plaque levels and frank gingivitis. This was the conclusion of Flötra (1973) and Usher (1975), who demonstrated significant reductions in plaque, debris, and gingivitis when chlorhexidine gel was applied in trays to the teeth of severely handicapped individuals for whom conventional cleaning methods were unacceptable. The efficacy of gel application in trays has recently been confirmed by Francis *et al.* (1987*a*) in a study of handicapped children, but most of the parents and house parents found the technique awkward and felt they would not be willing to continue the regimen for long periods (Francis *et al.* 1987*b*).

Spray

Some individuals, by virtue of physical or mental handicap, find mouth rinsing a difficult task. An alternative delivery system involving spray application of chlorhexidine has, therefore, been tested. Thus, although a low dose of chlorhexidine (1.5–2.0 ml of 0.2 per cent solution), applied in a spray to the teeth of handicapped children, was less effective than gel application in trays, and although its effect on plaque and gingivitis was minimal (Francis *et al.* 1987*a*), the spray method was considerably more popular among the care workers and parents responsible for its use than the mouthwash or gel (Francis *et al.* 1987*b*). It was later shown, in a 4-day plaque regrowth study, that, when chlorhexidine was sprayed under optimal conditions by dental professionals, there was a marked plaque inhibitory effect comparable to a standard 0.2 per cent mouthwash regimen (Kalaga *et al.* 1989*a*). Furthermore, there were considerable improvements in plaque and gingivitis in a 31-day trial when the spray was administered partly by dental professionals and partly by the handicapped individuals themselves or by their parents or guardians (Kalaga *et al.* 1989*b*). Therefore, if sufficient professional support is provided, spray application of chlorhexidine would appear to have some advantage over more traditional methods of chemical plaque control. These studies also show that, when teeth are targeted to receive the chlorhexidine, much lower doses are required for plaque control, the proportion of drug which becomes bound to the oral mucosa being minimized.

Safety and side-effects

Bacteriological studies conducted after long-term use of chlorhexidine mouthwash have shown that, although the number of salivary and plaque organisms were reduced, there was no detectable shift in microbial populations, no residual effects on salivary or plaque bacteria after cessation of rinsing (Schiött *et al.* 1976*a*; Briner *et al.* 1986*a*), and little evidence of bacterial mutation or selection of resistant strains (Schiött *et al.* 1976*b*; Briner *et al.* 1986*b*) Furthermore, after a 22-day period of twice daily mouth rinsing with 0.2 per cent chlorhexidine, the total salivary bacterial count increased to the control level within 48 hours (Schiött *et al.* 1970), and plaque formed at normal rates after 24 hours (Löe and Schiött 1970*a*).

Data accumulated over a period of 20 years concerning the safety of chlorhexidine in animal (Case 1977) and human (Rushton 1977) studies have been reviewed. It is known to have low irritancy and is most unlikely to produce sensitization. Absorption after oral ingestion is very low and long-term use has produced no changes in haematological or biochemical parameters. Prolonged application has failed to show carcinogenic or teratogenic effects.

The majority of side-effects are of a local nature. It has an unpleasant taste and produces disturbances in taste sensation which may last for several hours. Desquamative lesions of the oral mucosa occur in a small number of individuals, perhaps due to precipitation of acidic mucins and proteins that cover and protect mucous membranes (Flötra *et al.* 1971). This makes the epithelium vulnerable to mechanical trauma or to the cytotoxic effect of chemicals, including chlorhexidine itself (Almqvist and Luthman 1988). A few cases of unilateral or bilateral parotid gland swelling have been reported after use of chlorhexidine mouth rinses. The clinical features are suggestive of mechanical obstruction of the parotid duct (Rushton 1977). The unpleasant taste and mucosal effects can be diminished by reducing the concentration (and using a larger volume to maintain clinical efficacy).

Brown discoloration of teeth and fillings is common, both with mouthwash and gel preparations of chlorhexidine, a side-effect which is shared with other cationic antiseptics. Brown staining of the dorsum of the tongue occurs with the mouthwash but not with the toothpaste/gel. There is an interaction between locally adsorbed chlorhexidine and factors derived from diet such as the tannin-like substances in red wine, tea, and coffee (Jensen 1977; Addy *et al.* 1979; Praynito *et al.* 1979). This interaction is responsible for the characteristic stain. There is also a tendency for more supragingival calculus to be formed (Löe *et al.* 1976;

Grossman *et al.* 1986; Segreto *et al.* 1986) which counteracts the benefits of chlorhexidine. The mechanism for this effect may involve the suppression of acidogenic plaque bacteria; the pH at the tooth surface is raised, leading to precipitation of calcium and phosphate.

Stain and calculus formation are dose-dependent and cannot be reduced significantly without loss of antiplaque effects (Jenkins *et al.* 1989).

Clinical applications

Although the side-effects are minor, their existence has placed limitations on the application of chlorhexidine to clinical practice. Nevertheless, chlorhexidine has been shown to serve a useful function in the following circumstances.

1. The post-operative management of periodontal wounds.

2. The management of desquamative forms of gingivitis: individuals with painful gingival lesions may be placed on a chlorhexidine mouthwash regimen instead of tooth-brushing.

3. Plaque control during intermaxillary fixation.

4. Long-term plaque control in handicapped individuals or medically compromised patients.

Unfortunately, the success of chlorhexidine in these specific situations is not equalled by its effect on established periodontal disease. As previously noted, the standard mouthwash regimen will not remove existing supragingival plaque or penetrate below the gingival margin to remove subgingival plaque. Indeed, it is also apparent that chlorhexidine does not penetrate the interdental space sufficiently well to have any significant effect on interdental gingivitis (Bowsma *et al.* 1992; Caton *et al.* 1993). Furthermore, if chlorhexidine mouthwash is used during the initial phase of hygiene therapy, it will mask the effects of personal mechanical plaque control upon which successful long-term treatment of periodontal disease is dependent, and make proper evaluation of the patient's efforts impossible. Chlorhexidine, therefore, should be reserved for prevention of plaque accumulation only where mechanical plaque removal is impracticable.

PHENOLIC COMPOUNDS

Listerine, a combination of the phenol-related essential oils, thymol and eucalyptol, mixed with menthol and methyl salicylate in a hydroalcoholic vehicle, is a well-established commercial mouthwash. Early studies, both short- and long-term, reviewed by Mandel (1988), confirm moderate antiplaque and antigingivitis effects, with a bitter taste and occasional staining as the principal side-effects. More recent studies are reviewed by Ramberg *et al.* (1992) and show that, in short-term comparative studies, with chlorhexidine as a positive control, Listerine is less effective. There is no data on the substantivity of Listerine.

Triclosan, another non-ionic phenol, has been a common constituent of soaps and deodorants for the last 25 years. It is a broad-spectrum antimicrobial agent of moderate activity and substantivity. It has been formulated with a copolymer (Gantrez) to improve its substantivity and, in a 6-month study, a 0.03 per cent triclosan/Gantrez mouthwash achieved moderate reductions in plaque and gingivitis without side-effects when used as a pre-brushing rinse (Worthington *et al.* 1993). Being non-ionic, triclosan is compatible with toothpaste ingredients, and is now a common constituent of toothpaste in combination with Gantrez, or with pyrophosphate, or with zinc citrate. Pyrophosphate is a weak antimicrobial agent. It has low substantivity but acts synergistically with triclosan to give an enhanced antimicrobial effect *in vitro* (Marsh and Bradshaw 1993). Zinc, in common with other metal ions, is a highly substantive antimicrobial agent. It is formulated with citrate to reduce the metallic taste and, when combined with triclosan, exhibits synergistic action comparable *in vitro* to the triclosan/pyrophosphate combination (Marsh and Bradshaw 1993). Gantrez, zinc salts, and pyrophosphates are also crystallization inhibitors and are effective at preventing mineralization of supragingival plaque (White 1992). Considerable data is available, proving the efficacy of Gantrez/triclosan and zinc citrate/triclosan as inhibitors of plaque and gingivitis (Van der Ouderaa 1992). Comparative *in vitro* and clinical studies of toothpastes containing 0.3 per cent triclosan have been carried out to assess the relative merits of the various triclosan combinations. Thus, Creeth *et al.* (1993) found that significantly more triclosan was delivered to and retained on oral surfaces from a triclosan/zinc citrate toothpaste compared to a triclosan/copolymer or triclosan/pyrophosphate paste. Furthermore, in a 7-month tooth-brushing study, a triclosan/zinc citrate toothpaste provided significantly greater reductions in plaque, calculus, and gingival bleeding than other triclosan toothpastes formulated with copolymer or pyrophosphate (Svatun *et al.* 1993). Compared to controls, the zinc citrate formulation produced reductions of 33 per cent in plaque, 51 per cent in gingival bleeding, and 67 per cent in calculus formation; the toothpastes which were formulated with copolymer or pyrophosphate achieved only a 25 per cent reduction in gingival bleeding and showed no statistically significant effect on plaque or calculus.

It appears from numerous studies that triclosan in toothpaste does not reduce the bioavailability of fluoride or disrupt the natural microbial ecology of the mouth.

CONCLUDING REMARKS

Although periodontal disease accounts for 20–30 per cent of all extractions, the benefits of prevention of periodontal disease are not limited to tooth survival: bleeding gingivae and bad taste may be distressing; red, swollen gingivae, migrated teeth, and gingival recession may be unaesthetic, and halitosis is socially undesirable. As living standards improve and health expectations rise, an increasing number of individuals may be unwilling to accept mere tooth survival as a suitable yardstick of dental fitness. Freedom from periodontal symptoms and a sense of personal well-being must, therefore, be an important objective of preventive periodontal care.

Increasing the availability and utilization of present systems of restorative dental care is not an appropriate means to improve periodontal health. Indeed, it has been shown that periodontal disease may progress at the same rate in those receiving regular dental care of the traditional reparative variety as in those who attend sporadically (Björn 1974). Oral hygiene education and the provision of optimum conditions for self-performed plaque control form the basis of periodontal disease prevention.

Any population strategy which results in improved tooth-cleaning behaviour is certain to reduce the prevalence and severity of periodontal diseases. However, while public dental health education may be a relatively inexpensive way to deliver a preventive message, there is little evidence, so far, that such a population-based approach can produce a significant and sustained improvement in oral hygiene and periodontal health. Furthermore, because of the great variation in disease susceptibility and the differing needs of individuals, it follows that prevention of periodontal disease will be most effective when provided on a one-to-one basis in a dental surgery.

Practice-based periodontal care involves diagnosis and treatment of existing periodontal disease *before* proceeding with a preventive maintenance programme. This is because a maintenance schedule, comprising single-visit sessions of scaling and oral hygiene instruction at widely spaced intervals, is unlikely to restore periodontal health or prevent progressive attachment loss when a significant amount of disease was present at the outset. Instead, a sustained course of treatment should first be given, and continued until the patient achieves his peak level of plaque control, and all accessible deposits have been removed. Surgical intervention may also be necessary. Once treatment is complete, a needs-related maintenance programme based on oral hygiene re-instruction and scaling should be established to intercept new or recurrent disease while still at an early stage. The individual's subjective needs, level of motivation, susceptibility to periodontal disease, and response to treatment will determine the long-term treatment goal as well as the interval between visits.

If established disease is present and proves unresponsive to treatment because of inadequate personal oral hygiene or inaccessible subgingival deposits, the clinician is faced with a dilemma: how much and what kind of supportive care is appropriate? This question has still to be adequately addressed by appropriate clinical research. There is, so far, little evidence that periodontal disease can be 'contained' by repeated subgingival instrumentation at sites where subgingival deposits are not fully accessible or where the prevailing level of plaque control is insufficient to prevent pockets being recolonized. In fact, repeated subgingival débridement in these cases may be counter-productive in the long-term because of the high risk of attachment loss due to instrumentation trauma (Claffey *et al.* 1988).

With regard to the practical aspects of plaque control, the level of oral hygiene necessary to maintain periodontal health is likely to vary within the dentition as well as between individuals, and oral hygiene aids should be prescribed to suit individual needs and capabilities. While tooth-brushing is invigorating and, therefore, well accepted, most patients find little incentive for interdental cleaning, which is comparatively difficult and time-consuming, whatever means are employed. Nonetheless, thorough *daily* interdental cleaning is essential to maintain periodontal health in most individuals. Indeed, the establishment and maintenance of a good inter-

dental cleaning habit is the principal goal of education and instruction for periodontal patients.

Many chemical antiplaque agents are now available, their development promoted by lack of public enthusiasm for mechanical methods of plaque control. The broad-spectrum antiseptic, chlorhexidine, has been exhaustively tested and, in mouthwash form, remains the agent of choice in chemical control of supragingival plaque when effective mechanical plaque control is temporarily suspended. There is, however, little point encouraging long-term use of chlorhexidine, if only because of its undesirable side-effects, although an argument can be made for its long-term use in one form or another for special needs groups. Many other mouthwash solutions are now commercially available, although none are as effective as chlorhexidine. Furthermore, the long-term use of all mouthwashes, even those without side-effects, has major cost implications. Attention, therefore, is now being focused on toothpaste as a vehicle for chemical antiplaque agents, and toothpastes containing triclosan show some promise.

Clearly for the majority of individuals with a positive attitude towards oral health, the means already exist to maintain reasonably good periodontal conditions throughout life using comparatively simple forms of personal and professional care. There remains, however, a minority of individuals who are highly susceptible to the destructive effects of plaque accumulation.

SUMMARY

- Susceptibility to periodontal breakdown varies considerably within and between individuals, and must be professionally assessed before selecting a preventive strategy.

- In developed countries, where ritual toothbrushing is already practised, the establishment and maintenance of a good interdental cleaning habit is the principal goal of education and instruction for periodontal patients.

- Oral hygiene instruction must be periodically reinforced.

- Existing periodontal disease should be treated and optimal periodontal health established *before* embarking on a programme of preventive maintenance.

- Preventive procedures and the interval between recall visits should be related to individual needs and susceptibilities.

- Preventive maintenance should comprise, as necessary, re-instruction in plaque control methods, removal of factors which inhibit personal oral hygiene, such as calculus and restoration overhangs, and treatment of recurrent disease while still at an early stage.

- Chlorhexidine mouthwash is the antiplaque agent of choice when mechanical cleaning has been temporarily compromised or suspended. It will inhibit new supra-gingival plaque formation on exposed tooth surfaces.

- Long-term use of chlorhexidine as a mouthwash, gel, or spray, may be appropriate for special needs groups.

REFERENCES

Addy, M. and Bates, J.F. (1979). Plaque accumulation following the wearing of different types of removable partial dentures. *J. oral Rehabil.* **6**, 111–7.

Addy, M., Praynito, S.W., Taylor, L., and Cadogan, S. (1979). An *in vitro* study of the role of dietary factors in the aetiology of tooth staining associated with the use of chlorhexidine. *J. perio. Res.* **14**, 403–10.

Addy, M., Moran, J., and Wade, W. (1994). Chemical plaque control in the prevention of gingivitis and periodontitis. In *Proceedings of the 1st European Workshop on Periodontology* (Ittingen, 1993) (ed. N.P. Lang and T. Karring), pp. 244–57. Quintessence, London.

Agerbaek, N., Poulsen, S., Melsen, B., and Glavind, L. (1978). Effect of professional tooth cleansing every third week on gingivitis and dental caries in children. *Commun. Dent. oral Epidemiol.* **6**, 40–1.

Ainamo, J., Barmes, D., Beagrie, G., Cutress, T., Martin, J., and Sardo-Infrri, J. (1982). Development of the World Health Organisation (WHO) community periodontal index of treatment needs (CPITN). *Int. dent. J.* **32**, 281–91.

Almqvist, H. and Luthman, J. (1988) Gingival and mucosal reactions after intensive chlorhexidine gel treatment with or without oral hygiene measures. *Scand. J. dent. Res.* **96**, 557–60.

Anderson, R.J. (1981). The changes in the dental health of 12-year-old schoolchildren in two Somerset schools. A review after an interval of 15 years. *Br. dent. J.* **150**, 218–21.

Ashley, F.P. and Sainsbury, R.H. (1981). The effect of a school-based plaque control programme on caries and gingivitis. *Br. dent. J.* **150**, 41–5.

Axelsson, P. (1993). New ideas and advancing technology in preventive and non-surgical treatment of periodontal disease. *Int. dent. J.* **43**, 223–38.

Axelsson, P. and Lindhe, J. (1974). The effect of a preventive programme on dental plaque, gingivitis and caries in schoolchildren. *J. clin. Perio.* **1**, 126–38.

Axelsson, P. and Lindhe, J. (1977). The effect of a plaque control programme on gingivitis and dental caries in schoolchildren. *J. dent. Res.* **56** (special issue C), 142–8.

Axelsson, P. and Lindhe, J. (1978). Effect of controlled oral hygiene procedures on caries and periodontal disease in adults. *J. clin. Perio.* **5**, 133–51.

Axelsson, P. and Lindhe, J. (1981). Effect of oral hygiene instruction and professional toothcleaning on caries and gingivitis in schoolchildren. *Commun. Dent. oral Epidemiol.* **9**, 251–5.

Axelsson, P. and Lindhe, J. (1987). Efficacy of mouthrinses in inhibiting dental plaque and gingivitis in man. *J. clin. Perio.* **14**, 205–12.

Axelsson, P., Lindhe, J., and Nyström, B. (1991). On the prevention of caries and periodontal disease. Results of a 15-year longitudinal study in adults. *J. clin. Perio.* **18**, 182–9.

Badersten, A., Nilvéus, R., and Egelberg, J. (1984). Effects of non-surgical periodontal therapy. II. Severely advanced periodontitis. *J. clin. Perio.* **11**, 63–76.

Baelum, V., Manji, F., and Fejerskov, O. (1991). The distribution of periodontal destruction in the populations of non-industrialized countries: evidence for the existence of high risk groups and individuals. In *Risk markers for oral diseases*: Vol. 3. *Periodontal diseases*, (ed. N.W. Johnson), pp. 27–75. Cambridge University Press.

Bain, M.J. and Strahan, J.D. (1978). The effect of a 1% chlorhexidine gel in the initial therapy of chronic periodontal disease. *J. Perio.* **49**, 469–74.

Barnes, G.P., Stookey, G.K., and Muhler, J.C. (1971). *In vitro* studies of the calculus-inhibiting properties of tooth surface polishing agents and chelating agents. *J. dent. Res.* **50**, 966–75.

Bassiouny, M.A. and Grant, A.A. (1975). The toothbrush application of chlorhexidine. *Br. dent. J.* **139**, 323–7.

Bergenholtz, A. (1972). Mechanical cleaning in oral hygiene. In *Oral hygiene*, (ed. A. Frandsen), pp. 27–62. Munksgaard, Copenhagen.

Bergenholtz, A. and Brithon, J. (1980). Plaque removal by dental floss or toothpicks. An intra-individual comparative study. *J. clin. Perio.* **7**, 516–24.

Bergenholtz, A. and Olsson, A. (1984), Efficacy of plaque-removal using interdental brushes and waxed dental floss. *Scand. J. dent. Res.* **92**, 198–203.

Bergenholtz, A., Hugoson, A., and Sohlberg, F. (1967). The plaque-removing property of some oral hygiene aids. *Svensk Tand. Tidskr.* **60**, 447–54.

Bergenholtz, A., Bjorne, A., and Vikström, B. (1974). The plaque-removing ability of some common interdental aids. An intra-individual study. *J. clin. Perio.* **1**, 160–5.

Bergenholtz, A., Bjorne, A., Glantz, P.-O., and Vikström, B. (1980). Plaque removal by various triangular toothpicks. *J. clin. Perio.* **7**, 121–8.

Billier, I.R., Hunter, E.L., and Featherstone, M. (1980). Enamel loss during a prophylaxis polish in vitro. *J. Int. Ass. Child.* **11**, 7–12.

Bimstein, E., Delaney, J.E., and Sweeney, E.A. (1988). Radiographic assessment of the alveolar bone in children and adolescents. *Ped. Dent.* **10**, 199–204.

Björn, A.-L. (1974). Dental health in relation to age and dental care. *Odontologisk Revy*, **25**, supplement 29.

Björn, A.-L. (1982). Economy aspects of preventive dentistry. In *Dental health care in Scandinavia*, (ed. A. Frandsen), pp. 217–24. Quintessence, Chicago.

Blinkhorn, A.S., Fox, B., and Holloway, P.J. (1983). *Notes on dental health education*, Scottish Health Education Group, Edinburgh, and Health Education Authority, London.

Bowen, W.H. (1974). Effect of restricting oral intake to invert sugar or casein on the microbiology of plaque in *Macaca fascicularis (irus)*. *Arch. oral Biol.* **19**, 231–9.

Bowsma, O.J., Yost, K.G., and Baron, H.J. (1992). Comparison of a chlorhexidine rinse and a wooden interdental cleaner in reducing interdental gingivitis. *Am. J. Dent.* **5**, 143–6.

Boyde, A. (1971). The tooth surface. In *The prevention of periodontal disease*, (ed. J.E. Eastoe, D.C.A. Picton, and A.G. Alexander), pp. 46–63. Kimpton, London.

Brecx, M., Theilade, J., and Attström, R. (1980). Influence of optimal and excluded oral hygiene on early formation of dental plaque on plastic films. A quantitative and descriptive light and electron microscopic study. *J. clin. Perio.* **7**, 361–73.

Briner, W.W., *et al.* (1986*a*). Effect of chlorhexidine gluconate mouthrinse on plaque bacteria. *J. perio. Res.* **21** (suppl. 16), 44–52.

Briner, W.W., *et al.* (1986*b*). Assessment of susceptibility of plaque bacteria to chlorhexidine after six months oral use. *J. perio. Res.*, **21** (suppl. 16), 53–9.

Brown, L.J., Oliver, R.C., and Löe, H. (1990). Evaluating periodontal status of US employed adults. *J. Am. dent. Ass.* **121**, 226–32.

Brunsvold, M.A. and Lane, J.J. (1990). The prevalence of overhanging dental restorations and their relationship to periodontal disease. *J. clin. Perio.* **17**, 67–72.

Case, D.E. (1977) Safety of Hibitane. 1. Laboratory experiments. *J. clin. Perio.* **4** (extra issue), 66–72.

Caton, J.G., *et al.* (1993). Comparison between mechanical cleaning and an antimicrobial rinse for the treatment and prevention of interdental gingivitis. *J. clin. Perio.* **20**, 172–8.

Cercek, J.F., Kiger, R.D., Garrett, S., and Egelberg, J. (1983). Relative effects of plaque control and instrumentation on the clinical parameters of human periodontal disease. *J. clin. Perio.* **10**, 46–56.

Ciancio, S.G. (1992). Agents for the management of plaque and calculus. *J. dent. Res.* **71**, 1450–4.

Claffey, N., Loos, B., Gantes, B., Martin, M., Heins, P., and Egelberg, J. (1988). The relative effects of therapy and periodontal disease on loss of probing attachment after root débridement. *J. clin. Perio.* **15**, 163–9.

Clerehugh, V., Lennon, M.A., and Worthington, H.V. (1990). 5-year results of a longitudinal study of early periodontitis in 14 to 19-year-old adolescents. *J. clin. Perio.* **17**, 702–8.

Committee Report (1966). Oral health care for the prevention and control of periodontal disease. In *World workshop in periodontics* (ed. S.P. Ramfjord, D.A. Kerr, and M.M. Ash), pp. 444–53. University of Michigan Press, Ann Arbor.

Corbet, E.F. and Davies, W.I.R. (1993). The role of supragingival plaque in the control of progressive periodontal disease. A review. *J. clin. Perio.* **20**, 307–13.

Craft, M.H. (1984). Dental health education and periodontal disease: health policies, disease trends, target groups and strategies. In *Public health aspects of periodontal disease* (ed. A. Frandsen), pp. 149–60. Quintessence, Chicago.

Creeth, J.E., Abraham, P.J., Barlow, J.A., and Cummins, D. (1993). Oral delivery and clearance of antiplaque agents from Triclosan-containing dentrifices. *Int. dent. J.* **43**, 387–99.

Cumming, B.R. and Löe, H. (1973a). Optimal dosage and method of delivering chlorhexidine solutions for the inhibition of dental plaque. *J. perio. Res.* **8**, 57–62.

Cumming, B.R. and Löe, H. (1973b). Consistency of plaque distribution in individuals without special home care instruction. *J. perio. Res.* **8**, 94–100.

Cummins, D. and Creeth, J.E. (1992). Delivery of antiplaque agents from dentifrices, gels and mouthwashes. *J. dent. Res.* **71**, 1439–49.

Cushing, A.M. and Sheiham, A. (1985). Assessing periodontal treatment needs and periodontal status in a study of adults in north-west England. *Commun. dent. Health*, **2**, 187–94.

Cutress, T.W. (1986). Periodontal health and periodontal disease in young people: global epidemiology. *Int. dent. J.* **36**, 146–51.

Davies, R.M., Jensen, S.B., Schiött, C.R., and Löe, H. (1970). The effect of topical application of chlorhexidine on the bacterial colonization of the teeth and gingiva. *J. perio. Res.* **5**, 96–101.

De La Rosa, M.R., Guerra, J.Z., Johnston, D.A., and Radike, A.W. (1979). Plaque growth and removal with daily toothbrushing. *J. Perio.*, **50**, 661–4.

Douglass, C.W., Gammon, M.D., and Orr, R.B. (1985). Oral health status in the United States: prevalence of inflammatory periodontal diseases. *J. dent. Educ.* **49**, 365–7.

Egelberg, J. (1965). Local effect of diet on plaque formation and development of gingivitis in dogs. III. Effect of frequency of meals and tube feeding. *Odontologisk Revy*, **16**, 50–60.

El Ghamrawy, R. (1979). Qualitative changes in dental plaque formation related to removable partial dentures. *J. oral Rehab.* **6**, 183–8.

Flanders, R.A. (1987). Effectiveness of dental health educational programs in schools. *J. Am. dent. Ass.* **114**, 239–42.

Flötra, L. (1973). Different modes of chlorhexidine application and related local side effects. *J. perio. Res.* **8** (suppl. 12), 41–4.

Flötra, L., Gjermo, P., Rölla, G., and Waerhaug, J. (1971). Side effects of chlorhexidine mouthwashes. *Scand. J. dent. Res.* **79**, 119–25.

Flötra, L., Gjermo, P., Rölla, G., and Waerhaug, J. (1972). A 4-month study on the effect of chlorhexidine mouthwashes on 50 soldiers. *Scand. J. dent. Res.* **80**, 10–17.

Francis, J.R., Hunter, B., and Addy, M. (1987a). A comparison of three delivery methods of chlorhexidine in handicapped children. I. Effects on plaque, gingivitis and tooth staining. *J. Perio.*, **58**, 451–5.

Francis, J.R., Addy, M., and Hunter, B. (1987b). A comparison of three delivery methods of chlorhexidine in handicapped children. II. Parent and house-parent preferences. *J. Perio.* **58**, 456–9.

Frandsen, A. (1985). Changing patterns of attitudes and oral health behaviour. *Int. dent. J.* **35**, 284–90.

Garre, D., Rölla, G., Aryadi, F.J., and van der Ouderaa, F. (1990). Improvement of gingival health by toothbrushing in individuals with large amounts of calculus. *J. clin. Perio.*, **17**, 38–41.

Gibson, J.A. and Wade, A.B. (1977). Plaque removal by the Bass and roll brushing techniques. *J. Perio.* **48**, 456–9.

Gjermo, P.E. (1967). Effect of combined audiovisual motivation and individual instruction in oral hygiene (abstract). *J. perio. Res.* **2**, 248.

Gjermo, P. and Flötra, L. (1970). The effect of different methods of interdental cleaning. *J. perio. Res.*, **5**, 230–6.

Gjermo, P., Baastad, K.L., and Rölla, A. (1970). The plaque-inhibiting capacity of 11 antibacterial compounds. *J. perio. Res.*, **5**, 102–9.

Glantz, P.-O. (1969). On wettability and adhesiveness. *Odontologisk Revy*, **20** (suppl. 17).

Glavind, L., Christensen, H., Pedersen, E., Rosendahl, H., and Attström, R. (1985). Oral hygiene instruction in general dental practice by means of self-teaching manuals. *J. clin. Perio.*, **12**, 27–34.

Graves, R.C., Disney, J.A., and Stamm, J.W. (1989). Comparative effectiveness of flossing and brushing in reducing interproximal bleeding. *J. Perio.* **60**, 243–7.

Greene, J.C. (1963). Oral hygiene and periodontal disease. *Am. J. pub. Health*, **53**, 913–22

Greene, J.C. (1966). Oral health care for prevention and control of periodontal disease. In *World workshop in periodontics*, (ed. S.P. Ramfjord, D.A. Kerr, and M.M. Ash), pp. 399–443. University of Michigan Press, Ann Arbor.

Grossman, E. *et al.* (1986). Six-month study of the effects of a chlorhexidine mouthrinse on gingivitis in adults. *J. perio. Res.*, **21** (suppl. 16), 33–43.

Hamp, S.-E., Lindhe, J., Fornell, J., Johansson, L.Å., and Karlsson, E. (1978). Effect of a field program based on systematic plaque control on caries and gingivitis in school-children after 3 years. *Commun. Dent. oral Epidemiol.*, **6**, 17–23.

Hansen, F., Gjermo, P., and Eriksen, H.M. (1975). The effect of a chlorhexidine-containing gel on oral cleanliness and gingival health in young adults. *J. clin. Perio.* **2**, 153–9.

Health Education Council (1979). *The scientific basis of dental health education. A policy document.* Health Education Council, London.

Honkala, E., Nyyssonen, V., Knuuttila, M., and Markkanen, H. (1986). Effectiveness of children's habitual toothbrushing. *J. clin. Perio.* **13**, 81–5.

Horowitz, A.M., Suomi, J.D., Peterson, J.K., and Lyman, B.A. (1977). Effects of supervised daily dental plaque removal by children: 24 months' results. *J. pub. Hlth. Dent.*, **37**, 180–8.

Hoyos, D.F., Murray, J.J., and Shaw, L. (1977). The effect of chlorhexidine gel on plaque and gingivitis in children. *Br. dent. J.*, **142**, 366–9.

Hugoson, A. and Koch, G. (1979). Oral health in 1000 individuals aged 3–70 years in the community of Jönköping, Sweden. *Swed. dent. J.* **3**, 69–87.

Hugoson, A. and Rylander, H. (1982). Longitudinal study of periodontal status in individuals aged 15 years in 1973 and 20 years in 1978 in Jönköping, Sweden. *Commun. Dent. oral Epidemiol.*, **10**, 37–42.

Hugoson, A. *et al.* (1986). Oral health of individuals aged 3–80 years in Jönköping, Sweden, in 1973 and 1983. II. A review of clinical and radiographic findings. *Swed. dent. J.* **10**, 175–94.

Hugoson, A., Laurell, L., and Lundgren, D. (1992). Frequency distribution of individuals aged 20–70 years according to severity of periodontal disease experience in 1973 and 1983. *J. clin. Perio.* **19**, 227–32.

Jeffcoat, M.K. and Reddy, M.S. (1991). Progression of probing attachment loss in adult periodontitis. *J. Perio.*, **62**, 185–9.

Jenkins, S., Addy, M., and Newcombe, R. (1989). Comparison of two commercially available chlorhexidine mouthrinses. II. Effects on plaque reformation, gingivitis and toothstaining. *Clin. prev. Dent.* **11**, 12–16.

Jenkins, W.M.M. and Kinane, D.F. (1989). The 'high risk' group in periodontitis. *Br. dent. J.*, **167**, 168–71.

Jensen, J.E. (1977). Binding of dyes to chlorhexidine treated hydroxyapatite. *Scand. J. dent. Res.*, **85**, 334–40.

Joyston-Bechal, S., Smales, F.C., and Duckworth, R. (1979). The use of a chlorhexidine-containing gel in a plaque control programme. *Br. dent. J.*, **146**, 105–11.

Kalaga, A., Addy, M., and Hunter, B. (1989a). Comparison of chlorhexidine delivery by mouthwash and spray on plaque accumulation. *J. Perio.*, **60**, 127–30.

Kalaga, A., Addy, M., and Hunter, B. (1989b). The use of 0.2% chlorhexidine spray as an adjunct to oral hygiene and gingival health in physically and mentally handicapped adults. *J. Perio.* **66**, 381–5.

Kegeles, S.S. (1963). Why people seek dental care: The test of conceptual formulation. *J. Hlth hum. Behav.* **4**, 166–73.

Khocht, A., Simon, G. Person, P., and Denepitiya J.L. (1993). Gingival recession in relation to history of hard toothbrush use. *J. Perio.* **64**, 900–5.

Kiger, R.D., Nylund, K., and Feller, R.P. (1991). A comparison of proximal plaque removal using floss and interdental brushes. *J. clin. Perio.*, **18**, 681–4.

Lang, N.P. and Ramseier-Grossman, K. (1981). Optimal dosage of chlorhexidine digluconate in chemical plaque control when applied by the oral irrigator. *J. clin. Perio.* **8**, 189–202.

Lang, N.P., Cumming, B.R., and Löe, H. (1973). Toothbrushing frequency as it relates to plaque development and gingival health. *J. Perio.* **44**, 396–405.

Lang, N.P., Hotz, P., Graff, H., Geering, A.H., and Saxer, U.P. (1982), Effects of supervised chlorhexidine mouthrinses in

children. A longitudinal clinical trial. *J. perio. Res.*, **17**, 101–11.

Lindhe, J. and Axelsson, P. (1973). The effect of controlled oral hygiene and topical fluoride application on caries and gingivitis in Swedish schoolchildren. *Commun. Dent. oral Epidemiol.* **1**, 9–16.

Lindhe, J. and Koch, G. (1966). The effect of supervised oral hygiene on the gingivae of children. Progression and inhibition of gingivitis. *J. perio. Res.*, **1**, 260–7.

Lindhe, J., Koch, G., and Månsson, J. (1966). The effect of supervised oral hygiene on the gingiva of children. *J. perio. Res.* **1**, 268–75.

Lindhe, J. and Koch, G. (1967). The effect of supervised oral hygiene on the gingivae of children. Lack of prolonged effect of supervision. *J. perio. Res.* **2**, 215–20.

Lindhe, J. and Wicén, P.-O. (1969). The effects on the gingivae of chewing fibrous foods. *J. perio. Res.* **4**, 193–201.

Lindhe, J., Axelsson, P., and Tollskog, G. (1975). Effect of proper oral hygiene on gingivitis and dental caries in Swedish schoolchildren. *Commun. Dent. oral Epidemiol.* **3**, 150–5.

Löe, H. (1969). Present day status and direction for future research on the etiology and prevention of periodontal disease. *J. Perio.* **40**, 678–82.

Löe, H. and Schiött, C.R. (1970a). The effect of mouthrinses and topical application of chlorhexidine on the development of dental plaque and gingivitis in man. *J. perio. Res.* **5**, 79–83.

Löe, H. and Schiött, C.R. (1970b). The effect of suppression of the oral microflora upon the development of dental plaque and gingivitis. In *Dental plaque*, (ed. W.D. McHugh), pp. 247–55. Edinburgh, Churchill Livingston.

Löe, H., Theilade, E., and Jensen, S.B. (1965). Experimental gingivitis in man. *J. Perio.* **36**, 177–87.

Löe, H., Schiött, C.R., Glavind, L., and Karring, T. (1976). Two years oral use of chlorhexidine in man. I. General design and clinical effects. *J. perio. Res.* **11**, 135–44.

Löe, H., Anerud, A., Boysen, H., and Morrison, E. (1986). Natural history of periodontal disease in man. Rapid, moderate and no loss of attachment in Sri Lankan labourers 14 to 46 years of age. *J. clin. Perio.* **13**, 431–40.

Lövdal, A., Arno, A., Schei, O., and Waerhaug, J. (1961). Combined effect of subgingival scaling and controlled oral hygiene on the incidence of gingivitis. *Acta odont. Scand.* **19**, 537–55.

MacGregor, I.D.M. and Rugg-Gunn, A.J. (1985). Toothbrushing duration in 60 uninstructed young adults. *Commun. Dent. oral Epidemiol.* **13**, 121–2.

MacGregor, I.D.M., Rugg-Gunn, A.J., and Gordon, P.H. (1986). Plaque levels in relation to the number of toothbrushing strokes in unistructed English schoolchildren. *J. perio. Res.* **21**, 577–82.

Magnusson, I., Lindhe, J., Yoneyama, T., and Liljenberg, B. (1984). Recolonization of a subgingival microbiota following scaling in deep pockets *J. clin. Perio.*, **11**, 193–207.

Mandel, I.D. (1988). Chemotherapeutic agents for controlling plaque and gingivitis. *J. clin. Perio.*, **15**, 488–98.

Marsh, P.D. and Bradshaw, D.J. (1993). Microbiological effects of new agents in dentifrices for plaque control. *Int. dent. J.* **43**, 399–406.

McKendrick, A.J.W., Barbenel, L.M.H., and McHugh, W.D. (1968). A two year comparison of hand and electric toothbrushes. *J. perio. Res.* **3**, 224–31.

Muhler, J.C., Dudding, N.J., and Stookey, G.K. (1964). Clinical effectiveness of a particular particle size distribution of zirconium silicate for use as a cleaning and polishing agent for oral hard tissues. *J. Perio.* **35**, 481–5.

Murray, J.J. (1974). The prevalence of gingivitis in children continuously resident in a high fluoride area. *J. dent. Child.* **41**, 133–9.

Newcomb, G.M. (1974). The relationship between the location of subgingival crown margins and gingival inflammation. *J. Perio.*, **45**, 151–4.

Okamoto, H., Yoneyama, T., Lindhe, J., Haffajee, A., and Socransky, S. (1988) Methods of evaluating periodontal disease data in epidemiological research. *J. clin. Perio.*, **15**, 430–9.

Oliver, R.C., and Brown, L.J. (1993). Periodontal diseases and tooth loss. *Perio 2000*, **2**, 117–27.

Oliver, R.C., Brown, L.J., and Löe, H. (1991). Variation in the prevalence and extent of periodontitis. *J. Am. dent. Ass.* **122**, 43–8.

Papapanou, P.N., Wennström, J.L., and Grondahl, K. (1988). Periodontal status in relation to age and tooth type. A cross-sectional radiographic study. *J. clin. Perio.* **15**, 469–78.

Poulsen, S., Agerbaek, N., Melsen, B., Korts, D.C., Glavind, L., and Rölla, G. (1976). The effect of professional tooth cleansing on gingivitis and dental caries in children after 1 year. *Commun. Dent. oral Epidemiol.* **4**, 195–9.

Praynito, S., Taylor, L., Cadogan, S., and Addy, M. (1979). An *in vivo* study of dietary factors in the aetiology of tooth staining associated with the use of chlorhexidine. *J. perio. Res.* **14**, 411–7.

Ramberg, P., Furuichi, Y., Lindhe, J., and Gaffar, A. (1992). A model for studying the effects of mouthrinses on *de novo* plaque formation. *J. clin. Perio.* **19**, 509–20.

Ramberg, P., Lindhe, J., and Eneroth, L. (1994). The influence of gingival inflammation on *de novo* plaque formation. *J. clin. Perio.* **21**, 51–6.

Rethman, M. and Greenstein, G. (1994). Oral irrigation in the treatment of periodontal diseases. In *Current opinion in periodontology*, (ed. R.C. Williams, R.A. Yukna, and M.G. Newman), (2nd edn), pp. 99–110. Current Science, Philadelphia.

Rushton, A. (1977). Safety of Hibitane. II. Human experience. *J. clin. Perio.* **4** (extra issue), 73–9.

Saxton, C.A. (1973). Scanning electron microscope study of the formation of dental plaque. *Caries Res.* **7**, 102–19.

Sbordone, L., Ramaglia, L. Gulletta, E., and Iacono, V. (1990). Recolonization of the subgingival microflora after scaling and root planing in human periodontitis. *J. Perio.* **61**, 579–84.

Schiött, C.R., Löe, H., Jensen, S.B., Kilian, M., Davies, R.M., and Glavind, K. (1970). The effect of chlorhexidine mouthrinses on the human oral flora. *J. perio. Res.* **5**, 84–9.

Schiött, C.R., Briner, W.W., and Löe, H. (1976a). Two years use of chlorhexidine in man. II. The effect on the salivary bacterial flora. *J. perio. Res.* **11**, 145–52.

Schiött, C.R., Briner, W.W., Kirkland, J.J., and Löe, H. (1976b). Two years oral use of chlorhexidine in man. III. Changes in sensitivity of the salivary flora. *J. perio. Res.* **11**, 153–7.

Segretto, V.A., *et al.* (1986). A comparison of mouthrinses containing two concentrations of chlorhexidine. *J. perio. Res.* **21** (suppl. 16), 23–32.

Siegrist, B.E., Gusberti, F.A., Brecx, M.C., Weber, H.P., and Lang, N.P. (1986). Efficacy of supervised rinsing with chlorhexidine digluconate in comparison to phenolic and plant alkaloid compounds. *J. perio. Res.* **21** (suppl. 16), 60–73.

Silness, J. (1980). Fixed prosthodontics and periodontal health. *Dent. Clin. N. America*, **24**, 317–29.

Silness, J., and Røynstrand, T. (1985). Relationship between alignment conditions of teeth in anterior segments and dental health. *J. clin. Perio.* **12**, 312–20.

Sjödin B. and Matsson L. (1994). Marginal bone loss in the primary dentition. A survey 7–9-year-old children in Sweden. *J. clin. Perio.* **21**, 313–19.

Smith, J.F. and Blankenship, J. (1964). Improving oral hygiene in handicapped children by the use of an electric toothbrush. *J. dent. Child.* **31**, 198–203.

Söderholm, G. (1979). Effect of a dental care program on dental health conditions. A study of employees of a Swedish shipyard. Unpublished thesis. University of Lund, Sweden.

Stamm, J.W. (1986). Epidemiology of gingivitis. *J. clin. Perio.* **13**, 360–6.

Stoltze, K. and Bay, L. (1994) Comparison of a manual and a new electric tooth-brush for controlling plaque and gingivitis. *J. clin. Perio.* **21**, 86–90.

Strålfors, A. (1962). Disinfection of dental plaques in man. *Odont. Tid.* **70**, 182–203.

Suomi, J.D. and Barbano, J.P. (1968). Patterns of gingivitis. *J. Perio.* **39**, 71–4.

Suomi, J.D., Green, J.C., Vermillion, J.R., Doyle, J., Chang, J.J., and Leatherwood, E.C. (1971a). The effect of controlled oral hygiene procedures on the progression of periodontal disease in adults: results after third and final year. *J. Perio.* **42**, 152–60.

Suomi, J.D., West, T.D., Chang, J.J., and McClendon, B.J. (1971b). The effect of controlled oral hygiene procedures on the progression of periodontal disease in adults: radiographic findings. *J. Perio.* **42**, 562–4.

Suomi, J.D., Leatherwood, E.C., and Chang, J.J. (1973a). A follow-up study of former participants in a controlled oral hygiene study. *J. Perio.* **44**, 662–6.

Suomi, J.D., Smith, L.W., Chang, J.J. and Barbano, J.P. (1973b). Study of the effect of different prophylaxis frequencies on the periodontium of young adult males. *J. Perio.* **44**, 406–10.

Sutcliffe, P. (1972). A longitudinal study of gingivitis and puberty. *J. perio. Res.* **7**, 52–8.

Svatun, B., Saxton, C.A., Huntington, E., and Cummins, D. (1993). The effects of three silica dentifrices containing Triclosan on supragingival plaque, calculus formation and gingivitis. *Int. dent. J.* **43**, 441–52.

Swartz, M.L. and Philips, R.W. (1957). Comparison of bacterial accumulation on rough and smooth enamel surfaces. *J. Perio.* **28**, 304–7.

Theilade, E. and Theilade, J. (1976). Role of plaque in the etiology of periodontal disease and caries. *Oral sci. Rev.* **9**, 23–64.

Usher, P.J. (1975). Oral hygiene in mentally handicapped children. *Br. dent. J.*, **138**, 217–21.

Van der Ouderaa, F.J.G. (1992). Human clinical studies of antiplaque and anti-gingivitis agents dosed from a dentifrice. In *Clinical and biological aspects of dentifrices* (ed. G. Embery and G, Rölla), pp. 181–204. Oxford University Press.

Van der Velden, U., Abbas, F., and Hart, A.A.M. (1985). Experimental gingivitis in relation to susceptibility to periodontal disease. I Clinical observations. *J. clin. Perio.* **12**, 61–8.

Van der Weijden, G.A., Timmerman, M.F., Nijboer, A., Lie, M.A., and Van der Velden, U. (1993) A comparative study of electric toothbrushes for the effectiveness of plaque removal in relation to toothbrushing duration. Timerstudy. *J. clin. Perio.* **20**, 476–81.

Wade, A.B. (1971). Brushing practices of a group with perio-dontal disease. In *The prevention of periodontal disease*, (ed.) J.E. Eastoe, D.C.A. Picton, and A.G. Alexander), pp. 218–23. Kimpton, London.

Waerhaug, J. (1976). The interdental brush and its place in operative and crown and bridge dentistry. *J. oral Rehab.* **3**, 107–13.

Wennström, J.L., Papapanou, P.N., and Grondahl, K. (1990). A model for decision making regarding periodontal treatment needs. *J. clin. Perio.* **17**, 217–22.

White, D.J. (1992). Tartar control dentifrices: current status and future prospects. In *Clinical and biological aspects of dentifrices*, (ed. G. Embery and G. Rölla), pp. 277–92. Oxford University Press.

Wilcox, C.E. and Everett, F.G. (1963). Friction on the teeth and the gingiva during mastication. *J. Am. dent. Ass.* **66**, 513–20.

Wilson, M.A., Clerehugh, V., and Lennon, M.A. (1988). An assessment of the validity of the WHO periodontal probe for use with the Community Periodontal Index of Treatment Needs. *Br. dent. J.* **165**, 18–21.

Worthington, H.V., *et al.* (1993). A six-month clinical study of the effect of a pre-brush rinse on plaque removal and gingivitis. *Br. dent. J.*, **175**, 322–6.

Yates, R., Jenkins, S., Newcombe, R., Wade, W., and Addy, M. (1993). A 6-month home usage trial of a 1% chlorhexidine toothpaste. I. Effects on plaque, gingivitis, calculus and tooth-staining. *J. clin. Perio.* **22**, 130–8.

Yukna, R.A. and Shaklee, R.L. (1993) Evaluation of a counter-rotational powered brush in patients in supportive periodontal therapy. *J. Perio.*, **64**, 859–64.

Yuodelis, R.A., Weaver, J.D., and Sapkos, S. (1973). Facial and lingual contours of artificial complete crown restorations and their effects on the periodontium. *J. prosthet. Dent.* **29**, 61–6.

9. Oral health promotion

F.P. ASHLEY and C.D. ALLEN

INTRODUCTION

In the previous edition, this chapter was entitled 'Role of dental health education in preventive dentistry'. Whilst dental health education has an important part to play in preventive dentistry, to understand its role, it is important to appreciate the wider concept of oral health promotion. Oral health promotion has occasionally been described as dental health education plus factor 'x'—this is an oversimplification but acts as a useful starting point.

In the past, the dental profession has taken a didactic stance on the prevention of dental disease through the use of their highly specialized knowledge. This knowledge has been used in the development of preventive messages which have been passed to the layperson in the hope that they would effect a behaviour change that would bring about a reduction in the dental disease they suffered. The remit of dental health education was to use the accepted scientific research into the causes of dental diseases to produce educational material whose message was more accessible to the public at large.

The scientific basis for these educational messages is largely what this book is devoted to and is essential learning for all who would work in the arena of preventive dentistry. A significant proportion of this chapter is still devoted to the specific role of dental health education in the prevention of dental disease as it is the understanding of how to apply the knowledge gained from this book that may be most useful to the oral care worker. In addition, an appreciation of the role of dental health education in the wider scope of oral health promotion is helpful in understanding the changing emphasis of oral health programmes and why some are successful whilst others fail.

It was partly due to the frustrations of failed health education programmes that the public health movement became somewhat sceptical of the biomedical approach to prevention. Out of this dissatisfaction has grown the comparatively new study of health promotion.

WHAT IS HEALTH?

Within the medical model, health is regarded as a lack of any recognized pathology. Good health and ill health are, however, more to do with a relative state or feeling. Health has been described as a state of optimum capacity for effective performance of valued tasks (Parsons 1972).

It can be appreciated then that health promotion must take into account not only the prevention of the diseases of the oral cavity, caries and periodontal disease being the most prevalent, but also the aspects of the individual's life which can affect oral health. Thus the general aim of oral health promotion is no different to the aim of dental treatment, that is to achieve the lifelong maintenance of a dentition which is comfortable, functional, socially acceptable, and promotes good general health. Acceptability of comfort and function are largely determined by the individual, not necessarily being coincident with the normative need, as decided by the profession. Social acceptability relates to factors such as appearance, ability to speak clearly, and the absence of halitosis and bleeding gums associated with oral disease. The social acceptability of an individual's dentition is largely determined by the individual and the individual's contacts and not by the dentist or any other provider of dental health education.

Promotion of good health through a healthy dentition is a more general concept and includes aspects such as reducing the risk of infective endocarditis from bacteriaemias of oral origin in susceptible individuals, through to ensuring that the individual can eat an adequate diet and has a good self-image.

It has to be recognized that some individuals with a high susceptibility to disease may be incapable of maintaining a natural dentition over their lifetime. In addition, there are dental conditions such as severe malocclusions, impacted teeth, and so on, which are not amenable to normal preventive procedures. Therefore, perfect oral health may not be achievable. Oversimplification of a dental health education message may result in unnecessary and incorrect feelings of guilt or responsibility in the individuals with the disease or condition. In most cases such victim-blaming is entirely inappropriate.

DETERMINANTS OF HEALTH

In order to appreciate how health promotion fits into the prevention of dental disease, it is necessary to think a little about the factors that may influence oral health.

We know that bacterial plaque, sugar, and fluoride are inextricably linked to the two most common dental diseases of caries and periodontal disease. The control of plaque build-up, radical reduction of sugar in the diet, and the expedient use of fluoride would to a large extent prevent these diseases.

Were life so simple then the bulk of caries and periodontal disease would have been banished to the history books, along with scarlet fever and smallpox.

Unfortunately, there are many factors in our lives over which we do not have complete control. Food is often bought and prepared for us so we have no control over the amount of sugar consumed or when it is eaten. Political pressure or expense may result in the water supplies not being fluoridated, so many people have to forego the benefits.

Factors such as these have been described as the determinants of health. One suggested framework for consideration of the determinants of health was proposed by Lalonde (1974). He suggested that there are four basic elements or fields that have a role in the determination of health.

1. *Biological*: This is determined largely by genetic make-up. A phenomenon which is common to many of the chronic diseases afflicting mankind is the variation in individual susceptibility to the condition despite apparent similarities in their exposure to the recognized aetiological factors. This was illustrated in relation to periodontitis by the classic epidemiological study of Tamil tea labourers by Löe *et al.* (1986). All subjects had consistently high levels of plaque and gingivitis but a tremendous variation in the severity of periodontitis was found. This ranged from the worst 10 per cent, who had lost most of their teeth by the time they were 40 years old because of periodontal disease, to the least affected 10 per cent, who had virtually no bone loss. This latter group were presumably the dental equivalent of the 90-year-old who has smoked 40 cigarettes a day for all his or her adult life with no apparent adverse effects. The other major biological aspect over which we have no control is that of maturation and ageing and the effect these have on the oral tissues. As yet there is very little that can be done about this biological determinant. With future developments in genetics, however, this may be possible.

2. *Environment*: This concerns those factors that surround us in everyday life. The environment can have obvious effects on health if we consider aspects such as water and air pollution and the use of pesticides and drugs on non-manufactured foods, such as vegetables, dairy products, and meat. Environmental factors include the levels of fluoride in the water supply and the effect this has on caries. There is also the social environment in which we live. Socio-economic deprivation is linked to many diseases and morbidity states, dental disease being among them. This is covered in more detail elsewhere in this book.

3. *Lifestyle*: There is a general acceptance that lifestyle probably has the largest effect on health and disease and much of the traditional approach of dental health education has been targeted on this issue. In dentistry, this has mainly concerned the modification of diet and oral hygiene techniques. As will be seen later, however, health promotion is concerned with the wider aspects of lifestyle and not just behavioural practices. Recently, much of the government's 'health of the nation' policy (Department of Health 1992) has been concerned with the promotion of healthy lifestyles to bring about health gains.

4. *Health care services*: The quality, quantity, and equity of health care services and the provision of health care can affect the lives of many people. The basis of the National Health Service (NHS) was the provision of free health care paid out of taxation. It was designed to secure improvement in the physical and mental health of the people in the UK and to concern itself with the prevention, diagnosis and treatment of illness (Ministry of Health 1946). To date, the NHS has been concerned principally with the treatment of disease. Certainly in dentistry the provision of treatment has been the major focus, although no longer free. There are many who believe that there should be a shift in the balance of such a service in favour of the promotion and funding of a preventive health care service. Access to health services is also an important determinant of their use. For example, the lower socio-economic groups, who suffer the worst health problems, have the most difficulty in accessing preventive health care (Townsend and Davidson 1982).

It can be seen that it is important to appreciate all the factors that play a part in health and disease if we are to try and promote health and prevent ill health.

HEALTH PROMOTION

Health promotion has often been equated with health education but in fact has a wider remit. The basic concept of health promotion is the process of enabling individuals and communities to increase control over the determinants of health and thereby improve their health. It includes aspects of the individual's lifestyle, structure of the society, and a multi-disciplined approach to health.

One convenient model of health promotion has been suggested by Tannahill (1985) who describes three essential elements to health promotion. These three essential elements are: health education, prevention, and health protection. The interrelationship between these elements produce seven domains (Fig. 9.1). Each of these seven domains can be described within the remit of health promotion to illustrate the wide-ranging influences that can be utilized to achieve health gain (Downie et al. 1990). Even though, as will be appreciated, the boundaries to these domains become a little blurred, this model supplies a useful framework in which to discuss health promotion and its relation to dentistry.

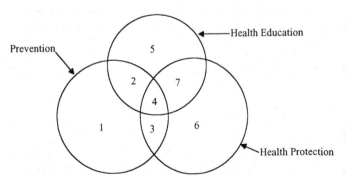

Fig. 9.1. Model of health promotion. [After Tannahill, in *Health promotion* by Downie, Fyfe, and Tannahill (1990), Chapter 4.]

The first four domains to be described mainly emphasize the prevention of disease. They involve many of the services that already exist within the hospital, community, and general dental services. The final three domains are concerned with the enhancement of positive health.

1. Preventive services and facilities.

Existing services include the school screening programmes that take place to identify children that may require dental help by referral to a general dental practitioner or clinic. Prevention can then be provided in the form of fissure sealant and topical fluoride applications to reduce future caries in these identified high risk groups. Another service is the professional cleaning of the teeth by dentists and hygienists as such treatment would hopefully reduce the incidence of periodontal disease. There is also room for expansion of these services for example in the development of screening programmes to detect early cancerous changes in the mouth, or other oral soft tissue conditions. It is accepted that the sooner oral cancer is diagnosed the better is the long term prognosis for the patient and also the associated reduction in morbidity means less expensive health care. Such screening programmes could be part of the dental examination or be included in health checks carried out in general medical practice.

2. Preventive health education

Preventive health education is aimed at influencing lifestyle and oral hygiene behaviours in the interest of preventing oral disease. It is also aimed at encouraging the use of the preventive services and facilities, previously described. The encouragement to look after the teeth and gums and discouragement from smoking and alcohol to prevent cancer, fall under this heading. Traditional dental health education as has been practised for many years falls within this domain, and the principles will be described later in the chapter. This type of health education often occurs on a one-to-one basis but it can take place in Dental Health Promotion Units and Schools. Packs such as the Health Education Authority's (HEA) Natural Nashers Schools Programme and various commercial programmes sponsored by toothpaste manufacturers already exist and are being used to great effect. There are also similar educational packs for adults available for use in the workplace, such as the 'Brush up your smile' programme developed by Elizabeth Towner and the HEA. Modern educational packs are better focused, researched and evaluated and can be used to great effect. An example for use in the dental surgery is the 'Look after your gums' pack, developed by the HEA from post-doctoral research. This pack contains a number of leaflets containing specific information for the patient. The idea is that the dentist or hygienist puts together a personalized pack containing information that is relevant to a particular patient. The patient does not then have to wade through irrelevant material.

3. Preventive health protection

Preventive health protection is the use of legal and fiscal controls and policies, or voluntary codes of practice to prevent disease or ill health, that grew out of the old regulatory public health measures. Fluoridation of the water supplies is an excellent example of this and the role of fluoride in the reduction of caries experience is widely accepted. The use of fluoride in salt has been effective in some of the Cantons in Switzerland and may offer a viable alternative to water fluoridation where water supplies are too limited for cost effective fluoridation or where political pressure stops the fluoridation of the water supplies. Another example from the recent past was the banning of 'Skoal Bandits'. These were oral snuff packs which were placed in the cheek. They came from the USA, were being made in the UK, and marketed to young people. Their outlawing has prevented a probable rise in oral cancer, especially in the young. As a further example, a voluntary code of practice by the retail trade could ensure retailing outlets remove sweets from supermarket checkouts and encourage them and manufacturers to provide healthy alternatives for snacks. Voluntary codes or legal controls could be used to ensure advertisers do not promote the eating of sweets at bedtime or encourage between meal snacking with sweets, promoting a more responsible attitude to snacking. Policies on food labeling are being developed, but it is unlikely that it will be made mandatory to list the amount of sugar in a product, separate from the carbohydrate content. Finally, preventive health protection is also about ensuring the infrastructure and legislation necessary to enable everyone to access preventive services from a dentist is in place.

4. Health education for preventive health protection

There is a need to ensure that those in the position to develop policy understand the importance of preventive health protection. The basis of health education for preventive health protection is aimed at influencing these decision makers. It has much to do with the lobbying of disparate political groups and other influential bodies to understand the need for preventive health protection as previously discussed. At times, health education alone is ineffective, for example, in the use of seat belts. Education campaigns were not having the desired effect and it was only after legislation was introduced that seat belt use was widespread. In the dental field much lobbying is required in educating decision makers to support a positive fluoridation policy. There is a need for greater legislation to enable fluoridation of most water supplies to become a reality. It is important to ensure that the decision makers and purchasers of health care understand why there must be money available for preventive and screening programmes and for the treatment of individuals identified as at high risk from developing oral disease. Health education aimed at health protection also involves fostering multi-agency awareness of the benefits of good oral health and securing support for fitting the message of oral health promotion into policies and programmes of other professionals. There is a duty to educate other professionals as to how they may promote positive attitudes to a healthy mouth by promoting a healthy lifestyle. One example would be to enrol the support of pharmacists. They could be encouraged to dispense sugar free medicines unless sugar containing medicine was specifically asked for, and they could give advice on 'tooth friendly' over the counter medicines. Another influential recruit would be the health visitor. Enlisting health visitors to scrutinize 'Bounty Packs' of free samples of infant food and drink, given to new mothers could reduce the amount of sugar containing foods and drinks given to newly born children. They could also advise on the importance of deciduous teeth and how to protect against tooth decay.

The remaining three domains focus on positive dimensions of health through the use of positive health messages and highlighting life benefits. They are concerned with the development of positive health attributes such as high levels of self esteem and decision making skills. In developing such skills and instilling self confidence, people are more likely to overcome societal expectations and peer pressure against change. It is by the empowerment of the individual or community that healthy choices will be made more easy.

5. Positive health education

Positive health education address the factors other than the purely biomedical causes of disease. It will allow individuals to make valued judgements and choose a course of action that they may feel will benefit them and at the same time reduce the risks of ill health. The use of positive health educational messages can indirectly help oral health and conversely the use of oral health messages can influence general health. For example, encouraging a healthy diet would probably involve a low sugar intake. The dental benefits of this would be obvious. Similarly, promoting the positive benefits of a sound healthy and aesthetic dentition could have an influence on sugar intake and so favour healthy eating practices.

6. Positive health protection

Positive health protection is about increasing the chance for people to live in a healthy environment. Examples are, a work place smoking policy in the interest of providing clean air, promoting the benefits to a healthy life of an aesthetic, functional dentition and ensuring accessibility to such care that was needed to attain this state. It is about making healthy choices easier choices.

7. Health education aimed at positive health protection

This involves raising awareness of, and securing support for, positive health protection measures among the public and policy makers.

Thus, Health Promotion comprises efforts to enhance positive health and prevent ill health, through the overlapping spheres of health education, prevention, and health protection.

A wider role for dental health promotion

Oral health workers do not have to be bound by the confines of the mouth to be involved in health promotion. For instance, they can help in the evolvement of general health programmes aimed at common risk factors and the development of health related life skills and through them also achieve gains in oral health. In recent years the Health of the Nation strategy (Department of Health 1992) has been interested in

developing ways of achieving the health targets set for the five 'Key Areas'. Dentistry can fit into many of these 'Key Areas'. The 'Key Area' of 'Coronary Heart Disease and Stroke' involves promoting a diet that is also beneficial to oral health. In the area of 'Cancer', for example, the reduction in smoking that is hoped for will benefit periodontal health and reduce oral carcinoma. The use of mouth shields can be promoted to reduce damage to the teeth in the Key Area of 'Accidents'. In the area of 'HIV and Sexual Health'; the first signs of conversion from HIV positive status to AIDS often appear in the mouth. Finally, the fifth Key Area of 'Mental Health' could benefit from a dental input in the development of high levels of self esteem that follow from a sound healthy and aesthetic dentition.

PRINCIPLES OF DENTAL HEALTH EDUCATION

The aim of this section is to take a more specific view of dental health education. Points which will be considered include the aims of dental health education, the selection of target groups, and the importance of the correct message, as well as current messages and the effectiveness of dental health education.

TARGET GROUPS

There are two basic approaches to targeting groups for prevention. A high-risk approach or a population approach. If individuals or groups could be accurately identified as likely to develop oral disease then preventive action taken with these high-risk groups could be very successful. If such high-risk groups are unable to be identified then any preventive programme has to be aimed at a larger target group which will inevitably include a number of people who will never develop the disease. Using such a population approach the immediate success of preventive programmes is not usually so apparent as in the high-risk approach. In the population approach, unlike in the high-risk situation, the individuals do not appear to benefit in any dramatic way. In the long term, however, there may well be larger overall reductions in the prevalence of disease within a population. This is the so-called 'preventive paradox' (Rose 1985).

These targeting problems abound in dentistry when developing preventive programmes. It could be argued that the resistant groups within the population are not in any need of dental health education to prevent, say, their periodontitis as their natural resistance will ensure that they retain sufficient periodontal support for their lifetime. A similar argument may be advanced in relation to dental caries. When 55 per cent of 5-year-olds are free from dental caries (O'Brien 1994), we should in theory be targeting our dental health education at the caries-prone group.

There are several objections to this approach. First, we are not yet in a position where we can assess the susceptibility of an individual to disease with sufficient accuracy to have great confidence in our selection of targets. Secondly, many of the methods or predictive tests which are being developed are relatively expensive to administer on a population basis. The commercially available kits which estimate salivary buffering capacity and counts of lactobacilli and *Streptococcus mutans* are expensive in relation to the current expenditure on dental health education. Thirdly, it is apparent that behavioural changes are far more likely to occur if the whole population is involved rather than just the highly susceptible sector.

This advocacy of a general population approach for dental health education rests on the continuing high prevalence of dental disease, and the need for changes in behaviour to achieve reductions in these diseases. It does not preclude some targeting of certain broad groups. Epidemiological data may be used to indicate which social, geographical, or age groups are most at risk to the various dental diseases. Other factors, such as the likely receptiveness of the target audience or their potential for influencing other people, may also be important.

The target groups identified by the former Dental Health Programme Planning Group of the Health Education Council (1986) were:

1. *The public*: although all of the public were considered to be potentially in need of dental health education, the proposed target groups were: young children (3 to 5-years-old); adolescents; young adults (16 to 20-years-old); middle-aged adults; and older people.

2. *Professionals*: all professionals, and in particular the members of the dental team.

3. *Decision-makers*: ranging from those involved in decisions on such matters as fluoridation to food manufacturers, who may need encouragement to develop non-cariogenic, nutritionally acceptable snacks and drinks.

Even if the whole population is to be the target of dental health education, the message should be tailored to take account of the different needs of the individuals within the population. This is more easily achieved when the approach is on a one-to-one basis rather than to a group. Further discussion of this point has been presented in the chapter on the prevention and control of chronic periodontal disease. In theory, use of mass media, such as television, radio, and newspapers, permits access to most of the population and is frequently advocated as the solution to all the problems of dental health education. There is very little evidence to support this opinion. Mass media campaigns can raise public awareness but their effect on behaviour seems limited (Shou 1987; Rise and Sogaard 1988). The one-to-one approach is possible every time a patient attends a dental surgery, and this is one reason why the dental team is singled out as a target group and why the former Health Education Council in its dental health programme sought 'to foster a preventive approach by dental professionals'. Decision-makers form another obvious target group—the most important decision made in recent years was probably that concerned with the marketing of fluoride toothpastes.

THE IMPORTANCE OF THE CORRECT MESSAGE

In a review of dental health education during the previous hundred years, Fox and Maddick (1980) noted that there had been three consistent messages during that time: (1) regular dental visits; (2) good oral hygiene; and (3) a properly balanced diet. However, they observed that there had been changes in the more specific recommendations and the reasons given for their justification. Some of the earlier messages, in particular concerning the relationship between diet, oral hygiene, and caries, are now considered to be incorrect. The previous emphasis on diet was concerned with ensuring the correct development of the tooth structure rather than limiting the number of occasions on which acid was formed in the plaque in response to a sugar intake. Similarly, tooth brushing was stressed as central to the prevention of caries, and apples were considered as nature's toothbrush. It would be naïve to suppose that changes in knowledge will not result in our successors in another fifty years finding some fault with our current messages.

The problems associated with changes in knowledge are compounded by the health educator's need for relatively simple messages. A message hedged around by too many 'ifs', 'buts', and 'howevers' ceases to be a message which can be easily understood and acted upon by the target audience. On the other hand, oversimplification of the facts may result in a message which will soon cease to be correct. This is particularly disturbing in view of the observation (I. Maddick and B. Fox, personal communication) that different generations retain the message which was in vogue during their school-days.

Cynics might argue that if there is any doubt at all about the message it is better to keep quiet. However, to do so may deprive people of knowledge which would enable them to make health choices. It should be emphasized that this problem is not unique to dental health education, indeed dental health education rests on a sounder scientific basis than most of health education.

The Health Education Authority (formerly the Health Education Council) published a policy document *The scientific basis of dental health education* (Levine 1989), which has played a major role in ensuring that the providers of dental health education are aware of what is currently seen as the correct message. However, as Towner (1987) points out: 'There is now a plethora of reports and studies available upon which dental health education can draw. Social science has revealed the complexity of developing, evaluating and disseminating effective materials and programmes. Perhaps paradoxically the self assurance demonstrated in the mass propaganda campaigns of the inter-war period is not so evident now and the way forward less certain'.

CURRENT MESSAGES IN DENTAL HEALTH EDUCATION

In *The scientific basis of dental health education* (Levine 1989), the statement is made that in the past the information presented to the public by dental health educators has been unnecessarily complicated, frequently contradictory, and sometimes wrong. It is suggested that advice should be based on four simple statements:

1. '*Reduce the consumption and especially the frequency of intake of sugar-containing food and drink*. The number of times sugar enters the mouth is the most important factor in

determining the rate of dental decay. Snacks and drinks should be free from sugars. The frequent consumption of acidic drinks should be avoided'.

One problem with suggesting 'safe snacks' is avoiding conflict with the general health education message. Cheese, crisps, and peanuts may be acceptable from a dental viewpoint but are open to criticism from a general health aspect because of their fat and salt content. It is important that we ensure that any dietary advice given as part of dental health education is consistent with the general health education guidelines. At the same time, the dental profession has to try and ensure that these guidelines are consistent with good dental health. Current dietary trends encourage the consumption of fruit and fruit juices, which if excessive, may predispose to erosion. It is important to make the public aware of this.

2. '*Clean the teeth and gums thoroughly every day with a fluoride toothpaste.* The removal of dental plaque is essential for the prevention of periodontal disease. The toothbrush is the only means of plaque removal that should be recommended on a public health basis, other oral hygiene aids, apart from disclosing agents, being a matter for personal professional advice. Thorough brushing, every day, is of more value than more frequent cursory brushing, and a careful scrub technique should be advised. The tooth-brush size and design should allow the user to reach all accessible tooth surfaces and gum margins easily and comfortably. Regular tooth brushing by itself will not prevent dental decay, but a definite benefit will be gained by the use of a fluoride toothpaste'.

This statement is clearly aimed at the prevention of both caries and periodontal disease, and by bringing the two aspects together it builds on the public perception that toothbrushing is of positive benefit to dental health. This belief owes much to the success of previous dental health education activities. These were based on the concept that 'a clean tooth never decays'. E. Theilade and J. Theilade (1976) date this back to Greenwood (1760–1815). Towner's (1986) survey of 296 factory workers aged 18–40 years, indicated that brushing was directed at the prevention of tooth decay rather than gum disease. She also found that knowledge of gum disease was less than that of caries and the perceived susceptibility was also less. It would appear unwise to be over-critical of the value of tooth brushing on its own in the prevention of caries as we wish people to continue to brush their teeth both to prevent periodontal disease and to deliver fluoride in toothpaste to reduce caries.

3. '*Water fluoridation.* Fluoridation of the water supply has a profound influence on the dental health of the community and should be implemented at the earliest possible time. Fluoride tablets or drops are an alternative for motivated parents.'

For many years, health educators were cautious about promoting fluoride tablets or drops as it was considered that their use tended to undermine the case for water fluoridation.

In addition, the relationship between caries and socio-economic status meant that the individuals most likely to benefit from their use would be least likely to take them on a regular basis unless they were administered at school. This latter comment is still true but the slow progress with water fluoridation and cost considerations in those water authorities serving small populations, means that promotion of fluoride tablets or drops is appropriate.

4. '*Regular dental attendance.* Studies on the control of periodontal disease have emphasized the importance of regular professional cleaning in addition to daily plaque removal. It is the dentist's responsibility to ensure that this is carried out effectively at intervals depending on the needs of individual patients. Once decay is established and a definite cavity is present, it cannot be remineralized, but the tooth can be restored and the importance of early detection and appropriate treatment makes regular attendance advisable. Other disorders can occur in the mouth which are unrelated to the presence of natural teeth and which may be life-threatening. For all these reasons, an examination at least once a year is recommended for everyone so that the health of the whole mouth can be monitored and appropriate dental health advice provided. However, children may need to be seen more frequently during the active stages of dental development, as may individuals prone to oral disease.'

The vagueness of the term 'regular dental attendance' reflects the state of the scientific literature in relation to attendance. In fact, if the emphasis were to be placed on periodontal health, one study (Axelsson and Lindhe 1978) would lead us to believe that oral hygiene reinforcement, scaling, and necessary root planing, should be carried out every two to three months in adults.

These comments on the statements in *The scientific basis of dental health education* (Levine 1989) are made to emphasize the point that they are open to debate and modification as the years pass. However, the statements are an excellent summary of the consensus view of experts in the UK in 1989.

EFFECTIVENESS OF DENTAL HEALTH EDUCATION

One approach to the assessment of the effectiveness of dental health education would be to say that the programme concerned is not worth implementing unless it results in a significant reduction in dental disease. This is perhaps a reaction to well-meaning but misguided efforts at dental health education, which in some cases were based on incorrect assumptions about methods of preventing dental disease. Such a hard-line approach underestimates the importance of achieving improvements in knowledge, attitudes, and behaviour. Indeed, it could be argued that dental health education is justified if it results in a significant gain in knowledge and understanding of both the causes of dental disease and its prevention. In theory, the individual is then able to make an informed choice but in fact, the choices available may be restricted because of economic or other constraints. Even if the argument that everyone has the right to some dental health education is accepted, questions arise as to how effective the education is and how much of our resources should be devoted to health education. Inevitably, we have to relate this to the overall cost of dental disease and the potential benefits of prevention. It is therefore customary to build evaluation into dental health education programmes.

Most programme initiatives have been related to children and the major effort in the UK has come from the Cambridge Dental Health Study of the Health Education Council. Between 1975 and 1986, the Dental Health Study Team, led by Michael Craft, carried out a range of studies into various aspects of dental health education. They developed, evaluated, and disseminated two programmes for children: 'Natural Nashers' for adolescents, and 'Good Teeth' for pre-school children (Craft and Croucher 1979; Croucher *et al.* 1985). Coincident with the development of these programmes others were being developed and evaluated either in response to local needs (Hodge *et al.* 1985), or nationally, supported by toothpaste manufacturers (Maddick and Fox 1982, Towner 1984; Dowell 1983). Although the HEA still supports the 'Natural Nashers', most health educational material tends to be supported by local initiatives through the community dental services or national bodies such as the British Dental Association, General Dental Council, the British Dental Health Foundation, and commercial bodies.

Assessment of the contribution of dental health education to the improvement in dental health in the last 25 years is almost impossible. It may well be argued that the decision of the toothpaste manufacturers to promote fluoride toothpaste was the most important factor. However, dental health education may have contributed to this decision and its acceptability by the public as well as promoting the more widespread and frequent use of such toothpaste. When the reduction in rampant caries in very young children, associated with dietary changes such as the more limited use of sweetened comforters, is considered (Holt *et al.* 1982) then we are on firmer ground, as it is doubtful that fluoride toothpaste would have affected this group, many of whom were not having their teeth cleaned on a regular basis.

It is unlikely that we will see such a rapid rate of overall improvement in the oral health of children in future years, although there is potential for improvement in those groups of people who still suffer high caries experience. We cannot be sure what level of oral health promotion is required even to maintain the present position. In any event it will always be necessary to balance the cost of effective oral health programmes against the potential benefits. In this context we are not just talking about savings in treatment costs but other benefits, such as the reduction in experience of pain and general anaesthesia, as well as the contribution made to the general well-being of the individual. Currently, public awareness of health issues is increasing, creating fertile ground for oral health promotion, which should help to bring about further improvements in oral health.

CONCLUSIONS

- Health is not just the absence of pathology but a state of optimum capacity for effective performance of valued tasks.

For oral health this means the lifelong maintenance of a dentition that is comfortable, functional, socially acceptable, and promotes good general health.

- The determinants of health are not always under an individual's control and may be categorized as biological, environmental, lifestyle, and health care services.

- Health promotion comprises efforts to enhance positive health and prevent ill health through the overlapping spheres of health education, prevention, and health protection.

- It is important to identify target groups when planning prevention programmes and to evaluate health gain.

- Oral health advice should be based on the four simple statements:
  - Reduce the consumption of sugar and especially the frequency of intake of sugar containing food and drink
  - Clean teeth and gums thoroughly every day with a fluoride toothpaste
  - Water fluoridation
  - Regular dental attendance.

REFERENCES

Axelsson, P. and Lindhe, J. (1978). Effect of controlled oral hygiene procedures on caries and periodontal disease in adults. *J. clin. Perio.* **5**, 133–51.

Craft, M.H. and Croucher, R.E. (1979). Preventive dental health in adolescents. Results of a controlled field trial. *Roy. Soc. lth, J.* **2**, 48–56.

Croucher, R.E., Rodgers, A.I., Franklin, A.J., and Craft, M.H. (1985). Results and issues arising from an evaluation of community dental health education: the case of the 'Good Teeth Programme'. *Commun. dent. Health*, **2**, 89–97.

Department of Health (1992). *The health of the nation. A strategy for health in England.* Cmnd. 1986. HMSO, London.

Dowell, T.B. (1983). Dental health education. Yours for Life Programme. *Dent. Advert. Hyg. For.* No. 22 (Feb.), 16–18.

Downie, R.S., Fyfe, C., and Tannahill, A. (1990). *Health promotion: models and values.* Oxford University Press, Oxford.

Fox, B. and Maddick, I. (1980). A hundred years of dental health education. *Br. dent. J.* **149**, 28–32.

French, J. (1985). To educate or promote health? *Hlth educ. J.* **44**, 115–16.

Health Education Council (1986). *Dental health programme plan.* Health Education Council, London.

Hodge, H., Buchanan, M., Jones, J., and O'Donnell, P. (1985). The evaluation of the infant dental programme developed in Sefton. *Commun. dent. Health*, **2**, 175–85.

Holt, R.D., Joels, D., and Writer, G.B. (1982). Caries in preschool children: the Camden Study. *Br. dent. J.* **153**, 107–9.

Lalonde, M. (1974). *A new perspective on the health of Canadians.* Minister of Supply and Services.

Levine, R.S. (1989). *The scientific basis of dental health education. A policy document*, (3rd edn). Health Education Council, London.

Löe, H., Anerud, A., Boysen, H., and Morrison, E. (1986). Natural history of periodontal disease in man. *J. clin. Perio.* 13, 431–40.

Maddick, I. and Fox, B. (1982). The assessment of a teacher-based programme of dental health education for 5–7 year olds. *J. dent. Res.* **61**, 540.

Ministry of Health (1946). *NHS Bill. Summary of the proposed new service.* Cmnd. 6761. HMSO, London.

O'Brien, M. (1994). *Children's dental health in the United Kingdom 1993*, HMSO, London

Parsons, T. (1972). Definitions of health and illness in light of American values and social structures. In *Patients, physicians and illness* (ed. E.G. Jaco), pp. 107–127. Macmillan, New York.

Rise, J. and Sogaard, A.J. (1988). Effect of a mass media periodontal campaign upon preventive knowledge and behaviour in Norway. *Commun. Dent. oral Epidemiol.* **16**, 1–4.

Rose, G. (1985). Sick individuals and sick populations. *Int. J. Epidemiol.* **14** (1), 32–8.

Schou, L. (1987). Use of mass-media and active involvement in a national dental health campaign in Scotland. *Commun. Dent. oral Epidemiol.* **15**, 14–18.

Tannahill, A. (1985). What is health promotion? *Health Educ. J.* **44**, 167–8.

Theilade, E. and Theilade, J. (1976). Role of plaque in the etiology of periodontal disease and caries. *Oral sci. Rev.* **9**, 23–64.

Towner, E.M.L. (1984). The 'Gleam Team' programme: Development and evaluation of a dental health education package for infant schools. *Commun. dent. Health*, **1**, 181–91.

Towner, E.M.L. (1986). *The adult dental health education study.* Research Report No. 9. Health Education Council, London.

Towner, E.M.L. (1987). *History of dental health education.* Occasional Paper No. 5. Health Education Authority, London.

Townsend, P. and Davidson, N. (1982). *Inequalities in health: The Black Report.* Harmondsworth, Penguin.

10. The prevention of dental trauma

R.R. WELBURY

TRAUMA to children's teeth occurs quite frequently (Todd and Dodd 1985). Moreover, in the UK there is evidence to suggest that the incidence is increasing. In the permanent dentition, damage increases with age into teenage years and then remains constant at about 25 per cent of all children. Traumatic injuries may be more common in boys in the UK (Todd and Dodd 1985) and in girls in Sweden (Crona-Larson and Noren 1989). The incidence of trauma to primary teeth is not so well documented but figures of between 11 and 30 per cent have been reported (Andreasen and Ravn 1972; Zadik 1976).

The major causes of these injuries vary considerably and include accidents in and around the home, injuries sustained during play including sport, and injuries as a direct result of violence (Crona-Larsen and Noren 1989; *Br. dent. J.* 1989). The main 'peak periods' for dental injury are described as being between the ages of 1 and 3 and again between the ages of 7 and 10. For children under 3 years old, who are usually both unsteady on their legs and lacking in a proper sense of caution, falls are the most common cause of injury. In school-age children, bicycle, skate-board, and road accidents are the most significant factors, while in adolescence there is another, although less marked, peak largely due to sports injuries. Most of these injuries result from participation in contact sports such as American football, rugby, soccer, boxing, wrestling, diving or stick sports (Gelbier 1967; Hedegard and Stalhane 1973; O'Mullane 1973; Sane and Ylipaavalnieni 1988; McNutt *et al.* 1989). However, other sports like skiing, skating, cycling, and horse riding, which do not necessarily involve player contact, may also place the participant at risk. The Fédération Dentaire International (FDI) have recently classified organized sport into two categories: (1) high-risk sports that include American football, hockey, ice-hockey, lacrosse, martial sports, rugby, football, and skating, and (2) medium-risk sports that include basketball, diving, squash, gymnastics, parachuting, and waterpolo (FDI 1990). In later adolescence a smaller percentage of injuries can be attributed to violence. An iatrogenic cause of trauma, particularly in younger patients where the anterior teeth are only partially erupted and root length is not complete, is avulsion reportedly caused by excessive pressure from a laryngoscope during intubation anaesthesia (Powell and Keown 1965).

As the aetiology of dental injuries is multi-factorial it is difficult to institute effective preventive measures. However, it has been shown that individuals who take part in contact sports (Gelbier 1967; Hedegard and Stalhane 1973; McNutt *et al.* 1989) and those who have an increased overjet and inadequate lip coverage have an increased prevalence (Lewis 1959; Eichenbaum 1963; McEwen *et al.* 1967; O'Mullane 1973; Todd and Dodd 1985), and injuries also tend to be more severe (Eichenbaum 1963). It has also been suggested that sportswomen may be more susceptible than men to injury as it has not been traditional for them to wear any form of mouth protection in sports (Olvera 1989).

The prevention of trauma can be either primary or secondary.

PRIMARY PROTECTION

PLAYGROUND SURFACES

The most common cause of tooth injury in children is falling on to a hard surface. The British Standard for new play equipment for permanent installation outdoors, BS 5696 (1990), strongly recommends that any organization responsible for the purchase of play equipment should ensure that an impact-absorbing surface is provided around the items from which children are most likely to fall. Studies of accidents to children in playgrounds have shown that the majority of the more serious cases were head injuries caused through striking hard ground (Illingworth *et al.* 1975). Playgrounds should be all about fun and be as safe as practically possible, however, no matter how safe the equipment or the playground's layout, there is always a risk that children will trip or stumble, run into each other or a piece of equipment, miss their footing or loose their grip or more seriously fall from a height. A fall onto an impact-absorbing surface means that a fall is cushioned and the child is less likely to be seriously hurt.

The ability of a surface to absorb an impact is measured by its Critical Fall height (CFH). British Standard 7188 (1991) gives details for CFH testing criteria as well as tests for a surface's resistance and ease of ignition. BS 7188 (1991) uses the Severity Index (SI) as a means of calculating CFH, but a new European standard for playground surfacing is currently being drafted which will used Head Injury Criteria (HIC) as its means of calculating CFH. The test which determines a human's tolerance to an impact SI is based on research into road vehicle design and the NASA manned space programme (Gadd 1966). They estimated the severity of a blow to the head by mathematical integration of the area under a plot of deceleration versus time for the entire duration of the impact event (Wayne State University Curve). This curve produces a theory of 'short duration, high acceleration' tolerance. If deceleration does not exceed 50 g the fall is more likely to be survivable. However, if deceleration exceeds 50 g the fall can be tolerated for a few milliseconds only.

Impact-absorbing surfaces are tested by dropping a head-form representation of a child's head from a series of heights on to the surface (BS 7188 1991). Accurate electronic deceleration measurements are taken during the period of impact in order to obtain the SIs for these falls which are then plotted. A surface's CFH represents the greatest height of a head-first fall from which a child, landing on a surface, could be expected to avoid sustaining a critical head injury. The height of the curve at which the SI or Head Injury Criteria is 1000 represents the surface's CFH.

In addition to the measurement of a surface CFH, BS 7188 (1991) also describes the measurement of four other parameters:

(1) the ability of the surface to resist abrasive wear;

(2) the slip resistance of the material;

(3) the resistance to indentation by part landing and recovery from sustained landing; and

(4) the response of the material to one particular source of ignition.

The resilient or compliant elastomeric composition of impact-absorbing surfaces is expensive. A cheaper alternative would be tree bark chippings, but these have the disadvantage of needing daily raking to remove, for example, broken glass and dog faeces. In addition to consideration of the playground surface, all playground equipment should meet British Standard safety criteria. Slides should not be free standing, but should be built into earth mounds. Supervision of small children at play (parental or professional) is very important, and probably the most effective way of preventing serious injury.

EARLY (MIXED DENTITION) TREATMENT OF LARGE OVERJETS

In the UK, the incidence of accidental damage to permanent incisors significantly increases with overjets greater than 9 mm (Table 10.1). Even though the proportion of children with an overjet of 7 mm or more never exceeds 9 per cent (Table 10.2), this is still a significant number of children at high risk from traumatic injury. It should be the aim of any caring society to prevent disfigurement from loss of or damage to a permanent incisor and therefore early treatment of large overjets is often justified.

Orthodontic treatment in the early mixed dentition is classically carried out in uncrowded arches using functional appliances or extra oral traction. Both treatments work best during active growth and, may have a favourable influence on growth in some cases. An early start to treatment does not always mean an early finish, and treatments can be prolonged. However, if treatment is done in crowded arches then it is inevitably longer and involves two stages:

Table 10.1. The percentage of children in the UK with accidental damage to permanent incisors by size of overjet and age (Todd and Dodd 1985)

Age (yrs)	Children with overjet < 5 mm	Children with overjet ≥ 5 mm	Children with overjet ≥ 9 mm
8–9	10	17	7
10–11	14	31	34
12–13	22	32	45
14–15	22	39	44

Table 10.2. The percentage of children by age with an overjet of 7 mm or more in the UK in 1983 (Todd and Dodd 1985)

Age (yrs)	Percentage with overjet ≥ 7 mm
8–9	9
10–11	9
12–13	8
14–15	5

1. Primary canine extraction and overjet reduction.

2. Relief of crowding in the permanent dentition by extraction followed by arch realignment with fixed orthodontic appliances.

Therefore, while it may be feasible to correct incisor oral relationship in the early mixed dentition, a number of problems may arise and treatment should not be attempted unless there are strong indications for doing so, and certainly not without a precise orthodontic diagnosis and treatment plan.

PROVISION OF MOUTH PROTECTION IN SPORTS

Dental injuries associated with sports in British children under 15 years of age account for only 10 per cent of all injuries (O'Mullane 1973; Winter and Kernahan 1986). The incidence in Sweden in the same age group is 25 per cent (Peterson and Renstrom 1986).

In the majority of cases it is the front teeth of the upper jaw that are affected, and usually more than one tooth has been damaged. It is rare that a dental injury heals spontaneously without treatment and such injuries in children should be considered as serious, since injuries to the teeth and jaws that are not fully developed can lead to their being adversely affected for life. The use of mouth protectors has been made mandatory by the controlling bodies of some sports in different countries. In 1962, it was made compulsory for American football players, high schools and junior colleges, to wear mouthguards, and in 1973 mandatory for university teams by the National Collegiate Athletics Association (NCAA). In addition, in 1990 the NCAA made it mandatory for all players to wear yellow mouthguards so that they were easily visible to all players, officials, and coaching staff. In 1986, it was estimated that 2.26 per cent of all American football wounds involved injuries to the dental or facial tissues. Earlier studies, following the mandatory introduction of face masks and mouth protectors for college footballers showed that the prevalence of injuries had been reduced to 0.3 per cent (Heintz 1968). However, more recent studies suggest that the prevalence of dento-facial injuries to football players is greater than previously reported (Garon *et al.* 1986). Studies in other sports have shown a dramatic reduction in the number of dental injuries when a mouthguard was worn (Garon *et al.* 1986; McNutt *et al.* 1989) and their advocation by the dental profession for all persons, especially children and adolescents involved in contact sports, is justified.

Impact to the maxilla and/or mandible during sport is usually by a direct blow from a fist, elbow or knee. The injury patterns sustained have led to the development of mouthguards, protective helmets, and faceguards. The different functions of mouthguards have been described by Stevens (1981):

1. They hold the soft tissues of the lips and cheeks away from the teeth, preventing laceration or bruising of the lips and cheeks against the hard and irregular teeth during impact.

2. They cushion the teeth from direct frontal blows and redistribute the forces that would otherwise cause fracture or dislocation of anterior teeth.

3. They prevent opposing teeth from coming into violent contact, reducing the risk of tooth fracture, or damage to supporting structures.

4. They provide the mandible with resilient support which absorbs impacts that might fracture the unsupported angle or condyle of the mandible.

5. They help prevent neurological injury by holding the jaws apart and act as shock absorbers to prevent upward and backward displacement of the mandibular condyles against the base of the skull. Under experimental conditions they may reduce intracranial pressure and bone deformation due to impact (Hickey *et al.* 1965).

6. They provide protection against neck injuries. It has been demonstrated on cephaloametric radiographs that repositioning of the mandibular condyle, cervical vertebrae, and other cervical anatomic structures takes place when a mouthguard is in place.

7. They are psychological assets to contact sport athletes (Walkden 1975).

8. They fill the space and support adjacent teeth so that removeable prostheses can be taken out during contact sports. This prevents possible fracture of the prostheses and accidental swallowing or inhaling of the fragments.

Criteria for mouthguard construction

The Fédération Dentaire Internationale has listed the following criteria for constructing an effective mouthguard (FDI 1990):

- The mouthguard should be made of a resilient material which can be easily washed, cleaned and readily disinfected.

- It should have adequate retention to remain in position during sporting activity, and allow for a normal occlusal relationship to give maximum protection.

- It should absorb and dispense the energy of a shock by:
  - covering the maxillary dental arch,
  - excluding interferences,
  - reproducing the occlusal relationship,
  - allowing mouth breathing,
  - protecting the soft tissues,

The FDI also recommends that mouthguards should, preferably, be made by dentists from an impression of the athlete's teeth.

Mouthguard design

The accepted design is based on that suggested by Turner (1977). The mouthguard is normally fitted to the maxillary arch except in Class III malocclusion. It should be close-fitting and should cover the occlusal surfaces of the teeth except where it is anticipated that the exfoliation of primary teeth or further eruption of teeth will occur. It should extend at least as far back as the distal surface of the first permanent molar.

The flanges of the mouthguard should extend beyond the gingival attachment, but short of the muco-buccal fold. The flange should be no greater than 2 mm thick over the labial mucosa to avoid stretching the lips which could lead to them splitting on impact. The buccal edge of the flange should be smooth and rounded and carefully relieved around the frena and muscle attachments.

The palatal aspect of the mouthguard should extend approximately 5 mm on to the palate and should be tapered to a smooth, thin, rounded edge to avoid interference with speech and breathing or stimulation of the 'gagging' reflex. The occlusal thickness of the guard should not exceed the width of the freeway space and should occlude evenly and comfortably with the opposing arch.

An alternative design advocated by Chapman (1985a) describes a bimaxillary mouthguard that covers both arches and holds the mandible in a position that allows maximum oral air flow. It is claimed that this design offers several advantages by allowing complete protection of the teeth, as well as the intra- and extra-oral tissues, from injury. It is also suggested that this mouthguard offers increased mandibular protection by giving it rigid support, reducing the likelihood of concussion by preventing the transmission of forces through the tempromandibular joint to the base of the skull.

Chandler *et al.* (1987) described a design which thickened the occlusal surface over the molar teeth in a maxillary guard so as to disengage the incisors. They suggested that this design provided protection equal to the bimaxillary type described by Chapman. Clearly, further studies are necessary to fully evaluate the design of mouthguards.

Mouthguard materials

The most commonly used material is polyvinyl acetate–polyethylene copolymer (PVAc-PE). Polyurethane (PU) was popular but is now less frequently used (Going *et al.* 1974; Chaconas *et al.* 1985.) The physical and mechanical properties of the materials vary with their chemical composition. The properties can be different with different brands of the same material and this may be due to a variation in the degree of cross-linking between polymer chains, the proportion of plasticizer present, and the volume of the filler particle (Chaconas *et al.* 1985; Godwin and Craig 1970).

Types of mouthguards

Mouthguards can be classified into three types: (1) stock, (2) mouth-formed, and (3) custom-made.

1. Stock mouthguards made of latex rubber or polyvinyl chloride, can be obtained in small, medium, and large sizes and are commonly used in the boxing profession. They can only be kept in place by biting the teeth together, have no inherent retentive properties, impede speech and breathing, and are a danger to the airway, especially when consciousness is impaired. There is no evidence that they are effective in redistributing forces of impact, and soft tissue injury may result from rough or sharp edges.

2. Mouth-formed guards are available in two types. The first is made with a firm white outer shell of a plasticized vinyl chloride plastic in the form of a dental arch, which is filled with a soft chemo- or thermosetting acrylic resin that is adapted to the teeth. The outer shell is fitted and trimmed, if necessary, around the frenal attachments prior to filling with soft lining and seating in the mouth. The resin sets in the mouth after 3–5 minutes and remains resilient at mouth temperature. Unfortunately, this appliance is extremely bulky and it makes normal speech virtually impossible. The margins of the outer shell may also be sharp unless protected by an adequate thickness of the lining material.

The second most commonly used type of mouth-formed guard is constructed from a preformed thermoplastic shell of PVAc-PE copolymer or PVC that is softened in warm water and then moulded in the mouth by the athlete using tongue and fingers. Even under professional supervision it is difficult to mould this type effectively. The temperature necessary to allow adequate adaptation for the teeth is fairly high and there is a risk of burning the mouth. In addition, if it is not centred correctly during moulding then it will be thinner in some areas thus reducing its effectiveness.

3. Custom-made mouthguards are made by a heating-vacuum unit on dental casts poured from impressions of the player's mouth. This is the most satisfactory mouthguard in terms of acceptability and comfort to the athlete (Dukes 1954; Nicholas 1969; Chapman 1985*b*, Stokes *et al.* 1987) but there is no evidence that they are more effective in preventing injuries (Upson 1985, Chapman 1985*b*, Stokes *et al.* 1987). Alginate impressions are taken of both arches together with a wax jaw registration with the mandible in a physiolog-

ical rest position. The mouthguard is constructed with an even occlusal imprint which enables the athlete to brace the muscles of the head and neck as the teeth come into uniform contact with the mouthguard (Walkden 1975). This increases the separation between the cranial base and the condyle and reduces the risk of brain concussion (Chapman 1985*a*). An optimal thickness of 4.5 mm for the occlusal surface has been recommended (Chapman 1985*a*). Proper extension of the mouthguard is very important but all fraenum attachments must be sufficiently relieved. It should be extended just short of the muco-buccal fold and distally to cover the second molars. The edges should be smoothed with a polishing stone, and flamed with an alcohol torch on the cast prior to placement in the mouth.

Care of mouthguards

Bacteriological studies have led to the recommendation that mouthguards should: (a) be washed with soap and water immediately after use, (b) be dried thoroughly and stored in a perforated box, and (c) be rinsed in mouthwash or mild antiseptic (e.g. 0.2 per cent chlorhexidine) immediately before use again (Render 1963). Practically, however, most dentists would advise that the mouthguard be thoroughly rinsed after use and stored in a sturdy identifiable container.

Life of mouthguards

A mouthguard constructed for a child in the mixed dentition, and up until about 15 years old, may need to be renewed once a year. Once the occlusion is established there is no reason why a polyvinyl acetate–polyethylene mouthguard, if well looked after, should not last for between two to three years.

Special considerations in mouthguard design

Partially dentate athletes should not wear removable prostheses while participating in sports, in order to prevent injury or aspiration of fragments if the appliance were to fracture. Occlusal rims may be constructed on a thermoplastic base to replace the missing teeth.

Athletes undergoing fixed orthodontic treatment can have a mouthguard constructed provided that the brackets and arch wires are covered with wax prior to taking an impression. Care should be taken not to place the lips or other soft tissues under tension by making the mouthguard too thick. While the design of mouthguards and the materials from which they are made need further investigation to produce more effective and inexpensive guards there can be little doubt that evidence to date suggests that a correctly made mouthguard reduces considerably the severity of oral injuries.

PROVISION OF MOUTH PROTECTION FOR SPECIAL GROUPS

Self-inflicted injuries have been reported in individuals who are intellectually compromised as a result of neurological damage. This may be due to brain anoxia at birth or congenital syndromes (Freedman *et al.* 1981; Turley and Henson

1983; Finger and Duperon 1991). The authors describe a number of methods for the treatment of self-induced oral injuries and these include processed hand acrylic splints, wire and acrylic splints, and double thickness soft vinyl mouthguards. Mouthguards have also been recommended for patients with Parkinson's disease whose involuntary movements may traumatize oral soft tissues (Hussein 1989), and comatose patients can be protected from intra-oral injury by wiring a tongue stent to the mandible (Hanson *et al.* 1975).

The use of laryngoscopes during intubation anaesthesia have been associated with dental injuries (Bamforth 1963; Wright and Manfield 1974; Nyek and Winnick 1976; McCarthy and Carlson 1977; Seals and Dorrough 1984; Lockhart *et al.* 1986). Teeth may be fractured or displaced by using the incisal edges of the anterior teeth as a fulcrum when inserting a laryngoscope, retractors or endoscopes. Mouth-formed and custom-made guards (Henry and Barb 1964; Davis *et al.* 1971; Nyek and Winnick 1977, and adhesive oral bandage (Evers *et al.* 1982) have been used to prevent these oral injuries.

Pre-term infants who need prolonged intubation may suffer long-term damage to their palates (Ash and Moss 1987). Damage may range from inducement of cleft palates (Blanc and Tremblay 1974; Duke *et al.* 1976) to dilaceration of primary incisor teeth (Seow *et al.* 1990). Appliances have been described which aim to protect the palatal tissue in this group of vulnerable neonates (Sullivan 1982; Ash and Moss 1987).

SECONDARY PREVENTION

Prompt intervention following accidental damage to teeth can have a secondary preventive effect by reducing the complications of trauma. The development of both the acid-etch technique and dentine bonding agents means that there can be no excuse for leaving exposed dentine for any length of time in coronal fractures. The recognition that non-setting calcium hydroxide is capable of allowing continued root growth and apexification in non-vital immature incisors has made both treatment and long-term prognosis more predictable for these teeth. The avulsed tooth is no longer a non-viable proposition and if stored correctly and replanted soon after injury may be retained as functioning member of the dentition for life.

CONCLUSIONS

- The prevention of oral trauma and the maintenance of a healthy complete dentition for life should be the aim of any caring parent and dental practitioner.

- Playgrounds and play areas should be carefully designed and constructed.

- Young children's play should be supervised.

- Large overjets should be treated in the mixed dentition.

- Correctly fitting 'custom-made' mouthguards should be worn for contact sports.

REFERENCES

Andreasen, J.O. and Ravn, J.J. (1972). Epidemiology of traumatic dental injuries to primary and permanent teeth in a Danish population sample. *Int. J. oral Surg.* **1**, 235–9.

Ash, S.P. and Moss, J.P. (1987). An investigation of the features of the preterm infant palate and the effect of prolonged orotracheal intubation with and without protective appliances. *Br. J. Orthod.* **14**, 253–61.

Bamforth, B.J. (1963). Complications during endotracheal anaesthesia. *Anaes. Analges.* **42**, 727–32.

Blanc. V.F. and Tenblay, N.A.G. (1974). The complication of tracheal intubation: a new classification with review of the literature. *Anaesth. Analges.* **53**, 202.

British Dental Journal (1989). Patient and practice newsletter, 15 April.

BS 5696. *Play equipment intended for permanent installation outdoors*: Part 1: Methods of Test, 1986. Amended 1990; Part 2: Specification for construction and performance, 1986. Amended 1990; Part 3: Code of practice for installation and maintenance, 1979. Amended 1990. British Standards Institution, London.

BS 7188. British Standard methods of test for impact absorbing playground surfaces, 1989. Amended 1991. British Standards Institution, London.

Chaconas, S.J., Caputo, A.A., and Bakken, K. (1985). A comparison of mouthguard materials. *Am. J. sports Med.* **13**, 193–7.

Chandler, N.P., Wilson, N.H.F., and Daber, B.S. (1987). A modified maxillary mouthguard. *Br. J. sports Med.* **21**, 27–8.

Chapman, P.J. (1985*a*). The bimaxillary mouthguard: Increase protection against orofacial and head injuries in sport. *Australian J. sci. med. Sport*, **17**, 25–9.

Chapman, P.J. (1985*b*). The prevalence of oro-facial injuries and use of mouthguards in rugby union. *Australian dent. J.* **30**, 364–7.

Crona-Larson, G. and Noren, J.G. (1989). Luxation injuries to permanent teeth—A retrospective study of aetiological factors. *Endod. dent. Traumatol.* **5**, 176–9.

Davis, F.O., Defreece, A.B., and Shroff, P.F. (1971). Custom made plastic mouthguards for tooth protection during endoscopy and endotracheal intubation. *Anaesth. Analges.* **50**, 203–6.

Duke, P.M., Coulson J.D., Santos, J.I., and Johnson, J.D. (1976). Cleft palate associated with prolonged orotracheal intubation in infancy. *J. Paediatr.* **89**, 990–1.

Dukes, H.H. (1954). Latex football mouthpieces. *J. Am. dent. Ass.* **49**, 445–8.

Eichenbaum, I.W. (1963). A correlation of traumatized anterior teeth to occlusion. *ASDCJ dent. Child.* **30**, 229–36.

Evers, W., Racz, G.B., Glazer, J., and Dobkin, A.B. (1967). Orahesive as a protection for the teeth during general anaesthesia and endoscopy. *Can. Anaes. soc. J.* **14**, 123–8.

FDI (Fédération Dentaire Internationale) (1990). *Commission on dental products.* Working Party No. 7. I.D.I. World Dental Press, London.

Finger, S. and Duperon, D.T. (1991). The management of oral trauma secondary to encephalitis: a clinical report. *ASDCJ dent. Child.* **58**, 60–3.

Freedman, A., *et al.* (1981). Neuropathologic chewing in comatose children: A case report. *Paediatr. Dent.* **3**, 334–6.

Gadd, C.W. (1966). Use of a weighted impulse criterion for estimating injury hazard. In *Proceedings of the 10th Stapp Car Crash Conference.*

Garon, M.W., Merkle, A., and Wright, J.T. (1986). Mouth protectors and oral trauma: A study of adolescent football players. *J. Am. dent. Assoc.* **112**, 663–5.

Gelbier, S. (1967). Injured anterior teeth in children. A preliminary discussion. *Br. dent. J.* **123**, 331–5.

Godwin, W.C. and Craig, R.G. (1970). Stress transmitted through mouth protectors. *J. Am. dent. Assoc.* **77**, 316–20.

Going, R.E., Loehman, R.E., and Chan, M.S. (1974). Mouthguard materials: Their physical and mechanical properties. *J. Am. dent. Assoc.* **89**, 132–8.

Hanson, G.E., Ogle, R.G., and Giron, L. (1975). A tongue stent for the prevention of oral trauma in the comatose patient. *Crit. care Med.* **3**, 200–3.

Hedegard, B. and Stalhane, I. (1973). A study of traumatized permanent teeth in children aged 7–15 years. Part 1. *Swed. dent. J.* **66**, 431–50.

Heintz, W.D. (1968). Mouth Protectors: A progress report. *J. Am. dent. Assoc.* **77**, 632–6.

Henry, P.J. and Barb, R.R. (1964). Mouth protectors for use in general anaesthesia. *J. Am. dent. Assoc.* **68**, 569–70.

Hickey, J.C., *et al.* (1965). The relation of mouth protectors to cranial pressure and deformations. *J. Am. dent. Assoc.* **74**, 735–40.

Hussein, S.B. (1989). Use of a gum shield for Parkinson's disease patients. *Br. dent. J.* **166**, 320.

Illingworth, C., Brennan, P., Jay, A., Al-Rawi, F., and Collick, M. (1975). Two hundred injuries caused by playground equipment. *Br. med. J.* **4**, 332–4.

Lewis, T.T. (1959). Incidence of fractured anterior teeth as related to their protrusion. *Angle Orthodont.* **29**, 128–31.

Lockhart, P.B., *et al.* (1986). Dental complications during and after tracheal intubation. *J. Am. dent. Assoc.* **112**, 480–3.

McCarthy, G. and Carlson, O. (1977). A dental splint for use during peroral endoscopy. *Acta Otolaryngol.* **84**, 450–2.

McEwen, J.D., McHugh, W.D., and Hitchin, A.D. (1967). Fractured maxillary incisors and incisal relationships. *J. dent. Res.* **46**, 1290, Abs. No. 87.

McNutt, T., Shannon, S.W., Wright, J.T., and Feinstein, R.A. (1989). Oral trauma in adolescent athletes. *Paed. Dent.* **11**, 209–13.

Nicholas, N.K. (1969). Mouth protection in contact sports *N.Z. Dent. J.* **65**, 14–24.

Nyek, A.M., and Winnick, A.M. (1976). An acrylic dental protector in oral endoscopy. *J. Otolaryngol.* **5**, 86–8.

Olvera, N. (1989). *8th Symposium on Sports Dentistry.* US Olympic Training Centre, Colorado Springs, Colorado, USA.

O'Mullane, D.M. (1973). Some factors predisposing to injuries of permanent incisors in school children. *Br. dent. J.* **134**, 328–32.

Peterson, L. and Renstrom, R. (1986). *Sports injuries, their prevention and treatment.* Martin Dunitz, London.

Powell, J.B., and Keown, K.K. (1965). Endobronchial aspiration of a tooth. An unusual anaesthetic complication. *Anaesth. analges. carr. Res.* **44**, 355–7.

Render, T.P. (1963). Mouth protector sanitation. *J. Am. dent. Assoc.* **66**, 709.

Sane, J. and Ylipaavalniemi, P. (1988). Dental trauma in contact team sports. *Endod. dent. Traumatol.* **4**, 164–9.

Seals, R.R. and Darrough, B.C. (1984). Custom mouth protector: A review of their applications. *J. prosthet. Dent.* **51**, 238–42.

Seow, W.K., Perham, S., Young, W.G., and Daley, T. (1990). Dilaceration of a primary incisor associated with neonatal laryngoscopy. *Paed. Dent.* **12**, 321–4.

Stevens, O.O. (1981). In *Traumatic injuries to the teeth*, (ed. J.O. Andreason), Chapter 12, The prevention of traumatic dental and oral injuries, p. 442. Munksgaard, Copenhagen.

Stokes, A.N.S., Croft, G.C., and Gee, D. (1987). Comparison of laboratory and intraorally formed mouth protectors. *Endod. Dent. Traumatol.* **3**, 255–8.

Sullivan, P.G. (1982). An appliance to support oral intubation in the premature infant. *Br. dent. J.* **103**, 191–5.

Todd, J.E. and Dodd, T. (1985). *Children's dental health in the United Kingdom, 1983.* HMSO, London.

Turley, P.K. and Henson, J.L. (1983). Self injurious lip biting; etiology and management. *J. Pedod.* **7**, 209–20.

Turner, C.H. (1977). Mouth protectors. *Br. dent. J.* **143**, 82–6.

Upson, N. (1985). Mouthguards, an evaluation of two types for rugby players. *Br. J. sports Med.* **19**, 89–92.

Walkden, L. (1975). The medical hazards of rugby football. *Practitioner*, **215**, 201–7.

Winter, G.B. and Kernahan, D.C. (1986). The importance of mouthguards. *Br. dent. J.* **120**, 564–5.

Wright, R.B. and Manfield, F.F.V. (1974). Damage to the teeth during the administration of general anaesthesia. *Anaes. Analges.* **53**, 405–8.

Zadik, D. (1976). A survey of traumatized primary anterior teeth in Jerusalem preschool children. *Commun. Dent. oral Epidemiol.* **4**, 149–51.

11. The prevention of malocclusion

P.H. Gordon

INTRODUCTION

Malocclusion of the teeth is not really a disease in the way that dental caries and periodontitis are diseases, it is more a reflection of the natural variation that occurs in any biological system. True prevention of malocclusion is difficult to envisage, as there is a strong genetic component in the make-up of most malocclusions (Mills 1978). Preventive measures may be effective in dealing with environmental factors, but are unlikely to influence the outcome in cases where the genetic background is one of the more important determining factors.

The interception and early treatment of developing malocclusions has come to be regarded as almost synonymous with the prevention of malocclusion, but interception is, of course, early treatment of malocclusion rather than prevention. True prevention is virtually impossible, but early treatment may prevent the full expression of a malocclusion or may result in easier treatment, or less treatment. On the other hand, it sometimes results in two courses of orthodontic treatment rather than one. The decision as to whether to treat a malocclusion early rather than late has to be taken bearing in mind the likely benefit to the child, balanced against the costs. In this review of the role of interceptive orthodontics the various situations will be considered in which interceptive or early treatment of a developing malocclusion is likely to prove helpful.

IDEAL OCCLUSAL DEVELOPMENT

The primary incisor teeth erupt at approximately 7 months of age (Foster and Hamilton 1969), followed by the primary first molars at approximately 16 months of age. These are followed by the primary canine teeth at around 19 months and the primary second molars at around 28 months. There are particular occlusal features that occur commonly in the primary dentition, as outlined by Friel (1954) and by Foster and Hamilton (1969). These are the presence of anthropoid spacing, mesial to the upper primary canine and distal to the lower primary canine, the presence of generalized spacing in the incisor region, and the molar teeth occluding so that the distal surfaces of the primary second molars are in the in the same vertical plane. Variation in the eruption sequence of the primary teeth is relatively uncommon, though there is considerable variation in the age at which the teeth erupt into the mouth. Variation in the occlusion of the teeth is

relatively common. Crowding of primary teeth is not usually a problem, although absence of spacing between the primary incisor teeth is a reliable indication that the permanent teeth in that area will be crowded in due course (Baume 1950; Leighton 1971). Variation in the occlusion of the molar teeth, either in the antero-posterior or the transverse plane, is commonplace, but is seldom treated in the primary dentition, as it does not seem to give rise to any functional problem.

The permanent teeth start to erupt at about the age of 6 years (Houston *et al.* 1992). The first tooth to erupt is generally the lower first permanent molar, followed by the upper first molar and the lower central incisor. The upper central incisor, lower lateral incisor, and upper lateral incisor usually erupt between the ages of 7 and 9 years. The lower canine and the four first premolar teeth erupt at about the age of 10 or 11 years, followed by the second premolars, the upper canine, and the second permanent molars.

The distal surfaces of the second primary molar teeth guide the erupting first permanent molars into a cusp-to-cusp occlusion with their opposing teeth (i.e. half unit Class II). The permanent upper incisors are more proclined than their primary predecessors and this allows some forward repositioning of the mandible, which encourages the formation of a Class I molar occlusion (Friel 1954). The lower second primary molar is larger than the corresponding tooth in the upper arch and when these teeth are shed, the lower first permanent molar moves mesially rather more than the upper first molar. This also encourages the establishment of a Class I molar occlusion.

The above account is very much simplified and idealized; in real life the occlusion is seldom so well organized and there are several factors, inherited and environmental, which can influence the development of the occlusion.

AETIOLOGY OF MALOCCLUSION

SKELETAL FACTORS

The skeletal pattern (i.e. the relationship of the mandible to the maxilla in the antero-posterior, transverse, and vertical dimensions) is one of the most important factors governing the presence or absence of a malocclusion of the teeth, being intimately related to both incisor overjet and overbite and to the occlusion of the teeth in the buccal segments. There are two aspects of the skeletal pattern which have to be taken into account: one is the size of the mandible, relative to the size of the maxilla; the other is the position of the mandible, relative to the maxilla.

Since the time of Pierre Robin, clinicians and research workers have made determined efforts to influence the developing skeletal pattern (Robin 1902). A variety of myofunctional appliances have been developed and exercises proposed, with the intention of modifying the muscular environment of the developing bones, in the hope thereby of influencing their final size and position. These determined efforts have met with some limited success. It does seem possible to modify the position of the mandible relative to the maxilla, mainly by restraining the downwards and forwards translation of the maxilla during growth, but this change in skeletal pattern occurs only to a minor extent. Even less are the alterations produced in the size of the maxilla or the mandible—these changes are barely measurable. Myofunctional orthodontic appliances can undoubtedly influence the developing dentition, but they seem to produce their effects mainly by inducing dento-alveolar changes rather than by modifying the underlying skeletal pattern.

Similarly, the use of head-gear to apply relatively high forces to the maxilla, during growth, can influence the position of the maxilla to a certain extent, but these forces are applied to the maxilla via the teeth. The teeth will move, under the influence of these forces, producing dento-alveolar changes rather than any substantial modification of the underlying skeletal pattern.

The changes in occlusion produced by the use of myofunctional appliances and head-gear are achieved only with a major expenditure of time and effort. It is probably more appropriate to regard the use of these appliances as active treatment of a developing malocclusion rather than as any kind of preventive or interceptive measure.

Soft Tissue Form and Function

Skeletal pattern is one factor that can influence the position of the teeth, but it is by no means the only factor. The dental arches and, indeed, the skeletal pattern itself, develop within a soft-tissue environment. Muscular activity in the lips, cheeks, and tongue, and in the muscles of mastication, has a profound effect on the occlusion of the teeth, influencing, as it does, the labio-lingual inclination of the anterior teeth and the development of buccal segment crossbites (Wilmott 1984).

Sucking Habits

Digit-sucking habits can cause malocclusion, though it is probably a less important cause than is perceived by the general public. The majority of young children have a sucking habit, either digit-sucking, or sucking on a dummy (Johnson and Larson 1993). The effect of this activity on the position of the teeth is very variable; in some cases a very determined habit will have no noticeable effect, in other cases the sucking habit will produce a change in the position of the teeth. The effect will vary according to what it is that is being sucked. Thumb sucking, if only one thumb is being sucked, will tend to produce a Class II division 1 type of incisor relationship, with an asymmetric increase in the incisor overjet,

produced by proclination of the upper incisors and retroclination of the lowers (Melsen *et al.* 1979). The incisor overbite will tend to be incomplete, and there will be a tendency towards a crossbite of the buccal segment teeth. While the child is indulging in the habit, there is a lowering of the intra-oral air pressure accompanied by a lowered tongue position (Day and Foster 1971). These are the two factors that tend to produce a buccal segment crossbite. Sucking both thumbs (at the same time) will tend to produce a more symmetrical increase in incisor overjet. Finger-sucking may have less effect on the incisor overjet.

The changes produced by the sucking habit are dentoalveolar changes, the angulation of the teeth is changed with little impact on the underlying skeletal pattern (Larsson 1972). When the sucking habit is continued into the mixed dentition it may start to give rise to concern. If the upper incisor teeth are proclined and the lower teeth retroclined, then the lower lip may start to function behind the upper incisors, maintaining the position of the teeth after cessation of the habit. This arrangement is not self-correcting and will require a course of orthodontic treatment to re-establish a Class I incisor occlusion. If the habit is producing an obvious proclination of the upper incisors, it would be sensible to discourage the habit before establishment of a lip-trap. Interceptive treatment of a sucking habit will only be useful in Class I cases—thumb-sucking is often blamed for an increased incisor overjet that is really the result of an underlying Class II skeletal pattern.

Interceptive measures usually involve the provision of some sort of intra-oral appliance, together with the application of a bit of psychological pressure. The appliance may be an acrylic baseplate, retained by Adam's clasps, possibly with a bulge of acrylic in the middle of the palate. This serves as reminder to the child that they should stop sucking their thumb and may reduce the satisfaction obtained by continuation of the habit. Psychological pressure, or encouragement, may be brought to bear by pointing out to the parent, in the presence of the child, that thumb-sucking is something that all young children do, and something that they tend to stop doing as they grow older and more mature.

Dento-Alveolar Factors—the Management of the Developing Dentition

Dento-alveolar factors, the *local* causes of malocclusion, are the causes that are most amenable to an interceptive approach. Early detection of an anomaly, followed by early treatment, can sometimes avoid the need for more complex treatment at a later date. The various factors that can adversely affect the development of an otherwise normal occlusion can be categorized according to the developmental age at which a problem becomes evident.

INTERCEPTIVE MEASURES

Primary Dentition

Relatively little interceptive orthodontic treatment is carried out in the primary dentition, before the eruption of any permanent teeth. The dental arches are generally well aligned. There may be an increased incisor overjet, or a Class III incisor relationship, but these occlusal features are seldom so pronounced that they give rise to comment. Crowding of the primary dentition is usually expressed as an absence of spacing—the primary teeth are well aligned and unspaced—and crowding will become evident when the permanent teeth erupt.

Early loss of a primary first molar may allow mesial drift of the second molar. This is difficult to prevent when the child is so young. The techniques employed are the same as those suggested for use in the mixed dentition, but the space maintainers have to be worn for an extended period of time. If the primary second molar is lost prior to the eruption of the permanent first molar, then it is very difficult, though not absolutely impossible, to prevent mesial movement of the unerupted permanent tooth (Fields 1992).

Early loss of a primary incisor should have little effect on the arrangement of the permanent teeth. If the primary incisors are spaced, then one would not expect much mesial movement of the teeth distal to the lost incisor. Some space closure may well take place if the primary incisors are not spaced, but it can be argued that, in this situation, the permanent incisors are already short of space and the early loss of the primary tooth has merely served to localize the pre-existing crowding of the permanent teeth.

MIXED DENTITION

It is in the mixed dentition that most attempts have been made to intercept the development of malocclusion, with the aim of simplifying later orthodontic treatment, or even of avoiding the need for orthodontic treatment at a later date.

EARLY LOSS OF PRIMARY MOLAR TEETH

The effect, in the mixed dentition, of early loss of primary molar teeth depends on the amount of crowding in the dental arches and on which tooth it is that has been lost (Richardson 1965). If the dentition is crowded, then the crowding tends to become apparent either in the incisor region, or else in the region of the permanent molar teeth. The cumulative size of the primary canine and molar teeth exceeds the cumulative size of the permanent canine and premolar teeth (Houston *et al.* 1992), so that if the primary teeth are retained until they are shed in the ordinary way as the permanent teeth erupt, then there will be sufficient space for the permanent canine and premolar teeth. If a primary molar tooth is lost prematurely, such as through caries, and if the teeth are crowded, the teeth adjacent to the tooth that is extracted will tend to drift into the space that has become available, reducing the amount of space available for the developing permanent canine and premolar teeth.

If a primary second molar is lost and the teeth are crowded, the first permanent molar will move forward into the space, reducing the space available for the second premolar. There may be some shift of the centre-line, with the crowded incisor teeth moving round to the side of the missing primary molar, but most of the space loss occurs by mesial movement of the first permanent molar. If a primary first molar or canine is lost and the teeth are crowded, then the permanent incisor teeth will move round to that side, resulting in a more pronounced shift of the centre-line (van der Linden 1990). There may be some forward movement of the first permanent molar, but more loss of space occurs as a result of drifting of the incisor teeth.

BALANCING AND COMPENSATING EXTRACTIONS

The shift in centre-line which occurs when a tooth is lost on one side, in a crowded dentition, is difficult to correct once established. A balancing extraction (extracting a second tooth, on the opposite side of the same dental arch) is sometimes recommended, in crowded arches, to prevent the centre-line shift (Ball 1993). The tooth extracted to balance the first extraction is not necessarily the same tooth on the opposite side—the operator is guided in the first instance by the condition of the teeth.

If the occlusion of the buccal segment teeth is Class I, with good interdigitation of the cusps, then the loss of a tooth in one arch will allow mesial drift of the posterior teeth in that arch, on that side, leading to disruption of the buccal segment occlusion. A compensating extraction, that is, the extraction of a tooth from the opposing arch, will allow both upper and lower buccal segment teeth to drift forwards together, maintaining the Class I occlusion. A compensating extraction may also be carried out in the case of the early loss of a lower first permanent molar from a dentition with a Class I occlusion, in which case the upper first molar may have no opposing tooth with which to occlude and will over-erupt.

Balancing extractions, to prevent centre-line shifts in occlusions with crowded teeth, are commonly carried out. No matter what the inter-arch relationship, centre-line discrepancies are difficult to correct once established; the prevention of a centre-line shift may prevent the need for quite comprehensive orthodontic treatment at a later stage. Compensating extractions are less frequently indicated; they are potentially useful mainly in Class I occlusions.

SERIAL EXTRACTIONS

Kjellgren (1948) proposed a treatment for crowded Class I occlusions that illustrates well the concept of balancing and compensating extractions. In the case of a crowded Class I occlusion, the occlusal problem generally becomes apparent following the eruption of the permanent lateral incisors, when it can be seen that there is insufficient space to accommodate the anterior teeth. Kjellgren suggested that the four primary canine teeth should be extracted in these cases, at around the age of 8 or 9 years. This would allow the four incisor teeth in each arch to move distally into the space made available by the extractions, thereby improving the alignment of these teeth. It would be anticipated that the buccal segment teeth would move mesially, to some extent, helping to close any residual space. This mesial movement would occur in both upper and lower arches, maintaining the Class I buccal segment occlusion.

The intention is to obtain good alignment of the teeth and relief of crowding by the eventual extraction of all four first premolars. Early loss of these teeth will afford the maximum opportunity for spontaneous alignment of the permanent canine teeth, and Kjellgren suggested that the four primary first molars should be extracted when their roots were approximately half resorbed, in order to encourage early eruption of the first premolars, so that they, in turn, could be extracted at the earliest possible moment.

The problem here is that there is no guarantee that the extraction of the first primary molars will lead to early eruption of the first premolars (Kerr 1980). In addition, it is unlikely that the roots of the primary molars will all be resorbing at the same rate, so the recommendation that these teeth be extracted at just the right moment, when their roots are half resorbed, is difficult to implement. Another difficulty lies in the fact that the eruption of the lower premolar occurs, on average, at approximately the same time as the eruption of the permanent canine in that arch. These teeth are competing for the same space and the canine tooth is often displaced labially, to the extent that it unlikely to align spontaneously following the extraction of the first premolar.

Serial extraction, as the technique became known, is not practised nowadays in the way originally described by Kjellgren. In particular, the primary first molars are not extracted, since it has been found that these extractions confer no additional benefit. Occasionally, if these teeth are in poor condition, the primary first molars may be extracted instead of the primary canine teeth. The alignment of the permanent incisors proceeds more slowly than if the primary canines had been removed, but the final alignment will be much the same. Extraction of primary canine teeth to allow alignment of the incisors is widely practised, especially if the maxillary lateral incisors are instanding, and if extractions are required in one arch, in a Class I case, then they are generally carried out in both arches. Spontaneous alignment will result in an improvement in the position of the incisors, but sometimes only to a limited extent. If perfect alignment is required, a fixed appliance will generally be necessary.

THE TREATMENT OF ANTERIOR CROSSBITES

An anterior crossbite (one or more maxillary incisors occluding lingually to the opposing teeth) may become apparent when the incisor teeth erupt. There may be dento-alveolar factors involved in the development of this anomaly, or the crossbites may be an indication of an underlying skeletal discrepancy. Crowding, resulting in the lingual displacement of the upper lateral incisors may possibly be treated with a modified serial extraction technique. An anterior crossbite may result from the prolonged retention of a primary incisor (possibly a non-vital tooth that has failed to undergo root resorption) and the subsequent lingual deflection of the permanent tooth. In this case the prompt removal of the offending primary tooth may allow spontaneous alignment of the erupting permanent incisor, providing that the incisor overbite has not produced an occlusal lock.

Early treatment of instanding upper incisor teeth may be indicated for a variety of reasons. The inevitable occlusal interferences can lead to mandibular displacement; the opposing lower tooth or teeth are liable to move labially, producing a marked gingival recession on the labial aspect of these teeth. In addition, the labial surface of the instanding upper incisor can undergo marked attrition, with the production of a noticeable facet or 'chisel edge' incisally. Treatment usually involves proclination of the instanding tooth, probably with a removable orthodontic appliance. If it is necessary to create space in the dental arch in order to accomplish this tooth movement, then a form of serial extraction treatment will probably be needed to provide sufficient space.

There are a number of pitfalls that may prevent the successful execution of these apparently simple tooth movements. If the teeth are crowded, then the unerupted permanent canine tooth may impede forward movement of the upper lateral incisor. More often, lack of incisor overbite may prevent the establishment of a stable Class I incisor relationship. This is particularly likely if there is an underlying Class III skeletal relationship, in which case interceptive measures are unlikely to prove successful and the malocclusion is best left for definitive treatment at a later date.

THE TREATMENT OF POSTERIOR CROSSBITES

Crossbites involving posterior teeth are generally associated with a discrepancy in width of the upper and lower dental arches. In the case of a buccal crossbite, the buccal cusps of the lower teeth occlude outside the buccal cusps of the upper teeth, with the lower arch being disproportionately wide, or the upper narrow. In the case of a lingual crossbite, the buccal cusp of the lower tooth occludes lingually to the palatal cusp of the opposing upper tooth, with the upper arch wide or the lower narrow. The discrepancy in width may be dento-alveolar in origin, or it may be a sign of a skeletal discrepancy. Buccal segment crossbites may be bilateral or unilateral and the two tend to be treated differently.

A unilateral buccal crossbite may be associated with a mandibular displacement. The discrepancy in arch widths produces a cusp-to-cusp transverse relationship between the dental arches when the teeth occlude in the retruded contact position. In order to achieve a better occlusion, the mandible is postured to one side when moving to the intercuspal position. This produces a normal buccal segment occlusion on one side and a buccal crossbite on the other. In such a case, if the maxillary arch were expanded in the transverse dimension until it was wide enough to accommodate the lower in the retruded contact position, then both the buccal segment crossbite and the mandibular displacement would be corrected. A narrowness of the upper arch may also be associated with lack of space for the incisor teeth and the expansion of the upper arch may also provide sufficient space to correct this problem. Early treatment of unilateral buccal segment crossbite may be indicated in the early mixed dentition, after the eruption of the first permanent molar, when it becomes apparent that there is insufficient space for the upper incisor teeth.

This line of treatment is attractive only if the skeletal pattern is Class I, so that there is no need to correct the incisor relationship and only if the expansion will provide sufficient space for the upper incisor teeth. This can be assessed by using the space available for the lower incisor teeth as a guide to the space available for the upper incisors.

If the incisor relationship requires correction, or the teeth are crowded, then an interceptive approach to correct the buccal crossbite will involve two courses of treatment rather than one. For the same reason the interceptive approach is more often indicated when the crossbite has a dento-alveolar basis rather than having its origin in the skeletal pattern. In the latter case there is likely to be some other orthodontic treatment needed at a later date and this reduces the benefit of an interceptive approach.

Bilateral crossbites are seldom amenable to treatment at an early age. There is usually a skeletal component in the aetiology of the condition; there is often no associated mandibular displacement and therefore less indication for treatment. In addition, the amount of correction required is considerably greater than is the case with a unilateral crossbite and the condition is more likely to relapse. If a bilateral crossbite is corrected at all, the correction is usually done as part of a comprehensive course of orthodontic treatment, rather than as an interceptive measure. In the same way, a lingual crossbite, if not due to the deflection of a single tooth by a retained primary predecessor, is generally associated with a marked Class II skeletal pattern and is not amenable to treatment using an interceptive approach.

SUPERNUMERARY TEETH

Supernumerary teeth can occur anywhere in the mouth, but are particularly common in the maxillary labial segment. They are usually classified by their shape, as supplemental, conical, or tuberculate (Taylor 1972). Supplemental teeth resemble those of the normal series found in that area of the mouth—it is often difficult to determine which is the supernumerary tooth. Conical supernumerary teeth have conical crowns and are usually found in the maxillary labial segment; they are sometimes inverted and may remain unerupted, more or less indefinitely. Supplemental and conical teeth seldom interfere with the eruption of the permanent teeth of the normal series. If the supernumerary teeth erupt, the teeth are usually crowded and extractions, with or without appliance therapy, will be needed to allow alignment of the remaining teeth.

Tuberculate supernumerary teeth, which occur palatal to the developing maxillary incisors, usually the central incisors, seem to prevent the eruption of the developing permanent teeth. It is very important that the presence of these teeth is recognized at an early age. The unerupted tuberculate supernumerary teeth should be extracted, surgically, as soon as possible. It is not necessary to uncover the unerupted permanent incisors; the mucoperiosteal flap should be replaced and the incisors left to erupt spontaneously. This is what is gained by early diagnosis—if detected early, the prompt removal of the tuberculate supernumerary teeth will allow spontaneous eruption of the permanent incisors. If detected late, then removal of the supernumerary teeth is less likely to result in spontaneous eruption of the central incisors. Their subsequent surgical exposure, followed by orthodontic alignment, produces a less satisfactory result. Orthodontic extrusion of unerupted teeth tends to leave a long clinical crown, with an unsatisfactory gingival margin and reduced periodontal support.

PLANNED LOSS OF FIRST PERMANENT MOLAR TEETH

Haphazard loss of first permanent molar teeth can have a detrimental effect on the developing occlusion. The worst effects are usually seen in the lower arch, when mesial tipping and mesio-lingual rotation of the second molar is usually evident, with a poor contact or no contact between the second molar and the second premolar (Crabb and Rock 1971). In addition, the upper first molar can over-erupt into the space left by the extraction of the lower tooth. In the case of early loss of an upper first molar, the upper second molar will usually move mesially, rotating about its palatal root, but with relatively little tipping. If it is evident at an early age that the first permanent molars have a poor long-term prognosis, then careful planning of the timing of the extraction of these teeth can help minimize the deleterious effects.

If the first molar is lost early, before the formation of the root of the unerupted second molar, than the second molar will generally move forwards before it erupts, coming through to replace the first molar (Thilander *et al.* 1963). If the extraction of the first molar is delayed until the second molar is erupted or is on the point of eruption, there will be little forward movement of the second molar, which will then proceed to tip and rotate in the manner described above.

It follows, then, that the timing of the extractions should be varied according to the space requirements of the case in question. If there is no malocclusion and the first permanent molars are being extracted simply because of caries or hypoplasia then early extraction of all four teeth, when the bifurcation of the roots of the lower second molar is just visible on a radiograph (at about the age of 10 years), will allow forward movement of the unerupted second molars, which in this case is just what is wanted. If the incisor overjet is increased, or the anterior teeth are crowded, so that the space created by the extraction of the first molars is needed for the alignment of the teeth, then the extractions should be delayed. In the case of the upper arch, in such a situation, it would be prudent to delay the extraction of the first molars until after the eruption of the second molars. It would then be possible to use an orthodontic appliance, incorporating the second molars, to make best use of the space created by the extractions.

ABNORMALITIES OF TOOTH POSITION

MALPOSITIONED MAXILLARY CANINE TEETH

Malpositioned canines are a considerable nuisance, from the point of view of both the patient and the practitioner. They are difficult to treat—the treatment is lengthy and demanding in terms of co-operation on the part of the patient and in terms of technical expertise on the part of the operator. The malpositioned tooth can be left alone, or it can be extracted; it can be aligned by means of orthodontic treatment, or it can be aligned surgically. Each of these remedies has its own disadvantages. Is it possible to intercept the developing problem and, by early intervention, persuade the malpositioned canine to erupt into the correct position?

The most common line of interceptive treatment that has been recommended is extraction of the primary canine tooth. This approach is usually justified on empirical grounds rather than scientific—clinical experience is cited as the authority rather than the results of any prospective randomized clinical trial. There have, however, been retrospective studies that have lent support to this line of treatment (Ericson and Kurol 1988). Cases in which the primary tooth has been extracted are compared to cases in which it has not and it is claimed that the extraction of the primary tooth has been beneficial. The treatment in these retrospective studies has never been randomized and the groups in which the primary tooth has been left *in situ* always contain cases in which the reason the primary tooth was left in place was that the permanent tooth was in a truly hopeless position and there was no prospect whatsoever of aligning it. The milder the displacement, the more likely it is that the primary tooth will have been extracted, on the grounds that the displacement of the permanent canine may be due in part to some failure of resorption of the root of the primary tooth.

The presence of a palatally displaced maxillary canine may be associated with the presence of a diminutive upper lateral incisor, or a missing lateral incisor. It would appear that the root of the lateral incisor may play some part in guiding the eruption of the developing canine. The maxillary canine teeth should be palpable in the labial sulcus from the age of 10 years onwards. If these teeth are not palpable at this age then radiographs should be taken, to determine the position of the unerupted teeth. If a permanent canine is palatally displaced to a relatively mild degree and there appears to be a lack of root resorption of the primary canine, then extraction of the primary canine would be an acceptable line of treatment provided that it is intended eventually to align the permanent tooth. This will probably involve the use of a fixed orthodontic appliance, possibly preceded by the surgical exposure of the tooth, should it fail to erupt spontaneously. The extraction of the primary tooth will seldom result in spontaneous alignment of the unerupted, displaced canine, but may allow some improvement in its position. The extraction of the primary tooth commits the operator to a particular line of treatment at a later date. If the root of the primary tooth has not started to resorb, then the primary canine may have a better long-term prognosis than a permanent canine that has been repositioned surgically.

DILACERATION OF INCISORS

Supernumerary teeth can prevent the eruption of upper central incisor teeth. Another reason these teeth may fail to erupt is that the developing tooth is dilacerated. This developmental anomaly produces an angle between the crown of the tooth and its root. This could be caused by trauma to the primary upper incisors causing their impaction; the primary teeth are driven up into the gum and displace the calcified crown of the developing permanent incisor, producing an angle between the crown of the tooth and its root, which continues to develop in its original position. The permanent tooth then fails to erupt. While this is a plausible explanation for the production of this anomaly, it has to be said that dilacerated incisors frequently develop in situations where there is absolutely no history of trauma to the primary

teeth and the aetiology of the condition is quite obscure (Stewart 1978).

There is not much that can be done to prevent the dilaceration of incisors, but early diagnosis of the reason for failure of eruption of the permanent incisor will allow proper planning of any subsequent treatment. The dilacerated tooth is usually extracted, though in some cases it may be possible to align the tooth orthodontically, following its surgical exposure. This may, however, produce a disappointing result. If there is a marked bend in the root of the central incisor it may be difficult to align the tooth without interfering with the position of its neighbours.

TRANSPOSITION OF TEETH

Transposition of teeth occurs when two adjacent teeth attempt to erupt with their positions interchanged. For some reason the teeth that are usually affected are the permanent canine and first premolar in the upper arch and the permanent canine and lateral incisor in the lower arch. Once again there is little that can be done to prevent the problem; early treatment is sometimes carried out in the lower arch where the lateral incisor is usually extracted, following its ectopic eruption.

HYPODONTIA

Hypodontia, when one or more of the teeth fails to develop, is a relatively common condition which is almost certainly hereditary in origin; as such, there is little scope for prevention. If we disregard missing third molars, the prevalence of which is difficult to assess, then approximately six per cent of people have one or more missing teeth (Grahnen 1956). Early treatment is seldom indicated, but if the teeth are crowded, then the absence of a permanent tooth will influence the decision as to which teeth are selected for extraction.

SCREENING

It has sometimes been suggested that children should be screened for the presence of occlusal anomalies, at about the age of 10 years (Chung and Kerr 1987). The argument has been that this would expedite the early detection of these anomalies, allowing any preventive action or early treatment to be taken at the appropriate moment. The type of screening process that has usually been advocated would involve a clinical orthodontic assessment and the taking of a pan-oral radiograph. Studies of the efficacy of such a screening process have indicated that routine screening of children for occlusal anomalies would not be a cost-effective exercise (Hiles 1985). There are two reasons for this: the occlusal anomalies tend to be detected in any case, whether or not the children are screened and if an anomaly is detected as a result of the screening process, there are relatively few cases in which the child would benefit from early interceptive treatment (Popovich and Thompson 1975; Ackermann and Proffit 1980). In other words, the screening process does not affect the outcome in the majority of cases.

Whether or not a screening programme would result in the early detection of occlusal problems that would otherwise go unnoticed depends on the level of provision and uptake of dental services. If a population of children is exposed to a high level of provision of dental services, then they are likely to receive a dental examination in any case. The 'screening' for malocclusion then becomes part of that process, and is the responsibility of the examining dentist. If the level of provision of dental services, or the uptake of services is low then the resources that could be spent on the provision of a screening programme for occlusal anomalies would probably be better directed at improving the general dental condition of the children, rather than on screening for malocclusion.

SCOPE AND LIMITATIONS OF INTERCEPTIVE ORTHODONTICS

- It is difficult to prevent malocclusion—most of the effort that is expended on interceptive orthodontics is directed towards early treatment rather than prevention.

- Careful timing of the extraction of poor quality first permanent molars can prevent the development of local malocclusions, as can prompt extraction of retained primary teeth that are deflecting the eruption of their permanent successors.

- Early treatment of tuberculate supernumerary teeth will certainly encourage spontaneous eruption of the permanent incisors, and greatly simplify their subsequent alignment.

- There are some situations in which early orthodontic treatment may be beneficial, resulting in a simpler treatment plan or in a more rapid course of treatment, but all too often, early treatment means more treatment, extending over a longer period of time, or the provision of two consecutive courses of treatment.

- The use of myofunctional appliances to correct developing Class II malocclusions is probably better regarded as a full-blown course of orthodontic treatment than as an interceptive measure.

- The distinction between interceptive treatment and prevention may not be helpful. The aim of both interceptive treatment and of preventive treatment is to minimize the total amount of treatment that needs to be provided.

REFERENCES

Ackerman, J.L. and Proffit, W.R. (1980). Preventive and interceptive orthodontics: a strong theory proves weak in practice. *Angle Orthod.*, **50**, 75–87.

Ball, I.A. (1993). Balancing the extraction of primary teeth: a review. *Int. J. Paed. Dent.*, **3**, 179–85.

Baume, L.J. (1950). Physiologic tooth migration and its significance for the development of occlusion. *J. dent. Res.*, **29**, 123.

Chung, C.K. and Kerr, W.J.S. (1987). Interceptive orthodontics: application and outcome in a demand population. *Br. dent. J.*, **162**, 73–6.

Crabb, J.J. and Rock, W.P. (1971). Treatment planning in relation to the first permanent molar. *Br. dent. J.*, **131**, 396–401.

Day, A.J.W. and Foster, T.D. (1971). An investigation into the prevalence of molar crossbite and some associated aetiological conditions. *Dent. Practit.*, **21**, 402–10.

Ericson, S. and Kurol, J. (1988). Early treatment of palatally erupting maxillary canines treated by extraction of the primary canines. *Eur. J. Orthod.*, **10**, 283–95.

Fields, H.W. (1992). Treatment of nonskeletal problems in preadolescent children. In *Contemporary orthodontics*, 2nd edn, (ed. W.R. Proffit), pp. 376–468. Mosby, St Louis.

Foster, T.D. and Hamilton, M.C. (1969). Occlusion in the primary dentition. *Br. dent. J.*, **126**, 76–9.

Friel, S. (1954). The development of ideal occlusions of the gum pads and the teeth. *Am. J. Orthod.*, **40**, 196.

Grahnen, H. (1956). Hypodontia in the permanent dentition. *Odont. Revy*, **7**, Suppl 3.

Hiles, A.M. (1985). Is orthodontic screening of 9-year-old school children cost effective? *Br. dent. J.*, **159**, 41–4.

Houston, W.J.B., Stephens, C. D. and Tulley, W.J. (1992). *A textbook of orthodontics*, 2nd edn, Table 3.1, p. 31 and Table 3.2, p. 37. Wright, Oxford.

Johnson, E.D. and Larson, B.E. (1993). Thumb-sucking: literature review. *J. dent. Child.* **60**, 385–91.

Kerr, W.J.S. (1980). The effect of the premature loss of deciduous canines and molars on the eruption of their successors. *Eur. J. Orthod.*, **2**, 123–8.

Kjellgren, B. (1948). Serial extraction as a corrective procedure in dental orthopaedic therapy. *Acta odont. Scand.*, **8**, 17–43.

Larsson, E. (1972). Dummy- and finger-sucking habits with special attention to their significance for facial growth and occlusion. 4. Effect on facial growth and occlusion. *Sven. Tandlak. Tidskr.*, **65**, 605–34.

Leighton, B.C. (1969). The early signs of malocclusion. *Trans. Eur. Orthod. Soc.*, 353–68.

van der Linden, F.P.G.M. (1990). *Problems and procedures in dentofacial orthopedics*, pp. 27–38. Quintessence, Chicago.

Melsen, S., Stensgaard, K., and Pedersen, J. (1979). Sucking habits and their influence on swallowing pattern and prevalence of malocclusion. *Eur. J. Orthod.*, **1**, 271–80.

Mills, J.R.E. (1978). The effect of orthodontic treatment on the skeletal pattern. *Br. J. Orthod.*, **5**, 133–43.

Popovich, F. and Thompson, G.W. (1975). Evaluation of preventive and interceptive orthodontic treatment between three and eighteen years of age. In *Transactions of the Third International Orthodontic Congress*, (ed. J.T. Cook), pp. 260–81. C.V. Mosby, St Louis.

Richardson, M.E. (1965). The relationship between the relative amount of space present in the deciduous dental arch and the rate and degree of space closure subsequent to the extraction of a deciduous molar. *Dent. Practit.*, **16**, 111–18.

Robin, P. (1902). Demonstration practique sur la construction et la mise en bouche d'un nouvel appareil de redressement. *Rev. Stomatol.*, **9**, 561–90.

Stewart, D.J. (1978). Dilacerate unerupted maxillary central incisors. *Br. dent. J.*, **145**, 229–33.

Taylor, G.S. (1972). Characteristics of supernumerary teeth in the primary and permanent dentition. *Dent. Practit.*, **22**, 203–8.

Thilander, B., Jakobsson, S.O. and Skagius, S. (1963). Orthodontic sequelae of extraction of permanent first molars. *Scand. dent. J.*, **71**, 380–412.

Wilmott, D.R. (1984). Thumb-sucking habit and associated dental differences in one of monozygous twins. *Br. J. Orthod.*, **11**, 195–9.

12. The prevention of oral mucosal disease

CRISPIAN SCULLY

MOST conditions that affect oral mucosal health are acquired. Various chemical, physical, and biological factors may act singly or in concert to cause disease, some of which is preventable. The genetic constitution may well influence the result of an onslaught by some environmental agent such as a microorganism. Central to mucosal integrity are adequate nutrition and intact immune and other defences, such as saliva.

This chapter considers oral cancer, mucosal infections, common immunologically mediated mucosal disorders, and nutritionally related oral mucosal disease; and highlights the major risk factors that need to be addressed if some of the oral mucosal diseases are to be prevented or reduced.

ORAL CANCER AND POTENTIALLY MALIGNANT LESIONS

Oral squamous carcinomas are uncommon in the UK, where about 2000 new cases are seen annually. World wide it is the eighth most common malignant tumour. In many areas, the incidence appears to be increasing (Boyle et al. 1990a, 1991). It can present as a lump, ulcer, red or white lesion, and spreads locally and to the cervical lymph nodes. Although there must be genetic influences on susceptibility or resistance to oral cancer, the evidence is that lifestyle can significantly influence the risk. Habits, such as tobacco and alcohol use, are the major risk factors. The effect of vitamins and essential elements in protecting against oral cancers is reviewed. In addition, risks associated with various occupations are considered.

HABITS

Tobacco and alcohol use

Tobacco contains nicotine and other alkaloids. N-nitrosamines are the compounds thought to be the major carcinogenic agents in tobacco. Volatile and other nitrosamines may be found. Non-volatile N-nitroso compounds include N-nitrosonornicotine (NNN), 4-(methylnitrosamino)-1-(3-pyridyl)-1-butanone (NNK), and N-nitroso-anatabine (NAT).

Tobacco is smoked as cigarettes, cigars or in a pipe and, in some instances may be treated in a variety of ways, or contain additives. Tobacco smoking can have a range of adverse effects on oral health, including predisposing to candida carriage, candidiasis, and to one of the main potentially malignant lesions—leukoplakia.

Tobacco is chewed either alone or in special forms which may contain additives such as slaked lime or be in a betel quid (see below). Snuff is usually finely powdered tobacco which is used alone or with additives and is placed nasally or orally.

By 1988, both tobacco smoking (IARC 1986) and alcohol consumption (IARC 1988) had been accepted as independent risk factors for oral cancer (oral squamous cell carcinoma). Convincing evidence also exists that the combined effect of alcohol and tobacco is greater than the sum of the two effects independently, although this has not been a consistent finding (Rothman and Keller 1972; Graham et al. 1977). Smokeless tobacco and betel quid are also risk factors (IARC 1985) and the use of mouth washes may be a risk factor in a small subgroup of non-smoking, non-drinking women (Blot et al. 1983).

Analytical studies strongly suggest that tobacco smoking of any type, but especially pipe smoking significantly increases the risk of lip cancer. Working outdoors also increases the risk of lip cancer and a fair complexion may be an additional co-factor. As regards intra-oral carcinoma, the sites of tongue, mouth, oropharynx, and hypopharynx are so often grouped together in analytical studies, or grouped in a variety of different combinations, that it is difficult to discuss these tumours individually. Studies which have considered individual subsites therefore may have resulted in apparent differences in risk estimates from those studies which have not presented subsite data separately.

The effect of smoking falls off soon after smoking ceases (Blot et al. 1989). Given the large attributable risk for the two habits of smoking and alcohol drinking, this dramatic reduction in risk (within 5–10 years of quitting) provides great hope for the prevention and control of the growing menace of oral cancer in Western countries. Some fairly recent studies have helped elucidate these areas. Blot et al. (1989), in a case-control study based on 1114 US cases and 1268 population-based controls, found the risk for oral (and pharyngeal) cancer to increase with increasing cigarette consumption and independently with increasing alcohol consumption. Risk among non-drinkers increased with the amount of tobacco smoked and risks among non-smokers increased with the level of alcohol intake. Among those who both smoked and drank, the risk tended to combine in a multiplicative fashion. Those who consumed daily two or more packs of cigarettes and had more than four alcoholic drinks had a 35-fold increase in risk compared to non-smokers/non-drinkers. After stopping smoking for 10 or more years, there was no excess risk.

A study from Italy (Franceschi *et al.* 1990) showed considerable risk increases with alcohol and tobacco use, with risk decreasing with increasing years since cessation of tobacco use. The risk of oral and pharyngeal cancer was increased 80-fold in the highest levels of smoking and alcohol consumption considered compared to abstainers. Similar findings were reported subsequently (Franceschi *et al.* 1992).

Details of tar yield of cigarettes and type of cigarette used for the longest period can be used as the basis of a classification to examine the effects of different types of cigarette. Cigarettes can be classified as low or medium if the tar yield is below 22 mg, and as high if tar yield is above 22 mg. Compared with non-smokers the risk of oral cancer for smokers using low- to medium-tar cigarettes in 8.5 and for high tar cigarettes is 16.4 (La Vecchia *et al.* 1990).

Examination of various forms of alcohol in a large study from two centres in Italy (Barra *et al.* 1990) investigated the risk of oral and pharyngeal cancer in an area where large quantities of wine are consumed. Among the heaviest alcohol drinkers (i.e. more than 84 drinks per week), the risk for consumption of wine alone was 11.2; for wine plus spirits 9.9, and for a combination of wine, spirits, and beer was 4.1. Alcohol, particularly in persons who smoked tobacco was also a risk factor in recent studies of 1569 males in Uzbekistan (Evstifeeva and Zaridze 1992), 6701 males in Hawaii (Kato *et al.* 1992), and a study of 465 oral cancer patients in Israel (Gorsky *et al.* 1992).

A case-control study from Uruguay based on 108 male cases of oral and pharyngeal cancer and 286 controls showed elevated risk associated with heavy consumption of wine (DeStefani *et al.* 1988). Dark tobacco was reported as having a risk more than three times that of light (blond) tobacco.

Smokeless tobacco

Smokeless tobacco and betel quid are also risk factors (IARC 1985). In a study of oral cancer in India, Sankaranarayanan *et al.* (1989) found, among males, significantly increased risks in relation to tobacco chewing, bidi smoking, and bidi plus cigarette smoking. Alcohol also emerged as a significant risk factor. Other recent studies from India confirmed the association between tobacco chewing and oral cancer. The strong association with tobacco chewing on oral cancer risk on the Indian subcontinent gives an obvious priority for prevention strategies.

In Indian patients aged less than 30 years, with oral cancer, a much lower frequency of habits recognizably associated with oral cancer risk (tobacco chewing, smoking, alcohol use) was seen, suggesting that other factors may be associated with oral cancer risk at least at younger ages.

Smokeless tobacco contains a number of carcinogens and, particularly in view of the fact that snuff can produce oral leukoplakia and carcinoma, its use is to be deprecated. There is concern about the possible carcinogenicity and other adverse effects of the snuff now sold in small 'teabag' pouches. The fact that this form of smokeless tobacco is held in the mouth for very long periods, and is popular with children and adolescents in the cause for concern, though there is limited evidence for an association between the use of such smokeless tobacco and oral cancer. There is no doubt,

however, that smokeless tobacco can induce oral keratosis and gingival recession (Little *et al.* 1992).

Betel use and other habits

There is some confusion over the use of the term betel. Betel leaf is derived from the betel vine while nuts from the betel palm are termed areca nuts. These two products may be used orally alone, together, or together with other material such as tobacco, slaked lime, and other additives. In Papua New Guinea slaked lime (but not tobacco) is a prominent component of 'betel': in other areas tobacco may be a main component.

While there is clear evidence of carcinogenicity from tobacco, the risk of oral cancer is also increased in persons who chew betel with or without tobacco (Gupta *et al.* 1982). Areca nut use clearly predisposes to oral submucosal fibrosis, a recognized pre-malignant condition (Pindborg *et al.* 1984), can cause cytogenetic changes whether tobacco is, or is not used, and can result in the appearance of N-nitroso compounds in the saliva including N-nitrosoguvacine and nitrosamines such as 3-(methyl nitrosamino) propionitrile—a powerful carcinogen in rats. Areca nut specific N-nitroso compounds can also cause epithelial changes *in vitro* and can enhance experimental carcinogenesis.

Although the diversity of constituents of betel has caused some difficulties in interpretation it is now clear that betel use can result in submucosal fibrosis where areca nuts are chewed (Bhonsle *et al.* 1987), leukoplakia and/or carcinoma where tobacco is included, and oral cancer, particularly where slaked lime is used (Thomas and MacLennan 1992).

Mouth wash use

In a study based on 125 cases of oral cancer in women and a control group of 107 (Kabat *et al.* 1989), both cigarette smoking and alcohol consumption were confirmed as independent risk factors but no association was found for mouth wash use. Patients with oral cancer reported more frequently than did controls that they used mouth wash to 'disguise the smell of tobacco . . . [and] . . . alcohol' and mouth wash use was found to be strongly associated with smoking and drinking. Thus, using a mouth wash appeared in these instances to be a proxy for exposure to tobacco or alcohol, themselves risk determinants of oral cancer. However, a recent major US study (Winn *et al.* 1991) re-examined the question of mouth wash use in a study on 866 cases and 1249 controls from four areas. After adjustment for tobacco and alcohol use, the risk of oral cancer among users of mouth wash was found to be increased by 40 per cent in men and 60 per cent in women. This increased risk was apparent only when using mouth washes of a high alcohol content (25 per cent or higher). Thus, it appears that the risk from alcohol in mouth washes is similar, at least qualitatively, to that of alcohol used for drinking, although in terms of attributable risk the contribution of mouth wash use to oral cancer remains small.

Marijuana use

There have been some reports of oral cancers in marijuana smokers (Donald 1986), but these have yet to be supported by an epidemiological study. For example, there has been a recent report of an unusual case of tongue cancer in a patient who was only 23 years old (Almadori *et al.* 1990). The patient was a regular user of marijuana but also a heavy cigarette smoker, and this factor, as well as alcohol consumption and other risk factors such as oral snuff use, have to be controlled for so that a clearer picture can emerge of this independent role of marijuana in the risk of the disease. The authors argue that the cigarette smoking was unlikely to be the 'cause' of the cancer in this case because the patient had only been smoking a short time. However, that argument would seem to apply equally to the marijuana habit.

EFFECT OF VITAMINS AND ESSENTIAL MINERALS

Both natural vitamin A precursors (carotenoids) and synthetic analogues (retinoids) may have some protective effect against cancers. Over the past few years there has been considerable interest in the role of vitamin A in oral cancers (Scully and Boyle 1992). Vitamin and provitamin A (β-carotene) levels are lower in patients with oral cancer than in controls, although this may, of course, be a secondary effect. The risk of oral cancer has been inversely associated with consumption of fruit and vegetables in many studies (e.g. Notani and Jayanet 1987; La Vecchia *et al.* 1991; Franceschi *et al.* 1992; Zheng *et al.* 1993) and with consumption of vitamin A (Marshall *et al.* 1982). Oral mucosal cells show nuclear enlargement with occasional binucleate or giant forms, and hyperchromatism. The epithelium is thinned and may show basal hyperplasia and increased mitoses in vitamin B_{12} deficiency, and this may sometimes amount to epithelial dysplasia (Theaker *et al.* 1989). These mucosal changes respond rapidly to vitamin B replacement therapy and there is no evidence for a predisposition to carcinoma.

There is a tenuous association of vitamin C with a protective effect against oral, pharyngeal and oesophageal cancers (Barone *et al.* 1992; Rossing *et al.* 1989).

There may be a relationship of vitamin E to carcinogenesis, since vitamin E, like β-carotene, is antioxidant and appears to inhibit experimental oral carcinogenesis and, in humans, higher serum vitamin E levels appear associated with a decreased risk of oral cancer (Knekt 1988). Vitamin E use may have some protective effect against leukoplakias (Benner *et al.* 1993) and carcinomas (Barone *et al.* 1992; Gridley *et al.* 1992).

There is a possible role of iron deficiency in carcinogenesis in view of the premalignant potential of the Plummer–Vinson syndrome. This syndrome, consisting of iron deficiency, dysphagia, and post-cricoid oesophageal stricture may be accompanied by glossitis and angular stomatitis, and may be associated, in up to about 15 per cent with carcinomas of the post-cricoid pharynx, oesophagus, stomach, and occasionally mouth. However, any significant role for iron deficiency in oral carcinogenesis has yet to be established and, in animal models, iron deficiency has had only equivocal effects on chemical oral carcinogenesis (Prime *et al.* 1986). There is equivocal evidence that zinc may influence oral carcinogenesis (Edwards 1976) and some evidence that selenium deficiency may predispose to oral cancer (Rogers *et al.* 1991).

Epidemiological evidence links a high intake of saturated animal fats with oral and pharyngeal cancer, at least in males (Carrroll and Khor 1975).

OCCUPATION AND ORAL HEALTH STATUS

Limited epidemiological evidence suggests increased risk for oral and pharyngeal cancer for workers exposed to formaldehyde (Vaughan *et al.* 1986), printers and pressman (Dubrow and Wegman 1984), workers with access to alcohol (such as bartenders and restaurant workers (Dubrow and Wegman 1984), electrical and electronics workers (Winn *et al.* 1982), textile and apparel workers (Blot and Fraumeni 1977), and man-made mineral fibre workers (Moulin *et al.* 1986). Most of this evidence comes from occupational disease surveillance studies and from retrospective cohort studies in which the number of cases of oral cancer is small.

A recent study surveyed many occupations for oral cancer risk (Huebner *et al.* 1992) which observed associations warranting further investigations, including a high risk for carpet installers, and a low risk for textile workers. The lack of findings for certain occupations with previously reported associations with oral cancer is probably explained by better measurement and control for confounding by tobacco and alcohol.

There is a higher incidence of lip cancer in outdoor and rural populations than in office workers or urban populations, a relationship thought to be due to exposure to sunlight (and ultraviolet irradiation). Other studies have shown fair-skinned people to be predisposed to lip cancer in sunny climates and the fact that lip cancer involves the more exposed lower lip rather than the upper lip also supports a relationship with actinic radiation. (Boyle *et al.* 1991).

A poor dentition, as reflected by missing teeth, emerged as a risk factor independent of other established risk factors in studies from China (Zheng *et al.* 1990b). Those who did not brush their teeth also had an increased risk of oral cancer over those who brushed. Generally, similar findings were reported from other case-control studies in Brazil with higher risk of oral cancer among those who reported tooth-brushing to be infrequent compared with those who brushed their teeth daily (Boyle *et al.* 1991). The overall message appears to be that poor oral hygiene is independently associated with an increased risk of oral cancer. Recently, the relationship between socio-economic status and oral cancer risk was explored (Greenberg *et al.* 1991). Three indicators of socio-economic status were considered (education, occupational status, and percentage of potential working life in employment). After adjustment for established risk factors, the third index only was found to have an independent association with oral cancer risk consistent with the hypothesis that behaviours leading to social instability, or social instability itself, are linked to an increased risk of oral and pharyngeal cancer.

POTENTIALLY MALIGNANT LESIONS

The main potentially malignant lesions are leukoplakias, erythroplasias, erosive lichen planus, and submucosal fibrosis.

The term leukoplakia is now usually restricted to those white patches for which a cause cannot be found, and therefore implies a diagnosis by exclusion (e.g. exclusion of lichen planus, candidosis, etc.). The term is also used irrespective of the presence or absence of epithelial dysplasia, although there is a premalignant potential to some keratoses.

Clinically, leukoplakias fall into one of two main groups. The most common are uniformly white plaques (homogeneous leukoplakias), prevalent in the buccal (cheek) mucosa and usually of low pre-malignant potential. Far more serious, are nodular and, especially, speckled leukoplakias, which consist of white patches or nodules in a red area of mucosa. Chronic candidal infection is common in speckled leukoplakias and may be associated with an increased risk of malignant change. Candidal leukoplakias are often found at the commissures.

Syphilitic leukoplakia seen in tertiary syphilis, although of little more than historical interest, may have had a high malignant potential.

Leukoplakia of the anterior floor of the mouth and undersurface of the tongue (sublingual keratosis) may have a particularly high risk of malignant change. The cause of this lesion is unknown but it is more common in women than men and has a typical 'ebbing-tide' appearance clinically.

Though years of pipe smoking can lead to a characteristic type of benign keratosis of the palate—stomatitis nicotina—this is not pre-malignant. Trauma occasionally causes keratosis, usually at the buccal mucosal occlusal line or on edentulous ridges when the patient does not wear a denture. Again this is not pre-malignant.

Erythroplasia (erythroplakia) is a rare, red and often velvety lesion. It affects patients of either sex in their sixth and seventh decades and typically involves the floor of the mouth, the ventrum of the tongue, or the soft palate. Unlike leukoplakias, erythroplasia does not form a plaque but is level with, or depressed below, the surrounding mucosa. The importance of erythroplasia is that some 75–90 per cent prove to be carcinoma or carcinoma-*in situ* or show severe dysplasia. Red oral lesions are generally more dangerous than are white lesion.

Lichen planus, particularly when erosive and involving the tongue may have a malignant potential approaching that of leukoplakia. Submucosal fibrosis appears clearly related to exposure to areca nut and thus is potentially preventable.

Prevention of potentially malignant lesions includes avoiding habits such as the use of alcohol, tobacco, and betel, improving the diet by increasing intake of fruit and vegetables, treating possible infections such as candidiasis or syphilis (see below), and avoiding excessive exposure to the sun (and using sun-blocking agents).

PREVENTION OF ORAL CANCER

The messages required for the prevention of, or reduction in, oral cancer parallel the general health education advice: eliminate tobacco use, reduce excessive alcohol consumption, ensure a healthy diet free from vitamin and nutritional deficiencies, eliminate specific habits, such as betel nut chewing, and excessive exposure to the sun.

Reductions in the prevalence and extent of oral cancer may also be achieved by the early detection of pre-malignant and malignant lesions, which can be detected by carrying out a thorough examination of the mouth and regional lymph nodes by a clinician trained in the diagnosis of oral disease.

The most common sites of cancer in the oral cavity are the lower lip, the lateral margin of the tongue, and the floor of the mouth. The 'coffin corner' at the posterior tongue/floor of the mouth is a common site for tumour, easily overlooked. The clinical appearance of oral cancer is highly variable. Some present as ulcers; others as a red or white area, a lump, or fissuring. Suspicious lesions must be palpated for induration and fixation to deeper tissues (Scully 1993).

Any chronic oral lesion should therefore be regarded with suspicion, especially if in an older patient or if there are appearances as above, induration, fixation to underlying tissues, any recent changes in appearance, associated lymphadenopathy, or no obvious explanation for the lesion. Features apart from chronicity which particularly suggest that a mucosal lesion is malignant or premalignant include:

- the presence of erythroplasia
- a granular appearance or raised exophytic margins
- induration (i.e. a firm infiltration beneath the mucosa)
- the presence of abnormal blood vessels
- regional lymph node enlargement, especially if this is hard.

Suspicious lesions should be carefully recorded, preferably on a standard topographical diagram (Roed-Peterson and Renstrup 1969).

The whole mucosa should be examined as there may be widespread dysplastic mucosa ('field change'), or even a second neoplasm—these are not uncommon in the head and neck, lung or oesophagus. Additional primary carcinomas are most likely to be seen in the mouth in patients with gingival, floor of mouth, lingual or buccal carcinoma. Additional primary carcinomas are possible in the oesophagus mainly in patients with lingual carcinomas, and lung carcinoma mainly in patients with gingival or floor of mouth carcinomas. Furthermore, where lingual carcinoma has associated leukoplakia, the risk of a second primary tumour is increased 5-fold (Shibuya *et al.* 1986).

Spread of oral cancer is predominantly local or to regional lymph nodes in the anterior neck and late dissemination occurs to the lungs, liver, or bones. The cervical lymph nodes must always be examined for enlargement, hard consistency or fixation to deeper tissue suggestive of malignancy. In up to 6 per cent of patients with oral carcinoma, lymph node enlargement is the presenting features. Enlarged nodes in a patient with mouth cancer may however be caused by infection, or reactive hyperplasia secondary to the tumour, as well as by metastatic or other disease. Lymph node examination is of paramount importance to detect metatases and general examination and possibly endoscopy may be indicated.

BIOPSY

Any suspicious oral mucosal lesion, including any ulcer not healing within two to three weeks, must be biopsied. An incisional biopsy is invariably required, usually under local anaesthesia. Since red rather than white areas are most likely to show dysplasia, a biopsy should always be taken of the former if both red and white lesions are present.

Where it is difficult to decide which is more appropriate area of biopsy, *in vivo* staining may help, particularly if there are widespread lesions. Staining with toluidine blue followed by a rinse with 1 per cent acetic acid and then saline may stain the most suspicious areas and indicate those which need to be biopsied. Oral carcinoma-*in situ* and early invasive carcinoma have an affinity to retain toluidine blue dye and although several false positive results may be encountered, these can be minimized by restaining after 14 days (Mashberg 1983). It is clear that toluidine blue is more effective in experienced hands (Silverman *et al.* 1984) and when used with clinical judgement. Counterstaining with Lugol's iodine (Epstein *et al.* 1992) may enhance the usefulness of toluidine blue staining.

The biopsy should be sufficiently large to include enough suspect and apparently normal tissue to give the pathologist a chance to make a diagnosis and not to have to request a further specimen. Most patients tolerate (physically and psychologically) one biopsy session, and most biopsy wounds, whether 0.5 cm (too small) or 1.5 cm long (usually adequate), heal within 7 to 10 days. Therefore it is better to take at least one ample specimen. Indeed, some clinicians always take several biopsies at the first visit in order to avoid the delay, anxiety, and aggravation resulting from a negative pathology report for a patient who is strongly suspected to have cancer. Biopsies should be fixed in 10 per cent formal saline, in order to prevent autolysis. If the pathologist denies malignancy, and yet clinically that is still the diagnosis, then a re-biopsy is indicated.

An excisional biopsy should be avoided unless the lesion is very small since this is unlikely to have excised an adequately wide margin of tissue if the lesion is malignant, but will have destroyed for the surgeon or radiotherapist clinical evidence of the site and character of the lesion—although this can be avoided by tattooing the site.

MUCOSAL INFECTIONS

The most common mucosal infections in immunocompetent or immunocompromised persons are candidiasis and herpesvirus infections. A range of infections can affect the oral mucosa but few are more devastating than HIV, which can result in oral and other fungal, viral or other mucosal infections, or neoplasms (Scully *et al.* 1991*a*, *b*).

ORAL INFECTIONS IN THE IMMUNOCOMPETENT PERSON

Candidiasis

Endogenous mucosal infections are not common, except for candidiasis—especially chronic atrophic candidiasis (denture-induced stomatitis). Candidiasis is predisposed to by xerostomia, the use of antibiotics and corticosteroids.

Denture-induced stomatitis typically presents as chronic mucosal erythema beneath an upper denture, mainly full dentures. The term, 'denture sore mouth' is a misnomer. It is most common in the elderly, especially females, and particularly if dentures are worn at night. The earliest lesions are pinpoint areas of hyperaemia which progress to diffuse uniform erythema of the hard palate, not extending beyond the limits of the denture-bearing area. Few patients have soreness unless there is also angular cheilitis (angular stomatitis; perleche) which affects 8–30 per cent (Budtz-Jorgensen 1981). The only other, and unusual, complication is develop-

ment of a granular or nodular benign hyperplasia in the vault of the palate. *Candida albicans* may be implicated and Candida species colonize the fitting surface of the denture. Removal of the denture plaque usually leads to resolution of the stomatitis (Walker *et al.* 1981). It is unclear why only some denture wearers get chronic atrophic candidiasis since *C. albicans* is a common oral commensal. Factors that may be important include the local environment beneath the denture, diet, the spectrum or type of organisms in denture plaque, and the host immune and other defences. Trauma may contribute to a small extent, but hypotheses such as allergy to denture materials have been discounted (Budtz-Jorgensen 1981).

Candida species are capable of adherence to denture materials as well as to oral epithelial cells possibly via mannans, and local factors such as the bacterial constituents of plaque and dietary sugars, may well increase the adherence and hence predispose to disease. There is no reliable evidence that host immune responses are abnormal in chronic atrophic candidiasis or conclusive evidence that smoking is a significant factor. However, it is possible that local defences, such as those mediated by saliva, might be important since xerostomia clearly predisposes to oral candidiasis.

Although there is no evidence that host defences play an important role in predisposition to chronic atrophic candidiasis in most cases (Budtz-Jorgensen 1981), a few patients are iron-deficient especially those with angular stomatitis, and correction of the deficiency may sometimes aid resolution of the lesions. Other deficiencies, for example of folic acid or B-complex vitamins are occasionally found, and are especially likely in the few patients who also have angular stomatitis and/or atrophic glossitis. This is discussed further below (p. 169).

Prevention

Denture-induced stomatitis usually resolves, or can be prevented, if the dentures are left out of the mouth at night, plaque is removed by brushing, and the dentures disinfected (Walker *et al.* 1981).

Yeast lytic enzymes and proteolytic enzymes are the most effective agents against Candida. Denture soak solution containing benzoic acid completely eradicates *C. albicans* from the denture surface as it is taken up into the acrylic resin and eliminates the organism from the fitting surface of the prosthesis (Iacopino and Wathen 1992). Chlorhexidine gluconate is an effective disinfectant and hypochlorite is probably effective but some proprietary peroxide cleaners are not. A solution of 0.12 per cent chlorhexidine gluconate can eliminate *C. albicans* on the surface of the denture, and reduce palatal inflammation. A protease-containing denture soak (Alcalase) is also an effective way of removing denture plaque, especially when combined with brushing (Odman 1992).

Chronic atrophic candidiasis which does not resolve (especially if there is an angular cheilitis) may require treatment with topical antifungals such as nystatin, amphotericin or miconazole. Fluconazole is also effective, particularly when administered concurrently with an oral antiseptic such as chlorhexidine.

Viral infections

Apart from high standards of personal hygiene, and the avoidance of contact with those with communicable diseases, little can be done to prevent exogenous primary infections with pathogenic agents that cause mucosal lesions, most of which are herpesviruses or enteroviruses. It may, however, be possible to inhibit or suppress recurrences of latent viruses such as the herpes viruses. Though recurrence of herpes simplex virus (HSV) infection is seen mainly on the lips and in adults, patients of all ages can be affected by recurrent herpes labialis. The lesions begin with a prodromal burning sensation followed by vesicles which change to pustules before they scan and heal over 7–14 days. Lesions vary in site and size and are infectious. Recurrences appear spontaneously or may be precipitated by trauma, fever, and/or another viral illness, sunlight, menstruation, and possibly other factors such as stress.

Avoidance of factors that precipitate viral reactivation may reduce the recurrence rate to a limited extent. The use of barrier creams to protect against ultraviolet irradiation (e.g. Uvistat) may be of some use for those about to go to sunny climes but cannot be guaranteed to reduce attacks. Antivirals are now generally used for prophylaxis only in immunocompromised patients (see below). The diagnosis is usually obvious from the clinical features, but if not straightforward a Tzanck smear can be made, or vesicle fluid can be sent for culture and (occasionally) electron microscopy. Serology is not very helpful: it will usually show a high titre of antibodies to HSV in the acute serum with little or no rise in the convalescent serum if the lesion is herpes labialis, and therefore is of no true value in diagnosis (Scully and Samaranayake 1992).

Most patients will benefit only marginally from treatment. Currently, the most effective antiviral is acyclovir. This has been used as a 5 per cent cream, which appears most useful if applied as early as possible in the development of the lesion. However, topical acyclovir produces only minimal benefit in immunocompetent persons. Oral acyclovir reduces the duration of pain and healing time. Whether acyclovir should be used in immunocompetent persons is controversial: it is not cheap and acyclovir-resistant viruses may appear.

ORAL INFECTIONS IN THE IMMUNOCOMPROMISED PERSON

There are dramatic increases in the numbers of immunocompromised persons both as a consequence of the effects of infection by HIV and of treatment with immunosuppresive agents (Peterson *et al.* 1992). Organ transplant patients and persons with HIV disease, the main groups of immunocompromised persons, are both characterized by a predominantly T lymphocyte immune defect. T cells are essential to protection against infection with fungi, viruses, and some bacteria—mainly mycobacteria: immunocompromised patients are thus liable to infection both with recognized fungal and viral pathogens (if they come into contact with them) and with opportunistic organisms (Peterson *et al.* 1992; Scully 1992) particularly candida species and herpesviruses.

Infections in immunocompromised persons tend to be recurrent or protracted, severe and sometimes resistant to treatment. Occasionally they disseminate. In general, the spectrum of infections is wider, and their severity greater, the more profound the immune defect.

Oral fungal infections

Superficial oral fungal infections (mycoses), especially candidiasis, are extremely common in immunocompromised persons. Candidiasis accounts for nearly 80 per cent of hospital-acquired serious fungal infections. Most candidiasis is caused by *Candida albicans* but other species are increasingly found. Candidiasis presents with or without soreness, as typical white or cream-coloured lesions of thrush on an erythematous background (pseudomembraneous candidiasis), or as erythematous candidiasis. Some patients may develop angular cheilitis.

Oral candidiasis is usually preventable with, or responsive to, standard topical antifungals but relapses are increasingly seen and there is consequently a trend towards the use of systemic imidazoles (ketoconazole) and bis-triazoles (fluconazole and itraconazole).

Prevention

If antibiotics or corticosteroids (oral or inhaled) are contributing causes, reducing the dose or changing the treatment may help. Intermittent or prolonged use of topical antifungals may be necessary where the underlying cause is unavoidable or incurable. Antifungal prophylaxis may well be indicated in immunocompromised persons.

Oral herpesvirus infections

Herpes simplex virus (HSV) infections are the most commonly recognized oral viral infections and up to 50 to 75 per cent of immunocompromised patients or those on chemotherapy develop oral HSV lesions. Chronic extensive and painful mouth ulcers affecting especially the keratinized mucosa are the most common intra-oral lesions, and severe herpes labialis may be seen (Scully and Samaranayake 1992). Most infections result from reactivation of latent viruses (e.g. in the trigeminal ganglion) and the viruses are often shed in saliva.

Although patients with HSV-induced oral lesions are managed mainly with supportive treatment, particularly maintenance of fluid intake, antipyretics, and analgesics, and topical antiseptics to prevent bacterial superinfection, antivirals are indicated in immunocompromised patients or in others where there are frequent severe recurrences or complications (Schubert 1991).

Prevention

Antiviral prophylaxis therefore may well be indicated in immunocompromised patients. Acyclovir is a potent acyclic guanosine derivative of very low toxicity. Adverse effects are rare and extremely minor although rashes, nausea, and other gastrointestinal effects have been reported in some patients receiving the drug orally, and rises in blood urea and creatinine levels may be seen after intravenous administration. Acyclovir has significant clinical benefit against HSV and is far more effective than previous nucleoside analogues such as idoxuridine or vidarabine.

Acyclovir resistance is now becoming a clinical problem, however (Epstein and Scully 1991) particularly in patients with leukaemia, after tissue and organ transplants, and with HIV disease. Most acyclovir-resistant HSV isolates are fortunately, sensitive to foscarnet (trisodium phophonoformate hexahydrate). The adverse effects of foscarnet are noted below.

Other viral infections

Varicella–zoster virus (VZV) oral infections are less common than are HSV infections. VZV is latent in sensory root ganglia and reactivation may cause zoster (shingles). The lesions are ulcerative and extremely painful, may lead to scarring and post-herpetic neuralgia, and occasionally result in dissemination of VZV.

Human cytomegalovirus (HCMV) is one of the leading causes of morbidity and mortality in immunocompromised patients. It is latent in salivary glands, but only recently has been recognized as causing oral lesions: these are usually chronic painful oral ulcers (Scully and Samaranayake 1992).

Epstein–Barr virus may, in immunocompromised patients, be responsible for hairy leukoplakia (Scully *et al.* 1989).

Prevention

Acyclovir is the most reliable therapy, and may reduce the incidence of post-herpetic neuralgia, but acyclovir-resistant VZV are now being identified. Vaccines against VZV are being developed.

No absolutely reliable effective vaccine is available against HCMV but the Towne vaccine—a live, passage HCMV—may confer useful protection in at-risk patients such as transplant recipients. Passive immunization using specific immunoglobulin with high-titre, anti-HCMV antibody after accidental exposure to the virus may provide a degree of protection against primary infection in seronegative subjects at risk. Interferon has not been found to be protective.

Low doses of acyclovir (250 mg/m^2 3 times a day or 5 mg/kg twice a day) have not been effective in treatment of HCMV reactivation in bone marrow transplant patients but oral acyclovir (200 mg 4 times a day) significantly reduces HCMV shedding and, high-dose acyclovir (450 mg/m^2 4 times a day) can prevent reactivation of latent HCMV.

The current principle antiviral for HCMV is ganciclovir (2-hydroxy-1-(hydroxymethyl) ethoxymethyl) guanine; DHPG). Unfortunately, ganciclovir can cause bone marrow suppression and this, together with effects such as fever, skin rash, nausea, vomiting, central nervous system toxicity, and hepatotoxicity precludes its use, except for serious HCMV infections such as retinitis and pneumonitis. HCMV may also develop ganciclovir resistance especially following the chronic administration of ganciclovir.

Fortunately, ganciclovir-resistant HCMV are sensitive to foscarnet. Renal toxicity is seen in up to 50 per cent of the patients taking foscarnet and nausea, malaise, vomiting, fatigue, headache, and other CNS toxicity and haematological toxicity and hepatotoxicity may occur. Foscarnet-resistant HCMV mutants have been seen and it is anticipated that resistance to both ganciclovir and foscarnet may develop *in vivo*.

Oral bacterial infections

A wide range of bacteria can, in immunocompromised patients, occasionally colonize the mouth and may sometimes cause oral infections, or be the portal for septicemia. Broad-spectrum antimicrobials can also cause shifts.

Bacteria that are typically found elsewhere, such as lower in the gastrointestinal tract (*Escherichia coli*, *Pseudomonas aeruginosa*, *Enterobacter cloacae*, *Klebsiella pneumoniae*, *Salmonella enteritidis*), may colonize the mouth, and septicaemias involving viridans streptococci, coagulase-negative staphylococci, capnocytophaga and other microorganisms originating in the mouth are increasing recognized in leukaemic, neutropenic or other immunocompromised patients (Van de Leur *et al.* 1992). Viridans streptococci have emerged as important pathogens (Guiot *et al.* 1992). Mucositis following X-irradiation involving the oral mucosa may also have a bacterial component (Martin 1993).

In addition to bacterial infections of the oral mucosa, neutropenic patients may develop acute periodontal infections and organisms commonly viewed as pathogenic, such as *Staphylococcus epidermidis*, *C. albicans*, *Staph. aureus*, and *Pseudomonas aeruginosa*, may be detected in high concentrations in subgingival plaque. Acute periodontal infections, when they occur, usually develop when the granulocyte levels fall below (< 1000/mm^3); and inflammatory signs are typically markedly diminished (Peterson *et al.* 1987) despite the seriousness of the infection.

Prevention

Dental plaque control may therefore be critical in the immunocompromised patient. Conventional tooth-brushing is typically contraindicated during periods of myelosuppression due to the risk of bleeding and infection but since foam-brush substitutes are not as effective in controlling plaque and gingivitis, chemical decontaminating regimens (e.g. aqueous chlorhexidine) are also required.

COMMON IMMUNOLOGICALLY MEDIATED MUCOSAL DISORDERS

APHTHAE

Recurrent aphthous stomatitis (RAS) is a common oral disorder, the aetiology of which remains elusive. Aphthae are rounded, shallow, painful oral ulcers recurring at intervals of a few days to a few months. The natural history is of amelioration or resolution in adult life in many cases.

Minor RAS (MiRAS) are the most common variety accounting for more than 80 per cent of RAS. They are round shallow ulcers of less than 5 mm diameter with a grey-white pseudomembrane bordered by a thin erythematous halo. MiRAS usually occur on the lip (labial), cheek (buccal) mucosa, and floor of mouth and rarely affect the gum (gingiva), palate or dorsum of the tongue. These lesions heal within 10 to 14 days without scarring.

Major recurrent aphthous stomatitis (MaRAS) is a rare severe form of RAS. The ulcers are round or oval and may exceed 1 cm in diameter, they may approach 3 cm. MaRAS have a predilection for the lips, soft palate, and fauces but can affect any site. The ulcers of MaRAS are painful and persist for up to 6 weeks, healing slowing with scarring. MaRAS usually has its onset after puberty and is chronic, persisting for up to 20 or more years.

The third and least common variety of RAS is herpetiform ulceration, characterized by multiple recurrent crops of small painful herpetiform ulcers (HU) that are widespread and may be distributed throughout the oral cavity. As many as 100 ulcers may be present at a given time, each measuring 1–3 mm in diameter, although they tend to fuse to produce large irregular ulcers. HU have a female predisposition and a later age of onset than other types of RAS.

The aetiology of RAS is unclear but a genetic basis underlies some varieties. There is, thus, no evidence of any single aetiological factor for RAS, rather it would seem that a variety of factors might predispose. Predisposing factors that may be susceptible to prevention include trauma, nutritional deficiencies, and endocrine or allergic factors (Porter and Scully 1991). Trauma may initiate ulcers in a minority of susceptible people and deficiencies of iron, folic acid or vitamin B_{12} (haematinics) have been demonstrated to be twice as common in RAS patients as controls. Overall, some 20 per cent or so of hospital patients with RAS appear to have a haematinic deficiency and not all RAS respond to replacement of the deficient haematinic.

Haematinic deficiencies in RAS are sometimes related to disease of the small intestine, particularly gluten-sensitive enteropathy (GSE) and studies have now demonstrated GSE in 3–5 per cent of outpatients who initially present with RAS. A minority of females with RAS have cyclical oral ulceration related to the luteal phase of the menstrual cycle, possibly modulated by changing levels of progestogens, as the appearance of RAS in these patients seems unrelated to psychological factors. Some patients correlate the onset of ulcers with exposure to certain foods but controlled studies have failed to prove a causal association despite the fact that certain foods causing positive skin-prick reactions will elicit pain when they are topically applied to aphthous ulcers. Dietary manipulation rarely significantly improves RAS.

Other factors are less convincingly associated with RAS, or not amenable to prevention. There are limited data concerning any association of RAS with psychiatric factors or stress. Some studies have suggested that certain personality traits predispose to RAS patients but the data are conflicting. Similarly, any association between psychological stress and occurrence of oral ulceration remains to be established. Lesions similar to RAS can be seen in various systemic disorders including Behcet's syndrome, Sweet's syndrome, cyclic neutropenia, some primary immunodeficiencies, and an aphthous-like ulceration described in HIV infection.

There is no specific or reliably effective investigation or prevention or management for RAS. The symptoms can be reduced, but it is not possible to reliably prevent recurrences. In many studies, patients have improved with placebo (Hunter *et al.* 1993). Such a placebo effect, plus the often limited nature of RAS, ensures that most affected patients ultimately have a reduction in symptoms. Good, controlled trials are rather few (Porter and Scully 1991).

Patients with RAS possibly secondary to systemic disease, require referral to an appropriate specialist for detailed evaluation and suitable therapy. Haematinic replacement can be of value in patients with haematinic deficiency, progestogens may help those with luteally related aphthae, and individuals with RAS possibly related to foodstuffs may occasionally benefit from dietary alterations.

Chlorhexidine gluconate aqueous mouth rinse does seem to have some effect in the management of RAS, possibly by reducing secondary infection and is often used in combination with topical corticosteroids. Chlorhexidine can reduce the number of ulcer days, increase ulcer-free days, and the interval between bouts of ulceration, but cannot prevent the recurrence of ulcers. Chlorhexidine is generally used as a 0.2 per cent w/w (weight in weight) mouth rinse, but the 0.1 per cent w/w mouth rinse or 1 per cent gel can also be beneficial. However, one recent study found little objective value of chlorhexidine gluconate mouth rinse over placebo in the management of RAS.

Benzydamine-hydrochloride mouth wash has also been shown to be of no more benefit than placebo. Nevertheless benzydamine hydrochloride mouthwash or spray or lignocaine gel can produce transient relief of pain in severe RAS. Topical tetracyclines can reduce the severity of ulceration, but do not alter the recurrence rate of RAS.

Topical corticosteroids are the mainstay of RAS treatment. Systemic corticosteroids, with or without azathioprine, or immunomodulatory agents, such as colchicine or thalidomide, are rarely indicated and are best restricted to specialist use.

LICHEN PLANUS AND LICHENOID REACTIONS

The aetiology of lichen planus remains obscure in most cases but factors identifiable in a few patients include various drugs (Robertson and Wray 1992), and reactions to dental restorative materials (Scully and Elkom 1985; James *et al.* 1987). A wide range of drugs have been implicated, most commonly the non-steroidal anti-inflammatory agents, antihypertensive agents, antidiabetic drugs, and antimalarials (Table 12.1).

Oral lichen planus may also appear in close relationship to dental restorative material, especially amalgams (Bolewska *et al.* 1990). Recent studies, however, have found little reliable evidence of hypersensitivity (Nordlind and Liden 1993), and the appearance of lichenoid reactions to some composite restorations (Lind 1988) should dampen the enthusiasm for the wholesale replacement of amalgams.

Management of lichen planus is similar to that of aphthae, focused mainly on topical corticosteroids.

ORO-FACIAL GRANULOMATOSIS

The group of disorders variously described as oral Crohn's disease or oro-facial granulomatosis, and the probably related Melkersson–Rosenthal syndrome, and Miescher's cheilitis (cheilitis granulomatosa), may sometimes be precipitated by identifiable agents (Scully and Eveson 1991).

There is no doubt that classic Crohn's disease can be complicated by oral lesions—especially oral ulceration and this may also be seen when gastrointestinal symptoms are

Table 12.1. Oral mucosal side-effects of drug treatment (most are rare) (Scully 1989)

Oral candidiasis	**Oral mucosal pigmentation**
Broad-spectrum antimicrobials	ACTH
Corticosteroids	Amodiaquine
Drugs causing xerostomia	Anticonvulsants
Immunosuppressive	Busulphan
	Chlorhexidine
Oral ulceration	Chloroquine
Cocaine	Contraceptive pill
Cytotoxics	Heavy metals
Emepromium	Mepacrine
Gold	Minocycline
Indomethacin	Phenothiazines
Isoprenaline	Smoking
Naproxen	
Pancreatin	**Lichenoid reactions**
Penicillamine	Amiphenazole
Phenindione	Chloroquine
Phenytoin	Chlorpropamide
Potassium chloride	Dapsone
Proguanil	Gold
	Labetalol
	Mepacrine
Erythema multiforme	Methyldopa
(and Stevens Johnson	Non steroidal
syndrome)	anti-inflammatory drugs
Barbiturates	Oxprenolol
Busulphan	Penicillamine
Carbamazepine	Phenothiazines
Clindamycin	Practolol
Codeine	Propranolol
Frusemide	Quinine
Penicillin	Quinidine
Phenytoin	Streptomycin
Sulphonamides	Tetracycline
Tetracyclines	Thiazides
	Tolbutamide
	Triprolidine
Angioedema	
Aspirin	**Lupoid reactions**
Essential oils	Ethosuximide
Penicillin	Gold
	Griseofulvin
	Hydralazine
Gingival hyperplasia	Methyldopa
Contraceptive pill	para-Aminosalicylate
Cyclosporin	Penicillin
Diltiazem	Phenytoin
Felodipine	Procainamide
Nifedipine	Streptomycin
Nitrendipine	Sulphonamides
Phenytoin	Tetracyclines
Pemphigus-like reactions	
Captopril	
Glibenclamide	
Penicillamine	**Pemphigoid-like reactions**
Rifampicin	Clonidine
	Frusemide
	Penicillamine
	Psoralens

absent (Scully *et al.* 1982). However, the constellation of manifestations that may be seen in any combination, and include oro-facial swelling, mucosal tags, gingival hyperplasia, mucosal cobblestoning, ulcers, and angular stomatitis, may also be seen in the total absence of detectable gastrointestinal disease, and the alternative term 'oro-facial granulomatosis' has therefore been suggested (Wiesenfeld *et al.* 1985). This may be helpful to avoid the stigma of the term 'Crohn's disease'. In some, there may be an allergic basis and patients may respond to dietary manipulation and avoidance of putative precipitants such as various flavourings and other additives (Sweatman *et al.* 1986). Also, in some patients, there appear to be specific food intolerances, such as to cinnamaldehyde, carvone, piperitone, cocoa, carmosine, sunset yellow or monosodium glutamate (Sweatman *et al.* 1986).

ALLERGIC AND AUTOIMMUNE REACTIONS

Proven allergic reactions in the mouth are extremely rare but it is likely that some manifestations have been overlooked and that food intolerances will, in the future, be recognized to be of greater importance than hitherto supposed. There have, for example, been clear examples of reactions to various dentifrices and other materials.

Gingival lesions that have been termed allergic gingivostomatitis or plasma cell gingivitis have been recognized for many years. An association with supraglottic plasmacytosis has now been described, though any possible allergic basis remains unproven (Timms and Sloan 1991). Allergic reactions producing cheilitis and gingival changes have been described, however, with tartar-control and some other dentifrices (Beacham *et al.* 1990; Lamey *et al.* 1990). Angio-oedema can result from a range of agents, for example, angio-oedema in response to rubber dam and to ethylene imine (in 'Scutan') has been reported (Blinkhorn and Leggate 1984). Hypersensitivity to local anaesthetics is rare. The paraben preservatives of local anaesthetic solutions may account for some allergic responses, and the introduction of preservative-free preparations should minimize this hazard.

Contact stomatitis may result from antibiotics, oils of casia and cloves, mercury, gold; flavouring agents, such as cinnamon in toothpaste, epoxy resins, acrylic, eugenol, polyether impression material, karaya gum, and nickel-containing and stainless-steel wire. Contact cheilitis has occurred with the fluorescein stains in some lipsticks, carmine, oleyl alcohol, methyl heptine carbamate, peppermint, carvone, spearmint, pineapple, mangoes, asparagus, and cinnamon oil.

A variety of different agents have been implicated as precipitating factors in the development of erythema multiforme (Table 12.2), the most well-recognized being herpes simplex. The drugs most frequently associated with erythema multiforme are antimicrobials, antiepileptics, and analgesics (Duxbury 1990). The most commonly reported in the literature are the sulphonamides, penicillins, nitrofurantoin, erythromycin, streptomycin, phenytoin, carbamazepine, barbiturates, acetylsalicylic acid and its derivatives, piroxicam, and isoxicam. Recurrences of drug-induced erythema multiforme are rare—unless the drug is re-administered.

The autoimmune disorders are discussed elsewhere (Scully and Cawson 1992).

Table 12.2. Some factors precipitating erythema multiforme (Porter and Scully 1990)

Infections
Herpes simplex virus
Epstein–Barr virus
Influenza
Adenovirus
Mycoplasma pneumoniae

Drugs

Antimalarials	Mercurials
Barbiturates	Penicillins
Busulfan	Phenothiazines
Carbamazepine	Phenytoin
Chlorpropamide	Piroxicam
Codeine	Salicylates
Digitalis	Streptomycin
Gold salts	Sulphonamides
Hydralazine	Vitamin E
Iodides	

Others
Radiotherapy
Acute alcoholism
Hepatitis vaccination
Menstrually related hormonal (progesterone) changes

Table 12.3. Oral mucosal features which may result from nutritional deficiencies

Nutrient deficient	Mucosal features that may result
Vitamin A (retinol)	Keratoses? pre-malignancies
Vitamin B complex	Angular stomatitis, glossitis, burning mouth syndrome, aphthae, ? epithelial dysplasia
Vitamin B_1 (thiamine)	
Vitamin B_2 (riboflavine)	
Vitamin B_6 (pyridoxine)	
Nicotinic acid (niacin)	
Pantothenic acid	
Vitamin B_{12} (cyanocobalamin)	
Folic acid	
Vitamin C (ascorbic acid)	Scurvy, delay in wound healing
Vitamin K	Haemorrhage
Iron	Atrophic glossitis, angular stomatitis, aphthae, burning mouth, atrophic mucosa, reduced resistance to infection, ? premalignancies, ? candidiasis

OTHER IATROGENIC ORAL DISEASE

The range of oral lesions now recognized as iatrogenic complications is increasing and undoubtedly will increase in the future. Xerostomia is commonly a consequence of the use of tricyclic agents and other antidepressants, and of other drugs with an anticholinergic or sympathomimetic effect, and it predisposes to oral candidiasis. Gingival hyperplasia is now a recognized complication of cyclosporin, nifedipine, and some other calcium channel blockers. Space precludes full discussion but some are summarized in Table 12.1.

ORAL MUCOSAL LESIONS IN NUTRITIONAL DEFICIENCIES

The role of nutrition in carcinogenesis is discussed above. Glossitis and stomatitis may result from vitamin B_{12} deficiency (Table 12.3). The tongue tip reddens in the early stages of deficiency and this eventually spreads with fissuring—the so-called beef tongue—and with papillary atrophy. Angular stomatitis, aphthae, and erosive lesions may also be seen (Schmitt *et al.* 1988). Some patients may have burning-mouth syndrome, even in the absence of recognizable mucosal disease. Oral hyperpigmentation may also be seen. A role for vitamin B in burning-mouth syndrome has been proposed (Lamey *et al.* 1986) although these findings have not been confirmed by others (Hugoson and Thorstensson 1991). Deficiency of vitamin B_2 is commonly dietary, is especially seen in alcoholics, and leads to seborrhoeic dermatitis, corneal vascularization and anaemia, and oral mucosal mani-

festations similar to those of vitamin B_{12} deficiency. Angular stomatitis, glossitis, and oral ulceration have been recorded in vitamin B_2 deficiency. Deficiency of vitamin B_6 leads to dermatitis and peripheral neuropathy and oral mucosal manifestations similar to those of vitamin B_{12} deficiency—with angular stomatitis and generalized stomatitis and sometimes ulceration.

Deficiency of nicotinic acid is seen mainly in the West in alcoholics, and causes pellagra (dermatitis and neurological disturbances), oral mucosal erythema, and papillary atrophy of the tongue. There may be a burning sensation in the tongue, and hypersalivation, and angular stomatitis.

The oral effects of folic acid deficiency in man are virtually indistinguishable from those of vitamin B_{12} deficiency and include ulcers, angular stomatitis, depapillation of the tongue or burning mouth syndrome (Porter and Scully 1991). These manifestations respond promptly to replacement therapy.

Iron deficiency may predispose to aphthae, glossitis, and angular stomatitis, and burning-mouth syndrome. Atrophic glossitis is found in up to 40 per cent of iron-deficient patients and angular stomatitis in 15 per cent and about one-third of patients have a sore tongue. Manifestations respond within a few weeks to replacement therapy.

Taste may be impaired in zinc deficiency but there are no specific changes in the taste buds. Oral candidiasis may be seen in zinc deficiency. Despite initial suggestions that zinc may influence aphthae, this has been refuted (Wray 1982).

CONCLUSIONS

- The prevention of oral cancer is best achieved by reducing risk factors known to cause cancer in the mouth and elsewhere in the body: tobacco, excessive alcohol consumption, betel use, and prolonged exposure to sunlight, are four of the most important risk factors implicated in the aetiology of oral cancer.

- The same risk factors are also implicated in the development of potentially malignant lesions.

- In addition, improving the diet by increasing intake of fruit and vegetables, treating possible infections, such as candidosis or syphilis, and improving oral hygiene, may reduce the prevalence of pre-malignant lesions.

- Denture-induced stomatitis can be prevented if dentures are not worn at night, plaque is removed by brushing, and the dentures disinfected.

- Apart from high standards of hygiene, and the avoidance of contact with those with communicable diseases, or their tissues, little can be done to prevent primary infections with viruses that can cause mucosal lesions.

- Oral infections in the immunocompromised person may be prevented by prophylactic therapy, particularly with antifungal and antiviral agents.

- Chlorhexidine gluconate aqueous mouth rinses may have an effect in the management of RAS, possibly by reducing secondary infection.

- Proven allergic reactions in the mouth can be prevented by identifying and avoiding the cause.

REFERENCES

Almadori, G., Paludetti, G., Cerullo, M., Ottaviana, F. and D'Alatari, L. (1990). Marijuana smoking as a possible cause of tongue carcinoma in young patients. *J. Laryngol. Otol.* **104**, 896–9.

Armstrong, B.K., McMichael, A.J., and MacLennan, R. (1982). In *Cancer epidemiology and prevention*, (ed. D. Scholtenfeld and D.F. Fraumeni), p. 429. W.B. Saunders, Philadephia.

Barone, J., Taioli, E., Hebert, J.R., and Wynder, E.L. (1992). Vitamin supplement use and risk for oral and esophageal cancer. *Nutr. Cancer*, **18**, 31–41.

Barra, S., Franceschi, S., Negri, E., Talamini, R., and La Vecchia, C. (1990). Type of alcoholic beverage and cancer of the oral cavity, pharnx and oesophagus in an Italian area with high wine consumption. *Int. J. Cancer*, **46**, 1017–20.

Beacham, B.E., Kurgansky, D., and Gould, W.M. (1990). Circumoral dermatitis and cheilitis caused by tartar control dentifrices. *J. Am. Acad. Dermatol.* **22**, 1029–32.

Benner, S.E., *et al.* (1993). Regression of oral leukoplakia with α-tocopherol: a community clinical oncology program chemoprevention study. *J. Nat. Cancer Inst.*, **85**, 44–7.

Bhonsle, R.B., *et al.* (1987). Regional variations in oral submucous fibrosis in India. *Commun. Dent. oral Epidemiol.* **15**, 225–9.

Blinkhorn, A.S. and Leggate, E.M. (1984). An allergic reaction to rubber dam. *Br. dent. J.* **156**, 402–3.

Blot, W.J. and Fraumeni, J.R. Jr (1977). Geographic patterns of oral cancer in the United States: etiologic implications. *J. Chron. Dis.* **30**, 745–57.

Blot, W.J. *et al.* (1989). Smoking and drinking in relation to oral and pharyngeal cancer. *Cancer Res.* **48**, 3282–7.

Blot, W.J., Winn, D.M., and Fraumeni, J.F. (1983). Oral cancer and mouthwash. *J. Nat. Cancer Inst.* **70**, 251–3.

Bolewska, J., Hansen, H.J., and Holmstrup, P. (1990). Oral mucosal lesions related to silver amalgam restorations. *Oral Surg.* **70**, 55–8.

Boyle, P., MacFarlane, G.J., and Maisonneuve, P. (1990). Epidemiology of mouth cancer. *J. Roy. Soc. Med.* **83**, 724–30.

Boyle, P., *et al.* (1991). Recent advances in the etiology and epidemiology of head and neck cancer. *Curr. Opin. Oncol.* **2**, 539–45.

Budtz-Jorgensen, E. (1981). Oral mucosal lesions associated with the wearing of removable dentures. *J. oral. Pathol.* **10**, 65–80.

Carroll, K.K. and Khor, H.T. (1975). Dietary fat in relation to tumorigenesis. *Prog. Biochem. Pharmaco.* **10**, 308.

De Stefani, E., *et al.* (1988). Black tobacco, wine and mate in oropharyngeal cancer: a case control study from Uruguay. *Rev. Epidemiol. Sante' Publ.* **36**, 389–94.

Donald, P.J. (1986). Marijuana smoking—possible cause of head and neck carcinoma in young patients. *Otolaryngol. Head Neck Surg.* **94**, 517–21.

Dubrow, R. and Wegman, D.H. (1984). Cancer and occupation in Massachusetts: a death certificate study. *Am. J. Int. Med.* **6**, 207–30.

Duxbury, A.J. (1990). Systemic pharmacotherapy. In *Oral Manifestations of systemic disease*, (2nd edn) (ed. J.H. Jones and D.K. Mason), pp. 411–79. Ballière Tindall, London.

Edwards, M.B. (1976). Chemical carcinogenesis in the cheek pouch of Syrian hamsters receiving supplementary zinc. *Archs. oral Biol.* **21**, 133–5.

Epstein, J.B., Scully, C., and Spinelli J.J. (1992). Toluidine blue and Lugol's iodine application in the assessment of oral malignant disease and lesions at risk of malignancy. *J. oral pathol. Med.* **21**, 160–3.

Epstein, J.B. and Scully, C. (1991). Herpes simplex virus in immunocompromised patients: growing evidence of drug resistance. *Oral Surg., oral Med., oral Pathol.* **72**, 47–50.

Evstifeeva, T.V. and Zardize, D.G. (1992). Nass use, cigarette smoking, alcohol consumption and risk of oral and oesophageal precancer. *Oral Oncol. Eur. J. Cancer, Part B*, **28**B, 29–36.

Franceschi, S., Barra, S., La Vecchia, C., Bidoli, E., Negri, E. and Talamini, R. (1992). Risk factors for cancer of the tongue and the mouth. *Cancer* **70**, 2227–33.

Franceschi, S., *et al.* (1990). Smoking and drinking in relation to cancers of the oral cavity, pharynx, larynx and esophagus in Northern Italy. *Cancer Res.* **50**, 6502–7.

Gorsky, M., Dayan, D., Marom, Z., and Silverman, S. (1992). Consumption of tobacco as an etiologic factor in a group of 465 oral cancer patients in Israel. *CA* **5**, 208–10.

Graham, S. *et al.* (1977). Dentition, diet, tobacco and alcohol in the epidemiology of oral cancer. *J. Nat. Cancer Inst.* **59**, 1611–18.

Greenberg, R.A., *et al.* (1991). The relation of socioeconomic status to oral and pharyngeal cancer. *Epidemiology*, **2**, 194–200.

Gridley, G., McLaughlin, J.K., Block, G., Blot, W.J., Gluch, M. and Fraumeni, J.F. (1992). Vitamin supplement use and reduced risk of oral and pharyngeal cancer. *Am. J. Epidemiol.* **135**, 1083–92.

Guiot, H.F.L., Van der Meer, J.W.M., and Van de Broek, P.J. (1992). Prevention of viridans group streptococcal septicaemia in oncophematologic patient: a controlled comparative study on the effect of penicillin G and co-trimoxazole. *Ann. Hematol.* **64**, 260–5.

Gupta, P.C., Pindborg, J.J., and Mehta, F.S. (1982). Comparison of carcinogenity of betel quid with and without tobacco: an epidemiological review. *Ecol. Dis.* **1**, 213–19.

Huebner, W.W., *et al.* (1992). Oral and pharyngeal cancer and occupation: a case control study. *Epidemiology*, **3**, 300–9.

Hugoson, A., and Thorstensson, B. (1991). Vitamin B status and response to replacement therapy in patients with burning mouth syndrome. *Acta odont. Scand.* **49**, 367–75.

Hunter, I.P., Ferguson, M.M., Scully, C., Galloway, A.R., Main, A.N.H. and Russell, R.I. (1993). Effects of dietary gluten elimination in patients with recurrent minor aphthous stomatitis and no detectable gluten enteropathy. *Oral Surg., oral Med., oral Pathol.* **75**, 595–8.

Iacopino, A. and Wathen, W. (1992). Oral candidal infection and denture stomatitis: a comprehensive review. *J. Am. dent. Ass.* **123**, 46–51.

IARC (International Agency for Research on Cancer) (1988). *Monographs on the evaluation of the carcinogenic risk to humans. Alcohol drinking*, Vol. 44. IARC, Lyon.

IARC (International Agency for Research on Cancer) (1986). *Monographs on the evaluation of the carcinogenic risk to humans. Tobacco smoking*, Vol. 38. IARC, Lyon.

IARC (International Agency for Research on Cancer) (1985). *Monographs on the evaluation of carcinogenic risks to humans. Tobacco habits other than smoking: betel-quid and areca-nut chewing and some related nitrosamines*, Vol. 37. IARC, Lyon.

James, J., *et al.* (1987). Oral lichenoid reactions related to mercury sensitivity. *Br. J. oral Maxillofac Surg.* **25**, 474–80.

Kabat, G.C., Hebert, J.R. and Wynder, E.L. (1989). Risk factors for oral cancer in women. *Cancer Res.* **49**, 2803–6.

Kato, I., Nomura, A.M.Y, Stemmermann, G.N., and Chyou, P.H. (1992). Prospective study of the association of alcohol with cancer of the upper aerodigestive tract and other sites. *Cancer Causes and Control*, **3**, 145–51.

Knekt, P. (1988). Serum vitamin E and risk of female cancer. *Int. J. Epidemiol.* **17**, 281–8.

La Vecchia, C.L., Negri, E., D'Avavnzo, B., Boyle, P., Franceschi, S. (1991). Dietary indicators of oral and pharyngeal cancer. *Int. J. Epidemiol.* **20**, 39–44.

Lamey, P.J., Hammond, A., Allan, B.F. and MacKintosh, W.B. (1986). Vitamin status of patients with burning mouth syndrome and the response to replacement therapy. *Br. dent. J.* **160**, 81–3.

Lamey, P.J., Lewis, M.A.O., Rees, T.D., Fowler, C. and Binnie, W.H. (1990). Sensitivity reaction to the cinnamonaldehyde component of toothpaste. *Br. dent. J.* **168**, 115–18.

Lind, P.O. (1988). Oral lichenoid reactions related to composite restorations. *Acta odont. Scand.* **46**, 63–5.

Little, S.J., *et al.* (1992). Smokeless tobacco habits and oral mucosal lesions in dental patients. *J. Publ. Health Dent.* **52**, 269–76.

Marshall, J., Graham, S., Mettlin, C., Shedd, D. and Swanson, M. (1982). Diet in the epidemiology of oral cancer. *Nutr. Cancer*, **3**, 145–9.

Martin, M.V. (1993). Irradiation mucositis: a reappraisal. *Oral. Oncol. Eur. J. Cancer, Part B*, **29B**, 1–2.

Mashberg, A. (1983). Final evaluation of tononium chloride rinse for screening of high-risk patients with asymptomatic squamous carcinoma. *JADA*, **106**, 319–23.

Moulin, J.J., Mur, J.M., Wild, P. Perreaux, J.P. and Pham, Q.T. (1986). Oral cavity and laryngeal cancers among man-made mineral fiber production workers. *Scand. J. Work Environ. Health*, **12**, 27–31.

Nordlind, K. and Liden, S. (1993). In vitro lumphocyte reactivity to heavy metal salts in the diagnosis of oral mucosal hypersensitivity to amalgam restorations. *Br. J. Dermatol.* **128**, 38–41.

Notani, P.N., and Jayanet, K. (1987). Role of diet in upper aerodigestive tract cancers. *Nutri. Cancer* **10**, 103–13.

Odman, P.A. (1992). The effectiveness of an enzyme-containing denture cleanser. *Quintess. Int.* **23**, 187–90.

Peterson, D.E., *et al.* (1987). Microbiology of acute periodontal infection in myelosuppressed cancer patients. *J. Clin. Oncol.* **5**, 1461–8.

Peterson, D.E., Greenspan, D. and Squier, C.A. (1992). Oral infections in the immunocompromised host. *J. oral pathol. Med.* **21**, 193–8.

Pindborg, J.J. (1980). Pathology of oral leukoplakia. *Am. J. Dermatopathol.* **2**, 277.

Porter, S.R. and Scully, C. (1991). Aphthous stomatitis: an overview of aetiopathogenesis and management. *Clin. exp. Dermatol.* **16**, 235–43.

Porter, S.R. and Scully, C. (1990). Primary immune defects. In *Oral manifestations of systemic disease*, (2nd edn.) (ed. J.H. Jones and D.K. Mason), pp. 112–61. Balliere Tindall, London.

Prime, S.S., MacDonald, D.G., Sawyer, D.R. and Rennie, J.S. (1986). The effect of iron deficiency on early oral carcinogenesis in the rat. *J. oral Pathol.* **15**, 265–7.

Robertson, W.D. and Wray, D (1992). Ingestion of medication among patients with oral keratoses including lichen planus. *Oral Surg., oral Med., oral Pathol.* **74**, 183–5.

Roed-Peterson, B. and Renstrup, G. (1969). A topographical classification of the oral mucosa suitable for electronic data processing. *Acta odont. scand.* **27**, 681.

Rogers, M.A.M., Thomas, D.B., Davis, S., Weiss, N.S., Vaughan, T.L. and Nevissi, A.E. (1991). A case-control study of oral cancer and pre-diagnostic concentrations of selenium and zinc in nail tissue. *Int. J. Cancer*, **48**, 182–8.

Rossing, M.A., Vaughan, T.L. and McKnight, B. (1989). Diet and pharyngeal cancer. *Int. J. Cancer*, **44**, 593–7.

Rothman, K.J. and Keller, A.Z. (1972). The effect of joint exposure to alcohol and tobacco on the risk of cancer of the mouth and pharynx. *J. Chron. Dis.* **25**, 711–16.

Sankaranarayanan, R., *et al.* (1989). A case control investigation of cancer of the oral tongue and the floor of the mouth in Southern India. *Int. J. Cancer*, **44**, 617–21.

Schmitt, R.J., Sheridan, P.J. and Rogers, R.S. (1988). Pernicious anaemia with associated glossodynia. *JADA* **117**, 838–40.

Schubert, M.M. (1991). Oral manifestations of viral infections in immunocompromised patients. *Curr. Opin. Dent.* **1**, 384–97.

Scully, C. *et al.* (1982). Crohn's disease of the mouth: an indication of intestinal involvement. *Gut* **23**, 198–201.

Scully, C. (1989). *Patient care: a dental surgeon's guide*. British Dental Journal, London.

Scully, C. (1992). Oral infections in the immunocompromised patient. *Br. dent. J.* **172**, 401–7.

Scully, C. (1993). Clinical diagnostic methods for the detection of premalignant and early malignant oral lesions. *Comm. dent. Health,* (suppl. 1), 43–52.

Scully, C. and Boyle, P. (1992). Vitamin A related compounds in the chemoprevention of potentially malignant oral lesions and carcinoma. *Oral Oncol. Eur. J. Cancer, Part B,* **28B**, 87–90.

Scully, C. and Cawson, R.A. (1992). *Medical problems in dentistry.* Butterworths, Oxford.

Scully, C. and Elkom, M. (1985). Lichen planus: review and update on pathogenesis. *J. oral Pathol.* **14**, 431–58.

Scully, C. and Eveson, J.W. (1991). Oral granulomatosis (leading article). *Lancet* **38**, 20–1.

Scully, C. and Samaranayake, L.P. (1992). *Clinical virology in oral medicine and dentistry.* Cambridge University Press.

Scully, C., Epstein, J.B. and Porter, S.R. (1989). Oral hairy leukoplakia (leading article). *Lancet* **ii**, 1194.

Scully, C., Laskaris, G., Pindborg, J., Porter, S.R. and Reichart, P. (1991a). Oral manifestations of HIV infection and their management: 1. More common lesions. *Oral Surg., oral Med., oral Pathol.* **71**, 158–66.

Scully, C., Laskaris, G., Pindborg, J., Porter, S.R. and Reichart, P. (1991b). Oral manifestations of HIV infection and their management: 2. Less common lesions. *Oral Surg., oral Med., oral Pathol.* **71**, 167–71.

Shibuya, H., *et al.* (1986). Leukoplakia-associated multiple carcinomas in patients with tongue carcinoma. *Cancer* **57**, 843–6.

Silverman, S.J.R., Migliorati, C. and Barbosa, J. (1984). Toluidine blue staining in the detection of oral precancerous and malignant lesions. *Oral Surg. oral Med. oral Pathol.* **57**, 379–82.

Sohaimi, R.L. and Moxham, J. (1990). *Textbook of medicine* Churchill Livingstone, Edinburgh.

Sweatman, M.C. *et al.* (1986). Orofacial granulomatosis. Response to elemental diet and provocation by food additives. *Clin. Allergy,* **16**, 331–8.

Theaker, J.M., Porter, S.R. and Fleming, K.A. (1989). Oral epithelial dysplasia in vitamin B_{12} deficiency. *Oral Surg oral Med. oral Pathol.* **67**, 81–3.

Thomas, S.J. and MacLennan, R. (1992). Slaked lime and betel nut cancer in Papua New Guinea. *Lancet,* **340**, 577–8.

Timms, M.S. and Sloan, P. (1991). Association of supraglottic and gingival idiopathic plasmacytosis. *Oral Surg., oral Med., oral Pathol.* **71**, 451–3.

Van de Leur, J.J.J.P.M., Dofferhoff, A.S.M., Van Turnhout, J.M., Vollaard, E.J., and Clasener, H.A.L. (1992). Colonisation of oropharynx with staphylocci after penicillin in neutropenic patients. *Lancet* **340**, 861–2.

Vaughan, T.L., Strader, C., Davis, S. and Daling, J.R. (1986). Formaldehyde and cancers of the pharynx, sinus and nasal cavity. I. Occupational exposures. *Int. J. Cancer* **38**, 677–83.

Walker, D.M., Stafford, G.D., Huggett, R.M. and Newcombe, R.G. (1981). The treatment of denture-induced stomatitis. *Br. dent. J.* **151**, 416–19.

Wiesenfeld, D.W., *et al.* (1985). Orofacial granulomatosis: a clinical and pathological analysis. *Quart. J. Med.* **54**, 101–13.

Winn, D.M., Blot, W.J., Shy, C.M., Pickle, L.W., Toledo, A. and Frauneri, J.F. (1981). Snuff dipping and oral cancer among women in the southern United States. *N. Engl. J. Med.* **304**, 745–9.

Winn, D.M., Blot, W.J., Shy, C.M. and Fraumeni, J.F. Jr (1982). Occupation and oral cancer among women in the South. *Am. J. Ind. Med.* **3**, 161–7.

Wray, D. (1982). A double blind trial of systemic zinc sulfate in recurrent aphthous stomatitis. *Oral Surg., oral Med., oral Pathol.* **53**, 469–72.

Zheng, T., *et al.* (1990). Dentition, oral hygiene and risk of oral cancer: a case control study in the People's Republic of China. *Cancer Causes and Control,* **1**, 235–42.

Zheng, T., *et al.* (1993). A case control study of oral cancer in Beijing, People's Republic of China. Associations with nutrient intakes, foods and food groups. *Oral Oncol. Eur. J. Cancer, Part B,* **29B**, 45–6.

13. Prevention in the ageing dentition

A.W.G. WALLS

It is well established that the structure of the population within the UK is changing. This is a result of an improvement in economic status, health care, and social environment during the last century which has produced a dramatic increase in average life expectancy. For those aged 65, life expectancy has only risen one year for men and four years for women during the same period.

This alteration in the life pattern means that more people are surviving into their 'old age', producing a major change to health and social services. As we age, our bodies undergo a number of alterations or 'age changes'. An age change can be defined as;

An alteration in form or function to a tissue or organ, as a result of biological activity associated with minor disturbances of normal cellular turnover.

As such, there is a limited number of age changes which affect the oral cavity, most of which have no bearing on the dentition. These changes are confined to alterations in the oral mucosa and connective tissue, including the periodontium. The oral epithelium is thinned and the density and intensity of the rete peg apparatus is reduced impairing epithelial attachment in the submucosa. Oral connective tissue reduces in quantity and there is an increase in collagen density with an associated decreased rate of collagen turnover. The elastin within the connective tissue becomes less elastic, reducing tissue flexibility.

There are significant changes in the structure of all of the salivary glands with increasing age. These changes are greatest in the submandibular and minor salivary glands and least in the parotid gland (Scott 1986). These changes result in a reduced number of secretory units, and a consequent increase in fibrous and fatty tissue within the gland. Studies on the alteration of salivary flow with age are complicated by the involvement of the salivary glands in systemic disease, and the influence of a wide variety of medications upon salivary function (Baker and Ettinger 1985). The results of a number of investigations into salivary function with age, in which the medical history of the participants has been carefully controlled, have been reported. It would appear that there is little alteration in functional capacity of the parotid gland with increasing age, either in terms of stimulated or resting flow rates (Baum 1986; Heft and Baum 1984; Smith *et al.* 1992; Närhi *et al.* 1992). There is, however, some diminution in flow from minor salivary glands (Gandara *et al.* 1985; Smith *et al.* 1992) and the submandibular gland (Pedersen *et al.* 1985) with increasing age. It would appear that these func-

tional changes are manifest in the predominantly mucus-secreting glands, where the acinar structure deteriorates with age.

There is a dichotomy between the structural changes in ageing glands with an apparent reduction in secretory ability, and relatively limited changes in salivary flow with increasing age. One explanation for this dichotomy is the suggestion that there is a significant 'functional reserve' within the salivary glands (Gilbert and Minaker 1990). The reduction in secretory capacity as a product of age changes is not sufficient in the healthy individual to impair the quantitative flow requirements for normal function. However, should any further challenge to the secretion occur then a reduction in flow is more likely in older individuals than in the young (Fig. 13.1). Some evidence to support this work has been produced by Rashid and Bateman (1990) who demonstrated a more profound reduction in salivary flow in older subjects when they were exposed to a single bolus dose of atropine when compared to a group of younger individuals.

There are also some alterations in salivary composition, notably reduction in protein content and IgA (Smith *et al.* 1992), alteration in the pattern of salivary mucins (Denny *et al.* 1991), and a reduced sodium content. These changes will have some influence on the functional characteristics of this important oral fluid, although the nature of these effects has yet to be described.

There is a continued surface maturation of enamel with increased crystal growth and altered orientation. This is a product of exposure in the oral environment, and not an age change. Conversely, both dentine and pulp undergo some alteration in structure. There is an increase in peritubular dentine formation and in secondary dentine deposition with ageing, giving a more highly mineralized tissue. This is associated with a reduced number of odontoblasts. The vascularity of the pulp is reduced with an increase in pulpal fibrous tissue, and ectopic calcifications within the pulp are common. There is some evidence that even these dentine/pulpal changes are a manifestation of oral function rather than ageing *per se*, as they do not occur in teeth that have failed to erupt but are fully formed within the alveolus.

Ageing is associated with alteration in patterns of disease in the mouth and in disease activity. There are also changes in dental status with age, characterized by loss of teeth as a result of disease and 'wear and tear' over the years, and by progressive loss of support for the remaining dentition. These alterations are mainly a result of length of service of the dentition, along with the presence of chronic dental disease.

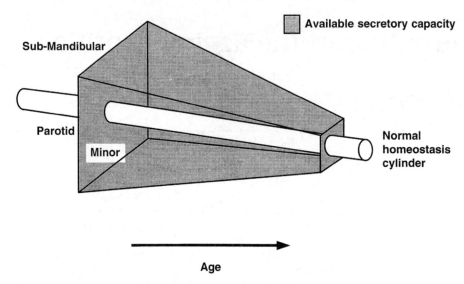

Fig. 13.1 A diagrammatic representation of changes in salivary secretory capacity (represented as the shaded cone) with age. The *normal* secretory capacity of the gland is less than the secretory capacity at all ages. (After Gilbert and Minaker 1990.)

As a consequence, there are alterations in the patterns of care provision and in the prevention of disease progression which are unique to an older population. It is to these problems that the remainder of this chapter will be addressed.

PERIODONTAL DISEASE

Loss of attachment increases with increasing age of the individual (Beck *et al.* 1984). The relationship between age and attachment loss seems to be related to long-term exposure to plaque rather than to any age changes within the periodontium. The rate of progression of periodontal disease is influenced by the body's immune response. It might be expected that the alterations in the immune response seen with age would result in a modification in the pattern of disease progression. There is some evidence for such change with shallow pockets being at reduced risk of progression in older populations when compared to deep pockets. (Grbic *et al.* 1991).

The often quoted sentiment that periodontal disease is the principal reason for tooth loss in the over-35s (Douglass *et al.* 1983; Kay and Blinkhorn 1986) does not hold true for the oldest adults (Chauncey *et al.* 1989). This may be a reflection of an innate resistance to periodontal destruction amongst older adults who retain some teeth, or simply that the teeth most likely to be lost as a consequence of periodontal destruction have already been extracted in the older cohorts.

The mainstay for prevention of further loss of attachment in the older patient is oral hygiene and non-surgical management (Lindhe and Nyman 1975). Unfortunately, oral hygiene in older patients is complicated by alterations in gingival architecture as a result of exposure of root surfaces, and the possible involvement of molar furcations.

In addition to these problems of an altered shape, an older person's ability to maintain an adequate standard of oral cleanliness may be impaired by reduced visual acuity, decrease in psychomotor skills, and possibly by physical handicap. It is often necessary to re-educate patients in their oral hygiene techniques, to include aids such as wood points and bottle-brushes to facilitate interproximal cleaning. Should such a change be required then the education process needs to be self-paced, rather than forced, to maximize its effectiveness in older people (Canestrari 1963). There will inevitably come a time when an older person can cope no longer with their own oral hygiene. When this occurs a decision has to be made whether to accept the inevitable sequelae of poor cleaning (gingivitis and caries) or whether to try to enlist the help of a carer, along with other aids, such as chemical plaque control, to try to maintain oral health. Teaching a carer how to brush well somebody else's teeth is often more difficult than brushing your own. In these circumstances the use of an electric tooth-brush can be of help.

ROOT CARIES

Caries on the root surface (Fig. 13.2) has been defined as:

A cavitation or softened area in the root surface which might, or might not, involve adjacent enamel or existing restorations (Hix and O'Leary 1976).

PREVALENCE

There is wide variation in the prevalence of root caries, from as low as 7.3 per cent (Burt *et al.* 1986), among individuals living in a community with high levels of natural water fluoridation, to 100 per cent (Fejerskov *et al.* 1985) in patients over the age of 60 attending a gerontology clinic. These differences probably represent a combination of some natural variation in prevalence in this disease, and marked variations in the diagnostic criteria used by the research workers in this field (Aherne *et al.* 1990). One source of variation is restored root surfaces. Restorations are placed on root surfaces for two clinical reasons, root caries and cervical tooth wear. It is not possible to decide why any given restora-

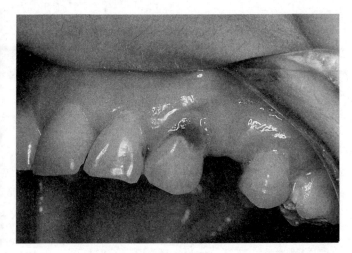

Fig. 13.2 An extensive active root surface caries lesion at the buccal cervical margin of an upper canine.

tion has been placed once it is in position. Thus, restorations placed because of cervical wear would inflate the 'filled' component of a root surface DMF score. This problem has been discussed in greater detail by de Paola *et al.* (1989). There are three possible solutions which have been adopted for this problem: firstly, restored surface can be discounted as far as caries prevalence is concerned (Vehkalahti *et al.* (1989); secondly, some allowance can be made for the problem (Hix and O'Leary 1976) or finally, all carious and restored surfaces can be included as 'root caries' (Beck *et al.* 1985). Each 'solution' brings with it further difficulties in terms of under- or overestimation of the prevalence of root caries.

The prevalence of root caries increases with increasing age of the population (Fig. 13.3). Whilst these figures give us an estimate of the total number of the population that have one or more root carious lesion, they do not give any indication of the magnitude of the problem within any given individual.

The mean number of lesions per person affected has been reported and varies, depending upon the age and nature of the population studied, from 0.2 for 28- to 29-year-olds from a non-fluoridated Western community (Katz *et al.* 1982) to 6.4 in primitive tribesmen over 30 years of age (Schamschula *et al.* 1974) (Table 13.1).

Once again these figures are useful, but they do not give any idea of the likelihood that any given individual will develop root caries. For a tooth to develop root caries, it is necessary that the root of the tooth is exposed in the oral cavity. A true 'attack rate' for root caries should relate the incidence of lesions to the number of surfaces at risk, i.e. exposed root surfaces. The root caries index (RCI) proposed by Katz (1984) computes an attack rate for root caries. The RCI for a number of population groups is given in Table 13.2. It can be seen that there is a trend for an increase in RCI with age. The numerical magnitude of these data may be somewhat misleading, in that restorations are counted within the RCI score. Notwithstanding this difficulty, there does appear to be an age-related increase in the attack rate for root surface caries demonstrated by these data. Steele (1994) reported that there was an uneven distribution of root caries/restorations within the population such that 70 per cent of the lesions/restorations were found in 30 per cent of the population. This concentration occurs despite the almost universal presence of root surface exposure in older individuals (Steele, 1994).

INCIDENCE

There is a growing body of evidence concerning the incidence of root caries derived from longitudinal studies of dental health amongst periodontally compromised patients and from studies of community dwelling adults (mainly in the USA) (Table 13.3). The annualized attack rates all fall in the region of 2 new carious surfaces per 100 surfaces at risk per year with the exception of data for chronically ill subjects (Banting

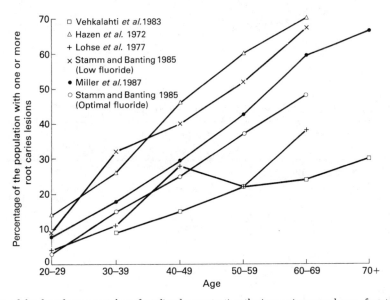

Fig. 13.3 A graphical presentation of the data from a number of studies demonstrating the increasing prevalence of root surface caries with age. This increase is independent of the nature of the population studied.

Table 13.1. Mean number of teeth with root caries and/or restorations in those with root caries by age in different population groups

Author	Population	Age					
		20s	30s	40s	50s	60s	70+
Katz *et al.* (1982)	Adult USA	0.2	0.6	1.9	3.0	3.4	
Todd and Lader (1991)	UK	0.3	0.8	1.2	1.9	1.9	
Miller *et al.* (1987)	USA	0.5	0.7	1.2	2.0	3.2	
Locker *et al.* (1989)	Community Canada				1.9	2.7	4.2
Fure and Zickert (1990)	Community Sweden				1.4	3.3	3.6
Luan *et al.* (1989)	Community China				1.0	1.8	1.5
Donachie and Walls (1991)	Community UK			2.1	3.2	3.8	3.3
Steele (1994)	Community UK					2.3	

Table 13.2. The root caries index by age in different population groups

Author	Population	Age					
		20s	30s	40s	50s	60s	70+
Katz *et al.* (1982)	USA	1	5	13	22	17	
Fure and Zickert (1990)	Sweden				13.8	16.1	21.5
Donachie and Walls (1991)	UK			14.6	18.9	21	21.1
Steele (1994)	UK					22.1	

Table 13.3. Incidence rates for root surface caries in older populations

Author	Population	Duration of study (months)	Attack rate	% developing new lesions
Banting *et al.* (1985)	Chronically ill	34	6.3[1]	36
Hand *et al.* (1988)	Community dwelling	36	1.8[2]	43
Wallace *et al.* (1988)	Community dwelling	12	1.6[2]	
MacEntee *et al.* (1993)	Community/institionalized	12	2.2[2]	66.7
Ravald *et al.* (1986)	Periodontal	48	1.1[2]	62

[1] Attack rate per 1000 surface months at risk.
[2] Attack rate per 100 surfaces at risk.

et al. 1985). If is of significance that most of the studies found that these new lesions occurred in a minority of the population.

DISTRIBUTION WITHIN THE MOUTH

There is a characteristic distribution for root caries lesions within the oral cavity (Fejerskov *et al.* 1985; Katz *et al.* 1985), with an increased prevalence in mandibular molar teeth, followed by maxillary anterior teeth, and maxillary posteriors. Mandibular anteriors seem to be least susceptible. The buccal and interproximal surfaces are more susceptible than the palatal or lingual aspects of affected teeth. This pattern of caries susceptibility has a marked similarity to the pattern of oral sugar clearance reported by Dawes and Macpherson (1993). Where sugar clearance is slowest, caries rates are raised.

This perceived pattern of attack may be distorted by two factors. Firstly, there is a well established pattern of tooth loss with increasing age (Fig 13.4) (van Wyk *et al.* 1977). It may be that those teeth that are lost would be the most susceptible to root caries, and those that are retained would have relatively low susceptibility, but are seen as carious in numbers out of proportion to their 'true susceptibility' as they are the only teeth present. Secondly, the high 'prevalence' rates recorded for buccal surfaces may be a reflection of filled surfaces, restored to repair cervical wear lesions, inflating the filled component of a root caries score.

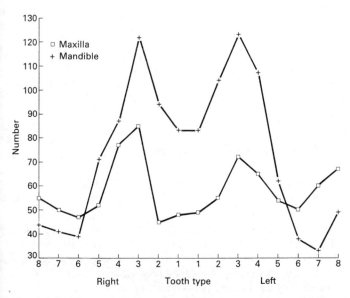

Fig. 13.4 The pattern of tooth retention in an ageing population. (After van Wyk *et al.* 1977.)

RISK FACTORS

The increasing prevalence of root caries with increasing age is probably a reflection of two factors acting together, increase in the number and extent of root surfaces exposed and an increase in disease activity with age.

There have been a large number of variables associated with the development of root caries. Beck *et al.* (1986) have proposed a multifactorial model which illustrates the intricate web of aetiological variables that may be associated with either the severity or progression of the disease (Fig. 13.5). As would be expected, subjects with periodontal disease have an increased level of root caries; however, the attack rate is greater for those with untreated periodontal disease compared with subjects after periodontal care (Hix and O'Leary 1976). Older individuals who demonstrate a good standard of oral hygiene have few root caries lesions (Locker *et al.* 1989).

Root surface exposure does not automatically lead to root caries. Indeed, one report from a developing country whose inhabitants exhibit extensive gingival recession with age found virtually no root caries (Muya *et al.* in Fejerskov and Nyvad 1986), whereas a second report from a primitive culture found very high levels of root caries, which correlated well with the high levels of periodontal destruction (Schamschula *et al.* 1974). It may be that the root surface within a periodontal pocket, or protected from the oral environment as a result of periodontal architecture, is at greater risk than when it is fully exposed.

High levels of root caries have also been reported in chronically ill, institutionalized, older adults (Banting *et al.* 1980), drug addicts, and in individuals with altered salivary function either as a result of a disease process (Fox *et al.* 1985), or radiation-induced damage to the salivary glands (Fig. 13.6) (Wescott *et al.* 1975).

The prevalence of root caries has been correlated with the number of 'fermentable carbohydrate assaults' (Hix and O'Leary 1976). There may be a relationship between coronal caries experience and root caries experience. The majority of workers have found that individuals with decayed or filled root surfaces had greater experience of decayed or restored coronal surfaces (Banting *et al.* 1980; Vehkalahti 1987). However, other workers (Sumney *et al.* 1973; Banting *et al.* 1985) have not been able to demonstrate a correlation with coronal caries experience. Previous root caries experience, either in the form of filled surfaces or decayed untreated lesions is also a potent risk factor for the development of new lesions (Banting *et al.* 1985; Scheinin *et al.* 1994). Two large studies have demonstrated slightly higher prevalence rates for males than females (Katz *et al.* 1985; Vehkalahti *et al.* 1983). There are a number of social attitudinal variables which are associated in both a positive and a negative manner with root caries. The number of remaining teeth and active social participation are both negative predictors for root caries (Beck *et al.* 1986). Whereas negative life events, low educational attainment, low income, recurrent chronic illness, infrequent oral hygiene, irregular attendance, and smoking are all positive predictors of the level of disease activity (Beck *et al.* 1986; Locker *et al.* 1989; Ravald *et al.* 1993).

It has been suggested that, for the over-65s, chronological age is of little significance in determining root caries activity. Whereas increased biological age, with associated medical/physical deterioration and disability is of great importance (Beck *et al.* 1986).

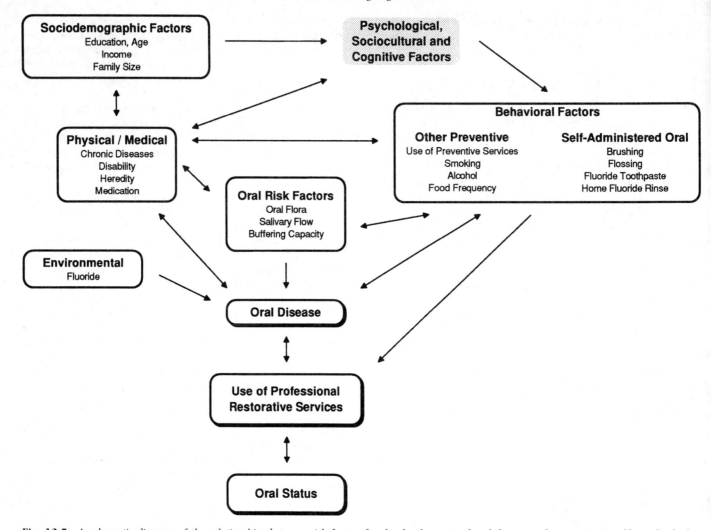

Fig. 13.5 A schematic diagram of the relationships between risk factors for the development of oral disease and root caries in older individuals (after Beck *et al.* 1986).

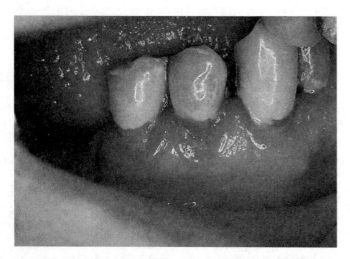

Fig. 13.6 Extensive and rapidly developing root surface caries lesions in an individual with radiation-induced xerostomia. This patient had a pharyngeal carcinoma; both parotid and submandibular glands were involved in the irradiated field.

MICROBIOLOGY AND HISTOLOGY

Coronal decay is a disease process of microbial origin. There is no doubt that bacteria have a similar part to play in root caries. *Streptococcus mutans* is of prime importance in initiating coronal caries, although other species may be of greater significance in extension of the carious lesion into dentine. There is, however, some debate concerning the species of bacteria that are responsible for root surface lesions in man. One reason for the possible broadening in the range of pathogenic bacteria for root caries is the somewhat elevated 'critical pH' for dentine and cementum when compared to enamel (Krasse 1984). As a consequence, bacteria of 'lesser acidogenicity' could contribute to demineralization of root lesions. The organisms most commonly associated with root caries are *Actinomyces viscossus/naeslundii*, *Strep. mutans*, Lactobacilli, and Candida species.

Actinomyces viscossus is one of the dominant species (Syed *et al.* 1975). Animal studies have also demonstrated that A. *viscossus* can cause both periodontal destruction and root

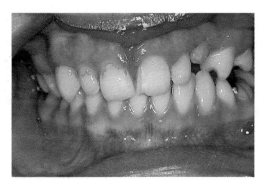

Plate 13.1 Extensive buccal tooth surface loss on the upper central and upper left lateral incisors. This subject chewed lemons as part of a 'diet'. The extensive wear occurred over a 2-year period.

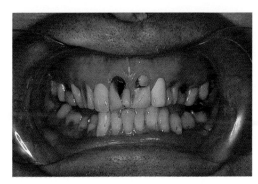

Plate 13.4 Marked tooth wear of the buccal surfaces of the upper anterior teeth. The two upper lateral incisors had been restored with porcelain bonded to metal crowns. Note the caries occurring in the exposed coronal dentine. This subject worked in a brick works and had not worn the protective mask provided by his employer. The abrasive dust laden atmosphere probably contributed to the buccal tissue loss. Eighteen months prior to this picture being taken, he had transferred to office work. This change in local environment allowed the carious lesions to develop on the exposed dentine surfaces.

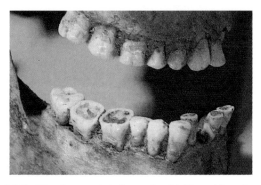

Plate 13.2 The characteristic flat occlusal table and broad contact areas of a 'primitive man'. This pattern of tooth wear is thought to be associated with a coarse, abrasive diet. (Illustration courtesy of Dr A.D.G. Beynon).

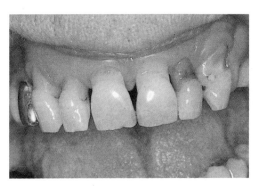

Plate 13.5 V- or U-shaped notching at the exposed cervical root surface, beneath the cement-enamel junction. This pattern of tooth wear may be associated with an improper oral hygiene technique.

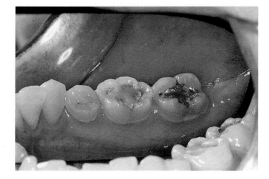

Plate 13.3 Extensive tooth wear of the lower right first molar in a 23-year-old man. There is also faceting of the lower first premolar and anterior teeth. This subject gave a history of recurrent regurgitation of stomach contents between the ages of 9 and 14 years, and admitted a clenching/grinding habit.

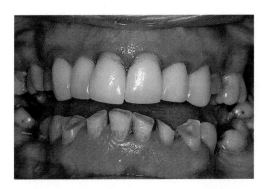

Plate 13.6 Gross destruction of the lower anterior teeth associated with rough, over-contoured, palatal surfaces on the porcelain bonded to metal restorations in the upper arch. The upper restorations had been in place for between 6 and 10 years.

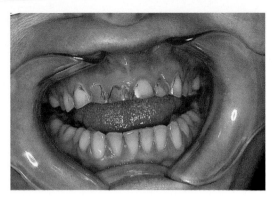

Plate 14.1 Heavily worn teeth in a young adult. There is extensive exposure of dentine on the functional surfaces and the teeth have lost a lot of their crown height. Treatment may be complex.

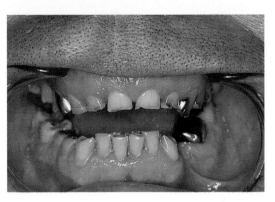

Plate 14.2 Heavily worn teeth in an older patient. The extent and severity of the wear is similar to that of the young adult in Plate 14.1, but the appropriate treatment is likely to be very different.

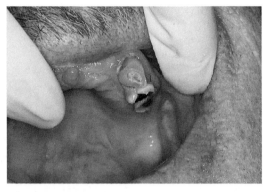

Plate 14.3 Widespread and unplanned tooth loss have led to a situation where the teeth remaining may be more of a hindrance than a help. There is little prospect for improving the patient's function.

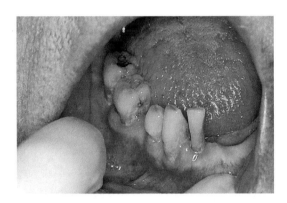

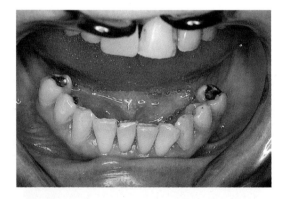

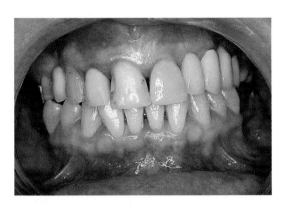

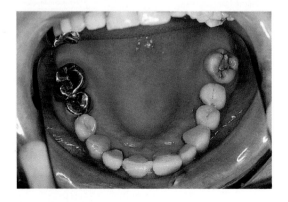

Plate 14.4 Example of a shortened dental arch, where an effort has been made to retain key teeth and maximize occlusal contacts. Even if several further teeth are lost there is still the scope for maintaining a satisfactory dentition if long-term priorities are set now.

caries in rodents (Socransky *et al.* 1970; Jordan and Hammond 1972). However, it has been demonstrated that, although Actinomyces species can frequently be isolated from root surface plaque, there is *no difference* in the prevalence or proportion of isolation of Actinomyces species between carious and caries-free root surfaces (Ellen *et al.* 1985*a*; Van Houte *et al.*1990). This may be a reflection of the predominance of *A. viscossus* in mature root surface plaque (Kmet *et al.* 1985).

Streptococcus mutans and Lactobacilli can also be isolated from root caries plaque in varying proportions (Ellen *et al.* 1985*a,b*). Ellen *et al.* (1985*b*) have correlated the detection of *Strep. mutans* and Lactobacilli, with the development of root caries within that individual. This pattern held true for the mouth as a whole, but was not site-specific.

The development of root caries, in periodontally involved subjects has also been correlated with the frequency of ingestion of fermentable carbohydrates (Hix and O'Leary 1976) and with high salivary Lactobacillus and *Strep. mutans* counts (Ravald *et al.* 1993).

Beighton and Lynch (1993) have used a novel sampling technique to remove small quantities of carious dentine from root lesions with varying degrees of clinical 'activity'. Microbiological culture of these dentine samples has demonstrated a strong positive relationship between caries activity (assessed on clinical criteria) and the frequency of isolation of both *Strep mutans* and Candida species. *Streptococcus mutans* were isolated more frequently from soft lesions, larger lesions, and those closest to the gingival margin. The Candida species, whilst isolated more frequently at similar sites, were present in low numbers. Their presence was though to be a reflection of their aciduricity rather than their acidogenicity. They hypothesize that Candida could be a marker organism for the most severe disease.

The macroscopic and microscopic appearance of root surface lesions will depend on the stage of progression of the disease. A root surface that is exposed in the mouth will take up mineral from oral fluids forming a hypermineralized surface layer. This phenomenon occurs whether the root surface is dentine or cementum (Westbrook *et al.* 1974; Hals and Selvig 1977). The early root caries lesion is characterized by demineralization beneath this hypermineralized surface. Demineralization is accompanied by dissolution of apatite crystals and splitting of the collagen bundles within the dentine matrix (Furseth 1970; Furseth and Johansen 1971). Softening of the root surface occurs at an early stage of the lesion, with surface breakdown at a number of discrete, localized sites (Fejerskov and Nyvad 1986). Bacterial penetration into the demineralized surface occurs quickly after the onset of decay, but the rate of progression of the lesion is slow, resulting in extensive, but shallow, carious lesions on the root surface. Obviously, such lesions can progress towards the pulp of the tooth and will lead to pulpal exposure.

PREVENTION

Long-term exposure to a water supply containing optimum levels (1 ppm or pro rata for the climatic conditions) of fluoride has a beneficial effect in reducing the prevalence of root caries (Stamm and Banting 1980; Brustman, 1986). The magnitude of the reduction in caries prevalence is not as great as that for coronal lesions. The preventive effect may be 'dose-related', as it has been reported that the attack rate amongst citizens in a population with 3.5 mg/l fluoride in their water supply is significantly less than that for subjects exposed to 0.7 mg/l. The RCI figures for the two populations were 1.22 and 6.68 per cent, respectively (Burt *et al.* 1986). One of the principal arguments on behalf of the anti-fluoridation lobby has been that the benefits of fluoride in the water supply are concentrated in childhood when teeth are developing, and that there is little benefit for adults. There are a number of studies which confound this conjecture in relation to root caries. These studies have examined the effect on caries prevalence and severity in adults who have moved into an area with fluoride in the water supply having lived during their childhood in communities with low-fluoride water. These studies suggest that 20–30 years of residence in an area with optimal fluoridation results in a reduced prevalence of root caries. Furthermore, individuals with 40 years or more residence in a fluoridated community have both a reduced prevalence and fewer root caries lesions compared to age-matched cohorts from non-fluoridated communities (Whelton *et al.* 1993; Brustman 1986; Hunt *et al.* 1989). These data are independent of the acknowledged preventive benefits from using a fluoride-containing dentifrice (Jensen 1988).

New carious lesions can be prevented, during the maintenance phase of periodontal treatment, by vigorous and regular individual and professional tooth-cleaning (Lindhe and Nyman 1975). It is debatable whether this level of motivation and professional support could be made available on a wide scale. In addition, such vigorous oral hygiene may lead to iatrogenic problems of its own (see below).

Monitoring salivary levels of Lactobacilli and *Strep. mutans* using simple surgery culture kits (Dentocult SM and LB; Vivacare, Vivadent: Schaan, Liechtenstein) has considerable prognostic value in terms of caries activity (Ravald *et al.* 1993).

Current preventive stratagems include the use of sodium or stannous fluoride mouth rinses, fluoride-containing prophylaxis pastes, and topical use of acidulated phosphate fluoride (APF) gels. This latter medicament is apparently useful in preventing dentine sensitivity and as well as radicular decay (Ramfjord 1987). Billings and Banting (1993) have pointed out that there is little information available currently about optimal delivery systems for fluoride when trying to prevent root caries. The variation in critical pH for dentine when compared to enamel and the relatively greater uptake of fluoride by dentine when compared to enamel (Banting and Stamm 1979) must affect the dose/response gradient for fluoride and the method of fluoride delivery (neutral/ acidulated, solution/gel/foam). The other chemotherapeutic agents used in an attempt to prevent root caries is chlorhexidine gluconate, either on its own or in combination with fluoride (Katz 1982). There are relatively few studies of the use of chlorhexidine in prevention of root caries, however, Ullsfoss *et al.* (1994) have recently demonstrated its efficacy in assisting in remineralization of artificial carious lesions in a human *in vivo* study. Chlorhexidine seems to be most effective in subjects with high levels of *Strep. mutans* colonization who use gel-type preparations over long time periods (Emilson 1994).

A variety of regimes have been described for the prevention and remineralization of root caries in individuals with

Table 13.4. Composition of a 'remineralizing mouth wash' (Johansen *et al.* 1987)

Calcium	5 mM
Phosphate	3 mM
Fluoride	0.25 mM (5 ppm)
Stabilized with sodium chloride at pH 7.0	

reduced salivary flow. All include the use of topical fluorides, either as a mouth rinse (Davis *et al.* 1985), or in gel form. (Wescott *et al.* 1975; Daly *et al.* 1972; Johansen and Olsen 1979) Johansen and Olsen (1979) took a different approach, with an initial daily application of APF gel for four weeks and a 'remineralizing mouth wash' (Table 13.4), followed by 'maintenance' using the mineralizing mouth wash alone (in conjunction with a fluoride-containing dentifrice and salivary stimulation with sugar-free chewing gum) for the duration of the study. This approach was modified to exchange neutral sodium fluoride for the APF gel in a later study (Johansen *et al.* 1987). All of these treatment modalities are of benefit in the xerostomic patient giving a reduction in caries prevalence. Davis *et al.* (1985) used a combined sodium fluoride and chlorhexidine-gluconate rinse, and found it to have similar benefit to a sodium fluoride preparation. It may be

that, in addition to their remineralizing role, many of these treatments act by reducing the *Strep. mutans* colonization of the root surface (Keene *et al.* 1984).

The second aspect of management for individuals with reduced salivary flow is either an attempt to stimulate residual salivary function or substitution with some form of oral lubricant (Fig. 13.7). Salivary flow can be enhanced using gustatory (although care needs to be taken in patients with teeth not to use acidic or sugar-containing agents), pharmacological or mechanical stimuli. The drugs used to enhance salivary flow must be cholinergic agonists and hence have the potential for causing systemic side-effects. Nevertheless, there are reports of good short-term success with low dose, oral, philocarpine hydrochloride in this role (Johnson *et al.* 1993). It has long been established that chewing gum stimulates salivary flow and enhances the rate of increase in pH of plaque after a cariogenic challenge (Edgar and Geddes 1990; Dawes and Macpherson 1993). There is some evidence of a learning effect in young adults where the improvement in salivary flow is enhanced with time (Jenkins and Edgar 1989). Consequently, chewing gum has been advocated as a preventive strategy for adults (Johansen *et al.* 1987), where there does seem to be a benefit in xerostomic subjects (Markovic *et al.* 1988). Chewing gums are available which contain fluoride to maximize the preventive effect (Fluorette, Tilkvervarde: Fertin, Vejle, Denmark).

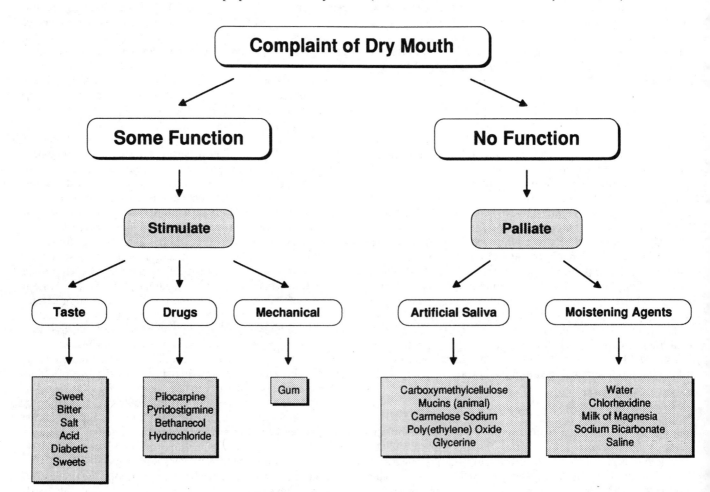

Fig. 13.7 Treatment options for subjects suffering from reduced salivary flow.

Improvement in perceived oral wetness can take the form os simple palliative such as saline or bicarbonate of soda, or attempts can be made to replace saliva using a salivary substitute. Their are a number of commercially available salivary substitutes, the effect of these agents on enamel *in vitro* have been reported by Joyston-Bechal and Kidd (1987). They found that two commercial products (Luborant and Saliva Orthana) contained 2 ppm fluoride with a pH in the region of 6.7. These agents proved to be very acceptable remineralizing media for enamel *in vitro*. Some artificial saliva attempt to increase salivary flow by incorporating an acid stimulus. These substances can cause demineralization of tooth tissue in their own right, and should not be used in partially dentate individuals (Kidd and Joyston-Bechal 1984).

MANAGEMENT OF ROOT CARIES

Root caries can provide the restorative dentist with a difficult clinical problem. There are three possible treatment modalities;

1. *Prevention/remineralization, using fluoride gels and/or mouth rinses, with or without a 'remineralizing' mouth rinse and/or chlorhexidine-gluconate mouth rinse.* There is little doubt that remineralization of a carious root surface lesion is practicable. One drawback of this approach is that the remineralized surface is dark brown or black with a leathery texture initially, and will eventually harden to give a polished highly mineralized surface. Some patients may not be prepared to tolerate this discoloration of the root surface. Such remineralized surfaces are reported to be more resistant to further carious attack than adjacent, otherwise sound, dentine. Nyvad and Fejerskov (1986) have reported that conversion from active to arrested lesions can be brought about using simple oral hygiene methods alone in appropriately motivated individuals.

2. *Surface recontouring.* It has been suggested that the earliest form of interceptive management for root caries should simply comprise removal of the softened dentine, followed by recontouring of the root architecture to give a smooth, cleansable surface. The freshly exposed dentine is treated with topical fluoride agents to stimulate the formation of a hypermineralized surface layer (Banting and Ellen 1976). This technique is attractive, but does, however, result in the removal of tooth tissue, which must produce some 'waisting' of the root contour. This approach is only applicable for shallow lesions, where excellent results have been reported (Billings *et al.* 1985).

3. *Restoration of the defect.* Once the carious lesion has become well established, repair using an appropriate restorative material will become necessary. A wide variety of materials, amalgam, gold, composite, resin and glass poly-alkenoate (ionomer) cements, have been used. Silver amalgam and gold require finite cavity form, and the cavity design must provide some form of mechanical retention. These two requirements result in destruction of sound tooth tissue beyond the margins of, and deep to, the lesion. In addition, neither material is 'tooth-coloured' which may not be acceptable to the patient.

There are two 'aesthetic' restorative materials that are commonly used in this situation, composite resin and glass ionomer cements. A number of commercially available 'dentine bonding agents' are available to provide a chemical bond between dentine and the resin. The medium-term durability of these systems appears to be satisfactory, although there remains some doubt about the long-term hydrolytic stability of some dentine bonding agents. It is likely that their success will be greatest in relatively shallow cavities where a large surface area of dentine is available for bonding and there is low bulk within the composite material. These criteria are met when restoring root caries.

Glass ionomer cements are also adhesive materials, which bind to the mineral component of dentine and enamel. Their physical properties are inferior to those of the composite resins, but are more than adequate for restoration of root caries (Walls 1986). The majority of the clinical trials of glass polyalkenoate cements have concerned their usage in restoration of cervical deficiencies in tooth substance (these have been summarized by Knibbs 1988). Recent results show acceptably good retention and aesthetics. These have been brought about as a result of modifications to the material, and greater awareness of the techniques required for use of an adhesive restorative material. One advantage of these cements is that they leach fluoride which has been shown to exhibit a caries inhibitory effect upon adjacent tooth substance *in vitro* (Kidd 1978; Hicks 1986), although there is no long-term clinical data available to support these suggestions. There are a number of disadvantages to their use, not least that nearly all of the commercially available, aesthetically acceptable materials are radiolucent, making the task of monitoring recurrent decay more difficult.

Root caries lesions can be inaccessible to conventional instrumentation. In such circumstances the chemo-mechanical removal of carious dentine using a hypochlorite agent may be a viable alternative to classical cavity preparation (Tavares 1988).

There have been some experimental studies into the use of lasers during the management of root caries, either to reduce the susceptibility of the surface to demineralization (Westerman *et al.* 1994), or as an adjunct to a restorative technique (Cooper *et al.* 1986). These techniques may offer a path for development for the future.

TOOTH WEAR

Tooth wear can be defined as:

The loss of mineralized tooth substance from the surface of the teeth, as a result of physical and/or chemical attack. The chemical assault must not be of bacterial origin.

It will occur as a natural phenomenon on all functional or contacting surfaces of the dentition. Consequently, it would be expected that the quantity of wear will increase with increasing age of the individual concerned. In certain individuals wear in excess of this norm occurs, under these circumstances the wear becomes unacceptable, warranting intervention to prevent further damage.

There is little published information concerning the prevalence of tooth wear within the community, or indeed the levels of wear that are 'normal' and/or acceptable for any age group. A number of indices have been described to attempt to quantify the severity of tissue damage. The majority of these focus upon one particular 'type' of war (i.e. cervical wear), and are only applicable for that specific pattern of tissue loss. One index (Smith and Knight 1984*a*) attempts to overcome this problem by subjectively scoring every visible surface of a tooth for wear. A set of approximate 'population norms' were established by examining a small group of patients (100 subjects in all). More recently these population norms have been shown to be an underestimate within the older age groups (Donachie and Walls, in press *a*). Smith and Knight (1984*b*) have described the use of their index as an adjunct during diagnosis for subjects with a worn dentition.

PREVALENCE

There is limited data available concerning the prevalence of tooth wear, particularly on the functional surfaces of teeth. Donachie and Walls (in press *b*) give data on a sample of over-45s. They reported minimal wear present on the smooth surfaces of the teeth (with the exception of the palatal surfaces of upper anteriors) in even their oldest age group (75 plus). However, more severe wear was usual on the occlusal/incisal surfaces and on the lingual aspects of the upper anteriors. Wear exposing secondary dentine on the incisal edges of anterior teeth was common. These findings support the data from Hand *et al.* (1987) who found dentine exposure in 72.9 per cent of their population of older Iowans, 4.5 per cent of whom had teeth worn down to the gingival margin. However, Hugoson *et al.* (1988) demonstrated a rather lower prevalence and severity of anterior tooth wear in their Swedish sample. Nevertheless, they did demonstrate increasing severity of wear with increasing age. Most workers in the field have also demonstrated that wear is more severe amongst males than females. In a recent study of younger adults, Silness *et al.* (1994) demonstrated a relationship between low Plaque and Gingival Index scores and increased wear of the incisal edges of teeth. This association may be related to oral hygiene practices.

There is some epidemiological data concerning the prevalence of cervical wear within the community. Sognnaes *et al.* (1972) examined nearly 11 000 extracted teeth, 18 per cent of which 'had typical patterns of erosion-like lesions'. They were unable to give an age-related breakdown of their results. Xhonga and Valdmanis (1983) found that approximately 25 per cent of their sample of adults exhibited cervical damage. This figure increases to 56 per cent amongst an elderly population (Hand *et al.* 1986). Todd and Lader (1991) demonstrated increasing numbers of teeth with cervical wear with increasing age. Donachie and Walls (in press *b*) found that cervical wear was almost universal in their sample of older adults, although the majority of the wear lesions were shallow. It should be remembered that the both the prevalence and severity of cervical wear will be underestimated in populations who attend for dental care as some worn surfaces are likely to have been restored in such groups.

Premolars are the most frequently involved teeth, followed by incisors in all age groups (Xhonga and Valdmanis 1983; Hand *et al.* 1986). In subjects with cervical tooth wear, the lesions progress at between 1 and 2 μm per day (Nordbo and Skogedal 1982).

AETIOLOGY

There are three mechanisms for physiological tooth wear:

1. *Erosion*. The progressive loss of hard tooth substance by chemical dissolution, not involving bacterial action.

2. *Attrition*. The progressive loss of hard tooth substance caused by mastication, or contact between occluding or approximal surfaces.

3. *Abrasion*. The progressive loss of hard tooth substance caused by mechanical factors other than mastication or tooth-to-tooth contacts.

Tooth wear is usually a product of all three mechanisms. Attrition and abrasion will occur, with sound tooth tissue. These two mechanical effects will potentiate the damage caused by an erosive component, as the softened surface produced after acid attack will be more readily removed by mechanical trauma. Whilst the definition of erosion precludes damage caused by bacterial acid production, it may be that this is of significance during wear of exposed root surfaces. The dentine of an exposed root surface is relatively soft and consequently is prone to mechanical damage, any further softening, via an erosive element which may include plaque acids, will only potentiate this phenomenon.

Excessive wear is normally the product of an exacerbation of one of the mechanisms responsible for 'physiological wear'. This tends to result in a pattern of tooth tissue loss that may be of use in determining the cause of wear (Table 13.5). A variety of aetiological factors have been implicated for wear.

Erosion

Sognnaes (1963) has postulated three linked 'mechanisms of hard tissue destruction' which may occur during erosion;

1. Absence or loss of a protective salivary organic coating on a tooth.

2. Loss of mineral form the tooth surface with a decalcifying agent (either extrinsic or intrinsic).

3. Destruction of decalcified tooth tissue with biochemical and/or biophysical and/or mechanical action.

Saliva has a number of roles in helping to prevent tooth wear. Not only does it buffer ingested acid and act as a remineralizing agent, but it also serves as a lubricant during oral function, thus minimising mechanical damage to tooth tissues. Excessive tooth wear is seen in subjects with impaired salivary function.

A number of sources of extrinsic or intrinsic acids or chelating agents have been described in the literature (Table 13.6) which may be responsible for tooth tissue loss. The

Table 13.5. Pattern of tooth loss with different aetiological agents

Erosion
The worn surface will be smooth with a dull surface finish. Acid-resistant restorations will stand proud of the surrounding tooth tissue.

Dietary
The pattern of loss will depend upon the dietary habit, e.g. an individual who chews citrus fruits will lose tissue from the incisal and labial aspects of the upper incisors (Plate 13.1).

Medicinal
Tissue loss from the occlusal surfaces of the lower molars and the occlusal and palatal surfaces of the upper molars.

Gastric reflux
Tissue loss from the occlusal surfaces of the molars and the palatal aspects of the upper anteriors and premolars.

Occupational
Tissue loss from the surfaces exposed to acid attack, classically the buccal surfaces of the upper and lower anterior teeth.

Attrition
Smooth polished surfaces with multiple facets that are mirror images of each other.

Pitting of the worn surface will occur when there is a significant element of erosion allied to the attrition (Plate 13.3)

Abrasion
Smooth polished defects in the mineralized surfaces of the teeth. The pattern of tissue loss will correspond to the abrasive stimulus.

Industrial
Loss of buccal contour from the surfaces exposed to environmental pollution. The appearance will be similar to that for erosive industrial damage.

Iatrogenic
Damage to tooth substance as a result of improper use of oral hygiene aids giving notching or waisting at the gingival margin. Use of abrasive dentifrices can cause marked damage to the buccal enamel of upper anterior teeth, giving dish-shaped wear facets.

Table 13.6. Possible demineralizing agents that have been implicated in the aetiology of erosive tooth wear

Dietary
Fruit (lemons, oranges, bananas, etc.)
Fruit juices
Carbonated beverages (both 'diet' and 'normal')
Fruit-flavoured infant drinks
Vinegar, pickles, pickled onions
Vitamin C

Medicinal
Hydrochloric acid replacement
Iron tonics
Vitamin C
Aspirin

Regurgitation
Hiatus hernia
Chronic alcoholism (recurrent vomiting)
Diabetes mellitus
Pregnancy
Drugs inducing nausea
Radiotherapy
Anorexia nervosa
Bulimia

Occupational
Industrial acid

Idiopathic
'Acid saliva'
Water from chlorinated swimming baths

pattern of tissue loss is not the same for all sources of decalcifying agent, indeed it can be almost pathognomic of a form of damage (Plate 13.1).

Järvinen *et al.* (1991) have attempted to establish the relative potency of a variety of factors in dental erosion. They computed the population attributable risk (PAR) (the percentage decrease in occurrence of erosion in the population if an erosive factor was eliminated) to compare the influence of variables on wear. The most important groups by far were reported vomiting and other gastric symptoms. However, consumption of citrus fruits (more than twice daily), soft drinks (four to six or more per week) and low salivary flow levels were important.

Attrition

Wear as a result of tooth to tooth contact will cause an increase in the area of teeth in contact, and may result in increased masticatory efficiency. The extent of attrition will depend on the use to which an individual puts their teeth. Attrition is increased in populations where the teeth are used as a tool (i.e. Eskimos, etc.) and in primitive tribal groups or early man where the diet has a greater abrasive component (Plate 13.2). Lavelle (1973) reported a marked decrease in attrition amongst the population of Britain when comparing Romano–British skulls to those of the nineteenth century.

Parafunctional clenching or grinding habits will produce abnormal patterns of wear (Pavone 1985). The aetiology of such habits is a complex mixture of psychological, emotional, dental, systemic, occupational, and idiopathic factors (see Pavone 1985). The systemic problems include tardive dyskinesias, which are more common in an elderly population (Karmen 1975). There may be an erosive component contributing to tooth tissue loss in a bruxist. If this is the case, exposed dentine surfaces will be worn away more rapidly than the enamel, producing 'cupping' of the contact surfaces (Plate 13.3).

There is some debate in the literature concerning the influence of residual tooth number on the severity of wear on the remaining teeth. There is a logical perception that as the number of contacting teeth decrease the functional load on the remainder would increase and hence the rate of functional surface wear on those teeth would also increase. There is evidence both in favour of this supposition (Ekfeldt *et al.* 1990), and against (Poynter and Wright 1990). Indeed,

Table 13.7 Adjusted odd ratios for factors influencing dental erosion (Jarvinnen *et al.* 1991)

Factor	Adjusted odds ratio	Population-attributable risk (%)
Citrus fruit (> twice daily)	37	26
Vomiting (weekly or more)	31	23
Other gastric (weekly or more)	10	67
Apple vinegar (weekly or more)	10	15
Soft drinks (>4 weekly)	4	26
Sports drinks (weekly or more)	4	15
Unstim. saliva (< 0.1 ml min^{-1})	5	19

Hand *et al.* (1986) reported that tooth wear increased with increasing numbers of teeth, rather than the opposite. Robb (1992) reported tooth wear data on over 1000 dental attenders. He states that there was no association within his data between wear and tooth loss, however in his oldest age group the correlation coefficient between wear and tooth loss was of the order of 0.6 which is likely to be of significance in a multi-factorial problem like tooth wear (Appleton *et al.* 1986).

Abrasion

There are two forms of attack which may be responsible for generalized abrasive wear of the dentition. First, individuals who work in an environment polluted by abrasive dust (i.e. coal mine, brick works), may suffer abrasive wear on any tooth surfaces exposed during speech (Plate 13.4). In addition, functional surface wear may result from the presence of an abrasive paste in their mouths during normal function. Secondly, the use and abuse of dental scaling instruments and/or oral hygiene aids by an individual (Bevenius *et al.* 1988). All of the 'normal' oral hygiene aids can produce abrasive wear. The most common site of damage is exposed root surface, where the softer dentine is easily damaged during oral hygiene. The classical picture is that of a V- or U-shaped defect immediately apical to the cemento-enamel junction (Plate 13.5). This is attributed to improper use of a toothbrush, with a horizontal scrubbing action, the use of excessive force, hard brush bristles, increased brushing frequency, or the use of an abrasive dentifrice.

The over-zealous or improper use of dental floss or inter-dental bottle-brushes, may produce grooving or waisting of the root surface. This is a complication during the maintenance of patients with periodontally involved teeth with extensive root surface exposure.

There is some correlation between the clinical signs of clenching or grinding habits (notably occlusal facetting) and the presence of cervical 'erosions' in the same patient (Xhonga 1977; Pavone 1985). It has been suggested that cervical wear could be exacerbated in upper teeth under functional load on their buccal cusps as a result of tooth flexure under loading and subsequent compression damage to the dentine at the amelo-cemental junction (Levitch *et al.* 1994).

Enamel will also be lost as a result of tooth-brush/dentifrice abrasion. This is unlikely to cause clinically significant damage unless a very abrasive dentifrice is used. Dentifrices designed to remove stain associated with smoking tobacco or those which 'whiten the teeth' are sufficiently abrasive to cause marked enamel damage. Their use should be discouraged.

Localized abrasive wear is usually the result of some form of habit. An example of this would be notching of the incisal edges of teeth as a product of holding pins or tacks between the teeth at work. It has been suggested that an active partial denture clasp may cause cervical abrasion if it rests on a dentine surface.

One final group of individuals for whom abrasive wear may be a problem is the quadraplegics, who often use their teeth as a tool, either for communication or artistic purposes. Great care must be taken to design any necessary appliances to minimize any damage to tooth tissue.

PREVENTION AND MANAGEMENT

The management of a patient presenting with a worn dentition falls into three areas: First, diagnosis, treatment planning, and the elimination of any aetiological factors (if possible). Secondly, the restorative reconstruction of the worn dentition, and thirdly, maintenance where the patient is taught how to care for their mouth without causing further, iatrogenic, wear. (The complexities of treatment planning and restorative reconstruction are beyond the scope of this chapter).

There are few measures, beyond instruction in 'correct' use of oral hygiene aids, which can be regarded as preventing tooth wear. However, there are a number of steps that can be taken, to prevent the condition from getting any worse. These procedures are designed to negate the aetiological factor which dominates the wear process.

Erosion

It is obvious that removal of the decalcifying agents in erosive wear will help to arrest its progress. It should be relatively easy to perform dietary counselling for a subject whose erosion was of dietary origin.

Achlorhydria is a condition where gastric acid secretion is either diminished, or fails. One treatment for this is ingestion of dilute hydrochloric acid, which can cause marked erosive damage. The acid should be sucked through a straw, to minimize contact with tooth surfaces. Two other preparations are now available in tablet form. Unfortunately, the tablets of betaine hydrochloride must be dissolved in water prior to use. This solution is also markedly acidic and must be sucked through a straw.

A number of other medications with low pH have been reported as producing erosive damage (aspirin, chewable Vitamin C, 'iron tonic') (Giunta 1983). The reports have usually involved excessive or abnormal use of these agents.

Erosion as a result of gastric regurgitation may present a more complex problem. Any preventative measures should begin with eliminating the aetiology if at all possible. Subjects who are suspected as suffering from anorexia nervosa with bulimia, or chronic alcoholism should be referred to a physician or psychiatrist for medical help. There are a number of medications which may cause nausea or vomiting as a side-effect. The patient's physician should be consulted to see if an alternative is available. Regurgitation as a result of incompetence of the cardiac sphincter at the base of the oesophagus can cause severe erosion. Once again, medical/surgical advice should be sought.

If there is an obvious time during which reflux/regurgitation occurs, then it may be possible to protect the dentition using a soft splint. This should extend well onto the palatal mucosae in the upper arch, and it may be of benefit to place a fluoride gel or antacid preparation inside the splint before use (Kleier *et al.* 1984).

If the acidic attack is of industrial origin, then appropriate measures should be taken to protect the mouth from acid vapour.

There is some evidence that topical fluoride therapy is of benefit in the control of erosive tooth tissue loss (Davis and Winter 1977).

Definitive reconstruction, utilizing full coronal restorations, should be delayed, in a case of erosive wear, until the aetiological factors involved have been identified and controlled. The marginal gaps around full coronal restorations would be highly susceptible to acid attack, leading to rapidly progressing recurrent decay beneath the restoration, if reconstruction is performed whilst the erosive challenge exists.

Attrition

Wear as a result of normal masticatory function cannot be eliminated, indeed, the current thinking that an increase in dietary fibre is beneficial may result, in time, in an increase in occlusal and interproximal wear. The most difficult problem to be surmounted in the care of a subject with attrition is deciding when the perceived wear is in excess of the physiological 'norm' and thus requires treatment.

The management of a subject with a bruxing habit is complex, depending up the aetiology of the condition. Management regimes can include occlusal splint therapy, either hard or soft, with or without occlusal adjustment, psychotropic medication, and psychological counselling. There is no evidence concerning the effect of any of these treatments upon wear *per se.* However, provision of some form of occlusal splint should be of benefit. Such splints would act as a buffer, preventing tooth to tooth contact. Any wear would be most likely to occur upon the splint itself, rather than the teeth.

It is important to recognize a bruxing habit in subjects who are undergoing restorative care, especially if full coronal restorations are being contemplated. Porcelain is a very hard material, and can have an abrasive surface, if poorly glazed or if it has been adjusted and not glazed. Regular contact with opposing tooth tissue will result in rapid wear of the tooth producing a complicated management problem (Plate 13.6). It is always desirable to produce tooth-to-artificial crown contacts on a metallic surface, or, a highly glazed porcelain surface.

Abrasion

Prevention should again be aimed at removing the cause of the damage. Consequently, the use of an appropriate mask in a dust-laden environment, teaching correct oral hygiene techniques, and an alteration in the habitual use of the teeth as a 'third hand' may all be of benefit in preventing the progression of abrasive wear.

CONCLUSIONS

- Root caries and tooth wear can pose problems in the ageing population, especially amongst certain 'at risk' group.

- Root caries is preventible with rigorous personal, and professional, oral hygiene, but there is a risk of iatrogenic tooth wear.

- Fluoride both in the water supply and as a topical agent reduces caries risk.

- Root caries lesions can be remineralized using flouride solutions, artificial salivas and *remineralizing solutions.*

- Those at high risk include subjects with poor salivary flow, those with high coronal caries scores and those with previous experience of root caries

- The operative management of root caries can be difficult, especially when access for retorative care is poor. Glass ionomer cements are the material of choice.

- Tooth wear is a normal functional phenomenon and can be expected to increase in magnitude with increasing age of the individual concerned.

- Wear is a product of MILD.

- Erosion: Decalcification of surface mineral from dietary acids.

- Attrition: As a result of normal tooth to tooth contact during mastication and deglutition, and from abrasive food substances. This will primarily occur on the occlusal and interproximal tooth surfaces.

- Abrasion: Routine use of a toothbrush and dentifrice will cause some loss of mineralised tissue.

- Excessive wear occurs when one or more of these mechanisms becomes abnormal in its expression.

- The perceived pattern of wear often gives a reasonable indication of the aetiological factors in any one individual.

- Since a degree of wear is normal, the prevention of wear is impracticable.

- Once wear is deemed excessive, progression can be prevented by eliminating, or counteracting, the aetiological factor(s) concerned.

REFERENCES

Aherne, C.A., O'Mullane, D., and Barrett, B.E. (1990). Indices of root surface caries. *J. dent. Res.* **69**, 1222–6.

Appleton, D.R., Rugg-Gunn, A.J., and Hackett, A.F. (1986). Interpretating the correlation coefficient when one of the variables is discrete. *J. dent. Res.* **65**, 1346–8.

Baker, K.A. and Ettinger, R.L. (1985). Intra-oral effects of drugs in elderly persons. *Gerodontics* **1**, 111–16.

Banting, D.W. and Ellen, R.P. (1976). Carious lesions on the roots of teeth: a review for the general practitioner. *J. Can. dent. Ass.* **42**, 496–502.

Banting, D.W. and Stamm, J.W. (1979). Effect of age and length of residence in a fluoridated area on root surface fluoride concentration. *Clin. prev. Dent.* **5**, 7–10.

Banting, D.W., Ellen, R.P., and Fillery, E.D. (1980). Prevalence of root surface caries among institutionalised older persons *Commun. Dent. oral Epidemiol.* **8**, 84–8.

Banting, D.W., Ellen, R.P., and Fillery, E.D. (1985). A longitudinal study of root caries: baseline and incidence data. *J. dent. Res.* **64**, 1141–4.

Baum, B.J. (1986). Salivary gland function during aging. *Gerodontics* **2**, 61–4.

Beck, J.D., *et al.* (1984). Risk factors for various levels of periodontal disease and treatment needs in Iowa *Comm. Dent. oral Epidemiol.*, **12**, 17–22.

Beck, J.D., *et al.* (1986). Root caries: Physical, medical and psychosocial correlates in an elderly population. *Gerodontics* **3**, 242–7.

Beighton, D. and Lynch, E.J.R. (1993). Relationships between yeasts and primary root-caries lesions. *Gerodontology*, **10**, 105–8.

Beighton, D., *et al.* (1991). Salivary levels of mutans streptococci, lactobacilli yeasts and root caries prevalence in non-institutionalized elderly dental populations. *Comm. Dent. oral Epidemiol.* **19**, 302–7.

Bevenius, J., Angmar-Mansson, B., and Thesander, M. (1988). An elderly patient with iatrogenic damage from repeated scaling. *Gerodontics*, **3**, 181–2.

Billings, R.J. and Banting, D.W. (1993). Future directions for root caries research. *Gerodontology* **10**, 114–9.

Billings, R.J., Brown, L.R. and Kaster, A.G. (1985). Contemporary treatment strategies for root surface dental caries. *Gerodontics* **1**, 20–7.

Billings, R.S., *et al.* (1982). *In vitro* studies on treatment of incipient root caries. *J. dent. Res.* **61** (Special issue) 210.

Brustman, B.A. (1986). Impact of exposure to fluoride-adequate water on root surface caries in the elderly. *Gerodontics*, **2**, 203–7.

Canestrari, R.E. (1963). Paced and self-paced learning in young and elderly adults. *J. Gerontol.*, **18**, 165–8.

Chauncey, H.H., Glass, R.L., and Alman, J.E. (1989). Dental caries. Principal cause of tooth extraction in a veteran population. *Caries Res.*, **23**, 200–5.

Cooper, F.F., *et al.* (1986). Shear bond strength of composite resin bonded to laser pretreated dentin. *J. dent. Res.*, **65**, 239.

Daly, T.E., Drane, J.B., and MacComb, W.S. (1972). Management of the problems of the teeth and jaws in patients undergoing irradiation. *Am. J. Surg.*, **124**, 539–42.

Davidson, C.L. and Bekke-Hoekstra, I.S. (1980). The resistance of superficially sealed enamel to wear and carious attack *in vitro*. *J. oral. Rehabil.*, **7**, 299–305.

Davis, B. and Winter, P.J. (1977). Dietary erosion of adult dentine and enamel. Protection with a fluoride toothpaste. *Br. dent. J.*, **143**, 116–9.

Davis, J., Harper, D.S. and Hurst, P.S. (1985). NaF and chlorhexidine for prevention of post-irradiation oral disease. *J. dent. Res.*, **64**, 206.

Dawes, C. and MacPherson, L.M.D. (1993). The distribution of saliva and sucrose around the mouth during the use of chewing gum and the implications for the site specificity of caries and calculus deposition. *J. dent. Res.*, **72**, 852–8.

Denny, P.C., *et al.* (1991). Age-related changes in mucins from human whole saliva. *J. dent. Res.*, **70**, 1320–7.

DePaola, M.S., Soparkar, P.M., and Kent, R.L. (1989). Methodological issues relative to the quantification of root surface caries. *Gerodontology*, **8**, 3–8.

Donachie, M.D., and Walls, A.W.G. (1991). Root caries experience and tooth retention in a group of ageing adults. *J. dent. Res.*, **70**, 684.

Donachie, M.D. and Walls, A.W.G. (in press *a*). The tooth wear index (TWI); A flawed epidemiological tool in an ageing population group *Commun. Dent. oral Epidemiol.*.

Donachie, M.D. and Walls, A.W.G. (in press *b*). An assessment of tooth wear in an ageing population. *J. Dent.*

Douglass, C.W. *et al.* (1983). National trends in the prevalence and severity of periodontal disease. *J. Am. dent. Ass.*, **107**, 403–12.

Ekfeldt, A. *et al.* (1990). An individual tooth wear index and an analysis of factors correlated to incisal and occlusal wear in an Adult Swedish population *Acta odont. Scand.* **48**, 343–9.

Edgar, W.M. and Geddes, D.A.M. (1990). Chewing gum and dental health; a review. *Br. dent. J.*, **168**, 173–7.

Ellen, R.P., Banting, D.W., and Fillery, E.D. (1985*a*). Longitudinal microiological investigation of a hospitalized population of older adults with a high root surface caries risk. *J. dent. Res.* **64**, 1377–87.

Ellen, R.P., Banting, D.W., and Fillery, E.D. (1985*b*). Streptococcus mutans and Lactobacillus detection in the assessment of dental root surface caries risk. *J. dent. Res.*, **64**, 1245–9.

Emilson, C.G. (1994). Potential efficacy of chlorhexidine against mutans streptococci and human dental caries. *J. dent. Res.*, **73**, 682–91.

Fejerskov, O. and Nyvad, B. (1986). Pathology and treatment of dental caries in the aging individual. In *Geriatric dentistry*, (ed. P. Holm-Pedersen and H. Loe), pp. 238–62. Munksgaard, Copenhagen.

Fejerskov, O., *et al.* (1985). Root surface caries in a population of elderly Danes. *J. dent. Res.*, **64**, 187.

Fox, P.C., *et al.* (1985). Xerostomia: evaluation of a symptom of increasing significance. *J. Am. dent. Ass.*, **110**, 519–25.

Fure, S. and Kickert, I. (1990). Prevalence of root surface caries in 55, 65, and 75-year-old Swedish individuals. *Commun. Dent. oral. Epidemiol.*, **18**, 100–5.

Furseth, R. (1970). Further observations on the fine structure of orally exposed and carious human dental cementum. *Archs. oral Biol.*, **16**, 71–7.

Furseth, R. and Johansen, E. (1971). The minimal phase of sound and carious human dental cementum studied by electron microscopy. *Acta odont. Scand.* **28**, 305–13.

Gandara, B.K., *et al.* (1985). Age-related salivary flow rate changes in controls and patients with oral lichen planus. *J. dent. Res.*, **64**, 1149–51.

Gilbert, G.H. and Minaker, K.L. (1990). Principles of surgical risk assessment of the elderly patient. *J. oral. maxillofac. Surg.* **48**, 972–9.

Giunta, J.L. (1983). Dental erosion resulting from chewable vitamin C tablets. *J. Am. dent. Ass.* **107**, 253–6.

Grbic, J.T., *et al.* (1991). Risk indicators for future clinical attachment loss in adult periodontitis. Patient variables. *J. Perio.* **62**, 322–9.

Hals, E. and Selvig, K.A. (1977). Correlated electron probe microanalysis and microradiography of carious and normal dental cementum. *Caries Res.* **11**, 62–75.

Hand, J.S., Hunt, R.J., and Reinhardt, J.W. (1986). The prevalence and treatment implications of cervical abrasion in the elderly. *Gerodontics*, **2**, 167–70.

Hand, J.S., Beck, J.D., and Turner, K.A. (1987). The prevalence of occlusal attrition and considerations for treatment in a non-institutionalised older population. *Spec. Care.*, **7**, 202–6.

Hand, J.S., Hunt, R.J., and Beck, J.D. (1988). Coronal and root caries in older Iowans: 36-month incidence *Gerodontics*, **4**, 136–9.

Hazen, S.P., Chilton, N.W., and Mumma, R.D. (1972). The problem of root caries; 3. A clinical study. *J. dent. Res.*, **51** (suppl), 219.

Heft, M.W. and Baum, B.J. (1984). Unstimulated and stimulated parotid salivary flow rate in individuals of different ages. *J. dent. Res.* **63**, 1182–5.

Hicks, M.J. (1986). Artificial lesion formation around glass-ionomer restorations in root surfaces: a histological study. *Gerodontics*, **2**, 108–14.

Hix, J.O. and O'Leary, T.J. (1976). The relationship between cemental caries, oral hygiene status and fermentable carbohydrate intake. *J. Perio.* **47**, 394–404

Hugosen, A., *et al.* (1988). Prevalence and severity of incisal and occlusal tooth wear in an adult Swedish population. *Acta odont. Scand.*, **46**, 255–65.

Hunt, R.J., Eldredge, J.B., and Beck, J.D. (1989). Effect of residence in a fluoridated community on the incidence of coronal and root caries in an older population. *J. publ. Hlth Dent.* **49**, 138–141.

Järvinnen, V.K., Rytöma, I.I., and Heinonen, O.P. (1991). Risk factors in dental erosion. *J. dent. Res.* **70**, 942–8.

Jensen, M. (1988). The effect of a fluoridated dentifrice on root and coronal caries in an older adult population. *J. Am. dent. Ass.* **117**, 829–32.

Jenkins, G.N. and Edgar, W.M. (1989). The effect of daily gum-chewing on salivary flow rates in man. *J. dent. Res.* **68**, 786–90.

Johansen, E. and Olsen, T. (1979). Topical fluoride in the prevention and arrest of dental caries. In *Continuing evaluation of the use of fluorides*. (ed. E. Johansen, D.R. Taves, and T. Olsen), AAS Selected Symposium 11. West View Press, Boulder, Colorado.

Johansen, E., *et al.* (1987). Remineralization of carious lesions in elderly patients. *Gerodontics*, **3**, 47–50.

Johnson, J.T., *et al.* (1993). Oral pilocarpine for post-irradiation xerostomia in patients with head and neck cancer. *N. Eng. J. Med.* **329**, 390–5.

Jordan, H.V. and Hammond, T.H. (1972). Filamentous bacteria isolated from human root surface caries. *Archs. oral Biol.* **17**, 1333–42.

Joyston-Bechal, S. and Kidd, E.A.M. (1987). The effect of three commercially available saliva substitiutes on enamel *in vitro*. *Br. dent. J.* **163**, 187–90.

Karmen, S. (1975). Tardive dyskinesia. A significant syndrome for geriatric dentistry. *Oral Med., oral Surg., oral Path.* **39**, 52–7.

Katz, S. (1982). The use of fluoride and chlorhexidine for the prevention of radiation caries. *J. Am. dent. Ass.* **104**, 164–70.

Katz, R.V. (1984). Development of an index for the prevelance of root caries. *J. dent. Res.* **63**, 814–8.

Katz, R.V., *et al.* (1982). Prevalence and intra-oral distribution of root surface caries in an adult population. *Caries Res.* **16**, 265–71.

Katz, R.V., Newitter, D.A., and Clive, J.M. (1985). Root caries prevalence in adult dental patients. *J. dent. Res.* **64**, 293.

Kay, E.J. and Blinkhorn, A.S. (1986). The reasons underlying the extraction of teeth in Scotland. *Br. dent. J.* **160**, 287–90.

Keene, H.J., *et al.* (1984). *Lactobacilii* and *S. mutans* in cancer patients using fluoride gels. *J. dent. Res.* **63** (special issue), 281.

Kidd, E.A.M. and Joyston-Bechal, S. (1984). Mouth lubricants and saliva substitutes. *Caries Res.* **18**, 155.

Kidd, E.A.M. (1978). Cavity sealing ability of composite and glass ionomer cement restorations. *Br. dent. J.* **144**, 139–42.

Kleier, D.J., Aragon, S.B., and Averbach, R.E. (1984). Dental management of the chronic vomiting patient. *J. Am. dent. Ass.* **108**, 618–21.

Kmet, P., Boyar, R., and Bowden, G. (1985). Microbial colonization of exposed root surfaces and enamel. *J. dent. Res.* **64** (special issue), 331.

Knibbs, P.J. (1988). Glass ionomer cement: 10 years of clinical use. *J. oral Rehabil.* **14**, 103–15.

Krasse, B. (1984). Can microbiological knowledge be applied in dental practice for the treatment and prevention of dental caries *J. Can. dent. Ass.* **50**, 221–3.

Lavelle, C. (1973). Alveolar bone loss and tooth attrition in skulls from different population samples. *J. Perio. Res.* **8**, 395–9.

Levitch, L.C. *et al.* (1994). Non-carious cervical lesion. (Review). *J. Dent.* **22**, 195–207.

Lindhe, J. and Nyman, S. (1975). The effect of plaque control and surgical pocket elimination on the establishment and maintenance of periodontal health. A longitudinal study of periodontal therapy in cases of advanced disease. *J. clin. Perio.* **2**, 67–79.

Locker, D., Slade, G.D., and Leake J.L. (1989). Prevalence of and factors associated with root decay in older adults in Canada. *J. dent. Res.* **68**, 768–72.

Lohse, W.G., Carter, H.G., and Brunelle, J.A. (1977). The prevalence of root surface caries in a military population. *Milit. Med.* **141**, 700–3.

Luan, W.M., *et al.* (1989). Dental caries in adult and elderly Chinese. *J. dent. Res.* **68**, 1771–6.

MacEntee, M.I., Clark, D.C., and Glick N. (1993). Predictors of caries in old age. *Gerodontology* **10**, 90–7.

McLean, J.W., Wilson, A.D., and Powis, D.R. (1985). The use of glass ionomer cements in bonding composite resins to dentine. *Br. dent. J.* **158**, 410–14.

Markovic, N., Abelson, D.C., and Mandel I.W. (1988). Sorbitol gum in xerostomics: The effects on dental plaque pH and salivary flow rates. *Gerodontology* **7**, 71–5.

Miller, A.J., *et al.* (1987). *Oral health of United States adults*. National Institute of Health Publications, No. 87–2868. United States Department of Health and Human Services. Washington DC, USA.

Muya, R.J., *et al.* (1986). Changing and developing dental health services in Tanzania 1980–2000. (Reported in Fejerskov and Nyvad 1986.)

Närhi, T.O., *et al.* (1992). Association between salivary flow rate and the use of systemic medication among 76-, 81-, and 86-year-old inhabitants in Helsinki, Finland. *J. dent. Res.* **71**, 1875–80.

Nordbo, H. and Skogedal, O. (1982). The rate of cervical abrasion in dental students. *Acta odont. Scand.* **40**, 45–7.

Nyvad, B. and Fejerskov, O. (1982). Root surface caries: clinical, histopathological and microbiological features and clinical implications. *Int. dent. J.* **32**, 311–26.

Nyvad, B. and Fejerskov, O. (1986). Active root surface caries converted into inactive caries as a response to oral hygiene. *Scand. J. dent. Res.* **94**, 281–4.

Pavone, B.W. (1985). Bruxism and its effect on the natural teeth. *J. prosthet. Dent.*, 692–6.

Pederson, W., *et al.* (1985). Age-dependent decreases in human sub-mandibular gland flow rates as measured under resting and post-stimulation conditions. *J. dent. Res.* **64**, 822–5.

Poynter, M.E. and Wright, P.S. (1990). Tooth wear and some factors influencing its severity. *Resr. Dent.* **6**, 8–11.

Ramfjord, S.P. (1987). Maintenance care for treated periodontitis patients. *J. clin. Perio.* **14**, 433–7.

Rashid, M.U. and Bateman, D.N. (1990). Effect of intravenous atropine in human submandibular gland flow rates as measured under resting and post-stimulation conditions. *Br. J. clin. Pharmacol.* **30**, 25–34.

Ravald, N., Hamp, S.E., and Birkhed, D. (1986). Long-term evaluation of root surface caries in periodontally treated patients. *J. clin. Perio.* **13**, 758–67.

Ravald, N., Birkhed, D., and Hamp S.-E. (1993). Root caries susceptibility in periodontally treated patients. Results after 12 years. *J. clin. Perio.* **20**, 124–9.

Robb, N.D. (1992). Epidemiological studies of tooth wear. D. Phil. Thesis. University of London.

Schamschula, R.G., Keyes, P.H. and Hornabrook, R. (1972). Root surface caries in Lufa, New Guinea. 1. Clinical observations. *J. Am. dent. Ass.* **85**, 603–8.

Schamschula, R.G., *et al.* (1974). Prevalence and inter-relationships of root surface caries in Lufa, Papua New Guinea. *Commun. Dent. oral Epidemiol.* **2**, 295–304.

Scheinin, A., *et al.* (1994). Multifactorial modelling for root caries prediction: 3-year follow-up results *Commun. Dent. oral Epidemiol* **22**, 126–9.

Scott, J. (1986). Structure and function in aging salivary glands. *Gerodontics*, 5, 149–58.

Sillness, J., Johansen, G., and Röynstrand, T. (1994). Longitudinal relationship between incisal tooth wear and periodontal condition. *Scand. J. dent. Res.* **102**, 1–4.

Silverstone, L.M. (1975). The acid etch technique: *In vitro* studies with special reference to the enamel surface and the enamel-resin interface. In *Proceedings of the International Symposium on the Acid Etch Technique*, (ed. L.M. Silverstone, I.L. Dogon), pp. 13–39. North Central Publishing, St Pauls, Minnesota.

Smith, B.G.N. and Knight, J.K. (1984*a*). An index for measuring the wear of teeth. *Br. dent. J.* **156**, 435–8.

Smith, B.G.N. and Knight, J.K. (1984*b*). A comparison of patterns of tooth wear with aetiological factors. *Br. dent. J.* **157**, 16–19.

Smith, D.J., *et al.* (1992). Effect of age on immunoglobulin content and volume of human labial gland saliva. *J. dent. Res.* **71**, 1891–4.

Socransky, S.S., Hubersak, C., and Propas, D. (1970). Induction of periodontal destruction in gnotobiotic rats by a human oral strain of *Actinomyces naeslundii*. *Archs. oral Biol.*, **15**, 993–5.

Sognnaes, R.F. (1963). Dental hard tissue destruction with special reference to idiopathic erosion. In *Mechanisms of hard tissue destruction*, p. 91. American Association for the Advancement of Science, Washington, D.C.

Sognnaes, R.F., Wolcott, R.B., and Xhonga, F.A. (1972). Dental erosion. 1. Erosion-like patterns occuring in association with other dental conditions. *J. Am. dent. Ass.* **84**, 571–6.

Stamm, J.W. and Banting, D.W. (1980). Comparison of root caries prevalence in adults with life-long residence in fluoridated and non-fluoridated communities. *J. dent. Res.* **59** (special issue), 405.

Steele, J.G. (1994). The dental status, needs and demands of the elderly in three communities. D. Phil. thesis. University of Newcastle-upon-Tyne.

Sumney, D.L., Jordan, H.V., and Englander, H.R. (1973). The prevalence of root surface decay in selected populations. *J. Perio* **44**, 500–4.

Syed, S.A., *et al.* (1975). Predominant cultivable flora from human root surface carious lesions. *Infect. Immun.* **11**, 727–31.

Tavares, M. (1988). Evaluation of a chemomechanical method of caries removal in root surface lesions. *Quintess. Int.* **19**, 29–32.

Todd, J.E. and Lader, D. (1991). *Adult dental health, 1988: United Kingdom*. HMSO, London.

Ullsfoss, B.N., *et al.* (1994). Effect of a combined chlorhexidine and NaF mouthrinse: an *in vivo* human caries model study. *Scand. J. dent. Res.* **102**, 109–12.

Van Houte J., *et al.* (1990). Association of the microbial flora of dental plaque and saliva with human root-surface caries. *J. dent. Res.* **69**, 1463–8.

Van Wyk, C.W., Farman, A.C. and Staz J. (1977). Tooth survival in institutionalized elderly cape coloreds from the Cape Peninsula of South Africa. *Commun. Dent. oral Epidemiol.* **5**, 185–9.

Vehkalahti, M.M. (1987). Relationship between root caries and coronal decay. *J. dent. Res.* **66**, 1608–10.

Vehkalahti, M.M., *et al.* (1983). Prevalence of root caries in an adult Finnish population. *Commmun. Dent. oral Epidemiol.* **11**, 188–90.

Wallace, M.C., Reteif, D.H., and Bradley, E.L. (1988). Incidence of root caries in older adults. *J. dent. Res.* **67**, 147.

Walls, A.W.G. (1986). Glass polyalkenoate (glass-ionomer) cements: a review. *J. Dent.* **14**, 231–6.

Wescott, W.B., Starcke, E.N., and Shannon, I.L. (1975). Chemical protection against post-irradiation dental caries. *Oral Surg., oral Med., oral Path.* **40**, 709–19.

Westbrooke, J.L., *et al.* (1974). Root surface caries: a clinical, histopathological and microradiographic examination. *Caries Res.* **8**, 249–55.

Westerman, G.H., *et al.* (1994). Argon laser irradiation in root surface caries: *in vitro* study examines laser's effects. *J. Am. dent. Ass.* **125**, 401–7.

Whelton, H.P., Holland, T.J. and O'Mullane, D.M. (1993). The prevalence of root surface caries amongst Irish adults. *Gerodontology*, **10**, 72–5.

Xhonga, F.A. (1977). Bruxism and its effect on the teeth. *J. oral Rehabil.* **4**, 65–76.

Xhonga, F.A. and Valdmanis, S. (1983). Geographic comparisons of the increase of dental erosion: a two centre study. *J. oral Rehabil.* 10, 269–77.

14. Ageing in perspective

J.G. STEELE

INTRODUCTION

The prevention of dental disease is a reasonable end in itself for younger subjects: dental caries in particular is associated with pain, morbidity and cost, and the benefits of disease prevention are obvious. Preventive dentistry for the elderly subject must be viewed in a different perspective. As age increases, the emphasis of prevention moves away from the diseases themselves and towards a wider strategy aimed at the prevention of a condition: dental disability, usually resulting from tooth loss. In addition, difficult questions have to be asked about how preventive and treatment resources can be used most efficiently, as the costs of care have the potential to rise while the benefits may diminish. This chapter will discuss prevention in the context of dental disability rather than the prevention of specific diseases (these are covered elsewhere in this book). In this context the term prevention may be primary (measures to prevent disease from occurring, such as fluoride use or oral hygiene), secondary (measures to prevent disease progressing by early detection and management, such as dental attendance for early treatment of caries) or tertiary (measures to avoid the disability resulting from disease, such as the placement of prosthetic tooth replacements).

The proportion of the population who are elderly is increasing all over the world (Craig 1983; Thompson 1987; OPCS 1991), whilst in most Western countries the proportion of them who retain a natural dentition is also increasing, in some cases rapidly (NIH 1987; Todd and Lader 1991; Willemsen 1994). Elderly people are more likely to be edentulous, and where they are dentate their number of teeth decreases with age. Root caries is more extensive and more prevalent (Katz 1980; Katz et al. 1982; Banting 1986), periodontal attachment loss increases with age (Goodson et al. 1982; Lindhe and Nyman 1984; Albander et al. 1986; Okamoto et al. 1988) and there may be an increased risk of continuing loss (Grbic et al. 1991; Grbic and Lamster 1992), whilst reduced salivary flow as a result of medication may exacerbate any existing problems. The differences between the elderly and the rest of the population are mostly of degree, and the strategies available for the prevention of such diseases are little different from those used for any adult at risk.

If the ultimate goal is to prevent disability as a result of dental problems, the prevention of dental disease is an essential step by which this can be realized, but it is not the only consideration. A number of side issues may determine what preventive strategies are most appropriate. These include individual variations in the risk of dental disease and limitations on the ability to receive care as a result of medical, social or economic constraints. Prevention of all disease in every case may not be an appropriate philosophy, and the concept of priority for different items of care may become increasingly important.

One further point should be made. Just as there is no age at which someone becomes officially elderly, any change in the emphasis of dental care is not sudden, occurring at some predetermined stage of life, but is gradual and dictated by individual considerations. Old age can last a long time. In most Western countries life expectancy is over 70 years and many individuals survive for considerably longer. As age increases so does life expectancy (OPCS 1994). Prevention of dental disability is required for the rest of a person's life. Table 14.1 shows life expectancy for adults at different ages and illustrates that the average years of life remaining, even for over-70-year-olds (11–14 years), is often considerably longer than the life of a conventional amalgam restoration. However, there is marked individual variation in the ageing process and biological ageing is still the subject of various theories (Martin 1992). The potential for discrepancy between biological and chronological age is well known and applies in dentistry as much as in any other aspect of health.

Table 14.1. Life expectancy at different ages: UK 1991

| Age | Life expectancy | |
	Males	Females
Birth	73.0	78.5
50	25.8	30.4
60	17.6	27.7
70	11.0	14.2
80	6.4	8.1

LONG-TERM CHANGES IN THE ORAL HEALTH OF OLDER ADULTS

In most Western countries patterns of oral health are changing. For most of this century, being over 60 years old has been associated with being edentulous and the need to prevent dental caries or periodontal disease was a priority of the young. Consequently the dental concerns of older adults were given little attention. In the last quarter of this century the combination of centrally subsidized dental treatment, preventive programmes, the widespread availability of fluoride toothpastes, increased personal wealth and changing attitudes to dental health have resulted in lower levels of disease (particularly caries) in young adults, and heavily restored but natural dentitions in middle-aged and older adults (Todd and Lader 1991). At the same time, life expectancy is increasing resulting in numerically more older adults. So change is occurring on two fronts, the number of older adults is increasing and the proportion of them who have natural teeth is also increasing.

Reliable national data collected over a long time scale are difficult to come by. However, in the UK data has been available over a 20-year period (1968–88) based on three national adult dental health surveys at 10-year intervals (Gray *et al.* 1970; Todd and Walker 1980; Todd *et al.* 1982; Todd and Lader 1991). Figure 14.1 shows the changes in edentulousness measured over this period and gives the statistical projections for the future based on these data. It shows that more and more people in each age band are retaining some natural teeth and are retaining them into later life. The overall incidence of edentulousness in all but the oldest groups will become very low. The UK data indicates not only that more elderly people are likely to have natural teeth in the future, but also, that they are likely to have more of them than dentate people in previous generations. Furthermore many of the standing teeth will be restored. Figure 14.2 gives the number of filled teeth in different age groups which indicates that the number of restorations in the over 65-year-olds may treble or quadruple over a 20-year period.

The statistical projections for edentulousness based on this data show a continuing reduction in the number of edentulous people well into the next century. However, a word of caution must be made about this forecast. The predictions are purely statistical and are based largely on the observed incidence of edentulousness in younger and middle-aged adults. It is still not certain whether the improved dental health of the young can be sustained through advanced age in the

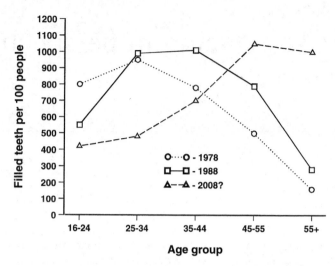

Fig. 14.2. Number of filled teeth per 100 people (dentate and edentulous combined) at different ages in 1978 and 1988, and an *eyeball* prediction for 2008 based on changes between 1978 and 1988.

whole population, particularly against a background of heavily restored teeth and enhanced dental risk. Furthermore, when edentulousness occurs (as it will continue to do, albeit at a reduced rate) little is known about the sequence of events which bring it about.

The trends which have been described for the UK are probably reflected in most other European and North American countries (Willemsen 1994). In other nations the demographic changes resulting from alterations in life expectancy and birth rate may provide sufficient stimulus in themselves to focus on the preventive needs in the elderly.

THE POSSIBILITIES FOR ORAL HEALTH IN OLDER ADULTS

The previous section gave some indication of the trends with age in terms of oral health. It is also important try to define our ultimate goal and to decide precisely what condition we want to prevent. It may often not be appropriate to attempt to prevent every tooth from being extracted or every millimetre of periodontal attachment from being lost. There will be limits on the provision of care; these may be economic or related to attitudes, medical or dental considerations. If an individual dentist or planner of health services is to make a decision about what constitutes appropriate care for the elderly, a clear long-term strategy with a defined oral health goal is required.

OPTIMUM ORAL HEALTH

Cohen (Cohen and Henderson 1991) has described the concepts of 'perfect health' and 'optimum health', and the distinction between the two is useful when trying to identify goals for the elderly. From a biological perspective 'perfect health' has been defined as 'the state in which every cell is functioning at optimum capacity and in perfect harmony with each other cell' (Twaddle 1974). An often quoted 1958

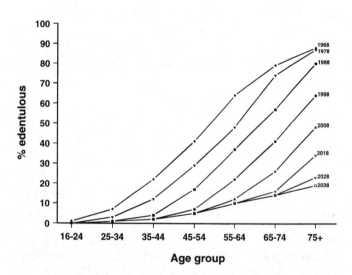

Fig. 14.1. Percentage of adults edentulous by age group in 1968, 1978, and 1988 (England and Wales) and predictions until 2038 (UK) based on the continuation of past incidence of edentulousness. (Data from Todd and Lader 1991.)

World Health Organization definition of health takes a much wider, less biological approach and describes health as 'a state of complete physical and mental well being' (WHO 1958). Whilst these definitions cover health in its widest sense, they could just as easily be applied to the narrower area of oral health. 'Perfect oral health' is not difficult to understand, but in itself it is not a particularly useful concept. According to the strictly biological definition, it would required 32 teeth which are totally undiseased in a mouth which harbours no disease and where the occlusion is ideal. To set this as an objective would be meaningless as it is unachievable by all but a tiny minority, and even where it was possible the cost of achieving and maintaining it would be prohibitive. The concept of 'optimum oral health' is useful. 'Optimum health' has been defined as 'that state where the cost of any improvement outweighs the value attached to the improvement' (Cohen and Henderson 1991). The terms 'cost' and 'value' may be interpreted purely in terms of economics, but could just as readily be applied to quality of life or any other major parameter by which health is assessed. 'Optimum oral health' is a useful concept for any age group but the change which occurs as age increases involves a shift in the balance between the cost and the value of the care, making it particularly appropriate for the elderly.

At this point it may be useful to give an example related to an individual case. Tooth wear is often quoted as a particular problem in the elderly, and this may be justified, but let us consider the same clinical condition in two adults with a 40-year age difference between them. A good example may be a mouth that contains between 20 and 24 teeth all of which are worn, with extensive exposure of dentine on posterior and particularly anterior teeth (see Plate 14.1). In a 25-year-old this may trigger extensive and expensive restorative treatment to protect the dentition from the wear which has clearly been progressing rapidly over the 15 years or so that the permanent dentition has been established. Crowns or onlays would be used which would involve the time and skill of an experienced dentist, the time and skill of an experienced technician, and the use of expensive and highly specialized techniques and materials (Watson and Tulloch 1985). In this case, the financial cost would be high, but the value may also be high. For example, the patient's aesthetics may be greatly improved at a time of life when this is likely to be of some importance, whilst further wear would also be prevented. Given that this dentition may have another 60 years or more of life left and has only taken about 10–15 years to reach its worn state, intervention to prevent further wear could be deemed to be essential to ensure the long-term future of a natural dentition.

A 65-year-old may have a similar pattern of wear (see Plate 14.2). If a set of study models and radiographs were consulted without reference to the patient's age the same treatment might be prescribed at the same cost. However, the value of the intervention may be considerably less. The patient's teeth have taken 50 years to reach this stage, the wear is not progressing rapidly, and will probably not threaten the dentition in the patient's lifetime. Discomfort, sensitivity, and possibly the risk of aesthetic complaints are less likely than they would be in the younger subject. Furthermore, the care may be more difficult or complex to

deliver and the subject may be less likely to demand complex treatment to prevent further wear.

This example illustrates some of the issues which should be considered in order to keep the preventive needs of elderly people in perspective. In the 65-year-old, optimum health resulting in equivalent value could have been obtained at a much lower cost, given the differences in terms of benefits to the quality of life and the required longevity of the dentition.

IS THERE A MINIMUM DENTITION CONSISTENT WITH FUNCTION AND SATISFACTION?

In order to prevent disability resulting from dental problems in the elderly it is important to know at what stage of functional impairment problems are likely to occur in most people. Much work has been done on the effect of tooth loss on normal and efficient function. Most has been based purely on mechanical considerations, and the following statements broadly sum up the findings:

1. Natural teeth are mechanically more efficient than complete dentures and the more natural teeth that are present the better is the mechanical function of the dentition (Manly and Braley 1950; Helkimo *et al.* 1978; Kayser 1981; Chauncey *et al.* 1984; Luke and Lucas 1985; Oosterhaven *et al.* 1988).

2. An artificial or a poor natural dentition may not function as efficiently as a full set of natural teeth, but this does not appear to affect the ability to digest food (Farrell 1956, 1957).

3. Limitation in dietary choice as a result of difficulty in chewing appears not to affect nutrition adversely, although there may be exceptions and there is scope for further research (Neill and Phillips 1970; Bates *et al.* 1971; Heath 1972, Hartsook 1974, Baxter 1984; Chauncey *et al.* 1984; Halling *et al.* 1988).

4. Around 20 or more teeth is consistent with adequate and comfortable function in most people, particularly where teeth are well positioned and form opposing pairs. Once again there will be individual exceptions (Agerberg and Carlsson 1981; Kayser 1981; Battistuzzi *et al.* 1987; Kayser 1990).

5. Despite their inferior mechanical function, many complete denture wearers are every bit as satisfied with their dental status and ability to function as their counterparts with natural teeth (Bergman and Carlsson 1972; Steele 1994).

If these points are distilled down further we get to a figure of 20 teeth as a realistic and reasonable minimum to provide satisfactory mechanical function, although the ability to function, dietary limitation, and satisfaction are subject to large individual variation. Kayser (1981) has suggested that this requirement may diminish further with age, although the evidence to support this is limited.

However, this approach has so far only given the teeth a mechanical role. Teeth have a number of other functions, particularly related to aesthetics and social interaction. Satisfaction with aesthetics has an important impact on oral health (Cushing *et al.* 1986) and missing anterior teeth are one of a number of possible sources of dissatisfaction with aesthetics. Speech impairment may also be associated with tooth loss or the replacement of missing teeth. Both aesthetics and speech have important social roles, so aesthetics and speech which are satisfactory (to the subject), or at least which are not impaired as a result of the loss of teeth, could be added as qualifiers to the minimum number of teeth.

One further qualification needs to be added. Dental pain and discomfort may have a substantial impact on people's daily life (Cushing *et al.* 1986). Furthermore, pain and discomfort are common in the elderly. Smith (Smith and Sheiham 1980) found that a third of a sample of over 65-year-old people reported pain from their mouths, whilst in another study 7–10 per cent of dentate over 65-year-olds had had pain in the previous 4 weeks and up to a quarter reported sensitivity (Steele 1994). In the same sample, mobile teeth, pain, and sensitivity were all found to contribute to dissatisfaction. Freedom from pain or discomfort, and a dentition where the likelihood of pain or discomfort occurring has been minimized, could be seen as a reasonable additional goal. In practice, this probably means a mouth which has been well maintained by both subject and dental personnel.

In summary, a minimum of 20 teeth, free from pain or discomfort and with no unrestored anterior spaces leading to impaired social functioning, is a reasonable goal for the population or for an individual. This may require modification in some cases, but would appear to be a sensible minimum for most. At present, this is unachievable by many people, whilst younger adults, who may only just achieve this minimum standard, risk dropping below it if further teeth are lost. In the long term, preventive strategies should be aimed at the widespread maintenance of this minimum level of oral health, for life where possible. Where the target is unachievable, as is the case with the majority of the present elderly population in the UK, strategies should be aimed at preventing the decline to late onset tooth loss or to minimizing the resultant disability where tooth loss occurs.

Furthermore, some tooth loss may be inevitable in old age, even where the dentition is apparently in good condition and well maintained, so this minimum standard of 20 teeth in good condition may be insufficient for the 'young old' (for example those in their 60s and early 70s). More teeth may be required in order to ensure that there is enough in reserve to accommodate further tooth loss later in life if necessary.

LIMITING FACTORS IN THE PURSUIT OF ORAL HEALTH IN OLDER ADULTS

The possibility of preventing oral disability and achieving a functional comfortable and satisfactory dentition based on 20 or more natural teeth may be limited by a range of complicating factors. These are discussed below.

Missed Targets

In the UK in 1988, only 21 per cent of over 65-year-old dentate adults (representing only 7 per cent of all over 65-year-old adults) had more than 20 teeth. A much smaller

Table 14.2. Percentage of adults in the UK with 21 or more standing teeth and 21 or more standing teeth with no spaces by different age groups: 1988

Age	Base	21 + teeth (%)	21 + teeth (and no spaces (%)
16–24	493	100	83
25–34	490	96	66
35–44	460	90	19
45–54	264	72	8
55–64	115	48	8
65+	42	23	3

proportion (only 2 per cent of dentate older adults) had these aligned in two good arches without spaces (see Table 14.2) (Todd and Lader 1991; Gordon *et al.* 1994). A random sample of older Dutch adults showed a similar distribution (Van Waas *et al.* 1993). Such individuals, those who are dentate but have few teeth, are the ones for whom it is most difficult to modify a target. The ultimate objective of preserving function, preventing disability, and providing satisfaction are unchanged, but this cannot usually be done with natural teeth alone and the circumstances will often preclude the provision of fixed prostheses. Partial dentures may provide a temporary solution by fulfilling the aesthetic and possibly the functional objectives. Restorative intervention (such as endodontic and periodontal treatment and the provision of complex restorations) may prevent further tooth loss for a time, but the need for such intervention may accelerate as increasingly complex problems arise from the ultimate failure of previous restorations. In the recent past, the situation may have been remedied by the provision of complete dentures, often at a young age. Whilst such a scenario would now be regarded as undesirable and is seen as a failure, it did ensure that denture wearers were provided with their first prostheses at a time when they were more able to adapt. Attitudes have changed and the present generations of dentate adults are more apprehensive about the prospect of edentulousness than in the past. The data presented in Table 14.3 provides a useful indication of how attitudes to edentulousness have changed (Todd and Lader 1991). The concern is that, in attempting to prevent edentulousness, we may be doing no more than delaying it, and slowing the process of tooth loss, so that edentulousness results at a time of life when the ability to adapt, both physiologically and psychologically, is diminished (Rabins 1992).

In those who are already edentulous the target is limited to the provision of satisfactory prostheses which will aid function, provide for the patients' aesthetic needs, and prevent the

Table 14.3. Percentage of dentate adults, in different age groups, who said that they would be very upset at total tooth loss: 1968–88

Age	1968 (%)	1988 (%)
16–34	27	60
35+	27	54

development of soft tissue lesions. Where dentures cannot be supported comfortably by the natural mucosa (and where finance can stretch to such a luxury) implant systems may help to prevent the disability and handicap which would otherwise result.

However, the first priority must be to look ahead and minimize the problem in future generations (those presently aged less than 60) by ensuring that adults arrive at old age still able to achieve a reasonable minimum standard of oral health based on natural teeth. As for the present, the best means of preventing disability, discomfort, and dissatisfaction will vary depending on individual circumstances. In some cases, it may be necessary to remove many or most of the remaining teeth and to provide complete overdentures, in others conventional primary prevention to try and retain every tooth may be in order. In all cases, the ultimate objective needs to be kept in sight: the long-term prevention of disability, discomfort, and dissatisfaction.

DENTAL FACTORS AS LIMITATIONS

Some older subjects are at substantially greater risk of dental disease than others, and this may limit the ability to achieve a minimum target for oral health based on natural teeth. Recent work in an older UK population has shown that teeth which are unsound as a result of root caries are concentrated in a minority of the older population, such that the most severely affected 20 per cent of the population account for 75 per cent of all of the active lesions (Steele 1994). Severe tooth wear problems are also restricted to a small proportion of the population (Robb 1992; Steele 1994), whilst the skewed distribution of severe periodontal disease has been recognized for some time (Johnson *et al.* 1988; Papapanou *et al.* 1988). The nature of such cases of enhanced risks is probably complex and will include interactions between a range of genetic, environmental, medical, and behavioural factors. For example, dry mouth (particularly as a result of the use of commonly prescribed medications) is clearly an important additional risk factor in the elderly. When combined with high levels of plaque (due to irregular tooth-brushing) and a diet high in fermentable carbohydrate, this risk will be further enhanced. Some dental conditions can also interact to enhance risks. Periodontal disease leading to attachment loss will predispose the development of root caries (by exposing vulnerable surfaces), whilst excessive wear can result in caries of exposed dentine on coronal surfaces (particularly in the presence of dry mouth).

Much of the increased risk of dental disease may be iatrogenic in origin. Overcut or poorly designed cavities may lead to fracture of tooth or restoration, or to irreversible pulpal damage. As many as 10–15 per cent of crown preparations have been found to be non-vital after 5–10 years (Bergenholtz and Nyman 1984; Felton *et al.* 1989). Overhanging restorations may act as plaque traps and predispose to periodontal attachment loss or caries at the margin. Partial dentures, often placed as an aesthetic imperative to restore the dentition after teeth have been lost, may significantly increase the risk of dental caries and periodontal disease. The issue of the risks presented to the remaining teeth by the placement of partial dentures deserves specific attention in the context of the elderly where such restorations are often required to counteract the effect of tooth loss. Bergman *et al.* (1982) showed that there was no difference between wearers and non-wearers where an aggressive prophylactic and self-care regime was instituted. However, these demanding criteria in terms of cleanliness are probably met only rarely outside clinical trials. In the real world, plaque control is not perfect. A number of recent studies have demonstrated the damaging effect of partial dentures, particularly with respect to root caries (Wright *et al.* 1992; Drake and Beck 1993). When a wide variety of factors are combined in a multivariate model, the presence of partial dentures are one of the major risk factors, doubling the odds of root caries being present (Steele 1994). It is ironic that a prosthesis placed to restore the function of teeth which have been lost as a result of disease, itself increases the chances of further teeth being lost and may accelerate the process of becoming edentulous. Seen against such a background, partial dentures could be viewed, in some cases, as little more than transitional restorations on the path to edentulousness. Preventive dentistry may involve the placement of alternative restorations, such as adhesive bridges which represent a simple and cost-effective alternative in many such cases.

For all these additional dental risks, effective prevention depends on recognizing the problem and tailoring individual strategies to reduce it. The interventions required in the situations described above will vary tremendously from conventional primary preventive measures, such as fluoride application or improved oral hygiene, through to secondary or tertiary measures such as modification or replacement of restorations. The point is that they all depend on the recognition of the specific problems and the additional steps required to address them.

MEDICAL AND PHYSICAL LIMITATIONS

Despite the common image of older people confined to sagging chairs or hobbling with the aid of zimmer frames, and the column inches in dental journals devoted to the provision of dental care to old people unable to leave home or to tolerate intervention, most older adults (over the age of 60, for the sake of argument) are mobile and self-reliant, especially in the developed world. Data from a random sample of older adults in the UK indicates that around a third of the over 60-year-olds had some sort of disability, but that in the majority of cases this was mild. Both the frequency of disability and its severity tend to increase with age, particularly over the age of 80 years. The range of disabilities is wide and their severity highly variable, but difficulties with locomotion and personal care are the most common forms, and both might have some bearing on the ability to maintain a reasonable standard of oral health (Martin *et al.* 1988*a*, 1988*b*).

Oral health problems may be complicated because of an inability to obtain care as a result of disability, for example, where a subject is housebound and unable to reach a dentist. Further insight into the scale of this problem may be obtained by examining the proportion who cannot leave home. Only 6 per cent of 60 to 74-year-olds and 18 per cent of over 75-year-olds who lived in a private household were unable to leave home at all, and most of those who could get out could manage without any assistance. It is reasonable to assume that a large majority of over 60-year-olds would be able to visit the dentist's surgery. In other circumstances, the subject may be able to reach a dentist but treatment is compromised, for example where the dentist has difficulty providing good-quality care because of the involuntary movements of Parkinson's disease, or where the patient cannot be treated supine due to musculoskeletal or cardiovascular problems. The scale of such problems in the community as a whole is unknown but they become more likely with increasing age.

It may be possible for the professional to provide, and the patient to receive quality treatment, but this may be compromised by the patient's inability to maintain the dentition in good condition because of difficulties with oral hygiene. A wide range of specific conditions may be responsible, for example, severe chronic arthritis, any neurological disturbances of motor function (stroke victims, Parkinson's disease, neuromuscular disease) and perhaps also painful oral mucosal conditions. However, among even the most severely disabled UK adults a majority are able to wash their hands and face (Martin *et al.* 1988*a*) and could perhaps be expected to perform the most basic oral preventive measures, such as fluoride mouth rinsing, even if brushing is not possible. Where there is a problem of this nature steps to address it can be taken. A range of alternatives to conventional tooth-brushes are available and may be appropriate for some elderly people, whilst straightforward regular prophylaxis may be enough to prevent deterioration of the oral condition in others: the provision of domiciliary care from a hygienist may be a cost-effective way of providing this. Education of carers is a priority for dependent elderly.

Medical conditions and their resultant disabilities can lead to an impaired ability to achieve oral health in one other way. Where medical problems are severe, or a chronic debilitating illness exists, there may be a tendency for oral health to seem trivial and 'not worth the effort'. In many circumstances this is understandable. On the other hand, if subjects reach this stage with a reasonable dentition the effort required to maintain at least one aspect of their own well-being in good condition may not be great. Where older adults can be empowered (by proper instruction and education) to take care of their own oral health the benefits in terms of self-esteem and general well-being, may extend well beyond the teeth themselves.

Disability and problems of mobility are common in the elderly, but most of the difficulties which may have an impact on oral health are experienced by the very old. If priority is given to ensuring that older adults arrive at this stage with a comfortable, functional, and satisfactory natural dentition, a minimum standard of oral health should be easy to maintain using simple primary preventive measures when problems of disability do arise (in the very old). Such measures are much easier to deliver in a domicillary setting than conventional restorative care.

DENTAL NON-ATTENDANCE AS A LIMITING FACTOR

Oral health in the elderly varies with age, gender, social, class and, in some areas, race (NIH 1987; Todd and Lader 1991).

Underpinning these observed variations are economic distinctions and cultural trends leading to differences in attitudes and ultimately behaviour. Dental attendance pattern is one of the most obvious manifestations of these behavioural variations and it is one that may limit significantly the possibility of maintaining a functional natural dentition.

Not everybody goes to the dentist for check-ups. This is not a profound statement which will come as a surprise to anybody reading it, but it is very important. Whether or not an older person visits the dentist for check-ups is probably one of the principal determinants of oral health in the dentate elderly. Attendance pattern may underlie much of the variation in the oral condition according to social and demographic variables, and it is something that it may be possible to modify. The importance of dental attendance pattern was shown in a recent study of UK adults. Steele *et al.* (Steele 1994) found that 16–18 per cent of over 60-year-old dentate subjects who visited the dentist only when they had problems had 21 or more standing teeth. This is in contrast to the subjects who attended for voluntary check-ups (even if these were not regular) of whom around 45 per cent had 21 or more teeth. The rate of untreated decay was at least double in the non-attenders what it was in the attenders, whilst moderate or severe tooth wear and widespread advanced attachment loss were both more frequent in non-attenders. Edentulous subjects were not included in the analysis reported above, but only a tiny proportion of them attended for check-ups.

Attendance pattern has shown some signs of improvement. In the UK, 50 per cent of all dentate adults over the age of 65 were regular dental attenders in 1988, compared with only 38 per cent in 1978. This is partly due to the fact that recent generations of younger adults have shown more regular attendance patterns than their predecessors. This is illustrated well by data from the Irish national survey which shows that younger dentate groups were more likely to have been regular attenders as children than the over 65-year-olds (O'Mullane and Whelton 1992). However, data from the past 25 years has suggested that it is not just a cohort effect we are witnessing, but that adults, particularly those who were young in the 1960s, have shown an increasing propensity to attend the dentist on a regular basis as they have aged. One cohort follow-up study in the Netherlands showed an increase of about 10 to 15 per cent in the proportion of adults who attended for a 6-monthly check-ups in the same cohorts between 1986 and 1992 (Willemsen 1994). It is possible to predict confidently that there will be a far larger number of dental attenders in future generations of elderly than there were in the past. Nevertheless, even in the current middle-aged in the UK, over a quarter only attend when driven by problems (Todd and Lader 1991). In the USA over a third of middle-aged dentate adults had not attended in the previous year and in Finland half said that they never attended for check-ups (NIH 1987; Vehkalhati and Paunio 1988).

If attendance is such a critical factor for oral health, dental non-attendance and the attitudes and circumstances which predispose to it, must be among the most important impediments to the goal of preventing oral disability. Before it is possible to change attitudes and attendance behaviours it is first necessary to understand what stops people attending, particularly the elderly. Three major categories of barrier have been identified: fear, image (of dentist and surgery), and cost (Finch *et al.* 1988; Todd and Lader 1991). Whilst a number of authors have identified these barriers as important, their relative importance varies (Fiske *et al.* 1990; Schou and Eadie 1991; Wilson 1991). Others have suggested additional barriers, such as the physical distances involved in a dental visit for rural communities, or simply negative attitudes (Kandelman and Lepage 1982). The effect of age is very difficult to clarify as some studies have looked at all age groups and others only at the elderly, and often there is no distinction made between dentate and edentulous. Both the 1988 UK national adult dental health survey and the 1989–90 Irish survey appeared to show that, in the dentate, *fear* barriers were less important in the elderly, whilst *image* and *cost* barriers were relatively more important, although the distinctions were subtle. For many older dentate non-attenders the most commonly reported reason for non-attendance was that many subjects felt that there was no need to go or that they simply could not be bothered (O'Mullane and Whelton 1992; Steele 1994). Of course, such reported reasons may conceal other barriers such as fear or cost.

Cost as a Limiting Factor in its Own Right

Cost has been widely reported as a reason for non-attendance in the elderly (Hoad-Reddick *et al.* 1987; Tobias and Smith 1987; MacEntee *et al.* 1988; Fiske *et al.* 1990; Todd and Lader 1991) However, Wilson (1991) noted that although fear was the most important reason for older adults not visiting the dentist, cost was the most important barrier to old people actually receiving the treatment they needed once they got there (Wilson 1991). So cost may present an obstacle to the prevention of dental disability in two ways. First, by reducing the likelihood of dental attendance (particularly when check-ups incur a cost), and secondly, by limiting the scope and complexity of treatment which can be afforded.

Comprehensive oral health care which is completely state-supported is now rare. Increasingly, the patient has to pay for most or all of the treatment either directly or through an insurance scheme. Financial considerations are therefore a major influence on the ability to meet the sort of minimum requirement for a natural dentition which has already been noted, so problems of economics will be discussed in more detail.

Because wealth is highly variable between individuals and populations it is difficult to make any bold and unequivocal statement about the disposable income of older adults. It will fluctuate continually depending on a wide range of factors: some people will always be rich and others relatively poor. However, the cost of the maintence which is required simply in order to prevent tooth loss has the potential to escalate in the elderly. As more tooth substance is lost through caries and the replacement of failed restorations, the work necessary to put it right becomes more complex. Where problems progress to involve the dental pulp, endodontics will be more difficult and time-consuming, and hence potentially more costly, than may be the case in a younger person. With the progressive loss of periodontal attachment the chance of treatment being complicated by involvement of furcations is increased.

The importance of wealth as a limitation to the provision of care also depends on the value placed by an individual or a population on oral health. As we have already seen, there is some evidence that natural teeth are becoming a commodity that is increasingly valued (Todd and Lader 1991). The role of the dental practitioner is to keep in sight the ultimate objective of care, that is the long-term prevention of disability, discomfort, and dissatisfaction. It is then the job of the professional to find a programme of prevention and treatment which can be managed within the financial limitations which prevail, but which still meet that objective. Appropriate management concepts, such as the shortened dental arch, which encompass preventive principles and take account of economic limitations, are available and will be discussed further in the next section.

APPROPRIATE MANAGEMENT CONCEPTS FOR THE DENTATE AGEING PATIENT

An oral health goal for the elderly has been identified: the prevention of disability resulting from dental problems. A minimum standard which would maximize the possibilty of this being achieved for most of the population has been identified: 20 or more natural teeth in good condition which provide satisfactory function and aesthetics to the patient without pain or discomfort. This may not be an ideal definition of a minimum standard but it is workable and backed up by some scientific evidence. This minimum would have to be present for an entire lifetime, which may mean that a greater number of teeth are required in middle or early old age in order to provide something in reserve. The factors which may limit the ability to maintain this level of health have also been discussed. It would be helpful if management strategies could be identified by which the the objectives may be achieved, given the limitations which have already been discussed.

In the case of subjects who are elderly or who are approaching old age there are two basic treatment planning approaches:

1. There is a short-term aim; to carry out treatment as dental problems arise or are forseen. Where resources can accomodate it this may result in the long-term aim of attempting to retain every tooth. Where this ideal is unachievable, teeth are treated on an individual basis according to the need and resources at the time.

2. Treatment is prioritized so that some teeth are always given priority over others as part of a defined long-term strategy. The long-term aim may be the same as in the first case (to retain every tooth), but where resources or the ability to deliver care are limited, certain teeth are specifically targeted as important and others may have to be abandoned. *Shortened dental arch* is an example of this approach.

Many dentists may use a bit of both, but often there is an absence of any long-term plan, other than perhaps the rather vague one of saving teeth. The risk of having no long-term aim or strategy is that, when resources cannot stretch or when the treatment cannot be delivered to every tooth, treatment is provided on a random basis and tooth loss may occur in a haphazard way leading to an early loss of function. This in turn may neccesitate the use of removable prostheses which could in turn result in generally increased levels of disease. Plate 14.3 shows an example of the dentition resulting where the former approach has been used. Teeth have been treated and ultimately removed as needs have arisen and although the patient is dentate in both arches there are no occlusal contacts and, function is seriously impaired to the point at which the patients quality of life is adversely affected. Partial dentures are required in order to provide some aesthetic and masticatory satisfaction and these may have a role in the continuing high level of disease. Plate 14.4, on the other hand, illustrates a case where a clear long-term strategy has been followed, in this case towards a shortened dental arch. This patient is also dentate in both arches, but here the tooth contacts have been maximized to give the optimum function given the limited number of teeth available and there is no need of a partial denture to provide aesthetic satisfaction.

The second strategy has the advantage of a long-term, clearly defined objective, although in many cases, the ultimate result (if all goes to plan) may be similar to that for the first (a complete dentition). However, it is underpinned by two fundamental principles. The first is that prevention (primary, secondary, or tertiary) must be appropriate to the ultimate objective, so there is no point going overboard to prevent the loss of teeth which are difficult to save or unimportant in the context of function. The second is that, like it or not, there will often be financial limitations to what is possible, and that care may need to be prioritized where resources are finite.

In 1981, Kayser described a treatment-planning philosophy which he called the 'shortened dental arch' (Kayser 1981). This is an example of the second approach, where there is a clear long-term strategy and prioritization of care.

Shortened Dental Arch

The shortened dental arch (SDA) treatment planning philosophy is based on the understanding that within a dentition some parts are of greater strategic importance than others. It acknowledges that a full functioning dentition is the theoretical ideal, but also takes into account some of the limitations which have already been identified, especially financial ones (Kayser and Witter 1985; Kayser 1990). It is based on the principle that the strategic parts of the dentition (the incisors and canines for aesthetics and the premolars for masticatory function) are given priority over the molars which are perceived to be of less strategic importance. This results from the finding that a minimum of four occlusal units (pairs of opposing teeth) are compatible with satisfactory occlusal function, and that molar teeth are the first to be lost, are more difficult and expensive to retain and have no more than a minimal influence on aesthetics. Resources are targeted from the front backwards; anteriors take priority over first premolars, which would normally take priority over second premolars, although the overall objective would be to maintain all eight premolars as an absolute minimum, and to retain two unbroken dental arches of reduced length. This,

incidently, would be a shortened arch of 20 teeth, so SDA philosophy is built around the minimum requirement described earlier in this chapter, except that SDA actually identifies which 20 teeth should be retained. Molar teeth only receive preventive care and restorative treatment if resources allow. Where the integrity of the arch is broken by missing teeth, spaces may be filled using fixed bridgework, the development of adhesive techniques would seem to be a particularly useful development in these conditions. Partial dentures appear not to improve function in shortened dental arches (Witter *et al.* 1989), and in view of their ability to cause further damage to the tissues it would seem sensible to avoid their use. One of the primary justifications for using this approach is to avoid the need for partial dentures.

It is important to regard shortened dental arch as much more than just 16 or 20 teeth in unbroken arches. It is not just a dental state but, predominantly, it is a way of planning dental management in the face of limiting factors (such as high disease risk, medical complications, poor attendance or cost). If the needs do not dictate it, there may be no loss of any teeth and no need to work towards a shortened arch, yet the philosophy may still be applied. A full dentition of 32 teeth with no immediate need for treatment is perfectly consistent with the application of the concept but would be unlikely to result in a shortened arch (at least in the short term).

Although it is most often discussed in the context of the older patient, the strategy is one which can be applied at any stage of the permanent dentition. For example, a child with a mixed dentition including grossly carious first molars may, if the options were limited by cost, or poor co-operation, benefit from their early removal so that second and third molars can erupt into favourable positions. Resources can then be targeted at primary prevention of the remaining teeth rather than treatment, re-treatment, and ultimately loss of the first molars at the cost of attention to the rest.

The principle is an attractive one. It is straightforward, pragmatic, and easy to understand with a clearly defined goal and strategy for achieving this. A number of cross-sectional studies of subjects with shortened dental arches and matched controls have been undertaken to investigate some of the criticisms of this form of management. These have concentrated on the potential for periodontal health to be compromised as a result of increased occlusal loads, that teeth may be more likely to drift, that SDA may predispose subjects to temporo-mandibular dysfunction, and that oral comfort and masticatory function may be impaired (Witter *et al.* 1987, 1988, 1990a, 1990b, 1992). On the whole, most of theses concerns have been demonstrated to be unfounded, but the research was cross-sectional and the results are not always easy to interpret. The findings of longitudinal studies are still awaited and the value of the philosophy has not been proven conclusively.

There are other potential problems with SDA. Sometimes, it may be more expedient to use simple early preventive measures on a molar with early disease than get involved in the complex treatment of a premolar with a limited prognosis. Of course, this does not prevent the adoption of an alternative long-term strategy. Another objection is that, if treatment fails and edentulousness results, it could be argued that the use of partial dentures would have been preferable to the adoption of a shortened dental arch. The experience of denture-wearing and the maintenance of posterior tongue space by using partial dentures may have been an advantage. This raises the question of the appropriateness of the technique in certain circumstances. In high-risk subjects with widespread severe disease which cannot be controlled easily, or where the ability to maintain the minimum dentition for life is in question, alternative strategies may be necessary.

On the whole, the shortened dental arch would seem to be an appropriate means of preventing dental disability for many people, but it is not a panacea. Individual considerations will always be the major consideration in determining the most appropriate strategy.

THE ROLE OF THE INDIVIDUAL

This chapter has concentrated on the role of the dental professional in providing care to older patients while keeping their overall needs in perspective. The dental team have a fundamental role to play in providing comprehensive but appropriate dental care to older people, but the patients themselves have a critical role to play.

The last 25 years have seen major changes not just in the dental status of adults but also in terms of attitudes and behaviour. In 1968, 27 per cent of dentate adults said that they would be very upset at the prospect of edentulousness: by 1988 this had increased to 57 per cent. Over the same period there was a 10 percentage point rise in the proportion of dentate regular dental attenders (from 40 per cent to 50 per cent) (Gray *et al.* 1970; Todd and Walker 1980; Todd *et al.* 1982; Todd and Lader 1991). It is important to note that these figures refer to the dentate, an altogether more dentally aware group than the edentulous, and one which is itself increasing rapidly, so the scale of such changes is multiplied further when this is taken into account. The increased expectations and demands of future generations of elderly people must be used positively in terms of oral self-care. Good oral hygiene is something that should be possible, and encouraged, for everyone. There are few physical difficulties which cannot be overcome. The widespread use of a variety of self-administered oral applications, such as those containing fluoride for control of root caries and others under development for the management of periodontal disease, may provide an extra dimension to preventive dental care for many older adults. Attitudes, behaviour, and general awareness of the value of oral hygiene may not be as surmountable.

CONCLUSIONS

- There have been increases in the total number of elderly people with natural teeth in most Western countries. This increase is likely to accelerate over the coming decades.

- The condition of teeth in these populations is often compromised by previous disease, and their retention into old age may bring problems of maintenance and subsequently impairment of function when they are lost.

- Where many teeth are lost late in life the functional impairment may be severe, particularly where complete dentures need to be provided.

- The dentist's priority in the elderly must be to prevent the disability which may result from dental disease, even if the disease itself cannot be eliminated.

- Minimum criteria for a natural dentition in the elderly which will allow satisfactory masticatory and social function, without the need for a partial denture, can be identified. The criteria include the requirement for 20 or more natural teeth, no unrestored anterior spaces, and freedom from pain or discomfort.

- A number of limitations in the ability to achieve or maintain this can also be identified. These include:

  - the large proportion of the present dentate elderly who already fall below the suggested target

  - an increased susceptibility to certain diseases, and the cumulative effect of others through a lifetime

  - medical or social problems which impair the ability to receive dental care

  - failure to utilize services as a result of social, cultural, or economic barriers.

- Long-term strategies for maintaining a functional dentition in the face of these limitations need to be developed.

- Shortened dental arch (SDA) is the best developed of these strategies and is based on the prioritization of resources to maximize the functional benefits over the long term.

- Shortened dental arch philosophy is not always appropriate, but the basic principles are open to modification in individual cases.

- Good quality oral self-care is important if a dentition dependent solely on natural teeth is to be maintained.

- Changes in the attitudes of adults to oral health can be identified, particularly an increasing desire to retain natural teeth, and these must be capitalized on if oral health is to be improved.

REFERENCES

Agerberg, G. and Carlsson, G.E. (1981). Chewing ability in relation to dental and general health. *Acta odont. Scand.* **39**, 147–53.

Albander, J.M., *et al.* (1986). Radiographic quantification of alveolar bone level changes. A 2-year longitudinal study in man. *J. clin. Perio.* **13**, 195–200.

Banting, D.W. (1986). Epidemiology of root caries. *Gerodontology*, **5**, 5–11.

Bates, J.F., *et al.* (1971). Studies relating mastication and nutrition in the elderly. *Geronto. Clin.* **13**, 227–32.

Battistuzzi, P.G.F.C.M., *et al.* (1987). Partial edentulism, prosthetic treatment and oral function in a Dutch population. *J. oral Rehab.* **14**, 549–55.

Baxter, J.C. (1984). The nutritional intake of geriatric patients with varied dentitions. *J. prosthet. Dent.* **51**, 164–8.

Bergenholtz, G. and Nyman, S. (1984). Endodontic complications following periodontal and prosthetic treatment of patients with advanced periodontal disease. *J. Perio.* **55**, 63–8.

Bergman, B. and Carlsson, G. (1972). Review of 54 complete denture wearers. Patients opinions after 1 year of treatment. *Acta odont. Scand.* **30**, 399–414.

Bergman, B., *et al.* (1982). Caries, periodontal and prosthetic findings in patients with removable partial dentures: a ten year longitudinal study. *J. prosthet. Dent.* **48**, 506–14.

Chauncey, H.H., *et al.* (1984). The effect of the loss of teeth on diet and nutrition. *Int. dent. J.* **34**, 98–104.

Cohen, D.R. and Henderson, J.B. (1991). *Health, prevention, and economics.* Oxford University Press.

Craig, J. (1983). The growth of the elderly population. *Pop. Trends,* **32**, 28–34.

Cushing, A.M., *et al.* (1986). Developing socio-dental indicators— the social impact of dental disease. *Commun. dent. Health,* **3**, 3–17.

Drake, C.W. and Beck, J.D. (1993). The oral status of elderly removable partial denture wearers. *J. oral Rehab.* **20**, 53–60.

Farrell, J.H. (1956). The effect of mastication on the digestion of food. *Br. dent. J.* **100**, 149–55

Farrell, J. (1957). Partial dentures in the restoration of masticatory efficiency. *Dent. Practit. Dent. Rec.* **7**, 375–9.

Felton, D., *et al.* (1989). Long term effects of crown preparation on pulp vitality. *J. dent. Res.* **68** (special issue).

Finch, H., *et al.* (1988). Barriers to the receipt of dental care. Report for the British Dental Association.

Fiske, J., *et al.* (1990). Barriers to dental care in an elderly population resident in an inner city area. *J. Dent.* **18**, 236–42.

Goodson, J.M., *et al.* (1982). Patterns of progression and regression of advanced destructive periodontal disease. *J. clin. Perio.* **9**, 472–81.

Gordon, P.H., *et al.* (1994). The shortened dental arch: Supplementary analyses from the 1988 adult dental health survey. *Commun. dent. Health* **11**, 87–90.

Gray, P.G., *et al.* (1970). *Adult dental health in England and Wales in 1968.* London HMSO.

Grbic, J.T. and Lamster, I.B. (1992). Risk indicators for future clinical attachment loss in adult periodontitis. Tooth and site variables. *J. Perio.* **63**, 262–9.

Grbic, J.T. and Lamster, I.B. (1991). Risk indicators for future clinical attachment loss in adult periodontitis. Patient variables. *J. Perio.* **62**, 322–9.

Halling, A., *et al.* (1988). Diet in relation to number of remaining teeth in a population of middle-aged women in Gothenburg, Sweden. *Swedish dent. J.* **12**, 39–45.

Hartsook, E.I. (1974). Food selection, dietary adequacy and related dental problems of patients with dental prostheses. *J. prosthet. Dent.* **32**, 32–40.

Helkimo, E., *et al.* (1978). Chewing efficiency and state of dentition. A methodologic study. *Acta odont. Scand.* **36**, 33–41.

Hoad-Reddick, G., *et al.* (1987). Knowledge of dental services provided: investigations in an elderly population. *Commun. Dent. oral Epidemiol.* **15**, 137–40.

Johnson, N.W., *et al.* (1988). Detection of high-risk groups and individuals for periodontal diseases. *J. clin. Perio.* **15**, 276–82.

Kandelman, D. and Lepage, Y. (1982). Demographic, social and cultural factors influencing the elderly to seek dental treatment. *Int. dent. J.* **32**, 360–70.

Katz, R.V. (1980). Assessing root caries in populations. The evolution of the root caries index. *J. pub. Hlth Dent.* **40**, 7–16.

Katz, R.V., *et al.* (1982). Prevalence and intra- oral distribution of root caries in an adult population. *Caries Res.* **16**, 265–71.

Kayser, A. (1981). Shortened dental arches and oral function. *J. oral Rehab.* **8**, 457–62.

Kayser, A.D. and Witter, D.J. (1985). Oral functional needs and its consequences for dentulous older people. *Commun. dent. Health,* **2**, 285–91.

Kayser, A.F. (1990). How much reduction of the dental arch is functionally acceptable for the ageing patient. *Int. dent. J.* **40**, 183–8.

Lindhe, J. and Nyman, S. (1984). Long-term maintenance of patients treated for advanced periodontal disease. *J. clint. Perio.* **11**, 504–14.

Luke, D.A. and Lucas, P.W. (1985). Chewing efficiency in relation to occlusal wear and other variations in the natural human dentition. *Br. dent. J.* **159**, 401–3.

MacEntee, M.I., *et al.* (1988). Oral health concerns of an elderly population in England. *Commun. Dent. oral Epidemiol.* **16**, 72–4.

Manly, R.S. and Braley, L.C. (1950). Masticatory performance and efficiency. *J. dent. Res.* **29**, 448–62.

Martin, J., *et al.* (1988a). *The prevalence of disability among adults.* London, HMSO.

Martin, J., *et al.* (1988b). *Disabled adults: Services, transport and employment.* London, HMSO.

Martin G.M. (1992). Biological mechanism of ageing. In *Oxford textbook of geriatric medicine,* (ed. J.G. Evans and T.F. Williams), pp. 41–8. Oxford University Press, Oxford.

Neil, D.J. and Phillips, H.J.B. (1970). The masticatory performance, dental state and dietary intake of a group of elderly army pensioners. *Br. dent. J.* **128**, 581–5.

NIH (National Institutes of Health) (1987). *Oral health of United States adults. National findings* Publication No. 87-2868. NIH, Betheseda.

O'Mullane, D. and Whelton, H. (1992). *Oral health of Irish adults 1989–1990.* The Stationery Office, Dublin.

Okamoto, H., *et al.* (1988). Methods of evaluating periodontal disease data in epidemiological research. *J. clin. Perio.* **15**, 430–9.

OPCS (Office of Population Censuses and Surveys) (1991). World population trends and projections. *Pop. Trends,* **63**, 36–9.

OPCS (Office of Population Censuses and Surveys) (1994). Mid 1993 population estimates for England & Wales. *OPCS Monitor* PP194/2. 1–5.

Oosterhaven S.P., *et al.* (1988). Social and psychological implications of missing teeth for chewing ability. *Commun. Dent. oral Epidemiol.* **16**, 79–82.

Papapanou, P.N., *et al.* (1988). Periodontal status in relation to age and tooth type. A cross sectional study. *J. clin. Perio.* **15**, 469–78.

Rabins, P.V. (1992). Cognition. In *Oxford textbook of geriatric medicine,* (ed. J.G. Evans and T.F. Williams), pp. 479–83. Oxford University Press.

Robb, N.D. (1992). Epidemiological studies of tooth wear. Ph.D. thesis, London.

Schou, L. and Eadie, D. (1991). Qualitative study of oral health norms and behaviour among elderly people in Scotland. *Commun. dent. Health* **8**, 53–8.

Smith, J.M. and Sheiham, A. (1980). Dental treatment needs and demands of an elderly population in England. *Commun. Dent. oral Epidemiol.* **8**, 360–4.

Steele, J.G. (1994). The dental status, needs and demands of the elderly in three communities. Ph.D. thesis, University of Newcastle-upon-Tyne.

Thompson, J. (1987). Ageing of the population: contemporary trends and issues. *Pop. Trends*, **50**, 18–22.

Tobias, B. and Smith, J. (1987). Barriers to dental care and associated treatment needs in an elderly population living in sheltered accomodation in west Essex. *Br. dent J.* **163**, 293–5.

Todd, J.E. and Lader, D. (1991). *Adult dental health 1988 United Kingdom.* London, HMSO.

Todd, J.E. and Walker, A.M. (1980). *Adult dental health.* Vol. 1, *England and Wales 1968–1978.* London, HMSO.

Todd, J.E., *et al.* (1982). *Adult dental health. Volume 2, UK 1978.* London, HMSO.

Twaddle, A.C. (1974). The concept of health statues. *Soc. Sci. Med.* **8**, 29–38.

Van Waas, M.A.J., *et al.* (1993). Oral function in dentate elderly with reduced dentitions. *Gerodontology*, **10**, 40–3.

Vehkalhati, M.M. and Paunio, I.K. (1988). Occurrence of root caries in relation to dental health behavior. *J. dent. Res.* **67**, 911–14.

Watson, I.B. and Tulloch, E.N. (1985). Clinical assessment of cases of tooth surface loss. *Br. dent. J.* **159**, 144–8.

WHO (World Health Organization) (1958). Constitution of the World Health Organization. Annex 1. *The first ten years of the World Health Organization.* WHO, Geneva.

Willemsen, W.L. (1994). Aspects of dental health in dutch adults. Ph.D. thesis, University of Nijmegen.

Wilson, M.C. (1991). An investigation of factors affectiong dental care for dentate older people. Ph.D. thesis, University of Manchester.

Witter, D.J., *et al.* (1987). Migration of teeth in shortened dental arches. *J. oral Rehab.* **14**, 321–9.

Witter, D.J., *et al.* (1988). Signs and symptoms of mandibular dysfunction in shortened dental arches. *J. oral Rehab.* **15**, 413–20.

Witter, D.J., *et al.* (1989). The effect of removable partial dentures on oral function in shortened dental arches. *J. oral Rehab.* **16**, 27–33.

Witter, D.J., *et al.* (1990*a*). Shortened dental arches and masticatory ability. *J. Dent.* **18**, 185–9.

Witter, D.J., *et al.* (1990*b*). Oral comfort in shortened dental arches. *J. oral Rehab.* **17**, 137–43.

Witter, D.J., *et al.* (1992). Shortened dental arches and periodontal support. *J. oral Rehab.* **19**, 203–12.

Wright, P.S., *et al.* (1992). Relationship of removable partial denture use to root caries in an older population. *Int. J. Prosthodont.* **5**, 39–46.

15. Preventing a dental handicap

J.H. NUNN

WITH few exceptions, handicap remains a 'Cinderella' area of medicine and dentistry. However, it would appear that handicapped children and adults are assuming such numbers that the problem of their care, including their dental care, can no longer be an issue to be side-stepped. Care of the chronically sick and of the handicapped, in particular, have always been neglected areas of the National Health Service, with dentistry the poor relation of medicine. Not unnaturally whilst numbers were small or demand non-existent, dentistry and the handicapped person were separate entities and only crossed paths on an emergency basis. Yet the need, if not the demand, is there. Dentistry in the past has relied too heavily on demand for its services so that the handicapped population has inevitably lost out. Much of what has been published in the way of provision of dental services to handicapped people has probably been dealing with the tip of the iceberg. The provision of dental care for those with special needs has now become even more complex with the move to 'community care' and the so-called normalization of children with special needs and adults in long-stay accommodation (DHSS: Department of Health and Social Security 1989a).

The increasing sophistication in medical care has meant that many more infants at risk now survive the neonatal period than would have done previously, so that the number of children handicapped by one or more conditions may therefore increase. The advances have also generated handicapping conditions. Those surviving may well do so with more severe or even multiple handicaps, often well into adulthood (Morton 1977). The life-span of children with Down's syndrome is only modestly decreased with many thriving to their 60s (Baird and Sadovnick 1987).

Higher standards of paediatric care, whilst increasing the survival rate of already handicapped children, are vital also in the primary prevention of disability, as is the increasing availability of genetic screening and counselling (Fitzimmons 1982). Regrettably, those most vulnerable are often the people to make least use of these services (HMSO 1976; The Children's Committee 1980).

TERMINOLOGY

It soon becomes apparent that there is a persistent dilemma in the terminology of handicap. Assigning a 'label' to a child is not without its pitfalls: because of the complexity of some conditions, the way that they manifest in one child may be different from that in another, or the child may meet the criteria of assessment on one occasion and not on another (Morgan 1979). The condition may well regress or worsen, thus making a static definition inappropriate.

Once the label has been placed, however, these changes may not readily bring about a re-categorization. To a certain extent, the label assigned to a child with a handicap is dependent upon the agency through which the disabilities have first been diagnosed; this in turn may depend more on chance social class and presenting symptoms than on the child's actual needs. Categorization in this way of children and the schools which they attend is often convenient only for administrative purposes, for within each category of handicap there are many degrees of severity of condition, and indeed some children will have more than one handicap, for example, the psychiatric disorders superimposed on physical handicap (Harding 1980). Further arguments against the use of such rigid categories have been put forward in the Report of the Committee of Enquiry into Education of Handicapped Children and Young People (HMSO 1978b); recommendations made in the report aim to abolish the statutory categorization of handicapped pupils, and to integrate such children more closely with the normal schoolchild, embodied now in the 1981 Education Act.

A number of authors (Harris *et al.* 1971; Swerdloff 1980) have addressed themselves to the problem of definition of terms, and attempted to distinguish between defect, disability, and handicap. The World Health Organization, which are currently revising the International Classification of Diseases, do not propose to alter the definitions of impairment, disability, and handicap for the Tenth Revision, but state that it is possible that more emphasis will be laid on the role of the environment in the future, especially as regards handicap (M.C. Thuriaux, personal communication). In the context of dentistry for handicapped people, the categories suggested by Soble (1974) have practical applications: 'dentally handicapped' refers to patients 'who have some gross condition or deficit in their oral cavities which necessitates special dental treatment considerations'; and, 'handicapped for dentistry' referring to patients 'whose oral health may be considered within the normal range, but who have some physical and/or mental or emotional condition which may prevent them from being treated routinely in the dental situation'. Neither of these two are mutually exclusive.

CLASSIFICATION

Classification of the different types of handicaps can be carried out either from an aetiological point of view (Morgan 1979) or from presenting symptoms (Kanar 1979). The procedure of categorizing children is complicated by those individuals who possess a number of handicaps (DHSS 1971). This is almost inevitable because profoundly retarded people nearly always have significant neurological involvement and are more vulnerable to chronic diseases (Morgan 1979). In addition, handicap may be imposed on disability by psychological and social defects (Franks 1969).

In 1976, the Department of Education and Science subdivided handicap with reference to special educational needs: physical handicap and delicate; educationally subnormal; deaf and hearing impaired; blind and visually handicapped; maladjusted; epileptic; speech defect; and autism (Harding 1980). These have been superseded by the 1981 Education Act where all such children are designated as children with learning difficulties. Although a number of other classifications are still used in the dental literature, for the purposes of comparison of oral health, the format in common usage would appear to be mental, physical, medical, and sensory handicaps. Despite the inadequacies, already explored, of such a classification it is in this format the dental health of mentally, physically, and medically compromised children will now be presented.

DENTAL HEALTH OF HANDICAPPED CHILDREN

Difficulties also exist in defining oral health in special groups. This has led Beck and Hunt (1985) to conclude that categorization by the diagnostic label of developmental disability may be inappropriate, as it may not be the disability itself that influences dental disease rates, but how profound is the level of the disease. However, very few authors actually categorize their study groups in such a way, so that data presented give only mean values of dental disease prevalence for each type of disability. The issue is beginning to be addressed in the dental literature with the realisation that disabled children are not a homogenous group (Nielsen 1990; Kendall 1992). Increasingly, authors are moving away from the concept of a static 'label' and acknowledging that what may be an important factor for the effective delivery of dental care is the way in which the individual's disability presents (Evans *et al.* 1991; Nunn *et al.* 1993).

What is also worth considering here is that many of the studies reported in the literature have been carried out in the 1960s and 1970s. This is of relevance because following on from this period there has been a marked decline in the dental caries experience of many children in developed countries. In addition, this time period has also seen a move to de-institutionalization or 'normalization' of many disabled people, particularly children, and the dental advantages or disadvantages of these changes are as yet poorly documented in many countries (Kamen 1981).

The largest group of disabled children encountered are those with a mental handicap, and it is their dental disease experience which will be discussed first.

MENTAL HANDICAP

The causes of mental handicap are legion but for many such affected children a reason for their condition may never be found. A significant proportion of males with severe to moderate learning difficulties have fragile X syndrome but have never been given this definitive diagnosis. This is of significance dentally since many patients with fragile X syndrome have congenital heart defects (Nunn 1990). The category as a whole consitutes the largest subgroup when considering the total number of children in receipt of special education, with 25 per 1000 of the child population affected. Included in this heterogeneous group of children with a known or unknown cause of their condition is a large group of children with learning difficulties with a well-defined aetiology, namely Down's syndrome children, whose dental health is sufficiently different for them to merit separate consideration.

There would, however, appear to be distinct sex and social class bias in the determination of the numbers of mentally disabled children with mild to moderate special educational needs (McCabe 1979). Indeed, of the prevalence figures quoted for children with mild to moderate mental disability per thousand of the child population only one-third will have evidence of central nervous system pathology. The number of more severely affected children is of the order of 4 per 1000 and occurs more uniformly across the social class spectrum and with distinct pathological involvement in its aetiology rather than socio-cultural factors. Of the affected children, a significant proportion are usually found to be male, as with most other types of handicap.

DENTAL HEALTH IN MENTAL HANDICAP

DENTAL CARIES

Rhodes (1884) was one of the first people to examine and report on the dental health of the 'insane'; of the 350 inmates of a mental hospital in Cambridge, compared with 350 patients from Addenbrooke's Hospital in the same city, he commented that relative to other people of similar class, tooth quality was good. From the studies which have followed Rhodes', it would seem that overall the prevalence of dental caries in the mentally handicapped is similar to that found in normal populations and, in many cases, lower. A number of the studies encompassed the mentally handicapped in institutions where stricter dietary control may have encouraged a lower prevalence of caries attack (Schwarz and Vigild 1987). However, there are exceptions to this general finding of lowered disease prevalence in institutions (MacEntee *et al.* 1985). It may be that dental disease levels in these patients are more a reflection of the degree of disability rather than the type of residential care, with more severely disabled patients accommodated in residential institutions until recently. Another factor to consider is that many institutions are situated in more remote areas, away from central, often fluoridated, water supplies (Nowak 1984).

When the individual components of the mean DMF values are examined, some disparities are apparent when comparing handicapped and normal children. Generally, the amount of decay may be similar or even greater for the normal group, but the handicapped group will have more missing and fewer filled teeth (Nunn and Murray 1987; Holland and O'Mullane 1990; Pope and Curzon 1991).

Although lacking a formal control group, the study by Mellor and Doyle (1987) is most encouraging in that it demonstrates the reductions in caries prevalence to be gained by a very comprehensive system of dental prevention and treatment, undertaken by the community dental service. A total of 49 13-year-olds showed a reduction in the mean number of decayed teeth from a value of 3.8 to 0.4 in a 4-year period, with a concurrent increase in the restorative provision, an 'F' value of 0.7 in 1977 rising to 3.8 in 1982. Evans *et al.* (1991) found similar improvements in dental health could be achieved through mobile dental facilities used by the community dental service. Although in this study dental caries experience was higher for disabled 5-year-olds than for normal schoolchildren reflecting poor levels of care for disabled pre-school children, the data for older children were encouraging; the percentage of untreated decay for disabled 12- and 14-year-olds was similar to children of these ages in state schools.

Periodontal disease

Periodontal disease was generally found to be prevalent, and oral hygiene poor, amongst mentally handicapped children, especially if they were insitutionalized (Nunn and Murray 1987). More recent studies comparing disabled groups over a period of time have reported disappointing results with respect to gingival health. Despite improvements in dental caries with programmes of enhanced service provision, there has been virtually no improvement in gingival health (Holland and O'Mullane 1990; Evans *et al.* 1991). Other authors have commented on the worsening gingival picture in cerebral palsy children who have a significant mental disability, as well as the increased prevalence of gingivitis with increasing age (Pope and Curzon 1991).

Malocclusion

The early study by Rhodes (1884) concluded that the group of patients he studied had ill-formed maxillae and more than usual overcrowding. He gave detailed measurements for inter-canine widths, which he stated were much narrower than in a normal population.

Gullikson (1969) found that 67 per cent of his study group of 3- to 14-year-olds had a malocclusion, with a greater predominance of Angle's Class III malocclusions than would be expected in the normal population.

A more recent study, found that nearly half of the mildly mentally handicapped and two-thirds of the severely mentally handicapped children had a handicapping malocclusion (Nunn and Murray 1987).

DENTAL HEALTH IN DOWN'S SYNDROME

Down's syndrome children

Down's syndrome is a chromosomal disorder with three distinct aberrations: trisomy, translocation, and mosaicism. There are marked physical features, and mental subnormality of varying degree is found in all patients. A major cause of morbidity and mortality in adulthood is Alzheimer's disease

(Franceeschi *et al.* 1990). Approximately 1 in 600 newborns have Down's syndrome, although there is a marked variation with maternal age (Stoll *et al.* 1990).

Dental caries

From the epidemiological data available to date there is conflict in the views over caries susceptibility in Down's syndrome children. The earlier literature (Nunn 1984) indicated that caries prevalence was lower in Down's syndrome children, with between 50 and 84 per cent reported as caries free (Maclaurin *et al.* 1985b; Ulseth *et al.* 1991). The reasons put forward for this relative caries immunity are various, ranging from alterations in tooth eruption and tooth form to biochemical differences in salivary buffering (Vigild 1986). Institutionalization may be important in that residents may in the past have had less access to sweetened foodstuffs (Kroll *et al.* 1970). The study by Orner (1975) of 212 Down's syndrome children and their siblings showed the reduced caries prevalence of Down's syndrome children. The Down's group had only one-third the caries experience of their siblings, although 100 of the Down's syndrome children were institutionalized. This study is particularly useful in that, unlike some others, the comparisons on caries prevalence were matched for stage of tooth eruption rather than just by the children's chronological ages. This meant that each group was at comparable risk of disease.

Periodontal disease

Periodontal disease tends to be more prevalent in children with Down's syndrome. Much of the periodontal problem found in children with Down's syndrome is localized to the lower incisor region initially, and many studies report worse oral hygiene, bone loss, acute ulcerative gingivitis, gross calculus, and evidence of tooth loss confined to this segment, in young Down's syndrome populations (Johnson and Young 1963).

Twelve- to 14-year-old children with mobile lower incisors, and 15- to 17-year-olds with missing lower incisors were not uncommon in the Johnson and Young (1963) study. In the study by Maclaurin *et al.* (1985b), double the proportion of Down's syndrome children required further assessment with a view to complex periodontal treatment than did other mentally handicapped children; a fraction which in turn was higher than for normal children. The authors felt that the increased prevalence of periodontal problems may be a function of immunodeficiency in Down's syndrome, and related to the congenital disorder rather than directly to the oral hygiene. Whilst other studies have shown poorer oral hygiene and periodontal health in institutionalized Down's syndrome children, this was not shown by Vigild (1985a) who found that socio-economic background was an important determinant of improved oral hygiene levels; the best, as well as the poorest, oral hygiene and periodontal health was found among subjects living at home. Nunn (1984) found that poor gingival conditions were almost equally prevalent between Down's syndrome and other mentally handicapped children, 61 per cent and 53 per cent, respectively.

Malocclusion

One of the more striking features of the facies of children with Down's syndrome is the relative under-development of the middle third of the face and the consequent tendency to a Class III skeletal base relationship. A high vaulted palate is a common finding along with other intra-oral anomalies (McIver and Machen 1979). Many researchers cite a tendency to an Angle's Class III malocclusion in Down's syndrome subjects, together with a posterior cross-bite (Vigild 1985*b*).

PHYSICAL HANDICAP

The main physical handicaps of particular concern to dentists are those of cerebral palsy, spina bifida, and muscular dystrophy, together with a range of other orthopaedic disabilities. However, not all thses children will have so severe a defect that they merit special dental care.

CEREBRAL PALSY

This is defined as a disorder of movement and posture resulting from a non-progressive lesion of the brainstem. The prevalence of cerebral palsy is of the order of 1 to 2 per 1000 children of school age, a figure which is said, by some, to be stable during the late 1960s and 1970s because of the improved survival of premature babies (Pharoah *et al.* 1987). Other authors feel that over the longer period between 1970 and 1990 the prevalence has increased slightly and there has been a change in the various subtypes. For example, with the decrease in kernicterus, choreoathetoid cerebral palsy has become much less common whereas spastic diplegia, associated with prematurity has increased (Mutch *et al.* 1992). Manifestation of the disability varies enormously, from the quadraplegic child with sensory and intellectual impairments to the monoplegic with a barely discernible disability (Nielsen 1990).

DENTAL HEALTH OF CEREBRAL PALSIED CHILDREN

Dental caries

Most studies have shown that, despite the higher proportion of cerebral palsied children who are caries-free, the amount of untreated decay and the number of missing teeth are higher when compared with normal controls (Nielsen 1990; Pope and Curzon 1991). The study by Nielsen (1990) in Denmark subdivides the children into the difference presentations of cerebral palsy, as well as considering the degree to which the children are handicapped mentally. The results of the study show that the lowest caries experience is in the most severely mentally and motor handicapped individuals, the reverse of the situation in the UK. Nielsen proposes that this may be because of the reduced opportunity for the more severely disabled children to gain access to sugary foods but that the difference may also be explained by the delayed eruption of permanent teeth seen in such children. This has implications for dental treatment in that the more disabled children are the ones who are more difficult to treat; a situation reflected in the quality of restorative care provided as documented in the UK study where the children of 11 years and over had significantly poorer restorations than similar aged control group children. The authors made the point that this may have been improved by the provision of dental care under general anaesthesia by specially trained clinicians (Pope and Curzon 1991).

Periodontal disease

Values for gingivitis and oral hygiene indices have been found to be similar for the cerebral palsied and normal controls in spite of the difficulties sometimes experienced by the former in carrying out the necessary oral hygiene measures. Even without constant parental back-up, it has been shown (Melville *et al.* 1981) that, through weekly visits to special schools by dental therapists, improvements in poor oral hygiene and gingival conditions could be made, despite the difficulties some of the more severely handicapped children had in effectively cleaning their teeth. By contrast, other authors have found periodontal disease and oral hygiene to be worse in children with cerebral palsy largely, it is assumed, because of the difficulties imposed by the motor defects (Pope and Curzon 1991). Indeed it was found that in a group of 92 children with cerebral palsy (Nunn 1984), 50 per cent had poor oral hygiene and 53 per cent had poor gingival health, using the Good, Fair, Poor index of James *et al.* (1960).

Malocclusion

Given the varying abnormal degrees of muscle tonicity, and the involuntary movements of structures influencing the dental arches, not unexpectedly, cerebral palsied children are found to have a high prevalence of malocclusion (Strodel 1987). In the spastic cerebral palsied child, hypertonic facial muscles and a tongue thrust predispose to a Class II division 2 type of malocclusion, often with a cross-bite and crowding, due to the constriction of the dental arches. The athetoid type suffer hypotonicity of the orbicularis oris muscle coupled again with tongue protrusion, tending therefore towards an Angle's Class II division 1 type of malocclusion in 90 per cent of cases, often with an anterior open bite. Pope and Curzon (1991) postulated that poor swallowing and other abnormal muscle activity may have contributed to the increased overjet in their group of 11 children with athetoid cerebral palsy. Whilst this feature of the occlusion, together with the higher prevalence of epilepsy in this group, may expose children to the risk of trauma to their teeth, restraints in the child's wheelchair may prevent this happening. The ataxic type present with a variety of malocclusions (Kastein 1957). No such data are available for the remaining two types of cerebral palsy.

Foster *et al.* (1974), using cephalometry and matched controls, investigated the effects of cerebral palsy in 33 patients with varying severity of the defect; they concluded that the cerebral palsy did affect the size and form both of the jaws and skull, but that the severity of the defect and the age at which the lesion occured were important variables in determining the effect. Stratifying groups according to these variables was vital if such differences were not to be masked in a large group.

DENTAL HEALTH OF CHILDREN WITH SPINA BIFIDA

In spina bifida, there is a defective fusion of one or more posterior vertebral arches, with or without protrusion of some or all of the contents of the spinal canal. It is estimated that in 50–60 per cent of cases the condition is inherited, but that environmental agents may be responsible for the remainder. Unlike most other malformations, it is more common in females. Hydrocephalus may be present in 95 per cent of cases. One-quarter of patients with associated hydrocephalus suffer from epilepsy, and between 30 and 40 per cent may have impaired intelligence (Stark 1977). Spina bifida, along with other central nervous system defects, is the most frequent congenital malformation found in this country, with a prevalence of 2.5 per 1000 total births.

Dental caries

In a small subgroup of a larger sample of handicapped children (Nunn 1984), it was found that relative to the group as a whole, caries experience in the 53 children with spina bifida was lower, a dmf of 1.8 for the spina bifida group of 6- to 9-year-olds compared to 2.7 for a similar age range of handicapped children. In the permanent dentition, this picture was repeated with a DMF of 1.6 for 10- to 14-year-old spina bifida children, and 2.3 for other handicapped children of the same age. However, for children with spina bifida the proportions of decayed, missing, and filled teeth occupying the DMF index were more unfavourable compared with the handicap group as a whole; 31. 25, and 43 per cent compared with 28, 20, and 52 per cent, respectively.

Periodontal disease

The oral hygiene status of children with spina bifida in one study of 53 children (Nunn 1984) was worse than that of other handicapped children, and more children with spina bifida had poor gingival health than did handicapped children generally; 59 per cent and 44 per cent, respectively. These figures highlight the danger of combining data for handicapped children as this practice often masks the range of disease values found in subgroups.

Malocclusion

No published studies are available on the occlusion of children with spina bifida.

MUSCULAR DYSTROPHY

This is a group of inherited disease characterized by weakness and degeneration of affected muscles. Males are exclusively affected in the Duchenne type. Facial musculature is always affected in the fascio-scapulo-humeral type, rarely in other forms (Walton and Nattrass 1954). Walton and Nattrass (1954) quoted a prevalence of 4 per 100 000 children for two areas in the north of England. There is scant information on the dental health of these children; little difference from normal in the prevalence of caries experiences and periodontal disease has been found (Henderson 1968). Other authors have found an increased prevalence of malocclusions due to abnormalities of oro-facial musculature (Cohen and Feldman 1978).

MEDICALLY COMPROMISED CHILDREN

Children who are medically handicapped fall into two groups; first, those whose general health may be further jeopardized if they were to develop dental disease; and secondly, those in whom the need for dental care in itself constitutes a risk (Hobson 1980). The dental effects which have been found to be specific to particular medical conditions are summarized in Table 15.1. There is however, very little published information on the oral health in medically compromised children and, for many of these conditions, it remains difficult to separate out the effects of treatment from those of the condition itself, leukaemia being a classic example.

THE NEED FOR PREVENTION OF DENTAL DISEASE IN SPECIAL GROUPS

BACKGROUND

In spite of the accumulated evidence on the lack of treatment and consequent poor dental health of many disabled children which has been detailed in the preceding pages, little has been done through official channels to actively bring about a change in this state of affairs.

Early reports, both specific to handicap (HMSO 1978*a*) and general to dental health (1977*a,b*) make, if at all, only fleeting reference to preventive dentistry and handicapped groups in the population. The Royal Commission of the National Health Service (DHSS 1979*b*) reiterated much of what the Court Report (HMSO 1976) started with respect to dentistry in general, but neither the former enquiry or the Government's immediate response to it, *Patients first* (DHSS 1979*a*), said anything about dentistry and the handicapped. A follow-up, *Handbook on policies and priorities* (DHSS 1981) merely states that services for the handicapped were poor, without being more specific. Amendment of the 1978 NHS Act to allow the Community Dental Service to treat handicapped adults must have been in part an acknowledgement that dental care for this group of patients was not being taken up in the General Dental Services.

Publication of the Dental Strategy Review Group's Report *Towards better dental health* (HMSO 1981) saw not only the highlighting of the inadequate care for special and priority groups, but also suggestions, like discretionary payments to general dental practitioners who treated handicapped individuals, for overcoming this problem. A few years later, a Scottish group (Scottish Home and Health Department 1984), addressing itself specifically to the subject of dentistry for the handicapped came up with specific proposals for remedying the identified shortfall in care. In the rest of the UK, further acknowledgement of the developing role of the Community Dental Service in providing care for disabled people came in the Government's white paper 'Promoting better health' and the Department of Health Circular (DHSS 1989*b*) which followed. It was suggested that the Community Dental Service should be in a position to offer care to those patients who

Table 15.1. Dental disease in medically compromised children

Condition (authors)	Prevalence	No. and age (yrs)	Caries	Periodontal disease	Orthodontics	Other
Asthma	22/1000					
Wotman et al. (1973)		25, 10–15	–	100% with calculus	–	Clinical examination and saliva samples
		25 controls	–	43% with calculus		
Hyppa and Paunio (1979)		15, 10–11	DMFS 6.9	53% with calculus	–	Increase in Lactobacilli counts in asthmatics due to steroid inhalation
		30 controls	DMFS 8.6	60% with calculus	–	
Attrill and Hobson (1984)		30, 5–17	DMFT 3.3	Segments with plaque: 3.0	–	
		30 minor orthopaedic conditions	DMFT 5.2	Segments with gingivitis: 1.2 plaque: 2.7 (0) gingivitis: 0.9 (0)		
Cystic fibrosis (CF)	1/2000				–	
Swallow et al. (1967)		63, 11	♂ DMFT = 0 ♀ = 1.8	3% with gingivitis 9.5% with calculus		Saliva samples 1.5% with hypoplasia 36.5% with discoloured teeth
		15 000 physically handicapped	♂ = 3.5 ♀ = 3.8	–	–	
Brooks et al. (1970)		52, 2½–8½	defs 2.9 DMFS 3.3	–	–	Clinical examination and full mouth X-rays
		Sibling controls	defs 6.8 DMFS 6.4			
Wotman et al. (1973)		25, 10–15	–	90% with calculus	–	Clinical examination and saliva samples
		25 control	–	43% with calculus	–	
Jagels and Sweeney (1976)		21, 10–12	deft 2.57 DMFT 2.52	OH[1] score = 1.5; 10% cystic fibrosis	C1.[2] I 82% CF 76% sibs C1. II div. 1 15% CF 18% sibs	5% with hypoplasia
		19 siblings, 10–12	deft 2.42 DMFT 4.26	22% siblings	C1. II div 2 4% CF 3% sibs C1. III 0% CF 3% sibs	1% siblings with hypoplasia
Blackharsh (1977)		42, 4–25	–	30 with mild gingivitis 26 with mild plaque	–	30% with stains of clinical crown; no specific agent identified
		10 sibling controls	–	4 with mild gingivitis 2 with mild plaque	–	
Primosch (1980)		39, 16–19	DMFS 11.54	–	–	24% with discoloured teeth
		Controls	DMFS 15.92	–	–	42.7% with enamel defects

Table 15.1. *continued*

Condition (authors)	Prevalence	No. and age (yrs)	Caries	Periodontal disease	Orthodontics	Other
Attrill and Hobson (1984)		30, 5–17	dmft/DMFT 3.5	Segments with plaque 3.6 Segments with gingivitis 1.8	–	–
		30 minor orthopaedic (0)	dmft/DMFT 5.2	plaque 2.7 (0) gingivitis 0.9		
Kinirons (1985)		118 children mean age 3.45 $n = 42$	All ages: dmf 0.5	21% with calculus	–	Salivary pH 6.89 (resting);
		mean age 8.15 $n = 35$	DMF 1.54	69 mild gingivitis	–	buffering capacity of stimulated saliva, 1.5 ml
		mean age 12.22 $n = 39$ 85 siblings	DMF 3.07	63 mild plaque	–	
		mean age 3.02 $n = 30$	dmf 1.7	5% with calculus	–	Salivary pH 6.79
		mean age 8.38 $n = 26$	DMF 2.04	32 mild gingivitis	–	Buffering capacity of stimulated saliva, 1.34 ml
		mean age 12.61 $n = 26$	DMF 5.38	26 mild plaque		
Mahaney (1986)		50 females mean age 12.38	–	–	–	Dental age 0.84 yrs behind chronological age
		50 control females	–	–	–	Dental age 0.04 yrs behind chronological age
Epilepsy (EP) Gingis *et al.* (1980)	5–10/1000	46 (mean age 28) mentally retarded	–	Gingival overgrowth related to serum phenytoin levels	–	Abnormally short roots not related to high serum phenytoin
		45 mentally retarded	–	–	–	

Lundstrom *et al.* (1982)

No. and age (yrs)	Caries	Plaque frequency per individual	Increased probing depth (≥ 0.75 mm) GU³
21, 9–17 (I) carbamazepine	(I) DFS 5.7	60%	8.7
10, 8–17 (II) phenytoin	(II) DFS 8.0	41%	24.7
19, 7–22 (III) previous phenytoin	(III) DFS 13.2	58%	15.6
15, 8–14 (IV) epileptic, no medication	(IV) DFS 4.7	42%	7.8

Table 15.1. *continued*

Condition (authors)	Prevalence	No. and age (yrs)	Caries	Periodontal disease	Orthodontics	Other
Robinson *et al.* (1983)		229 medicated children 144 controls (c)	–	Gingival hyperplasia in 40% epileptics	–	Premolar volume 0.47 mm (Ep) 0.56 mm (c) Intercuspal width reduced in early-onset epileptics. Delayed shedding and eruption of teeth? due pseudohypopara-thyroidism effect of anticonvulsants.
Modeer *et al.* (1986)		30 phenytoin-treated	DFS 5.5	Visible plaque index (VPI): 42.8% Gingival bleeding index (GBI): 15.1% Increased probing depth (IPD) > 4 mm: 8.9%	–	Lysozyme activity in saliva increased significantly in phenytoin group
		25 other anticonvulsants	DFS 6.3	VPI: 48.5% GBI: 10.6% IPD: 1.9%		
Cardiac disease Kaner *et al.* (1946)	6–8/1000		Increase in carious lesions	Cyanotic soft tissues	Anterior open-bite in some patients	Delayed eruption; dilation and engorgement of pulp vessels
Gould and Picton (1960)		30 with cyanosis 30 without cyanosis (controls)	–	23% normal gums 43% overall redness 33% deep maroon 6% controls with overall redness Pocketing: 8% cyanotics > 2 mm 3% controls > 2 mm Oral hygiene: Good—14% cyanotics 24% controls Bad—5% cyanotics 3% controls	Cyanotics: Cl. III = 5 Controls: Cl. III = 2	
Hakala (1967)		65 cyanotics, 6.1	dmf 2.7 (deciduous molars	MG[4] 45.4% Cal[5] 26.8%	Cl. I 92.4% Cl. II 1.8% Cl. III 1.8%	Enamel hypoplasia: 16.9%
		180 acyanotics 6.9	dmf 3.1	MG 2.1% Cal 3.1%	Cl. I 90% Cl. II 6.2% Cl. III 1.0%	Enamel hypoplasia: 10.0%
		177 control hospital inpatients, 6.5	dmf 3.8	MG 2.5% Cal 4.0%	Cl. I 88.4% Cl. II 7.9% Cl. III 5.2%	Enamel hypoplasia: 5.2%

Preventing a dental handicap

Table 15.1. *continued*

Condition (authors)	Prevalence	No. and age (yrs)	Caries	Periodontal disease	Orthodontics	Other
Backman *et al.* (1990)		38 acyanotics, 6–7 76 control children, 5–7 12 acyanotics, 10–13 Control children, 10–13	dmft 3.8 dmfs 7.0 dmft 4.0 dmfs 5.5 DMFT 3.5 DMFS 5.0 DMFT 4.5 DMFS 8.0			Caries incidence reduced after cardiac surgery
Pollard and Curzon (1992)		32 heart defect children, 2–4	dmft 1.81	Segments with gingivitis = 0	–	*Strep. mutans* count positively correlated with number of decayed teeth in study group
		32 Control children, 2–4 31 heart defect children, 5–9 31 control children, 5–9 37 heart defect children, 10–16 37 control children, 10–6	dmft 1.6 dmft 4.3 dmft 2.7 DMFT 1.8 DMFT 1.6	Segments with gingivitis = 0 Segments with gingivitis = 1.1 Segments with gingivitis = 0.4 Segments with gingivitis = 1.8 Segments with gingivitis = 4.6		
Diabetes (D)	1/1600					
Sheppard (1936)		10, 10–19	–	80% minimal bone resorption 20% complete bone resorption	–	Full mouth radiographs Disease controlled by insulin and diet
Rutledge (1940)		20, 8–19	3 caries-free 11 'lower than expected caries'	16, gums of normal colour 10, evidence of bony changes	–	Life caries index (Bodecker)
Wegner (1971)		312, 10–18 388 matched controls	DMFT 12.6 DMFT 9.2	– –	– –	Included incipient lesions
Matsson and Koch (1975)		33, 9–16 Matched controls	DFS 13.4 DFS 20.5	–	–	Children treated by diet and insulin
Wegner (1975)		13–15 Controls	DMFT 1.88 DMFT 5.51	–	–	For diabetics diagnosed after 6 yrs of age
Faulconbridge *et al.* (1981)		94, 5–15 Matched controls (c)	Males: 16% with caries Females: 19% with caries Males: 16% with caries Females: 17% with caries	Males PLQ[6] = 0.57 Females PLQ = 0.55 Males PLQ = 0.42 Females PLQ = 0.28	–	Bay and Ainamo's Quantitative Index PLQ (1974)
Goteiner *et al.* (1986)		169, mean 11.3 80 controls mean 12.0	def/DMF 4.53 def/DMF 4.46	G1[7]: 1.39 (D) 1.34 (C) PDI[8]: 0.01 (D) 0.03 (C)	–	Children with family history of diabetes have lower caries prevalence

[1]OH, oral hygiene, [2]C1.; Class in Angle's classification; [3]GU, gingival units; [4]MG, marginal gingivitis; [5]Cal, calculus; [6]PLQ, stained plaque index; [7]GI, gingival index; [8]PDI, periodontal disease index.

were either unable or unwilling to obtain their care from a general dental practitioner. Despite the seeming increasing awareness in official circles that dental care for disabled people needs special provision, groups looking at the general health and related needs of such people often omit any mention of dental care (DHSS 1984, 1988; Royal College of Physicians 1987; Mansell 1992; Chamberlain 1993). A recent view from the Department of Health, after conferring with regional contacts, was that following on the publication of the Department's Health Circular (DHSS 1989b) this client group were being adequately served (B. Mouatt, personal communication).

REASONS FOR INADEQUATE DENTAL CARE

In spite of the recommendations just considered there is agreement that the dental health of disabled children is still neglected (Pollard and Curzon 1992; Nunn et al. 1993) and whilst dental health in healthy children has improved dramatically over the last 20 years, the same cannot be said for disabled children (Pope and Curzon 1991). Why this is so seems to arise from a number of factors, singly or in combination. Dentistry is largely a demanded service relying on sufficient motivation on the part of potential recipients to seek out such care. Not suprisingly then, people with disabilities in many instances have lost out. Other factors have been, and to an extent still are, the attitudes of provider, patient, and parents, as well as dental education and finance.

Many dentists have unfounded fears about providing dental care for handicapped people which culminate in negative attitudes in this sphere of their work (Ferguson et al. 1991; Gallagher 1991). Many parents and guardians have low expectations of dentistry which, when coupled with the often overwhelming, competing needs of their handicapped child, result in only emergency attendances for dental treatment (Finger and Jedrychowski 1989; Lo et al. 1991). In the past, very little attention, either didactic or practical, has been given to the topic of dentistry for handicapped people in undergraduate or even postgraduate education (Soto Rojas and Cushing 1991). This has meant that dental practitioners with a plentiful supply of work on normal patients are able to ignore the special groups. In addition, many dentists feel that providing such care is inadequately reimbursed and that these patients should be treated under the auspices of the salaried services, either community or hospital. The advent of fees on the general dental services fee scale (with prior approval) for the application of topical fluorides and fissure sealants for those with special needs, had little impact on the numbers of these items being provided. Likewise, the enhancement in fees paid to general dental practitioners for children whose treatment time is extended, is unlikely to be sufficient to encourage more practitioners to take on such care (Wilson 1992). More optimistically, annual returns for the community dental services indicate that more treatment is being provided for adults with disabilities (Murray and Nunn 1993). Whilst in the UK a lot of this care is provided by dentists with little formal training but much experience, other countries have had well-established training programmes for under- and postgraduates from which there are favourable

outcomes (Bedi and O'Donnell 1989; Ferguson et al. 1991; Marinelli et al. 1991).

Whilst dental care is free for children and young adults in full-time education, as well as for those in receipt of certain state benefits, parents and guardians may incur other expenses, like loss of time from work and in travel, which make dentistry less accessible.

NEED FOR SPECIAL DENTAL CARE

The need for good quality dental services in such special groups is necessary for many reasons but three in particular are of prime importance. There is some evidence that provision of dental treatment may markedly alter the habits and appearance of handicapped children (Ohmori et al. 1981), but there is general agreement that this on its own is not enough. Secondly, for a number of handicapped children, the need for dental treatment may impose a further handicap, and thirdly, the medical condition of some children is such that dental disease could be fatal (HMSO 1981). Part of these dental services must include preventive measures because of the difficulty of providing alternatives to the natural dentition for many of those patients (Burtner et al. 1991).

NEED FOR PREVENTION

In a memorandum submitted to the Royal Commission on the National Health Service, the British Dental Association (1977) stated that *prevention* of dental disease for handicapped patients was of vital importance and should receive absolute priority. Following on this, others (Ashton 1992; Holloway and Downer 1979; Richardson et al. 1981) have made the point that such preventive measures are justified for special groups although they may not be cost-effective for the population as a whole. Yet others have emphasized this point by stating that there is a case for the dental care of handicapped children to be at least as good (HMSO 1976), if not better, than that given to ordinary children.

This must be especially so in the light of such specific problem areas, common to many with disabilities, of, for example, the need to take medication long term. Such therapy is often given in a syrup vehicle, with disastrous consequences for the dentition (Hobson and Fuller 1987; Maguire 1994), although strenuous efforts are now being made by both the dental profession and the pharmaceutical industry to overcome this. Other authors have highlighted the particular risk that handicapped children face from dentally unsafe dietary practices (Palin-Palokas et al. 1987; Randell et al. 1992).

PREVENTIVE PROGRAMMES

With this and other such difficulties in mind, a number of authors have stressed the importance of a vigorous approach to prevention, including fluoride supplements, dietary advice, oral hygiene instruction, and the importance of regular professional dental care (Goodman 1981; Cooley and Sobel

1982; Pool 1982). However, prevention is not just up to the patient and/or parent but has to be the responsibility of the dentist. Indeed, many disabled children are further disadvantaged by poor preventive dental practices (Randell *et al.* 1992) or comprehensive restorative care not maintained if emphasis is not placed on prevention at follow-up (Mitchell *et al.* 1985). Unhappily, some parents who perceive a need for dental care want curative treatment rather than preventive procedures (Lo *et al.* 1991), although others are more positive about the benefits of preventive dental care for their child (Arch *et al.* 1994).

Aside from the one-to-one relationship, there are studies which have documented the establishment and success of programmes for groups of handicapped individuals. These programmes include supervised brushing by professional or lay staff, topical application of anti-bacterial agents, and the effects of tooth-brush modifications on oral hygiene programmes to target specific groups who are thought to require special dental care. These will be considered in turn.

The results from programmes of supervised brushing utilizing professional or lay staff are equivocal: regular daily brushing of the teeth of mentally handicapped patients does not always lead to long-term improvements in oral health when assessed over a period of years (Ogasawara *et al.* 1990; Shaw and Shaw 1990). However, closer supervision by care staff or supervised brushing gave more encouraging results (Lunn and Williams 1990; Dicks and Banning 1991). The study by Nicolaci and Tesini (1982) is interesting in that the steady improvement in oral hygiene was maintained over 18 months despite the loss of 45 per cent of the sample to placements in the community. Many of these latter group were the higher functioning residents and their loss could have been expected to bias the results in the opposite direction. Other studies do not report results but comment that the spin-off from the programmes is heightened awareness of oral health among all in the institutions, serving to maintain a high profile for dental health, particularly if senior administrators are involved (Fenton *et al.* 1982; Prosser, 1989).

Loesche (1981) summarized the use of topical agents to control specific plaque infections in handicapped people. Since that time other authors have reported positive effects from the use of topical agents, usually chlorhexidine. Many of the studies have been a double bind cross-over design and were run for a minimum of one month to a maximum of one year. Significant reductions in plaque and gingival indices were reported in studies using chlorhexidine mouth wash (McKenzie *et al.* 1992). Chlorhexidine spray, potentially easier to use in disabled populations than other vehicles, also produces significant reductions in periodontal scores (Francis *et al.* 1987; Chikke *et al.* 1991). Other easier to use techniques which also report significant results are chlorhexidine swabbing (Stiefel *et al.* 1992) and chlorhexidine toothpaste (Russel and Bay 1978). An innovation reported recently is chlorhexidine as a varnish to control dental plaque bacteria (J.I. Hogan, personal communication). Whilst this clinical trial is not yet complete, the evidence from laboratory studies is promising.

Modifications to manual tooth-brushes appear frequently as case reports in the literature; how much of the reported success is due to the mechanical modification and how much to the heightened awareness that such change brings is unclear (Soncini and Tsamtsouris 1989; Williams and Schuman 1988; Spratley 1991). The comparison of efficiency of manual versus electric tooth-brushes concludes similarly (Bratel and Berggren 1991).

Finally, the early targeting of special needs groups is fundamental to the success of any preventive programme. Identification of babies at risk and their subsequent follow-up dentally is now being investigated in a number of areas and an audit of one programme has shown promising results (J.G. Whittle, personal communication). Others allude to the potential spin-offs, as, for example, in the prevalence study by Jones and Blinkhorn (1986) of children at special schools in Glasgow. This study highlighted again the lower prevalence of dental caries relative to a control group, attributing the difference to the publicity given to fluoride supplements for handicapped children. However, in that study, only eight out of 34 special schools distributed fluoride supplements and, of those 34 schools, only 10 had organized tooth-brushing programmes.

Fluoride supplements for handicapped children have been dealt with only briefly. Dowell and Joyston-Bechall (1981) and Murray and Rugg-Gunn (1982), discussing fluoride supplement dosages, comment only that these may need to be altered for special groups.

A small number of texts, whilst supposedly addressing themselves to the topic of prevention for handicapped people, on the whole only discuss standard, accepted preventive techniques as used for non-handicapped groups in the population. However, there are a number of locally based preventive dental programmes underway in the UK for special groups of children and young adults which, as yet, have no published results. Other studies, with more detailed results are given in Table 15.2. For some of the programmes (Brown 1975) it is difficult to separate out the benefits to be gained from treatment and preventive efforts in terms of improvements in dental health. An additional problem encountered with some preventive schemes for special groups is that of using retrospective controls in a time of changing caries prevalence (Stephen and MacFadyen 1977).

CONCLUSIONS

● For many disabled children, dental care may not be perceived as important by parents or carers, yet dental disease or its consequences may pose further threats to already compromised children. The prevention of dental disease is thus a high priority for vulnerable groups in the population.

● In the UK, general dental services within the NHS accord a priority to children, as well as additional fees for the care of those with a disability. Practitioners are, however, unwilling to provide care for many such individuals, because of inadequate remuneration, training and experience with disabled people in general.

● The other main source of primary dental care for disabled people, the community dental service, is sometimes seen as inappropriate in an era of normalization, paradoxically *because* of its very specialist role.

Table 15.2. Preventive programmes for handicapped children

Study	Condition	Programme	Oral health		Other
			Dental caries	Periodontal disease	
Ripa and Cole (1970)	91 severely mentally retarded, 5–10 yrs	Cyanoacrylate fissure sealant applied under rubber dam, with body restraints, to 278 Ds, Es, 6s	84.3% reduction in permanent teeth (5 became carious, 32 in control teeth)	—	At 12 m one-third teeth sealed, one-third partly sealed, one-third lost all sealants; 63 teeth had some evidence of caries initially
Brown (1975)	53 children 7–18½ yrs, with variety of handicaps	Routine dental care plus home care to include fluoride supplements, diet control, oral hygiene measures, topical fluorides	DMFT increment over 18 m in 8–10-yr-olds = 0.6 (1.9 in normal controls)	Increments for 7–11 yr-olds over 18 m: debris: 12 → 0.7 gingivitis: no change pocketing: 4 → 3 segments involved	Maintenance required less than half the time and one-third of the cost of the initial restorative programme
Richardson et al. (1977)	160 retarded children, 5–21-yrs-old: IQ 30–80	UV-polymerized fissure sealant, half-mouth controls, 812 1° + 2° molars		—	2-yr results: 40% retained primary teeth: 61% retained on permanent teeth
Stephen and MacFadyen (1977)	57 cleft palate children, 3–5 yrs, 34 cleft palate children (retrospective control)	Dietary and oral hygiene advice, fluoride therapy and fissure sealing (Nuva-Seal)	defs after 3 yrs: 1.44 test 13.5 control Caries free: 74% test 0% control	—	Total costs: prevention for test group: £438; treatment for control group £426–£490. (Treatment 65%–90% more costly than prevention)
Dowell and Teasdale (1978)	Medical handicap 4 yrs 8 m	Health visitor and dental officer visits to home, fluoride tablets, OHI[1]. Surgery visits/4–6 m, topical fluorides and OHI.	80% caries-free; dmf 0.6	—	—
Loesche (1981)	Trisomy-21 and non-trisomy 21 children	Suspension of OH procedures and 5% Kanamycin (K) 3 × day or placebo (P) applied over 5 days at 5-wk intervals	—	Plaque weight (as % of initial value) K: 48% P: 114%, after 10 wks. Gingivitis (as % of initial value): K 87% P 106%, after 10 wks	Systemic metronidazole may also be useful for treatment of periodontitis

Table 15.2. *continued*

Study	Condition	Programme	Oral health — Dental caries	Periodontal disease	Other
Richardson et al. (1981)	103 mentally retarded children (IQ 30–80); 5–21 yrs; 64% male	5-yr follow-up of UV polymerized fissure-sealant resin (half-mouth controls)	Less than 50% of the decay in test teeth compared with controls		
Attril and Hobson (1984)	30 asthmatics (A), 30 cystic fibrosis (CF) 5–16 yrs 9 m 30 orthopaedic (O) controls	Dental treatment, OHI, fluoride tablets.	1st visit / 2nd visit d + D 1.5 (A) 0.4 1.7 (CF) 0.6 2.6 (O) — f + F 1.1 (A) 1.9 1.2 (CF) 2.4 1.5 (O) —	1st visit / 2nd visit plaque (segments) 3.0 / 1.3 3.6 / 1.3 2.7 / — gingivitis (segments) 1.2 / 0.6 1.8 / 0.4 0.9 / —	Fluoride tablet uptake continuing for 90.4% (28) children at 2nd visit. Uptake of care: 77% asthmatics; 87% cystic fibrosis by 2nd visit
Mellor and Doyle (1987)	Special schools children (1977) n = 106, 14 yrs (1982) n = 49, 14.3 yrs	Home visits, fluoride tablets, school brushing, comprehensive dental treatment	1977 / 1982 D 3.8 / 0.4 M 1.4 / 0.8 F 0.7 / 3.8 similar in 1982 to other Rochdale children	—	Uptake of treatment in community dental service: 1978 80% 1982 79% GA^2 requirements for ESN (S) children: 1977 34.8% 1982 7.0%
Schwarz and Vigild (1987)	329 mentally retarded, 6–9-yr-olds (resident and non-residents)	Community and personal preventive measures quarterly, bimonthly or not available, plus comprehensive dental care	40% caries-free (i) Non-residents had 25% more caries than normal individuals of same age (ii) 40% 13–19-yr-olds DMFS >8 with preventive programme; 60% DMFS >8 without preventive programme	(Non-residents) severe gingivitis: Supervised tooth-brushing 12% Unsupervised tooth-brushing 28%	

^{1}OHI = oral hygiene instruction. ^{2}GA = general anaesthesia.

- The advent of the purchaser/provider model of care provision in the NHS could remove the preventive focus for special children, if contracts for their care are taken up by the general dental services.

- Heightened awareness of the fundamental need for effective prevention from the earliest age, through paediatricians, health visitors, and others in primary care teams, is the only means whereby the disappointing dental health statistics for these disabled people will be improved.

REFERENCES

Arch, L.A., Jenner, A.M., and Whittle, J.G. (1994). *Int. J. paed. Dent.* **44**, 127–32.

Ashton, T. (1992). The purchaser–provider split: Implications for dental services. *N.Z. dent. J.* **88**, 121–25.

Attrill, M. and Hobson, P. (1984). The organisation of dental care for groups of medically handicapped children. *Commun. dent. Health*, **1**, 21–7.

Backman, T.K., Larmas, M.A., Kaar, M-L., and Paavilainen, T. (1990). Evaluation of stannous fluoride and chlorhexidene sprays on plaque and gingivitis in handicapped children. *J. Clin. Ped. Dent.* **15**, 51–4.

Baird, P.A. and Sadovnick, A.D. (1987). Life expectancy in Down syndrome. *J. Paediatr.* **110**, 849–54.

Beck, J.D. and Hunt, R.J. (1985). Oral health status in the United States: problems of special patients. *J. dent. Educ.* **49**, 407–26.

Bedi, R. and O'Donnell, D. (1989). Long term effects of a course on dental care for handicapped persons. *J. dent. Educ.* **53**, 722–4.

Blackharsh, C. (1977). Dental aspects of patients with cystic fibrosis: A preliminary clinical study. *J. Am. dent. Ass.* **95**, 106–10.

Bratel, J. and Berggren, U. (1991). Long term oral effects of manual or electric toothbrushes used by mentally handicapped adults. *Clin. prev. Dent.* **13**, 5–7.

British Dental Association (1977) Memorandum to the Royal Commission on the National Health Service Editorial: *Br. dent. J.* **142**, 53–63.

Brooks, H.T., Zacherl, W.A., and Rule, T.T. (1970). Caries prevalence in children with cystic fibrosis. *IADR*, Abstr. No. 338.

Brown, J.P. (1975). Dental treatment for handicapped patients. (1) The efficacy of a preventive programme for children. (2) The economics of dental treatment—a cost benefit analysis. *Australia dent. J.* **20**, 316–25.

Burtner, A.P., Low, D.W., McNeal, D.R., Hasse, T.M., and Smith, R.G. (1991). Effects of chlorhexidine spray on plaque on gingival health in institutionalized persons with mental retardation. *Spec. care Dent.* **11**, 97–100.

Chamberlain, M.A. (1993). *An assessment of health and related needs of physically handicapped young adults.* HMSO, London.

Chikke, U.M., Pochee, R., Rudolph, M.J., and Reinach, S.G. (1991). *J. clin. Perio.* **18**, 281–6.

Cohen, M.M. and Feldman, B.S. (1978). *Oral aspects of muscular dystrophy.* Proceedings of the 4th International Association of Dentistry for the Handicapped, London.

Cooley, R.O. and Sobel, R.S. (1982). Dental treatment considerations for the medically compromised child. *Ped. Clin. N. Am.* **29**, 613–29.

DHSS (Department of Health and Social Security) (1977a). *Prevention and health*, Cmnd. 7047. HMSO, London.

DHSS (Department of Health and Social Security) (1977b). *The way forward. Priorities in the health and social services.* HMSO, London.

DHSS (Department of Health and Social Security) (1979a) *Patients first.* HMSO, London.

DHSS (Department of Health and Social Security) (1979b). *Royal Commission of Enquiry into the National Health Services*, Cmnd. 7615. HMSO, London.

DHSS (Department of Health and Social Security) (1981). *Care in action. A handbook of policies and priorities for the health and personal social services in England.* HMSO, London.

DHSS (Department of Health and Social Security) (1984). *Helping mentally handicapped people with special problems. Report of a DHSS study team.* HMSO, London.

DHSS (Department of Health and Social Security) (1988). *Information needs of disabled people, their carers and service providers.* HMSO, London.

DHSS (Department of Health and Social Security) (1989a). *National Health Service and Community Care Bill.* HMSO, London.

DHSS (Department of Health and Social Security) (1989b) *Health services management: the future development of community dental services.* Health Circular (89)2. HMSO, London.

Dicks, J.L. and Banning, J.S. (1991). Evaluation of calculus accumulation in tube-fed, mentally handicapped patients: the effects of oral hygiene status. *Spec. Care Dent.* **11**, 104–6.

Dowell, T.B. and Joyston Bechall, S. (1981). Fluoride supplements age related dosages. *Br. dent. J.* **150**, 273–5.

Dowell, T.B. and Teasdale, J. (1978). Haemophilia and dental treatment. *J. Am. dent. Ass.* **144**, 177–8.

Evans, D.J., Greening, S., and French, A.D. (1991). A study of the dental health of children and young adults attending special schools in South Glamorgan. *Int. J. paed. Dent.* **1**, 17–24.

Faulconbridge, A.R., Bradshaw, W.C.L., Jenkins, P.A., and Baum, J.D. (1981). Dental status of a group of diabetic children. *Br. dent. J.* **151**, 253–5.

Fenton, S.J., DeBiase, C., and Portugal, B.V. (1982). A strategy for implementing a dental health education program for state facilities with limited resources. *Rehab. Lit.* **43**, 290–3.

Ferguson, F.S., Bernstsen, B., and Richardson, P.S. (1991). Dentists willingness to provide care for patients with developmental disabilities. *Spec. Care Dent.* **11**, 234–7.

Finger, S. and Jedrychowski, J.R. (1989). Parents' perception of access to dental care for handicapped children. *Spec. Care Dent.* **8**, 195–9.

Fitzimmons, J.S. (1982). The provision of regional genetic services in the United Kingdom. *The Times*, 19 March, London.

Foster, T.D., Griffiths, M.I., and Gordon, P.H. (1974). The effect of cerebral palsy on the size of the skull. *Am. J. Orthodont.* **66**, 40–9.

Franceeschi, M., Comola, M., and Piattoni, F. (1990). Prevalence of dementia in adult patients with trisomy 21. *Am. J. Med. Genet.* **7** (suppl.), 306–8.

Francis, J.R., Hunter, B., and Addy, M. (1987). A comparative survey of 3 delivery methods of chlorhexidene in handicapped children. *J. Period.* **58**, 451–5.

Gallagher, F.E. (1991). Professional attitudes towards the developmentally disabled patient. *J. Mass. dent. Soc.* **40**, 19–21.

Gingis, S.S., Staple, P.H., Miller, W.A., Sedranks, N., and Thompson, T. (1980). Dental root abnormalities and gingival overgrowth in epileptic patients receiving anti-convulsant therapy. *J. Perio.* **51**, 474–82.

Goodman, J.R. (1981). Dental treatment of children with congenital heart disease. *Proc. Br. paedodont. Soc.* **11**, 15–17.

Goteiner, D., Vogel, R., Deasy, M., and Goteiner, C. (1986). Periodontal and caries experience in children with insulin-dependant diabetes mellitus. *J. Am. dent. Ass.* **113**, 277–9.

Gould, M.S.E. and Picton, D.C.A. (1960). the gingival condition of congenitally cyanotic individuals. *Br. dent. J.* **109**, 96–100.

Guillikson, J.S. (1969). Oral findings of mentally retarded children. *J. dent. Child.* **34**, 59–64.

Hakala, P.E. (1967). Dental and oral changes in congenital heart disease. *Suom. Hammaslaak. Toim.* **63**, 284–324.

Harding, T.W. (1980). *The role of a constructional furniture system in special schools.* Handicapped Persons Research Unit, Newcastle-upon-Tyne Polytechnic.

Harris, A.I., Cox, E., and Smith C.R.W. (1971). *Handicapped and impaired in Great Britain.* HMSO, London.

Henderson, P. (1968). Changing patterns of disease and disability in school children in England and Wales. *Br. med. J.* **2** 259–63.

HMSO (1976). *Fit for the future.* The Report of the Committee on Child Health Services, Vol. 1, Cmnd. 6684, HMSO, London.

HMSO (1978a). *Development team for the mentally handicapped, first report, 1976–1977.* HMSO, London.

HMSO (1978b). *Special educational needs.* Report of the Committee of Enquiry into Education of Handicapped Children and Young People. HMSO, London.

HMSO (1981). *Towards better dental health.* Report of the Dental Strategy Review Group. HMSO, London.

Hobson, P. (1980). The treatment of medically handicapped children. *Int. dent. J.* **30**, 6–13.

Hobson, P. and Fuller, S. (1987). Sugar based medicines and dental disease—progress report. *Commun. dent. Health,* **4**, 169–76.

Holland, T.J. and O'Mullane, D.M. (1990). The organisation of dental care for groups of mentally handicapped persons. *Commun. dent. Health,* **7**, 285–93.

Holloway, P.J. and Downer, M.N. (1979). The benefit of preventive procedures for high risk groups. *Int. dent. J.* **29**, 118–24.

Hyppa, J. and Paunio, K. (1979). Oral health and salivary factors in children with asthma. *Proc. Finn. dent. Soc.* **75**, 7–10

Jagels, A.E. and Sweeney, E.A. (1976). Oral health of patients with cystic fibrosis and their siblings. *J. dent. Res.* **55**, 991–6.

James, P.M.C., Jackson, D., Slack, G.L., and Lawton, F.E. (1960). Gingival health and dental cleanliness in English school children. *Archs. oral Biol.* **3**, 57–66.

Johnson, N.P. and Young, M.A. (1963). Periodontal disease in mongols. *J. Perio.* **34**, 41–7.

Jones, M.G. and Blinkhorn, A.S. (1986). The dental health of children attending special schools in Glasgow. *J. paed. Dent.* **2**, 61–6.

Kamen, S. (1981). Dental management of patients with mental retardation and related developmental disorders. *J. Can. dent. Ass.* **47**, 663–6.

Kaner, A., Losch, P.K., and Green, H. (1946). Oral manifestations of congenital heart disease. *J. Paed.* **29**, 269–76.

Kastein, S. (1957). Oral dental and orthodontic problems of speech in cerebral palsy. *J. dent. Child.* **24**, 243–6.

Kendall, N.P. (1992). Differences in dental health observed within a group of non-institutionalized mentally handicapped adults attending day centres. *Commun. dent. Health,* **9**, 31–8.

Kinirons, M.J. (1985). Dental health of children with cystic fibrosis: an interim report. *J. paed. Dent.* **1**, 3–8.

Kroll, R.G. Budnick, J., and Kobren, A. (1970). Incidence of dental caries and periodontal disease in Down's syndrome. *NY State dent. J.* **36**, 151–6.

Lo, G.L., Soh, G., Vignehsa, H., and Chellappah, N.K. (1991). Dental service utilization of disabled children. *Spec. Care Dent.* **11**, 194–6.

Loesche, W.J. (1981). Plaque control in the handicapped. The treatment of specific infections. *Can. dent. Ass. J.* **47**, 649–86.

Lundstrom, A., Eeg-Olofsson, O., and Hamp, S.E. (1982). Effect of anti-epileptic drug treatment and carbamazepine or phenytoin on the oral state of children and adolescents. *J. clin. Perio.* **49**, 482–8.

Lunn, H.D. and Williams, A.C. (1990). The development of a toothbrushing programme at a school for children with moderate and severe learning difficulties. *Commun. dent. Health,* **7**, 403–6.

MacEntee, M.I., Silver, J.G., Gibson, G., and Weiss, R. (1985). Oral health in a long term care institution equipped with a dental service. *Commun. dent. oral Epidemiol.* **13**, 260–3.

Maclaurin, E.T., Shaw, L., and Foster, T.D. (1985b). Dental caries and periodontal disease in children with Down's syndrome and other mentally handicapping conditions. *J. paed. dent.* **1**, 15–20.

Maguire, A. (1994). Problem areas in liquid oral medication. In *Proceedings of the symposium: Sugarless—Towards the year 2000,* (ed. A.J. Rugg-Gunn) Royal Society of Chemistry, Cambridge.

Mahaney, M.C. (1986). Delayed dental development and pulmonary disease severity in children with cystic fibrosis. *Archs. oral Biol.* **31**, 363–7.

Mansell, J.L. (1992). *Services for people with learning disabilities and challenging behaviour or mental health needs.* HMSO, London.

Marinelli, R.D., Ferguson, F.S., Berentsen, B.J., and Richardson, P.S. (1991). An undergraduate dental education program providing care for children with disabilities. *Spec. Care Dent.* **11**, 110–13.

Matsson, L. and Koch, G. (1975). Caries frequency in children with controlled diabetes. *Scand. J. dent. Res.* **83**, 327–32.

McCabe, M. (1979). Handicap in Newcastle-upon-Tyne. Submitted B. Ed. (Hons) thesis. University of Newcastle-upon-Tyne.

McIver, F.T. and Machen, J.B. (1979). Prevention of dental disease in handicapped people. In *Dentistry for the handicapped patient.* Postgraduate dental handbook series, 5, (ed. K.E. Wessels), pp. 77–93. John Wright, Boston.

McKenzie, W.T., Forgas, L., Vernins, A.R., Parkes, D., and Lunestall, J.D. (1992). Comparison of a 0.12% chlorhexidine mouthrinse and an essential oil mouth rinse on oral health in institutionalized mentally handicapped adults. One year results. *J. Period.* **63**, 187–93.

Mellor, J. and Doyle, A.J. (1987). The evaluation of a dental treatment service for children attending special schools. *Commun. dent. Health.* **4**, 43–8.

Melville, M.R.B., Pool, D.M., Jaffe, E.C., Gelbier, S., and Tully, W.J. (1981). A dental service for handicapped children. *Br. dent. J.* **151**, 259–61.

Mitchell, L., Murray, J.J., and Ryder, W. (1985). Management of the handicapped and the anxious child: a retrospective study of dental treatment carried out under general anaesthesia. *J. paed. Dent.* **1**, 9–14.

Modeer, T., Dahllof, G., and Theorell, K. (1986). Oral health in non-institutionalized epileptic children with special reference to phenytoin medication. *Commun. Dent. oral Epidemiol.* **14**, 165–8.

Morgan, S.B. (1979). Mental retardation. In *Dentistry for the handicapped patient*. Postgraduate dental handbook series, 5, (ed. K.E. Wessels), pp. 21–28. John Wright, Boston.

Morton, M.E. (1977). Dental disease in a group of adult mentally handicapped patients. *Publ. Hlth.* **91**, 23–32.

Murray, J.J. and Rugg-Gunn, A.J. (1982). Fluoride tablets and drops. In *Fluorides in caries prevention*. Dental Practitioner Handbook, p. 95. Wright, Bristol.

Murray, J.J. and Nunn, J.H. (1993). Trends in the community dental service 1980–1990. *Commun. dent. Health*, **10**, 335–342.

Mutch, L., Alberman, E., and Hagberg, B. (1992). Cerebral palsy epidemiology. Where are we now and where are we going? *Dev. Med. Child. Neurol.* **34**, 547–55.

Nicolaci, A.N.B. and Tesini, D.A. (1982). Improvements in the oral hygiene of institutionalized mentally retarded individuals through training of direct care staff: a longitudinal study. *Spec. Care dent.* **2**, 217–21.

Nielsen, L.A. (1990). Caries among children with cerebral palsy: relation to CP-diagnosis, mental and motor handicap. *J. dent. Child.* **57**, 267–73.

Nowak, A.J. (1984). Dental disease in handicapped persons. *Spec. Care. Dent.* **4**, 66–9.

Nunn, J.H. (1984). The dental health of handicapped children in the Northern Region and the resources available to them for dental care. Ph.D. thesis. University of Newcastle-upon-Tyne.

Nunn, J.H. (1990). Fragile X (Martin Bell) syndrome and dental care. A case report and review of the literature. *Br. dent. J.* **168**, 160–2.

Nunn, J.H. and Murray, J.J. (1987). The dental health of handicapped children in Newcastle and Northumberland. *Br. dent. J.* **162**, 9–14.

Nunn, J.H., Carmichael, C.L., and Gordon, P.H. (1993). Dental disease and current treatment needs in a group of physically handicapped children. *Commun. dent. Health*, **10**, 389–96.

Ogasawara, T., *et al.* (1990). Oral findings in severely handicapped patients participating in the periodic dental check-up system for five years. *Shiroui, Shikagaku, Zusshi*, **28**, 732–40.

Ohmori, I., Awaya, S., and Ishikawa, F. (1981). Dental care for severely handicapped children. *Int. dent. J.* **31**, 177–84.

Orner, G. (1975). Dental caries experience among children with Down's syndrome and their siblings. *Archs. oral Biol.* **20**, 627–34.

Palin-Palokas, T., Hausen, H., and Heinonen, O.P. (1987). Relative importance of caries risk factors in Finnish mentally retarded children. *Commun. Dent. oral. Epidemiol.* **15**, 19–23.

Pharoah, P.O.D., Cooke, T., Rosenbloom, I., and Cooke, R.W.I. (1987). Trends in birth prevalence of cerebral palsy. *Archs. dis. Child.* **62**, 379–84.

Pollard, M.A. and Curzon, M.E.J. (1992). Dental health and salivary streptococcus mutans levels in a group of children with heart defects. *Int. J. paed. Dent.* **2**, 81–5.

Pool, D. (1982). Dental care for the handicapped adolescent. *Int. dent. J.* **32**, 194–202.

Pope, J.E.C. and Curzon, M.E.J. (1991). The dental status of cerebral palsied children. *Paed. Dent.* **13**, 156–62.

Primosch, R.E. (1980). Tetracycline discoloration, enamel defects and dental caries in patients with cystic fibrosis. *Oral. Surg.* **50**, 301–8.

Prosser, H. (1989). *Evaluation of the second phase workshop on dental care* (2). MENCAP, London.

Randell, O.M., Harth, S., and Seow, W.K. (1992). Preventive dental health practices of non-institutionalized Down syndrome children: a controlled study. *J. Clin. paed. Dent.* **16**, 225–9.

Rhodes, W.A. (1984). The mouths of the insane. *J. Br. dent. Ass.* **5**, 413–15.

Richardson, B.A., Smith, D.C., and Hargreaves, J.A. (1977). Study of fissure sealants in mentally retarded Canadian children. *Commun. Dent. Oral Epidermiol* **5**, 220–6.

Richardson, B.A., Smith, D.C., and Hargreaves, J.A. (1981). A 5-year clinical evaluation of the effectiveness of a fissure sealant in mentally retarded Canadian children. *Commun. Dent. oral Epidemiol.* **9**, 170–4.

Ripa, L.W. and Cole, W.W. (1970). Occlusal sealing and caries prevention: results after 12 months, after a single application of adhesive resin. *J. dent. Res.* **49**, 171–3.

Robinson, P.B., Harris, H., and Harvey, W. (1983). Abnormal skeletal and dental growth in epileptic children. *Br. dent. J.* **154**, 9–13.

Royal College of Physicians (1987). Physical disability in 1986 and beyond. *J. Roy. Coll. Phys.* **20**, 3–37.

Russell, B.G. and Bay, L.M. (1978). Oral use of chlorhexidine gluconate toothpaste in epileptic children. *Scand. J. dent. Res.* **86**, 52–7.

Rutledge, L.E. (1940). Oral and roentgenographic aspects of the teeth and jaws of juvenile diabetes. *J. Am. dent. Ass.* **27**, 1740–50.

Schwarz, E. and Vigild, M. (1987). Provision of dental services for handicapped children in Denmark. *Commun. dent. Health*, **4**, 35–42.

Scottish Home and Health Department (1984). *Dental services for the handicapped.* HMSO, London.

Shaw, M.J. and Shaw, L. (1990). The effectiveness of differing dental health education programmes in improving the oral health of adults with mental handicaps attending Birmingham training centres. *Commun. dent. Health*, **8**, 139–45.

Sheppard, I.M. (1936). Alveolar resorption in diabetes mellitus. *Dent. Cosmos*, **78**, 1075–9.

Soble, R.K. (1974). Sociological and psychological considerations in special patient care: the dentist, the patient and the family. *Dent. Clin. N. Am.* **18**, 554–6.

Soncini, J.A. and Tsamtsouris, A. (1989). Individually modified toothbrushes and improvement of oral hygiene and gingival health in cerebral palsy children. *J. Pedod.* **13**, 331–44.

Soto Rojas, A.E. and Cushing, A. (1992). Assessment of the need for education and/or training the dental care of people with handicaps. *Commun. dent. Health*, **9**, 165–70.

Spratley, M.H. (1991). A toothbrushing aid for a quadraplegic patient. *Spec. Care Dent.* **11**, 114–15.

Stark, G.G. (1977). *Spina bifida. Problems and management.* Blackwell, Oxford.

Stephen, K.W. and MacFadyen, E.E. (1977). Three years of clinical caries prevention for cleft palate patients. *Br. dent. J.* **143**, 111–16.

Stiefel, D.J., Truelove, E.L., Chin, M.M., and Mandel, L.S. (1992). Efficacy of chlorhexidine swabbing in oral health care for people with severe disabilities. *Spec. Care Dent.* **12**, 57–62.

Stoll, C., Alembik, Y., and Dott, B. (1990). Epidemiology of Down syndrome in 118, 265 consecutive births. *Am. J. med. Genet.* **7** (suppl.), 79–83.

Strodel, B.J. (1987). The effects of cerebral palsy on occlusion. *J. dent. Child.* **54**, 255–60.

Swallow, J.N., Dehallis, J., and Young, W.F. (1967). Side effects of antibiotics in cystic fibrosis: dental changes in relation to antibiotic administration. *Archs. dis. Child.* **42**, 311–18.

Swerdloff, M. (1980). The problems and concerns of the handicapped. *J. dent. Educ.* **44**, 131–5.

The Children's Committee (1980). *Second Annual Report, 1979–1980.* Mary Ward House, London.

Ulseth, J.E., Hestnes, A., Storner, L.J., and Storhaug, K. (1991). Dental caries and periodontitis in persons with Down syndrome. *Spec. Care Dent.* **11**, 71–3.

Vigild, M. (1985b). Prevalence of malocclusion in mentally retarded young adults. *Commun. Dent. oral Epidemiol.* **13**, 183–4.

Vigild, M. (1986). Dental caries experience among children with Down's syndrome. *J. ment. Def. Res.* **30**, 271–6.

Walton, J.M. and Nattrass, F.J. (1954). On the classification, natural history and treatment of the myopathies. *Brain,* **77**, 169–231.

Wegner, H. (1971). Dental caries in young diabetics. *Caries Res.* **45**, 188–92.

Wegner, H. (1975). Increment of caries in young diabetics. *Caries Res.* **9**, 91–6.

Williams, N.J. and Schuman, N.J. (1988). The curved-bristle toothbrush: an aid for the handicapped population. *J. dent. Child.* **55**, 291–3.

Wilson, K.I. (1992). Treatment accessibility for physically and mentally handicapped people—a review of the literature. *Commun. dent. Health,* **9** 187–192.

Wotman, S., Mercadente, J., Mandel, D.K., Goldman, S.R., and Denning, C. (1973). The occurrence of calculus in normal children, children with cystic fibrosis and children with asthma. *J. Perio.* **44**, 278–80.

16. Social factors and preventive dentistry

J.F. BEAL

These things one ought to consider most attentively... the mode in which the inhabitants live, and what are their pursuits, whether they are fond of drinking and eating to excess, and given to indolence, or are fond of exercise and labour, and not given to excess in eating and drinking (Hippocrates c.400 BC)

One of the most common criticisms that teachers at dental schools make of their students is that the students treat the individual tooth rather than the mouth as a whole. In reality that comment only goes half way. It is essential that we recognize that we are responsible not just to a mouth but to a patient. We are, therefore, required to consider what makes the patient 'tick'. What are his or her attitudes to their teeth? How were those attitudes formed, can they be changed, and if so how? Often it is necessary to go a step further. For example, if we consider water fluoridation we are concerned not for the dental health of an individual patient, but for that of a community which may include more than one million people. Again we must know something about that community. We must learn how public opinion is formed, how it can be measured, why some people are against fluoridation and how we can influence the decision-making process in order to promote the fluoridation of the water supply.

It can be seen, therefore, that preventive dentistry is not a mechanistic matter based purely on a knowledge of clinical techniques. It requires an understanding of the society in which we live. We need to know what social factors are relevant, how individuals are influenced by their upbringing, how we can best communicate with different groups and so on. This chapter examines the relationship between such social factors and dental health, and tries to suggest ways in which traditional approaches in preventive dentistry might be modified in the light of this extra dimension.

SOCIAL CLASS

Before looking at the relationship between social status and dental health, it is necessary to examine the concept of social stratification. In all societies members are divided into various social strata or layers. Some are recognized as 'superior' and other as 'inferior'. Each person, therefore, has a social *status* which is the position he or she occupies within the social system. There are, broadly speaking, two types of status, *ascribed* and *achieved*. An ascribed status is one which is determined at birth such as sex or caste. An achieved status on the other hand is gained during the lifetime of the person and may, for instance, be based upon the occupation of the indi-

vidual. A status group may be either *open* or *closed*. An open form of stratification is found in the Australian aborigines where status is related to age and where each man becomes successively a hunter, a warrior, and eventually reaches the heights of elderhood. Every man passes through each social position. The caste system, conversely, is an example of a closed status grouping. It is a permanent rank and determines one's whole lifestyle including what type of occupation one can have, with whom one can mix, and even who one can marry. Contact between those of different castes is limited and governed by predetermined rules, and movement from one caste to another is not allowed.

In Western society, social status is based upon the class system. This is a relatively open system in which mobility from one group to another is not automatic, as with the aborigines, but it is permitted and can be made with comparative ease. There are numerous systems of dividing the population in to social classes, ranging from the early classifications of Marx and Weber to the more generally used one of the Registrar General's Social Class (OPCS 1980), although this has recently been further modified by publication of the Standard Occupational Classification (SOC) for use by government departments (OPCS 1990). The Registrar General's Social Class, which is still widely used, is based upon the occupation of an individual and divides the population into five groups or classes. Table 16.1 shows the type of occupation allocated to each social class together with examples for each class. One of the disadvantages of this particular classification is that about a half of the population falls into class III. This class is, therefore, frequently subdivided into non-manual and manual categories.

The advantage of this type of classification is that it enables us to make generalizations about the lifestyles, behaviour, and attitudes of others, based on the pattern for that group as a whole. Of course, not everyone from a social class will share the same lifestyle, but the differences between those from the various classes are often great enough to identify patterns and trends. A number of these differences between the social classes have an important bearing on preventive dentistry. Mention will be made later of various other sociological factors which are themselves associated with social class. However, two of these factors are fundamental in understanding the relationship between social status and health. The first factor is income, where those in the higher social classes in general receive a higher income. The other factor is education. Most of those in social class I have a university or college education. At the other end of the scale the

Table 16.1. The Registrar General's Social Class

Social class	Description	Examples
I	'Professional' and top managerial occupations	Doctor, dentist, university lecturer, company secretary
II	'Intermediate' occupations, i.e. minor professions and lower managerial	Teacher, nurse, chiropodist, supermarket manager
III	'Skilled' occupations:	
	—non-manual	Draughtsman, clerk, policeman
	—manual	Plumber, tool-maker, coalminer
IV	'Semi-skilled' occupations	Gardener, storekeeper, postman
V	'Unskilled' occupations	Labourer, kitchen hand, office cleaner

majority of subjects in social class V left full-time education at the minimum school leaving age and went straight into a job or at least started looking for work.

Even though social class is a status which is achieved during the lifetime of an individual, it also has an ascribed component as a minor takes the social class of his or her father. In fact, the whole family is recognized as a unit of social class, a married woman being classified according to the social class of her husband.

In many cases there is a social gradient from those in social class I to those in social class V. However, it is often simpler to divide the population into just two groups in order to make broad statements about social differences. For the sake of convenience, classes I, II, and sometimes class III non-manual, are combined under the title of 'middle class' whilst classes III manual, IV, and V form the 'working class'.

SOCIAL CLASS AND DISEASE

It has long been recognized that there are a number of health inequalities related to social class. Edwin Chadwick in 1842 published a series of tables illustrating the connection between mortality and social class. This pattern is still found today. The infant mortality statistics in England and Wales (OPCS 1993) show that babies whose fathers had unskilled jobs run twice the risk of stillbirth and more than one and a half times the risks of death under one year than babies whose fathers worked in the professions. Exactly the same relationship is found in the mortality rates of men aged 16–64 years in England and Wales (OPCS 1986). Further, the Black Report (Report of a Research Working Group 1980) states that 'an extraordinary variety of causes of death such as cancer, heart and respiratory disease differentiate between classes'. In spite of the widely held expectation that the social gradient would reduce following the formation of the National Health Service, the differences not only remain (Eames *et al.* 1993), but the gap has, in fact, widened and is still widening (Whitehead 1992).

It is not only in death that inequalities exist between the rich and poor. Although the data is more limited it is clear that the pattern of morbidity is also strongly related to social status. North *et al.* (1993) reported that both short- and long-term sickness absence was more frequent in the poorer paid grades of the civil service. Many diseases are more associated with those from the working classes whilst a few are found more commonly in the middle classes. Examples of diseases in which the incidence is higher in the lower social classes are bronchitis, pneumonia, tuberculosis, rheumatic heart disease, ulcer and cancer of the stomach. Although overall rates for the infectious respiratory diseases have fallen, the differences between the classes have widened over the past 50 years. Conversely, a number of the diseases of affluence, formerly associated with those from the higher social groups, are now found to show no differences between classes, or even a reverse trend with the incidence being higher in the lower social groups (Blaxter 1976). One such example is coronary heart disease, which in the 1930s was a 'disease of the rich'. Now it is more commonly a cause of death among the least affluent sections of the community. The main reason for this reversal has been a fall in its incidence in the higher social groups (Marmot and McDowall 1986).

In 65 of the 78 disease categories used for men (OPCS 1986; Townsend *et al.* 1988) social classes IV and V had a higher mortality than either class I or class II. Only one cause, malignant melanoma, showed the reverse trend. In women, a similar social gradient was found in 62 of the 82 categories, with only four categories more common in social classes I and II. The rest are neutral. Clearly so-called 'diseases of affluence' have all but disappeared and what is left is a general health disadvantage of the poor (Whitehead 1992).

A knowledge of the social distribution of disease can be important, for example, in refuting allegations by anti-fluoridationists when they claim that fluoridation causes some particular disease. It was suggested at one time that as the incidence of cancer of the stomach was higher in Slough, where the natural level of fluoride was one part per million, compared with nearby fluoride-free Gerrards Cross, that the cause of this difference must be the fluoride. In fact, Slough is a large industrial town, whereas Gerrards Cross is a London commuter community with a much higher social-class composition. As cancer of the stomach is found more frequently in those from the lower social classes it would be expected that Slough would have a higher incidence of the disease. The only way of accurately making comparisons of disease levels in different communities is to use the process of *standardization*, a statistical technique which can be used to eliminate the effect of differences in the age, racial and social composition of the populations concern.

SOCIAL CLASS AND DENTAL DISEASE

As with many other diseases, social class differences exist in the prevalence of dental disease. Until about a century ago, dental caries was confined largely to the better off sections of the community. In the second half of the nineteenth century, however, dental caries increased considerably (Corbett and Moore 1976) following the 400 per cent increase in sugar consumption during the reign of Queen Victoria. Refined sugar was no longer the privilege of the rich but became cheap and available to all (James 1981).

A number of studies have demonstrated the present relationship between social status and dental caries. One of the largest dental surveys was the national study of child dental health carried out in England and Wales in 1973 (Todd 1975). Table 16.2 shows that those from the higher social classes were more likely to have no experience of dental decay and less likely to have widespread decay. Children from social classes IV and V were more likely to have had toothache than those from the higher groups.

Table 16.2. Decay experience of 5-year-old children according to social class (Todd 1975)

Social class	Percentage of children with no deciduous decay experience	Five or more deciduous teeth involved
I, II and III non-manual	38	30
III manual	24	41
IV and V	23	43

In a subsequent survey in 1983, Todd and Dodd (1985) showed that a similar pattern continues to exist. Five-year-olds from social classes IV and V had twice as many teeth with decay experience as their counterparts from professional households. Thus, in both the prevention of decay and the control of it, children of parents from the top social class group do significantly better than the others. A similar pattern is found with regard to gingival disease in adults (Cushing and Sheiham 1985; Todd and Lader 1991), see Table 16.3. Addy *et al.* (1990) found that the social class gradient was present for tooth-brushing frequency, oral hygiene scores, and periodontal health. Thus, the need for treatment for both dental caries and periodontal disease is greater in the lower social classes. A measure of the total met and unmet need for full dentures is indicated by the proportion of the population who are edentulous. In the case of partial dentures, an approximation of the relative need between groups may be ascertained from the proportion of dentate people who have less than 21 natural teeth, a level which has been termed 'the shortened dental arch' (Kayser 1981) and which is commonly accepted as providing a 'functional dentition' (WHO 1982). Table 16.4 shows that for both of these

Table 16.3. Percentage of dentate adults with no, 1–4, and 5–6 sextants free from periodontal disease (Todd and Lader 1991)

Social class	Number of health sextants		
	None	1–4	5 or 6
I, II, and III non-manual	31	56	13
III manual	38	54	8
IV and V	41	56	3

Table 16.4. An indication of the need for full and partial dentures according to social class (based on Todd and Lader 1991)

Social class	% edentulous	% with less than 21 natural teeth	% who need full or partial dentures
I, II, and III non-manual	14	17	31
III manual	24	21	45
IV and V	32	24	54

indicators, the lowest social classes have the greatest need for treatment (Todd and Lader 1991).

SOCIAL CLASS AND MEDICAL TREATMENT

In 1968, Titmus drew attention to differences in the use of health services and concluded that middle-class members of the community were more efficient in the use of the National Health Service and were receiving greater benefits from it. Although in general the lower social classes make less use of medical services there are differences in the utilization of the various parts of the service. For instance, the crude rate of visits to general medical practitioners by middle-aged adults is higher in the working class groups. However, if this is adjusted to take into account the differences in chronic morbidity, then those from the higher social classes are found to visit their general practitioner more than twice as much as those from social classes IV and V. An even greater disparity of utilization in relation to actual need is found in the hospital outpatient consultation rates (Blaxter 1976). Preventive services generally are used much more by the middle classes (Blaxter 1984; Nutbeam and Catford 1987). These include early attendance for antenatal care, child welfare clinics, and immunization and vaccination services.

SOCIAL CLASS AND DENTAL TREATMENT

All of the indicators already described show that those from the lower social classes have more dental disease and thus need more dental treatment than those from the higher social classes. In view of this, it might be expected that those from the lower social classes would visit the dentist more frequently in order to obtain this greater amount of treatment. The frequency of dental visits according to social class has been investigated at each of the UK national surveys of adult dental health. Table 16.5 shows that in 1988 (Todd and Lader 1991), in contrast to their respective dental needs, nearly six out of ten from the highest social group had been attending the dentist on a regular basis, whereas only a third of the subjects from social class IV and V attended for regular check-ups. Only one quarter of those from social class I, II, and III non-manual, wait until they are having trouble with their teeth compared to over a half of those in classes IV and V. A similar trend was found by Todd (1975) and Todd and Dodd (1985), who reported that not only were mothers from the highest social groups more regular in their own dental

Table 16.5. Percentage of dentate adults with different dental attendance patterns according to social class (Todd and Lader 1991)

Social class	Regular check-ups	Occasional check-ups	Only with trouble
I, II, and III non-manual	59	15	26
III manual	44	13	43
IV and V	34	14	52

attendance, but also that they took their children to the dentist at an earlier age. This social differential in the pattern of regular dental visits is consistent with the pattern already described for the usage of preventive health services generally. Even the choice of dental service is found to differ between the social groups. Middle class mothers take their children to their own general dental practitioner who is a 'family dentist'. In contrast, many more working-class mothers, who are less likely to go to a dentist themselves, send their children to the community dental service after receiving a note informing them that a school screening inspection has indicated a need for treatment (Todd 1975). Gratrix *et al.* (1990) showed that the dental attendance pattern of the mother was a good predictor of children's dental attendance. The vast majority of the mothers who attended a dental practitioner also took their 10 to 11-year-old child. However, less than 4 out of 10 mothers who did not attend a dentist themselves sent their child to a dental practitioner, while approximately the same proportion reported that the child attended a community dental service clinic. The study demonstrated clearly that the general dental service and community dental service treat different sections of the population. Crawford and Lennon (1992) carried out a similar investigation in an area of social deprivation. They found a smaller proportion of mothers who were dental attenders. A smaller proportion of children went to the dentist in both the 'attender' and 'non-attender' groups of mothers. In this study, fewer children went to the community dental service while more did not attend either a practitioner or clinic.

Todd and Lader (1991) investigated some of the barriers to dental attendance to see whether there were differences between the social groups. The results showed that a higher proportion of those from classes III manual, IV, and V agreed with each statement depicting a barrier to dental care. More of those from the lower social groups felt anxious about going to the dentist, and said that if they had toothache they would rather take painkillers than go to the dentist. A greater number said that they found National Health Service (NHS) dental treatment expensive, they did not want fancy, or intricate, dental treatment, would like to be able to pay in instalments and felt that it would cost less in the long run if they only went to the dentist when having trouble with their teeth.

It was also found in the national study that, overall, a lower proportion of those from higher social groups and those who were regular attenders had 18 or more sound teeth (such groups having more filled teeth). The exception to this pattern was in the young adults aged 16–24 years. This may indicate that dentists are now adopting a more preventive approach to the management of the young permanent dentition, especially in those from social classes I and II with their lower decay experience (Murray 1994).

Such social class differences are found not only with attendance patterns for routine dentistry but also with referrals for specialist treatment such as orthodontics. Jenkins *et al.* (1984a,b) reported more referrals for orthodontic advice and treatment from the higher social groups, who were also more likely to seek treatment for minor malocclusions, a finding confirmed by Kenealy and Shaw (1989).

Not only are attendance patterns different, but the mother's attitude and choice of treatment for her child differs from one social class to another. It has been shown (Beal and Dickson 1974b) that in the West Midlands those from social classes I and II were more than twice as likely to favour the restoration of carious primary teeth than the mothers from the lower social classes. Table 16.6, however, shows that even amongst mothers in the higher social groups only just over a half of the sample wanted primary teeth filled. In contrast, the treatment preference for decayed permanent teeth is, from the dentist's point of view, much more favourable. Nine out of ten mothers from classes I and II favoured fillings. Even so, as many as 54 per cent of social class IV and V mothers wanted the teeth extracted. More recently, Todd and Dodd (1985) found a rather higher overall percentage (88 per cent) of mothers of 5-year-old children who wanted decayed permanent teeth to be filled. The social gradient rose from 78 per cent in social class IV and V to 95 per cent in classes I and II.

Attendance at the dentist brings differences in the dental treatment actually received by different social groups. Table 16.7 shows that, in both studies, of those 5-year-old children who have visited the dentist, a greater proportion of those from the highest social group had never had to have any treatment. This social group were also found to have been less likely to have had teeth extracted.

The situation with regard to fillings is, however, changing. In 1973 those from the highest social group were more likely to have had fillings whereas in 1983 they were less likely to have received restorative treatment. In a study into the dental health of adults, Sheiham and Hobdell (1969) showed that, in the younger age groups, those in social class I had on average three times as many teeth filled as those in class V, whilst the latter had four times as many teeth both extracted and decayed as the former.

Table 16.6. Percentage of mother's choosing different types of treatment for 5-year-old children with decayed primary and permanent teeth according to social class (Beal and Dickson 1974a)

Social class	Primary teeth		Permanent teeth	
	Fill	Extract	Fill	Extract
I and II	54	46	90	10
III	40	60	58	42
IV and V	24	76	46	54

Table 16.7. Percentage of 5-year-old children who have been to the dentist and who have different treatment experience according to social class (Todd 1975; Todd and Dodd 1985)

Social class	No fillings No extractions		Had fillings		Had extractions	
	1973	1983	1973	1983	1973	1983
I, II, and III non-manual	38	61	38	26	17	7
III manual	20	49	35	29	28	12
IV and V	23	37	22	39	23	15

Cooper (1975) stated that the most important determinant of demand for medical services is the availability of resources. O'Mullane and Robinson (1977) compared the uptake of dental services in two towns, one where the dentist to population ratio was favourable and the other where it was unfavourable. They found that in the unfavourable area there was considerably greater utilization by the higher social classes, whilst in the favourable area there was a more similar pattern of usage throughout the social scale with only a slight bias in favour of the higher social groups. The net effect of having a greater availability of dentists seemed to be that only slightly more social class I and II individuals sought treatment whereas the percentage of patients from social class IV and V greatly increased. These results suggest that an increase in the availability of dental resources does not lead to an even greater utilization by the middle classes, but to an equalization between the classes.

Taylor and Carmichael (1980) have shown, in Newcastle, that general dental practitioners are more numerous in areas of high social class. The Community Dental Service, which should be complementary to the General Dental Services, does not always have clinics located in the dentally deprived areas. One way of providing dental services to those communities in lower social class areas is by the use of mobile dental caravans by the community service. As with medical services, the supply would then create its own demand (Carmichael 1981).

Carmichael (1991) has addressed the problems associated with inequalities of care. After a consideration of the reasons he outlines alternative options for achieving a redistribution of dental manpower. These include financial incentives in the form of a premium rate of fee-per-item in areas of under-provision, deprivation payments to dentists working in poor localities, grants to locate in undeserved areas, financial encouragement for single-handed practitioners in such areas to offset the savings which group practices are able to enjoy, control of practice location comparable to that for medical practitioners and changes in the admission policies of dental schools to positively discriminate in favour of accepting students from underprovided regions. More recently, the government has suggested that health authorities might 'purchase' the provision of primary dental care according to a locally agreed strategy. Such decisions must be based on sound epidemiological evidence so that the resources of the NHS are targeted towards areas of greatest need (Secretary of State for Health 1994; Department of Health 1994).

In summary, then, it can be seen that those from the higher social classes have less dental disease but are more regular attenders at the dentist, they are also less likely to have had any dental treatment. Conversely, those in the lower social groups have more dental disease but visit the dentist less frequently. They are more likely to have teeth extracted and, until recently, were less likely to have fillings although this situation is changing.

SOCIAL CLASS AND DENTAL KNOWLEDGE, ATTITUDES, AND BEHAVIOUR

Although a number of studies investigating social differences in knowledge, attitudes, and behaviour have been carried out in the USA, fewer UK studies have been conducted.

It is, however, possible to identify differences between those from various socio-economic backgrounds to their level of knowledge, dental attitudes, and behaviour patterns.

In general, as might be expected, those from the higher social classes, who have a higher level of education, are more knowledgeable about dentally related matters.

A demonstration of the different levels of knowledge is related to awareness that blackcurrant juice can be harmful to the teeth of young children. In a study of the mothers of 5-year-old children in the West Midlands, it was shown (Beal and Dickson 1974a) that twice as many mothers from social classes I and II knew that blackcurrant juice could be harmful to the teeth compared with the number of classes IV and V. The importance of this can be seen from the fact that the level of knowledge was closely related to reported behaviour. It was found that those who knew about the harmful potential were twice as likely to not give blackcurrant juice to their children, or if they did provide it, then it was given much less frequently.

There are a number of respects in which the general cultural patterns differ between the middle class and working class sections of the community. A number of these differences affect attitudes toward dentistry and the prevention of dental disease. It is most important that these should be understood by the dental practitioner in order to help the patient to improve his or her dental health.

The life orientation associated with the working classes is one of *immediate gratification*, whereas that more commonly found in middle class individuals is of *deferred gratification*. This means that the middle class person sees value in foregoing the pleasures of today in order to gain greater benefit in the future. Those from this group place great emphasis on education and training. They encourage their children to spend their evenings doing homework and studying for examinations, with the expectation that this will result in a 'better job'. They also save and invest their money in order to purchase what they want in the future or perhaps provide a pension after retirement. Those from the lower social groups, however, tend to be less interested in education. They do not buy so many books for their young children, and make fewer visits to the public lending library. Their children are not given the same encouragement to do their homework, or stay on at school in order to take examinations leading to attendance at college or university. Indeed, the working class boy or girl with a father in a unskilled or semi-skilled occupation may find great difficulties in studying at home. Not only are they less likely to receive parental support, especially if a girl, but the facilities at home may not be particularly conducive to study, and she or he may have to work in the room in which siblings and parents are watching television. In addition, the working class child is often subjected to a conflict of cultures between the school and home environments. Whilst the child will have been socialized into a working class culture, the teachers communicate using the speech and ideas appropriate to their own middle-class background and experience.

Saving is also less common in working class families, partly because they tend to have a lower income, and expensive items have to be bought on hire purchase. The children, are not encouraged to save a proportion of their money, but are allowed to spend it all without making any conditions as to its 'sensible use'. This results in more money being available for the purchase of snacks and sweets.

The patient's occupation and circumstances relating to his or her employment are factors which should be borne in mind by every dentist preparing a treatment plan whether or not it includes preventive therapy. Many middle class employees are paid a salary. When they are absent from work to visit the dentist they suffer no loss of income. The working class person, however, is often paid an hourly wage or 'piece work', whereby remuneration depends on productivity. Absence from work will, therefore, result in financial loss. Especially during times of economic recession and high unemployment some patients may be reluctant to undergo long courses of treatment involving many visits to the dentist for fear of losing their job. This may well influence the treatment plan in such a way as to require the minimum number of visits. On the other hand, it may also serve as an incentive for the patient to practice the self-help aspects of preventive dentistry in order to reduce the future need for dental treatment.

Dentists have been granted a protected monopoly in the provision of dental treatment and this privilege carries with it the responsibility of ensuring that an appropriate service is offered to the community. This should include making the service available when it is reasonable for patients to attend. Rogers *et al.* (1984) found that pre-school children whose parents worked were less likely to visit the dentist, especially if the parents would lose money if absent from work. A survey of adults in Leeds (Beal and Prendergast 1993) showed that, whilst those who were aged over 65 years found daytime appointments convenient, one in three of the younger respondents would prefer evening appointments and one in seven wanted to visit the dentist on Saturday morning.

Although some groups of skilled manual workers have narrowed the gap in recent years there remains a differential in the income of middle class and working class persons. There is also a difference in the income curve of the two classes. Those in the working classes can expect, after any initial training, to get the set rate for the job which will, apart from cost-of-living rises, remain the same until retirement. Many middle class persons earn nothing during training, which is often carried out full-time at places of higher education. After qualification they frequently enter posts in which they become *spiralists*, that is they are graded at the bottom of a hierarchical ladder. They can, however, expect annual increments as well as the cost-of-living rises. In addition, they seek promotion up the hierarchy, usually involving further training and qualifications, and will earn a higher salary with each successive step up the ladder. It is frequently not before they are well into middle age, or even older, that they earn their maximum income. It is interesting to note that dentists in the General Dental Services of the NHS have more in common with the working class in this respect, for they are not eligible for promotion within the service, do not get annual increments, and they cannot, because of the set fee per item of treatment, charge more because of greater experience as can professional groups like barristers or their own counterparts in wholly private dental practice.

One of the problems associated with using a classification of social class based on the occupation of an individual is that this relates only to present achieved status and provides no information about social origin. It has, however, already been stated that social class is a relatively open system, that is, movement from one status group to another can be achieved during a person's lifetime. *Social mobility* may be either horizontal or vertical. Horizontal mobility takes place when someone changes from one occupation to another within the same social class. Vertical mobility is exhibited by a person who changes from an occupation classified in one social class to another which falls in a different social class.

The results of studies in other fields have indicated that those who have shown vertical social mobility have attitudes and behaviour which are different from their socially static contemporaries (Rosser and Harris 1965). As a group they fit neither into the culture pattern of the social class into which they were born and brought up, nor into that into which they have moved. Goldthorpe *et al.* (1968) have described the conflict between their past and their present, and between their background and their aspirations that is found in these individuals. Blau (1956) describes this 'pattern of acculturation' in the following way: 'Both groups exert some influence over mobile individuals since they have, or have had, social contacts with members of both, being placed by economic circumstances amidst the one while having been socialized among the other. Hence their behaviour is expected to be intermediate between that of the two non-mobile classes.' This coincides with findings in the sphere of dental health (Beal and Dickson 1975*a*). As a group, the pattern of preference for restoring or extracting decayed teeth, of mothers' dental attendance, of a child's first dental attendance, of the child's tooth-brushing regularity, and of the amount spent on sweets, falls mid-way between the social group they had left and the one they had joined. Whether girls born into those working class families with 'middle class attitudes' are more likely to marry a middle class husband, or whether a working class girl who marries into the middle class changes her own attitudes to conform to those of her husband's social peers, and vice versa for downward mobility, is uncertain. The work of Goldthorpe *et al.* (1968, 1969) suggests that it is the former.

Some sociologists have suggested that with increasing affluence of the working class they will begin to adopt the cultural patterns which are traditionally associated with the middle classes, a process developed as the thesis of the *embourgeoisement* of the working class. Goldthorpe *et al.* (1969) have examined this in a study of automobile workers at Luton. They concluded that the differences they found in some sub-groups of car workers were much more likely to be due to factors such as social mobility than to the process of embourgeoisement. Although increasing affluence and education of the working class may well eventually lead to changes in dental attitudes and behaviour, it is essential that any dentist responsible for providing treatment to a working-class community is constantly aware, albeit subconsciously, of the different cultural background of many of his or her patients.

OTHER SOCIAL FACTORS RELATED TO DENTAL HEALTH

In this chapter so far the Registrar General's Social Class has been the only indicator of status that has been examined in relation to dental health. There are, however, many other factors associated with the concept of class by various social scientists. These include income, education, type of housing, and voting behaviour. All are found to be related to social class and they have each shown a social gradient in dental attitudes. However, dental behaviour is much more strongly related to area of residence than to any of the individual social variables. It may be that the area differences reflect a combination of the other differences. People living in one area may tend to be from the higher social classes, have a higher income, longer full-time education, and live in their own

house, whilst in another area there may be a tendency for the residents to be nearer to the lower end of all the social scales. Alternatively it may reflect a form of group learning, a process whereby members of the community are influenced in their attitudes and behaviour by others who live near to them even if they are not in the same social class. Certainly many of the factors associated with their environment are shared. For example, in areas with more people from the higher social groups there are often more dentists. It would, therefore, be easier even for working class mothers in that area, to go to the dentist for regular check-ups and to have children's teeth filled, whilst in other areas the mothers tend to wait until emergency extractions are necessary.

A summary of some differences in beliefs and values in working-class and middle-class persons are presented in Table 16.8. The dentally related beliefs and values have been added to general ones which are based on the work of Goldthorpe *et al.* (1969). A word of caution must be made at this point. The findings of many of the studies quoted have been based on the answers to a questionnaire. Leaving aside the thorny question as to whether the respondents have given honest answers, or merely reflected what they thought the researcher wanted, it is important to realize that non-response may bias the results. By examining a group of 5-year-old children, irrespective of whether their parents had returned a questionnaire on the child's past dental experience, it was found that the children of non-responders had poorer oral hygiene and higher caries levels (Prendergast

Table 16.8. Social class and dental health. A summary of differences in beliefs and values in working class and middle class persons. (Adapted from Goldthorpe *et al.* 1969)

	Working class perspective	Middle class perspective
General beliefs	The social order is divided into 'us' and 'them'; those who do not have authority and those who do	The social order is a hierarchy of differentially rewarded positions; a ladder containing many rungs
	The division between 'us' and 'them' is virtually fixed, at least from the point of view of one man's life chances	It is possible for individuals to move from one level of the hierarchy to another
	What happens to you depends a lot on luck; otherwise you have to learn to put up with things	Those who have ability and initiative can overcome obstacles and create their own opportunities. Where a man ends up depends on what he makes of himself
Dental beliefs	Tooth decay is inevitable. If you are born with weak teeth they will rot whatever you do	Tooth decay and loss of teeth signifies failure to look after them properly
	By the time you are in your 30s or 40s they will fall out or have to be pulled out anyway	It is up to each one of us to care for his or her teeth and get regular treatment. If you look after them they will last into old age
General values	'We' ought to stick together and get what we can as a group. You may as well enjoy yourself while you can instead of trying to make yourself 'a cut above the rest'	Everybody ought to make the most of their own capabilities and be responsible for their own welfare. You cannot expect to get anywhere in the world if you squander your time and money. 'Getting on' means making sacrifices
Dental values	I don't like going to the dentist so I won't go until I have pain, then I will have them out. I am not interested in prevention	It is worth the time, money and discomfort of going for regular check-ups and treatment—and for having preventive treatment
	The children enjoy their sweets—it is cruel to stop them	It is important to control the children's sweets so they don't get a lot of decay
	They can spend their pocket money on sweets if they like	I control how they spend their pocket money, so they won't buy lots of sweets

et al. 1993). Clearly, the children of responders and non-responders are different. It must, therefore, be recognized that if the non-response rate is high a bias of unknown magnitude may be introduced into the results.

The use of the social class measure or one of the above alternative single-item indicators has proved very valuable for developing an understanding of the differences between groups with respect to health and associated behaviour. However, they are not ideal and there are difficulties with their use. First, they require the researcher to obtain sensitive information, such as income, for each subject in the study. Secondly, they do not identify groups that are homogenous. There may be wide variations between individuals falling into the same occupational, educational, housing or income category. For example, there could be large differences in income within a given educational category or vice versa. Thirdly, they do not take into account the effect of the broader social environment referred to above. Perhaps the most important disadvantage is that they do not identify the localities where the people in the separate groups live (Locker 1993). Those responsible for the planning of services need to know where developments should be targeted. It is useful to know that many children in the lower social groups do not visit the dentist regularly but where should the dental health education campaign be undertaken to try to improve the situation? For these reasons a number of area-based indicators have been developed. These include ACORN (A Classification of Residential Neighbourhoods, CACI 1983), the Jarman Index (Jarman 1983), Super Profile Group codings (Charlton *et al.* 1985), the Overall Deprivation Index (Townsend 1988), and deprivation indices by Carstairs and Morris (1989) and Curtis (1990). The only information which has to be sought from the subjects of the study is their postcode, or their address from which the postcode may be obtained. This is then used to derive the relevant census information required for the calculation of any particular index of deprivation. The variables used in the various indices include households with no car, housing tenure, overcrowding, unemployment, semi-skilled or unskilled manual occupations, single parent families, children under five, elderly people living alone, ethnic minorities, and so on. Each index uses a different combination of these and other similar variables to calculate a score or classification for every locality. The relationship between the health attribute and the deprivation scores may then be computed. The result not only provides information about the association between the social variables and health but also allows the geographical location of the subjects to be plotted. This area-based approach may therefore be a valuable supplement to the traditional use of social indicators for the targeting of services to those most in need of them.

It is clear from numerous studies that dental health is poorer in areas of social deprivation. Whilst it is important to regularly monitor the level of dental disease in a community such as a health district, it is not always necessary to carry out detailed and costly epidemiological studies to identify areas of greatest dental need. For the planning of dental services, for example, targeting dental health education programmes, a study of the readily available census data will provide sufficient information to enable the health authority to make the necessary decisions without vast expense.

One of the unfortunate results of the social differences described is that those children who most need the dental services are the very ones who are least often taken to the dentist. The less educated and less well-off are not only least likely to take steps to prevent dental disease from occurring, but when it does occur, they do not take steps to seek dental treatment until it is too late to treat them conservatively. Hence, they regard the dentists as providing an emergency service only, and they have decayed teeth extracted and eventually replaced by dentures.

It is, therefore, this group who most need and in the past have obtained the greatest benefit from water fluoridation. Prior to the widespread use of fluoride in toothpaste the prevalence of dental caries was perhaps the only social or health indicator in which children from fluoridated inner city areas, such as Birmingham, were as well-off or even better than nearby children in high class but unfluoridated residential areas (Beal and James 1970, 1971). However, there is some doubt about whether this is still the case (French *et al.* 1984: Bradnock *et al.* 1984). The general improvement in dental health (see Chapter 00) has been found in all social groups, and there is evidence that even with the additional benefit of water fluoridation, children in the lower social groups may have more dental decay than those from the higher social groups living in non-fluoridated communities (Murray *et al.* 1991). The fact remains, however, that even if fluoridation does not totally obviate the influences of social background, it is the deprived sections of the community which gain the greatest improvement in absolute terms, especially in the reduction of the proportion of children with a high caries experience.

In addition to those factors associated with social status, there are others which are related to dental health. Obviously, the prevalence and severity of both dental caries and periodontal disease is related to age. The relationship between general and oral health, especially periodontal health, has been demonstrated on numerous occasions. Among children, girls are found to have cleaner teeth and less gingivitis (Todd 1975). In adults, females are shown to have better oral cleanliness (Sheiham 1969), less calculus, and less periodontal disease (Todd and Lader 1991). This latter study also found that females make more regular visits to the dentist, have more teeth filled but fewer teeth which were sound and untreated, and fewer teeth with active decay. Women also become edentulous at an earlier age. Todd and Dodd (1985) demonstrated that girls had a slightly lower experience of tooth decay in both primary and permanent dentitions.

Ethnic origin is another factor for which not only dental health but also attitudes and behaviour are found to vary from group to group. Studies conducted in the UK in the late 1960s and early 1970s found that children of Afro-Caribbean origin tended to have less caries experience than other ethnic groups (Downer 1970; Varley and Goose 1971; Beal 1973).

The position with Asian children was more confused with studies giving conflicting results, although in general they seemed to have a similar caries experience to white children. More recent studies have shown changes in the relative caries status of those from different ethnic groups. Paul and Bradnock (1986) found that Asian children of 4 and 5 years had more caries than white children, a finding confirmed by Bradnock *et al.* (1988) and Perkins and Sweetman (1986), who also reported that Afro-Caribbean children had a similar total caries experience to the white group. A similar pattern for 5-year-olds was reported by Beal (1990) but the situation in 14-year-olds was quite different. In this age group, the Asian children had less caries than the white sample. Such findings could be related to different patterns of sugar consumption in Asian children at different ages. For example, it has been shown that a higher proportion of Asian children are given bottles containing sweetened liquids than white children (Williams 1986). With the exception of the few who continue this habit after the age of about 6 years this would only affect the primary dentition. The sugar consumption in older Asian children may be more similar to that of white children. Alternatively it may be that different subgroups of Asians predominate in the younger and older samples, depending on the patterns of immigration over the past couple of decades. Gelbier and Taylor (1985) have pointed out that 'Asians' are not a homogeneous group. Like 'Europeans' the group comprises a number of subgroups. They may be broadly divided into those from India, Pakistan, and Bangladesh, although even these need to be subdivided into groups with different languages, religions, and cultural patterns, and some of these factors will affect behaviour related to dental health (Williams *et al.* 1987, Prendergast *et al.* 1989, Bedi and Elton 1991). Todd and Gelbier (1991) have shown that Vietnamese children living in London have a greater caries experience in the permanent dentition than white, Afro-Caribbean or Asian children.

Studies have shown that in the primary dentition the Asian children have the lowest proportion of affected teeth which have received treatment. In older children it is the Afro-Caribbean group which has least treatment relative to the need but who exhibit the highest proportion of extracted teeth (Beal 1990).

Other differences relate to the standards of dental cleanliness. In 5-year-olds, Paul and Bradnock (1986) found white children to have cleaner teeth than Asians, whilst Saxby and Anderson (1987), have found that dental cleanliness in teenagers was of a better standard in both Afro-Caribbean and Asian children than in white children of the same age.

Recent studies have also reported an association between ethnic background and both periodontal health and dental visiting patterns. Booth and Ashley (1989) found that the prevalence of periodontal disease in 15- to 17-year-olds was lowest in the white subjects, the proportion of the Asian group affected was nearly five times and the Afro-Caribbean group seven times as great. Mattin and Smith (1991) showed that, even though they had a high level of need for periodontal treatment, few Asian people aged over 55 years attended the dentist, preferring to wait until they had pain. This contrasts with the finding by Donaldson (1986) that elderly Asian people were high users of general medical services. Rogers (1991) reported that Muslim women had the lowest level of attendance at a dentist during pregnancy.

The dental attitudes and behaviour of the various ethnic groups have been studied. By the age of 5 years the majority of white children are regular attenders at the dentist. A lower proportion of Afro-Caribbean children and even fewer Asian children visit a dentist regularly. By the age of 14 the visiting pattern is much improved in the Afro-Caribbean group. Whilst there is a small increase in the proportion of Asian children who attend regularly there remains a majority who only go occasionally. There is, however, a difference in the service from which parents seek dental treatment for their children. The majority of white children are taken to a general dental practitioner whereas Asian children are more likely to go to a community dental service clinic, if they go anywhere (Paul and Bradnock 1986; Beal, 1991). It is clear that although the dental services are equally available to all groups, they are not equitable, being more appropriate for the white population. The findings indicate that there is a need to ensure, not only that the Asian community is aware of the dental services that are available and that they are encouraged to utilise the services, but also that these services are provided in a way that is culturally acceptable and takes into account the needs of their community.

One factor which is bound to influence the availability of preventive dentistry, and thus how much is carried out, is the attitudes of the dental profession itself. Craft and Sheiham (1976) found that general dental practitioners in the north of England were more negative in their knowledge, attitudes, and behaviour towards prevention than their colleagues in the south. The northern dentists were also much less likely to employ dental hygienists, a finding confirmed by Rock and Bradnock (1976). If a patient's own dentist is not positively orientated towards prevention, not only will it reduce the amount of preventive therapy that is carried out, but it is less likely that the patient will be inspired to practise those aspects of self-care prevention which are necessary on a daily basis at home.

The results of the national study of children's dental health (Todd 1975) highlighted a difficult problem for dental policymakers and planners. Although treatment from the General Dental Services of the NHS is, in theory, provided from an open-ended budget, in reality the total resources, including manpower, available for dental treatment are limited and are certainly insufficient to cope with the total need for treatment. Some form of rationing is therefore necessary. This has been done, not by restricting dental treatment to those who need it most, or to basic forms of treatment such as the relief of pain and simple operative procedures, but by providing comprehensive treatment to the self-selected group who demand it. In practice, this has meant that restorative dentistry has, for the most part, been restricted to those with the most favourable attitudes and behaviour. The dental visiting patterns of children are found, not surprisingly, to be influenced by the mothers. A very high proportion of children whose mothers are regular attenders are themselves regular attenders (Todd and Dodd 1985). Similarly, the mothers of children who only attend when they have trouble are more likely themselves to attend only when having trouble with their teeth, hence continuing the cycle of deprivation.

In order to produce any major breakthrough, it is necessary either to prevent a large proportion of dental disease, or to persuade those who do not at present demand dental treatment for themselves and their children to do so in future—or better still a combination of both. The recent reduction in the prevalence of dental caries in children (OPCS 1994; Pitts and

Palmer 1994), the increase in the number of dentists over the past couple of decades, and an increase in research into dental health education may all help to provide the conditions in which the required break in the cycle can be made. The British Government has recently set targets for the further improvement in oral health (Department of Health 1994).

Probably one of the most important factors will be to make sure that the maldistribution in dental manpower is further reduced so that those who at present have less easy access to the dentist no longer suffer from living in dentally deprived areas. Whether this might best take place by market forces encouraging dentists to open new practices in areas where there are few if any dentists; by financial or other incentives to dentists to work in these areas; or by some other method should be considered by the profession and those responsible for the planning of dental services. The Dental Strategy Review Group (1981), set up to advise the British Government on future dental policy, was in no doubt that the minimizing of the social and geographical differences in dental health will require a co-ordinated manpower policy and cannot be left to chance. As Davis (1980) states: 'once people are actually in the dental system—in other words, once the hurdle of access has been surmounted—neither education nor income exert much influence on the volume of care received, a finding that suggests that ease of entry into the dental system is the 'crucial contingency'. This has been confirmed by Eddie and Davies (1985).

However, in planning dental services it must be remembered that those living in deprived areas have greater needs. Carmichael (1985) has pointed out that 'equality means equal shares. Equity means fair shares. If two groups of dental patients have needs, a policy of equality will give each group half; but if one group has a large unmet need compared with the relatively smaller needs of the other group, a policy of equity would give the first group priority. Those living in inner city Britain deserve better than they get at present'.

SOCIAL FACTORS AND WATER FLUORIDATION

The fluoridation of water differs from most other methods of preventive dentistry, in that it is neither a clinical technique carried out by the dentist nor a matter which is the individual responsibility of each member of the population. The decision on its implementation or otherwise is, therefore, neither a matter for the clinician exercising the right of clinical freedom, nor one in which there is individual freedom for each person to decide for himself. It is a public health measure and the decision on whether to fluoridate or not is one which must be taken by the community. The method of making this decision differs from one community to another. It has been decided nationally in Eire: by local government in many parts of the USA; by health authorities in the UK; and by public referenda in other American communities.

In democratic communities, even if the decision is made without the direct involvement of the public by holding a referendum, it is usually necessary for there to be some indication of public support for such a measure before it is likely to be implemented. A number of surveys have been undertaken in order to ascertain the proportion of the population in

favour of, or opposing fluoridation. The results of national polls in the USA have been summarized by Frazier (1980). All of the studies conducted since 1959 have shown that over 70 per cent of the adult population have heard about fluoridation. In many of the studies only a half of the respondents knew why it is added to the water supply. However in a more recent national survey in the USA a sample of over 41 000 respondents were asked the purpose of fluoridation. 62 per cent correctly identified the reason. The level of knowledge was best among those with the highest levels of education and in the age groups 25–44 years (Centers for Disease Control 1992).

In the UK, many of the studies have been conducted in specific areas. However, several national samples have been asked about fluoridation. The earlier surveys showed that 46 per cent in 1968 (Jackson 1972); 49 per cent in 1971 (Jackson 1972); and 67 per cent in 1980 (West Midlands Regional Health Authority 1980) were in favour compared to 16, 14, and 16 per cent respectively who were opposed. The trend has been for an increasing level of support. Two studies for which the National Association of Health Authorities commissioned independent market research firms to conduct the investigation showed 71 per cent in favour in 1985 and 76 per cent in 1987. A third study, carried out in 1992, found 79 per cent supported fluoridation. The opposition was 17, 15, and 15 per cent respectively (British Fluoridation Society 1992). Recent local studies conducted in the north of England indicated support ranging from 54 to 92 per cent whilst opposition ranged from 5 to 23 percent. Several of the UK studies have shown a social gradient, those from the higher social classes being generally more knowledgeable and more likely to believe fluoridation to be desirable than those from the lower social classes.

Frazier (1980) notes that, although opinion polls in the USA consistently show a large majority in favour of fluoridation, when it is voted upon in public referenda it is often defeated. It is, therefore, necessary to investigate why some people are opposed to fluoridation, what sort of people they are and what factors influence how an individual casts his or her vote in a referendum. There has been little research in this field in the UK and it is to the American literature that one must turn for much of the evidence. It is important to bear in mind, therefore, that some of the findings may not apply to Britain.

Although there are conflicting results from various studies, there is fairly general agreement about some of the factors associated with opposition to fluoride (Frazier 1980). Frequently anti-fluoridationists are found to be older, without young children, and with low levels of income, occupational status, and education. When their attitudes to fluoridation have been studied in relation to other beliefs, opponents have been described as anti-science, anti-authoritarian, politically conservative, and against government intervention. They have also been found to be those unable to cope with the world, poorly integrated into the social and organizational life of the community, and to have feelings of political powerlessness and deprivation, these factors producing the so-called 'alienation hypothesis' to explain anti-fluoridation stances.

Sapolsky (1969) described how a generally favourable public opinion can be converted into one of opposition during the arguments and debate associated with a referendum campaign. It is suggested that this change takes place because doubts and anxiety are introduced by the anti-fluoride lobby. Many people simply become confused by the conflicting evidence produced by two sets of so-called 'experts'. This has given rise to the 'confusion hypothesis' of anti-fluoride attitudes. When leading anti-fluoridationists claim, for instance, that fluoride causes cancer, most members of the public are not equipped with the medical and scientific training necessary to interpret the data and form a reasoned opinion. Their subsequent confusion results in them voting against fluoridation, as they are unable to identify the scientific shortcomings in the anti-fluoridationists' argument. Often this decision is rationalized by suggesting that there are other less contentious and more effective methods of preventing dental decay which can be applied by each person individually. It is likely, therefore, that the alienation hypothesis fits more closely to the leaders of the anti-fluoride movement and the confusion hypothesis to the voters. It is certainly true that the anti-fluoridationists can form a small vociferous pressure group which can be very effective in generating conflict, doubt and subsequent rejection by the community.

Earlier in the fluoride controversy, those against fluoridation often suggested that it was not effective in reducing dental decay or that it only delayed the onset of caries (National Pure Water Association 1969). As there is abundant evidence that fluoridation is a true preventive measure this argument is heard less often now although some people claim that because of the general improvement in dental health fluoridation is no longer needed. Currently, the two most common objections to fluoridation are claims that it is harmful to general health, for example, that it causes cancer, bone disorders or allergic reactions and that it is mass medication or infringes personal liberty (Gibson 1993). These allegations have been analysed by Lowry *et al.* (1995).

Frazier (1980) reviews a number of investigations into the most important factors in the acceptance and implementation of fluoridation. Crain *et al.* (1969) have shown that fluoridation is most likely to be adopted where there is a degree of centralization of decision-making authority; top-level support from the mayor and other high-status, politically active leaders; and active support from health and non-health organizations.

Frankel and Allukian (1973) stated that the most important factor is the level of pro-fluoride activity. Where the pro-fluoridationists out-campaigned opponents, the ballot was more likely to show a majority in favour of fluoridation. In the UK, the part of the country which has been most successful in implementing new fluoridation schemes has been the West Midlands, where the Regional Health Authority set up an action group which initiated and co-ordinated activity amongst the dental and medical professions, members of health authorities, community health councils, teachers, the media, and key local politicians.

One group who might be expected to be providing information about fluoridation is school teachers. Much emphasis has been placed on the role of teachers in dental health education. A study carried out by Loupe and King (unpublished data), which is quoted by Frazier (1980), reveals in teachers a lack of knowledge about fluoridation, and little understanding of its importance. Responding to the challenge the British Fluoridation Society recently commissioned the production of a teachers' pack for use in secondary schools.

As already indicated, many of the studies on the social/psychological aspects of fluoridation have been conducted in the USA. Those studies which have been carried out in the UK have tended to confirm their findings. It is an area in which more research is needed. This must not, however, stop the dental profession from actively propagating the information about fluoridation in order to counter the misleading and inaccurate claims of anti-fluoridationists. It must be remembered that the opponents of fluoride are constantly sending leaflets and other materials giving their point of views to members of parliament, local authorities, and health authorities. The pro-fluoride case must not be allowed to go by default.

SOCIAL FACTORS AND DENTAL HEALTH EDUCATION

All too often in the past, dental health education programmes have been carried out without any evaluation into their effectiveness. Any measurement has usually consisted solely of the number of leaflets handed out, or the number of people contacted during the programme. Those projects in which a proper evaluation has been carried out have often produced disappointing results. Before focusing on some of the possible reasons for the comparative failure of much dental health education it is important to bear in mind some of its successes. One of the main messages of dental health educators has been concerned with the importance of regular toothbrushing. In a national child dental health survey, Todd and Dodd (1985) reported that 96 per cent of the mothers of 5-year-olds claimed that their child brushed at least once a day. Traditionally, the public has been told to brush their teeth because it will prevent dental decay, and this was given as the reason for brushing by over 70 per cent of the mothers. In fact, the message communicated by the dental profession, even if not totally accurate, was known by the vast majority of those questioned.

But what of the failures? What can be learnt from the mistakes of the past so that future programmes do not fall into the same errors?

Too often, those responsible for carrying out dental health programmes do not start by setting out exactly what they are hoping to achieve. It is essential before any planning takes place that the objectives of the project are identified. One of the first tasks must then be to decide to which group or groups the message should be provided. Obviously, a single campaign cannot hope to reach all sections of the community. It is important to bear in mind that the interests and problems of one group will be quite different from another. Something suitable for one particular group, say those in an old persons' home, will be totally irrelevant to others, such as groups of expectant mothers. Clearly we must first decide to whom we are aiming our programme, that is we must define our *target group* or groups. Usually our resources, both manpower and finance, are limited so we must consider which of the potential target groups are most likely to benefit from our programme. With which section of the population do we stand most chance of success in improving dental health? Is it pre-school children, primary school children, secondary school children, young adults, expectant mothers, old people's clubs, or some other section of the community?

In order to make this assessment we need first to look at how everyday attitudes and behaviour in such matters as oral hygiene and diet, are formed. Most people do not consciously make a logical decision each day about whether they should clean their teeth or what sort of snacks they are going to eat. It is something that they have grown up with, a habit which they continue unless they are activated into changing their behaviour. The key to this is the process known as *socialization*. Little of people's behaviour is purely instinctive, rather it is learned behaviour. Each society, or group, has its own culture or set of shared values, norms and beliefs. Socialization is the process by which culture is transmitted and a person learns the rules and practices of his or her social group. Just as we learn a game by playing it, so we learn life by engaging in it; we are socialized in the course of the activities themselves. For example, if we are untutored in manners, we learn the 'correct' manners for our society through the mistakes that we make and the disapproval that others display. We receive reinforcement and support for appropriate behaviour whilst being subjected to sanctions for deviance.

In the early years of life socialization takes place mainly within the family. It is the mother particularly who is responsible for training the young child and teaching the correct way to behave. This early learning is known as *primary socialization*, and it is during this period that many of our attitudes and styles of behaviour are formed and much of this will remain with us all our life. However, the process of socialization continues as we pass through successive stages of our life. When a child starts school, the teachers and other schoolchildren play an important role in the process. During adolescence, the young adult develops more and more as an independent person and begins to formulate his or her own beliefs, attitudes, and behaviour. This continuing process of adaptation to different social expectations is known as *secondary socialization*.

How does this relate to dental health and the messages we wish to communicate? In childhood the main dental problem is that of dental caries. Apart from water fluoridation, the most effective way of preventing decay is by controlling sugar intake. In this respect of course, parents have a big influence. They provide most of the food that is eaten and also the pocket money which is often used for the purchase of sweets or snacks. Unfavourable habits, such as the craving for sugar (a condition known as 'having a sweet tooth'), are often established very early in life. It is known to be much harder to change these habits later in life. It is, therefore, important to try to avoid their formation in the first place. As the mother is the main agent of primary socialization, an important target group for dental health education will be mothers of pre-school children.

It should, however, be remembered that there are a number of sociological barriers to changing the pattern of sugar intake, even in persuading a mother to control the sugar she gives to her child. Sweet eating is accepted as the social norm within our society. It may be possible to convince a few mothers that they should be different from everyone else for the benefit of their children's dental health, but it is a much more difficult matter to try to change the accepted way of behaving so that it is the deviant mother who gives her child sweets between meals. One of the problems is that sweet-eating is perceived by adults as differing from other foods. Sweets are consequently used in a number of different ways. Sometimes they are indeed used as a foodstuff, either as part of a main meal or as a snack: at other times they are used as a gift, a treat, or a token of affection given by parents, or other relatives or friends: in other circumstances they are used as a means of reinforcement, either as a reward for good behaviour or a bribe. In babies and young children, sweets and sugar drinks are also used as pacifiers. We thus find that when we suggest a modification of sweet-eating habits, we are in fact trying to change a practice which is deeply ingrained in our society. We are often seen as depriving children of something special or depriving adults of a method of showing affection to their children. An indication of this problem can be found in the answers given by mothers to two questions in the national survey of child dental health (Todd 1975). The mothers were first asked 'What do you think makes teeth decay—or go bad?' They were not prompted but their reply was written down verbatim. The next question asked 'What do you think can be done to stop teeth decaying?' Again their answer was recorded. The results are shown in Table 16.9. As more than one answer could be given the numbers total to more than 100 per cent. It can be seen that most mothers recognized that the eating of sweet things was the cause of dental caries. A slightly smaller percentage mentioned lack of cleaning. However, the situation changed when the mothers were asked about preventing decay. Clearly, although they recognized the role of sugar in the cause of the disease, they did not perceive the control of sugar as a reasonable way of preventing decay. We are thus faced with the difficult problem of having to change the social norms in our community and this will involve an approach not just to individual mothers, but to all those in the group or subculture to which this target population belongs.

Perhaps we are also too negative in our message relating to sugar consumption. The dentist is frequently seen as someone who admonishes patients and tells them *not* to have sweets, and *not* to have sugary snacks. Possibly a more positive attitude would be helpful. Advice should be given on controlling the frequency of sucrose consumption, suggesting that if sweets are to be eaten, then instead of eating them at intervals throughout the day, they should be eaten altogether, preferably at mealtimes when they will do least harm. Positive information should be given on less harmful and reasonably priced alternative snacks. It is also sometimes possible to associate the behaviour we are recommending with other

Table 16.9. The percentage of mothers of 5-year-old children giving eating/avoiding sweets and not brushing/brushing teeth as the cause/prevention of dental decay (Todd and Dodd 1985)

	Sugar sweets	Tooth-brushing
Cause	78	72
Prevention	48	74

motivations which already exist in an individual. For example, the patient who is concerned about a weight problem can be informed about the link between sugar and obesity and advised to reduce sweet consumption in order to control his or her weight.

After the teenage years, dental caries frequently becomes less of a problem whilst periodontal disease increases in severity. The main factor in the prevention of periodontal disease is regular and thorough oral hygiene. From the dental health educator's point of view, this is fortunate because the recommendation that individuals should brush their teeth coincides with the social norm. This time the health educator is supported by social pressure rather than working against it. It is a matter of trying to refine a technique rather than introduce a new form of behaviour. As young adults are often more motivated to perform an action for social or cosmetic reasons than for health reasons the social benefits of tooth-cleaning can be stressed. However, it is necessary to bear in mind that the purpose of brushing the teeth is to clean them. In the child dental health study, Todd and Dodd (1985) showed that while 94 per cent of mothers of 15-year-olds claimed that their child brushed at least once a day on clinical examination only 51 per cent of the children in that age group had clean teeth. The traditional message exhorting individuals to clean their teeth regularly is therefore not sufficient. Information on how to clean, and more importantly, how to check the efficiency of the cleaning must be provided. It is the thoroughness of cleaning which must be stressed.

Of course, providing information does not necessarily result in a change in behaviour or improvement in dental health. Nevertheless, if we wish people to use disclosing agents we must first make sure that they know about them and how to use them. However, even if a person believes that disclosing agents are a valuable aid in tooth cleaning it does not follow that he will use them. It is common for someone to believe in something which he or she does not practise, or to practise something they do not believe. Nurses who smoke are a good example. They know the evidence which shows that smoking is injurious to health. They believe that smoking is a major cause of ill health but they adopt a behaviour which seems to conflict with this belief. This separation of practice from belief has been called *cognitive dissonance* (Festinger 1957). When there is strong internal conflict between beliefs and attitudes, on the one hand, and behaviour on the other, then this may sometimes lead to a change taking place. This change can be either in the belief or the behaviour. We find, therefore, that behaviour may influence belief as well as beliefs influencing behaviour. In practice, if a person does not use disclosing tablets for any of a variety of reasons, he or she may justify their behaviour by adopting an unfavourable attitude to the value of disclosing agents. Conversely, children who already use disclosing tablets because they are told to by parents, may well adopt a favourable attitude to their role in oral hygiene. Despite all these difficulties we do have the advantage, in the prevention of periodontal disease, that we are building on already established social norms rather than trying to modify them, and this social support should be our most vital asset.

Another reason for the lack of success in many campaigns is the complexity of the language used both in the spoken word and printed materials. Dentists are, by definition, 'middle class' and most others in the field of dental health education also have middle class backgrounds. One of the attributes of the middle classes is their use of an *extended code* or wide vocabulary, often with the use of long words in lengthy complex sentences. Conversely, those from the working class use a *restricted code* composed of fewer and simpler words. Sentences are short. There are a number of methods of calculating reading age, one of which was devised by Gunning (1952). The Gunning index is based upon the number of difficult words (having three or more syllables) and the average length of the sentences. By using the prescribed formula, a number is calculated which represents the age at which a person could be expected to read and understand the passage concerned. It has been found that the materials produced for dental health education are often more difficult to read than the type of reading matter to which many people are accustomed. When leaflets are used it is, of course, essential that the recipient is able to read and understand them. One of the problems has been that most dental health leaflets are written by dentists who, naturally, use dental jargon. They use the word 'gingivitis' for 'gum disease'; 'dental caries' for 'tooth decay'; 'orthodontic appliance' for 'braces'. It must be remembered that materials produced for the lay person must be in lay language if they are to be understood. All too often we end up with dentists seeking to transmit middle class behaviour in middle class terminology to working class people who speak another language. If the recipient of the message does not then adopt the behaviour recommended by the dentist, he or she is then criticized as being apathetic, not caring about their teeth, or just plain 'thick'. Dental health educators fail to understand that they do not pour their messages, exhortations, and appeals into a void, but rather into an existing culture in which, at minimum, some displacement must take place—what Polgar (1962) has termed the 'fallacy of the empty vessel'. Similarly five years at dental school have ensured that dentists can instantly recognize and comprehend a section through the jaw showing erupted and unerupted teeth, or a section through a tooth exposing its various components. Most members of the population are not able easily to understand the meaning of such diagrams.

Dentists and dental health educators earn their living from people's mouths. A major part of their lives is devoted to dental matters. Too often, they forget that dental health is not of such vital importance to most other people. It is much lower down most people's order of priorities. It is, therefore, doubly essential that leaflets on dental health are attractive and easy to read. Otherwise most people will not bother to struggle through them. It is important also to recognize that, however well the materials are produced, they cannot take the place of personal contact and should be used as a back-up or *reinforcement* of a face-to-face communication.

Mention has already been made of incorrect or misleading information being included in dental health communication. Even when the message is scientifically accurate, it is important to make sure that it is not capable of misinterpretation by the reader. It is a wise measure to test draft materials with a selection of members from the target population in order to identify potential problems and misunderstandings. This should be carried out before the materials are produced so that the necessary modifications can be made.

Earlier in this chapter, reference was made to the social inequalities in oral health. It might be hoped that health education would improve the relative position of those from the more deprived communities. However, Baric (1989) has argued that health education, as currently practised, is not a means of reducing inequalities in health but, on the contrary, is something which contributes to the perpetuation of these inequalities. Schou and Wight (1994) reported the results of a dental health education programme aimed at improving the oral hygiene and gingival health of 5-year-olds. They compared the results for schools in deprived and non-deprived neighbourhoods. The findings showed that prior to the campaign there was no difference in oral cleanliness or gingivitis between the two groups of schools. After the completion of the project they found a significant improvement in both oral hygiene and gingival health in the non-deprived schools but no change in the children in the deprived schools. This inequality had been created by the dental health education campaign. The study underlines the need to take into account the appropriate needs and strategies for different populations. It also suggests that passive public health initiatives, such as water fluoridation, are more likely to benefit the children from deprived communities than dental health messages which require action in changing lifestyles.

It is often claimed that the most effective dental health education is on a one-to-one basis in the dental surgery. There is no real evidence for this claim, and in fact, it ignores a number of factors which suggest that it may not be true. It must be remembered that most patients in the dental chair are not at ease; they are anxious and apprehensive and are thus not in the best frame of mind for understanding the new information they are being given, or learning the details of new techniques they are being taught. They are also receiving this information in isolation from their friends and those to whom they relate in their day-to-day life. They may not, therefore, be subject to the social support of others. Short visits to the dentist will do little by themselves to change a patient's ingrained habits (Blinkhorn 1981). In contrast, dental health education aimed at a group is able to utilize the peer group pressures which are exerted on members of that group. It therefore becomes possible for individuals within the group to influence each other and, it is to be hoped, help to re-socialize deviant members of the group. This is not to argue, however, that the one-to-one relationship is of no value. Many people expect the dentist to give advice on how to care for their teeth. The dentist is able to adapt the message to the patient's individual needs and answer any questions which arise. It is also important for the dentist to be able to give his or her professional support and reinforcement to the advice which may have been given by others such as health visitors or teachers.

In every community there are certain key people who are opinion-formers. it is to these persons that others turn for advice. In the field of dental health these include, besides dentists, the other members of the dental team, doctors, health educators, health visitors, midwives, teachers, and journalists. Such persons must, therefore, be kept informed of the correct messages to communicate, and encouraged to use their contacts with mothers, children, and others to give dental advice whenever appropriate. The influence of these health and education personnel is not limited to those to whom they talk because the message becomes passed on to others in a *two-step* communication.

Finally, it is unrealistic of the organizers to expect to achieve major changes in behaviour and health status by single, short-term campaigns. As already described, behaviour patterns are built up over a considerable period of time and handed down from one generation to another. Dental health educators must ensure that periodic *reinforcement* of the message is received by constant repetition. It is only in this way, like the wearing away of stone by constantly dripping water, that changes in a community level will be achieved.

THE ROLE OF COMMERCE AND POLITICS

In considering the promotion of oral hygiene, much support may be received from the manufacturers of products such as dentifrices and tooth-brushes. Commercial activity, including the use of the mass media for advertising campaigns, has undoubtedly contributed significantly to the increasing use of fluoride toothpastes and the more frequent replacement of tooth-brushes. In this respect, some of the interests of the manufacturers coincide with those of the dental profession. In addition to the advertising of their own branded products, the manufacturers of dental-health aids have given financial and other support to a number of dental-health education initiatives. The manufacturers of sugar products, however, may find that their commercial interests conflict rather more often with the message of the dental-health educator. In the past, these companies have provided finance for the production of dental-health materials, but this has provoked the accusation that the dental-health message has been distorted and the role of sugar in the aetiology of dental caries not fully explained. Whilst any producer of dental-health education materials should be free to accept help from any available source, it is essential for the credibility of the material that the message should be consistent with the scientific facts, and that the content of the materials must be decided by those involved in dental-health education without interference from commercial sponsors.

The Black Report (Report of a Research Working Group 1980) recommended a number of social and political policies which could be taken in order to benefit the general health of the population, especially those in the lower socio-economic groups. Similarly, some have suggested, in relation to dental health, that political action should be taken in the control of sugar. Advocates of political action point to the commercial interests of the so-called 'sugar lobby' and the large sums of money spent annually on advertising in order to persuade the population to consume more sugar. This product, they point out, is responsible not only for dental caries, but is also associated with disorders such as obesity and heart disease. Various legal sanctions have been suggested including the taxation of sugar products, banning of advertising, and the printing of health warnings on wrappers and packets. Opponents of this point of view believe that these measures are either unworkable, ineffective, or infringe personal liberty in an unacceptable way. The dental profession has been reluctant to become involved in this type of political debate, but if all possible measures to reduce dental disease are to be considered then the merits and disadvantages of such political action will need to be discussed.

CONCLUSIONS

- Some of the most important social factors which are relevant to the practise of dentistry and, in particular, preventive dentistry, have been identified:
  - open and closed social status
  - manual and non-manual occupations
  - immediate and deferred gratification
  - horizontal and vertical social mobility
  - social deprivation and area-based indicators
  - attitudes and behaviour (cognitive dissonance)
  - alienation and confusion hypotheses
  - primary and secondary socialization
  - restricted and extended vocabulary.

- Dental caries should be considered as a disease of social deprivation. Many of those with the most dental disease receive the least treatment.

- Differences in disease levels and service usage by ethnic groups is described.

- Factors affecting attitudes to fluoridation are reported.

- If technical expertise in prevention is to be converted into reality the dentist needs to understand the attitudes and behaviour of his/her patients.

- Only by taking these social factors into account can the dental health of the community be improved.

REFERENCES

Addy, M., Dummer, P.M.H., Hunter, M.L., Kingdon, A., and Shaw, W.C. (1990). The effect of toothbrushing frequency, toothbrushing hand, sex and social class on the incidence of plaque, gingivitis and pocketing in adolescents: a longitudinal cohort study. *Commun. dent. Health*, **7**, 237–47.

Baric, L. (1989). Inequalities in health (education). *J. Inst. Hlth Educ*. **27**, 30–3.

Beal, J.F. (1973), The dental health of five-year-old children of different ethnic origins resident in an inner Birmingham area and a nearby borough. *Archs. oral Biol*. **18**, 305–12.

Beal, J.F. (1990). The dental health of minority ethnic groups. In *Good practices in the health care of black and minority ethnic groups*, (ed. F. Estein), Public Health Report, Occasional Papers, No. 2. Yorkshire Health Authority.

Beal J.F. (1991). Dental health in Leeds, In *Annual Report of the Director of Public Health*. Leeds Healthcare.

Beal, J.F. and Dickson, S. (1974*a*). Diet and dental health. *Hlth Educ. J*. **33**, 8–12.

Beal, J.F. and Dickson, S. (1974*b*). Social differences in dental attitudes and behaviour in West Midland mothers. *Publ. Hlth* **89**, 19–30.

Beal, J.F. and Dickson, S. (1975). Dental attitudes and behaviour related to vertical social mobility by marriage. *Commun. Dent. oral Epidemiol*. **3**, 174–8.

Beal, J.F. and James, P.M.C. (1970). Social differences in the dental conditions and dental needs of 5-year-old children in four areas of the West Midlands. *Br. dent. J*. **129**, 313–18.

Beal, J.F. and James, P.M.C. (1971). Dental caries prevalence in 5-year-old children following five and a half years of water fluoridation in Birmingham. *Br. dent. J*. **130**, 284–8.

Beal, J.F. and Prendergast, M.J. (1993). *Adult dental health in Leeds 1992*. Leeds Health Authority.

Bedi, R. and Elton, R.A. (1991). Dental caries experience and oral cleanliness of Asian and white Caucasian children aged 5 and 6 years attending primary schools in Glasgow and Trafford, UK. *Commun. dent. Health*, **8**, 17–23.

Blau, P.M. (1956). Social mobility and interpersonal relations. *Am. Soc. Rev*. **21**, 291–5.

Blaxter, M. (1976). Social class and health inequalities. In *Equalities and inequalities in health. Proceedings of the Twelfth Annual Symposium of the Eugenics Society*, London, 1975. (ed. C.O. Carter and J. Peel). pp. 111–25, Academic Press, London.

Blaxter, M. (1984). Equity and consultation rates in general practice. *Br. Med. J*. **288**, 1963–7.

Blinkhorn, A.S. (1981). Dental health education. In *Dental public health*, (ed. G.L. Slack), Wright, Bristol.

Booth, V. and Ashley, F. (1989). The oral health of a group of 15–17 year old British school children of different ethnic origin. *Commun. dent. Health*, **6**, 195–205.

Bradnock, G., Jadoua, S.I., and Hamburger, R. (1988). The dental health of indigenous and non-indigenous infant school children in West Birmingham. *Commun. dent. Health*, **5**, 139–50.

Bradnock, G., Marchment, M.D., and Anderson, R.J. (1984). Social background fluoridation and caries experience in a 5-year-old population in the West Midlands. *Br. dent. J*. **156**, 127–31.

British Fluoridation Society (1992). *Briefing on public attitudes towards fluoridation*. BFS, Liverpool.

CACI Market Analysis Group (1983). *ACORN. A new approach to market analysis*. CACI, London.

Carmichael, C.L. (1981). Social and geographical factors affecting the role and provisions of community dental services in Newcastle AHA(T). *Proc. Br. Ass. Study Commun. Dent*. **3**, 38–44.

Carmichael, C.L. (1985). Inner city Britain: A challenge for the dental profession. A review of dental and related deprivation in inner city Newcastle-upon-Tyne. *Br. dent. J*. **159**, 24–7.

Carmichael, C.L. (1991). A 10-year comparison of general dental service care in the northern region 1979–1989. *Br. dent. J*. **171**, 97–101.

Carstairs, V. and Morris, R. (1989). Deprivation and mortality: an alternative to social class? *Commun. Med*. **11**, 210–9.

Centers for Disease Control (1992). Knowledge of the purpose of community water fluoridation—United States, 1990. *Morb. Mort. Wkly Rep*. **41**, 919, 925–7.

Charlton, M., Openshaw, S., and Wymer, C. (1985). Some new classifications of census enumeration districts in Britain: a poor man's ACORN *J. Econ. soc. Measur*. **13**, 69–96.

Cooper, M.H. (1975). *Rationing health care*. Croom Helm, London.

Corbett, E.M. and Moore, W.J. (1976). Distribution of dental caries in ancient British populations, 4. The 19th century. *Caries Res*. **10**, 401–14.

Craft, M. and Sheiham, A. (1976). Attitudes to prevention amongst dental practitioners: a comparison between the north and south of England. *Br. dent. J.* **141**, 371–6.

Crain, R.L., Katz, E., and Rosenthal, D.B. (1969). *The politics of community conflict: the fluoridation decision.* Bobbs-Merrill, New York.

Crawford, A.N. and Lennon, M.A. (1992). Dental attendance patterns among mothers and their children in an area of social deprivation. *Commun. dent. Health,* **9**, 289–94.

Curtis, S. (1990). Use of survey data and small area statistics to assess the link between individual morbidity and neighbourhood deprivation. *J. Epid. comm. Health,* **44**, 62–8.

Cushing, A.M. and Sheiham, A. (1985). Assessing periodontal treatment needs and periodontal status in a study of adults in north-west England. *Commun. dent. Health,* **2**, 187–94.

Davis P. (1980) *The social context of dentistry.* Croom Helm, London.

Dental Strategy Review Group (1981). *Towards better dental health.* Department of Health and Social Security, London.

Department of Health (1994). *An oral health strategy for England.* Department of Health, London.

Donaldson, L.J. (1986). Health and social status of elderly Asians: a community survey, *Br. med. J.* **293**, 1079–82.

Downer, M.C. (1970). Dental caries and periodontal disease in girls of different ethnic groups: a comparison in a London secondary school. *Br. dent. J.* **128**, 379–85.

Eames, M., Yoav, B., and Marmot, M.G. (1993). Social deprivation and preventive mortality: regional comparison across England. *Brit. med. J.* **307**, 1097–1102.

Eddie, S. and Davies, J.A. (1985). The effect of social class on attendance frequency and dental treatment received in the General Dental Service in Scotland. *Br. dent. J.* **159**, 370–2.

Festinger, L. (1957). *A theory of cognitive dissonance.* Row Peterson, Evanston.

Frankel, J.M. and Allukian, M. (1973). Sixteen referenda on fluoridation in Massachusetts: an analysis. *J. publ. hlth Dent.* **33**, 96–103.

Frazier, P.J. (1980). Fluoridation: a review of social research. *J. publ. hlth Dent.* **40**, 214–33.

French, A.D., Carmichael, C.L., Furness, J.A., and Rugg-Gunn, A.J. (1984). The relationship between social class and dental health in 5-year-old children in the north and south of England. *Br. dent. J.* **156**, 83–6.

Gelbier, S. and Taylor, S.G.B.W.S. (1985). Some Asian communities in the UK and their culture. *Br. dent. J.* **158**, 416–18.

Gibson, S.L.M. (1993). *The dark side of fluoride.* North West Councils Against Fluoridation, Lancashire.

Goldthorpe, J.H., Lockwood, D., Bechhofer, F., and Platt, J. (1968). *The affluent worker; political attitudes and behaviour.* Cambridge University Press.

Goldthorpe, J.H., Lockwood, D., Bechhofer, F. (1969). *The affluent worker in the class structure.* Cambridge University Press.

Gray, P.G., Todd, J.E., Slack G.L., and Bulman, J.S. (1970). *Adult dental health in England and Wales in 1968.* HMSO, London.

Greatrix, D., Taylor, G.O., and Lennon, M.A. (1990). Mother's dental attendance patterns and their children's dental attendance and dental health. *Br. dent. J.* **168**, 441–3.

Gunning, R. (1952). *The technique of clear writing.* McGraw-Hill, New York.

Hippocrates (c. 400 BC). On Airs, Waters and Places. Translated by F. Adams. In *Great books of the Western world. No. 10, Hippocrates and Galen.* (ed. R.M. Hutchins). pp. 9–19. Encyclopaedia Britannica, Chicago (1952).

Infante, P.F. and Russell, A.L. (1974). An epidemiologic study of dental caries in pre-school children in the United States by race and socio-economic level *J. dent. Res.* **53**, 393–6.

Jackson, D. (1972). Attitudes to fluoridation: a survey of British housewives. *Br. dent. J.* **132**, 219–22.

James, P.M.C. (1981). One hundred years of dental public health. *Br. dent. J.* **151**, 20–3.

Jarman, B. (1983). Identification of underpriviledged areas. *Br. med. J.* **286**, 1705–9.

Jenkins, P.M., Feldman, B.S., and Stirrups, D.R. (1984a). The effect of social factors on referrals for orthodontic advice and treatment. *Br. J. Orth.* **11**, 24–6.

Jenkins, P.M., Feldman, B.S., and Stirrups, D.R. (1984b). The effect of social class and dental features on referrals for orthodontic advice and treatment. *Br. J. Orth.* **11**, 185–8.

Kayser, A.F. (1981). Shortened dental arches and oral function. *J. oral Rehab.* **8**, 457–62.

Kenealy, P. and Shaw, W. (1989). The effects of social class on uptake of orthodontic treatment. *Br, J. Orth.* **16**, 107–11.

Locker, D. (1993). Measuring social inequality in dental health services research: individual, household and area-based measures. *Commun. dent. Health,* **10**, 139–50.

Lowry, R.J., Beal, J.F., Jones, S., Thomas, D., Dewhirst, W., and Robinson, C. (1995). A critical appraisal of an anti-fluoridation publication. In preparation.

Marmot, M.G. and McDowall, M.E. (1986). Mortality decline and widening social inequalities. *Lancet,* **ii**, 274–6.

Mattin, D. and Smith, J.M. (1991). The oral health status, dental needs and factors affecting utilisation of dental services in Asians aged 55 years and over, resident in Southampton. *Br. dent. J.* **170**, 369–72.

Murray, J.J. (1994). The secular decline in dental caries in children and its effect on the dental needs of young adults. *Univ. Malaya Ann. Dent.* **1**, 16–27.

Murray, J.J., Breckon, J.A., Reynolds, P.J., and Nunn, J.H. (1991). The effect of residence and social class on dental caries experience in 15–16-year-old children living in three towns (natural fluoride, adjusted fluoride and low fluoride) in the north east of England, *Br. dent. J.* **171**, 319–22.

National Pure Water Association (1969). *11 years of fluoridation: ineffective and unsafe: errors and omissions in government report.*

North, F., Syme, S.L., Feeney, A., Head, J., Shipley, M.J., and Marmot, M.G. (1993). Explaining socioeconomic differences in sickness absence: the Whitehall II study. *Br. med. J.* **306**, 361–6.

Nutbeam, D. and Catford, J. (1987). Pulse of Wales social survey supplement. *Heartbeat Report No. 7.* Heartbeat, Wales, Cardiff.

OPCS (Office of Population Censuses and Surveys) (1980). *Classification of occupations.* HMSO, London.

OPCS (Office of Population Censuses and Surveys) (1986). *Registrar General's decennial supplement on occupational mortality 1979–83.* HMSO, London.

OPCS (Office of Population Censuses and Surveys) (1990). *Standard occupational classification.* HMSO, London.

OPCS (Office of Population Censuses and Surveys) (1993). *Mortality statistics, perinatal and infant: social and biological factors for 1991.* Series DH3 No. 25. HMSO, London

OPCS (Office of Population Censuses and Surveys) (1994). Dental caries among children in the United Kingdom in 1993. *OPCS Monitor.* OPCS, London.

O'Mullane, D.M. and Robinson, M.E. (1977). The distribution of dentists and the uptake of dental treatment by school children in England. *Commun. Dent. oral Epidemiol.* **5**, 156–9.

Paul, P.F. and Bradnock, G. (1986). The dental health of Asian and Caucasian four- and five-year-old children resident in Coventry. *Commun. dent. Health*, **3**, 275–85.

Perkins, P.C. and Sweetman, A.J.P. (1986). Ethnic differences in caries prevalence in 5-year-olds in north-west London. *Br. dent. J.* **161**, 215–16.

Pitts, N.B. and Palmer, J.D. (1994). The dental caries experience of 5-, 12- and 14-year-old children in Great Britain. Surveys coordinated by the British Association for the Study of Community Dentistry in 1991/92, 1992/93 and 1990/91. *Commun. dent. Health.* **11**, 42–52.

Polgar, S. (1962). Health and human behaviour: areas of interest common to the social and medical sciences. *Curr. Anthrop. J.* 159–79.

Prendergast, M.J., Williams, S.A., and Curzon, M.E.J. (1989). An assessment of dental caries prevalence among Gujurati, Pakistani and white caucasian five-year-old children resident in Dewsbury, West Yorkshire. *Commun. dent. Health*, **6**, 223–32.

Prendergast, M.J., Beal, J.F., and Williams, S.A. (1993). An investigation of non-response bias by comparison of dental health in 5-year-old children according to parental response to a questionnaire. *Commun. dent. Health*, **10**, 225–34.

Report of a Research Working Group (1980). *Inequalities in health.* HMSO, London.

Rock, W.P. and Bradnock, G. (1976). The employment of dental hygienists within the General Dental Service in the United Kingdom. *Br. dent. J.* **140**, 351–2.

Rogers, J. Gelbier, S., Twidale, S., and Plamping, D. (1984). Barriers faced by parents in obtaining dental treatment for young children: a questionnaire evaluation. *Commun. dent. Health*, **1**, 207–12.

Rogers, S.N. (1991). Dental attendance in a sample of women in the UK. *Commun. dent. Health* **8**(4), 361–8.

Rosser, C. and Harris, C. (1965). *The family and social change.* Routledge and Kegan Paul, London.

Sapolsky, H.M. (1969). The fluoridation controversy: an alternative explanation. *Pub. Opinion Q.* **33**, 240–8.

Saxby, M.S. and Anderson, R.J. (1987). Dental cleanliness in a West Midlands population aged 14–19 years according to sex, ethnic origin and the presence of 1 ppm fluoride in the drinking water. *Commun. dent. Health.* **4**, 107–15.

Secretary of State for Health (1994). *Improving NHS dentistry.* HMSO, London.

Schou, L. and Wight, C. (1994). Does dental health education affect inequalities in dental health? *Commun. dent. Health*, **11**, 97–100.

Sheiham, A. (1969). The prevalence and severity of periodontal disease in British populations: dental surveys of employed populations in Great Britain. *Br. dent. J.* 115–22.

Sheiham, A. and Hobdell, M.H. (1969). Decayed, missing and filled teeth in British adult populations. *Br. dent. J.* **126**, 401–4.

Taylor, P.J. and Carmichael, C.L. (1980). Dental health and the application of geographical methodology. *Commun. Dent. oral Epidemiol.* **8**, 117–22.

Titmuss, R.M. (1968). *Commitment to welfare.* Allen and Unwin, London.

Todd, J.E. (1975). *Children's dental health in England and Wales 1973.* HMSO, London.

Todd, J.E. and Dodd, T. (1985). *Children's dental health in the United Kingdom 1983.* HMSO, London.

Todd, R. and Gelbier, S. (1991). Dental caries and dental attendance patterns in Vietnamese children aged 11–12 years resident in three inner London boroughs, UK. *Commun. dent. Health*, **8**, 163–5.

Todd, J.E. and Lader, D. 1991). *Adult dental health 1988, United Kingdom* HMSO, London.

Townsend, P., Phillimore, P., and Beattie, A. (1988). *Health and deprivation: inequality and the North.* Croom Helm, London.

Varley, T.F. and Goose, D.H. (1971). Dental caries in children of immigrants in Liverpool. *Br. dent. J.* **130**, 27–9.

West Midlands Regional Health Authority (1980). Summary of opinion survey on fluoridation. Mimeograph.

Whitehead, M. 1992). *The health divide* (2nd edn.) Penguin Books, London, Harmondsworth.

Williams, S.A. (1986). Behaviour patterns affecting the dental health of infants. *Dent. Hlth* (Lond.) **25**, 3–4, 6.

Williams, S.A., Fairpo, C.G., and Curzon, M.E.J. (1987). An enquiry into the dental caries experience of pre-school children in an inner-city area. Abstract. *J. dent. Res.* **66**, 853.

WHO (World Health Organization) (1982). *A review of current recommendations for the organization and administration of community oral health services in northern and western Europe.* Report on a WHO workshop, Oslo, May 1982. World Health Organization, Geneva.

17. Oral health policy and prevention

A. SHEIHAM

INTRODUCTION

The central subject of this chapter is policy-making, the task of making and analysing policy, and examining alternative proposals for attaining desirable goals in both the long and short term. Policy-makers determine what works or has the greatest chance of working and if it does good and provides benefits, how much good, and who benefits and who loses. They need to concentrate their money on what is known to bring the most benefit. Success is not possible without planning but not all planning succeeds. There is a significant gap between the ways dental institutions make policy and current knowledge on the subject. Although some therapies are effective there may not be a policy to apply the measure. For example, there are no official policies in Britain on control of sugars consumption, professionally applied fluorides, fissure sealants or dental health education, and on prevention of trauma to teeth and jaws, oral cancers, and temporo-mandibular joint dysfunction. There are policies on water fluoridation and in the USA on fluoride mouth rinsing. Despite the lack of explicit policies numerous uncoordinated implicit untested schemes exist for preventing caries and periodontal diseases.

In this chapter, policy will be defined and an outline given of the dominant philosophy underlying the World Health Organization's 'Health for all', health promotion, and the intersectoral approach. The epidemiological basis for strategy is explored and the application of an integrated approach to chronic disease control, and the common risk approach examined. Case studies using food and periodontal health policies will illustrate the relevance to oral health.

ORAL HEALTH POLICY

WHAT IS POLICY?

Policy is a consensus on the ideas forming the basis for co-ordinating plans for actions which, in turn, ensure that services are provided equitably and healthy environments are maintained. It underlies decision-making at the international and national level, the provincial and municipal levels, and at the individual health unit or agency level (Labonte 1989; Dickson 1993). It is a complex, dynamic process whose various components make different contributions to it. Policy decides major guidelines for action directed at the future, mainly by government organs. These guidelines (policies) formally aim at achieving what is in the public interest by the best possible means (Dror 1974). Health policy is the sys-

tematic approach to the evaluation and management of the quality and quantity of health care, including prevention and health services. The quality of health care is usually measured as the structure, process, or outcome and quantity is related to utilization costs of services.

THE NEED FOR POLICY

For many, the slogan 'prevention is better than cure' is grossly over-used. Yet, despite the availability of the scientific epidemiological basis for preventing caries and periodontal diseases and the utilization of water fluoridation, topical fluorides, and fissure sealants, high levels of dental diseases persist. The DMF in American 12-year-olds was 1.7 in 1987 (OHCC 1993). Even in areas of the UK where the drinking water has been fluoridated and where nearly all toothpastes contain fluoride, 50 per cent of 5-year-olds had tooth decay, and 16 per cent of these children had 5 or more decayed teeth (Rugg-Gunn *et al.* 1988). These and other studies (Weaver 1950) indicate that 'caries risk can be reduced by non-dietary means, particularly the use of fluoride, but these methods can be expensive and are not completely effective'. (DoH 1989). The Committee on Medical Aspects of Food Policy (COMA) (DoH 1989) concluded that '[if] the prevalence of dental caries in the UK (which is similar to the prevalence in North America, Scandinavia and Australia) is to be reduced further it will be necessary to reduce the amount and frequency of consumption of non-milk extrinsic sugars'.

The persistence of high levels of dental diseases highlights the need for a broad community perspective which tackles the causes. Caries cannot be treated away. It can be prevented. Dental science has provided numerous effective dental preventive methods that have been extensively reviewed in this book. 'There is no clinical reason why dental decay in children should not be virtually eliminated' (DoH 1991b; Sharp 1993). That is more than can be said about any other chronic disease. We know the causes of dental caries and there are effective preventive methods readily available. Why then is caries still so prevalent and severe in 1994? A probable answer is that there is no policy to tackle the determinants of dental caries—non-milk extrinsic sugars. Secondly, there is no concerted policy on how to prevent caries. The approaches that have been used are best described by Lindlom (1965) as 'muddling through'—slow evolution of policies by cautious incremental changes.

A number of countries, such as Ireland, Malaysia, and Brazil, have government policies for water fluoridation. In others, there is permissive legislation but no policy. In the UK, progress on introducing fluoridation has been painfully slow. Fifty years after the first trials of fluoridation, less than 15 per cent of the population consume the optimum levels of fluoride. Policies to introduce fluoridation have been outlined by Castle (1987). There are no official policies on the use of any of the other tested caries preventive measures. Some professional bodies have published guidelines but that is merely one aspect of a policy process. Guidelines are necessary but not sufficient conditions for policy.

The central focus for preventing periodontal diseases is health education by dental health professionals. The shortcomings of that approach have been outlined by Croucher (1993). The emphasis is on imparting information without much regard to the substantial body of knowledge on health education. A move away from reliance on professional expertise (authoritarian health education) towards more supportive approaches valuing lay competence is required. This provides one explanation as to why many planned health education interventions are largely unsuccessful.

The present dominant dental approach to prevention is recognizable in the following allegory. A man was standing by the side of a river and heard a cry of a drowning person. He jumped in to rescue him, pulled him to the bank and applied artificial respiration. Just as the rescued man was recovering there were more cries from other drowning people. In jumped the rescuer, brought some back and resuscitated them. The rescuer could not cope on his own so he got some helpers and machines. Still he could not cope. So they worked faster in teams—four-handed and six-handed—with more complex equipment. The numbers of drowning people become so numerous that some could not be rescued before permanent damage occurred. How could he stop them from drowning? Swimming lessons were the solution. These rescuing and training activities kept him so busy that a no time did he stop to consider why people who could no swim were in the river. Who was pushing them in upstream? (McKinlay 1974; Cowell and Sheiham 1981).

The dentist's concentration on 'downstream' victim-blaming distracts attention from the 'upstream' activities of the confectionery, food, and drink companies who are 'pushing people into the water'. Health workers usually intervene only after the damage has been done. Instead of concentrating so much effort on downstream and midstream activities, more efforts should be directed at making the river shallower so that people do not have to learn to swim—making healthier choices the easier choices (Milio 1986)—and controlling the activities of those pushing people into the water—a direct attack on the determinants of health.

The need for policy is justified because oral diseases are important public health problems (Table 17.1). They are very prevalent and the impact of individuals are significant. Pain, disability, and handicap from oral diseases are common (Cushing *et al.* 1986: Locker 1988).

THE DOMINANT PHILOSOPHY, PRIMARY HEALTH CARE AND HEALTH PROMOTION

At the level of public policy, the influence of the World Health Organization in the 1980s was substantial. The publication of

Table 17.1. Public health importance of oral diseases

- High prevalence
- Impact on individuals and society is great
- Pain, discomfort, functional limitation and handicap are common, they affect the quality of life
- Financial cost to individuals and the community is considerable. Dental diseases are more expensive to treat than heart diseases and cancers
- Preventable: simple and cheap public health methods should be available to prevent and control
- Causes are known—diet, dirt, and cigarettes
- Easy to evaluate treatment
- Easy to detect
- Treatment relatively ineffective

the Declaration of Alma Ata (WHO 1978) and the subsequent development of the WHO strategy for 'Health for all by the year 2000' effectively set the agenda for the new public health. The principles in the Declaration of Alma Ata can be summarized by five principles:

1. *Equitable distribution.* Governments must endeavour to distribute equitably those variables which influence health.

2. *Community participation.* Individuals and communities should participate in all decisions which affect their health.

3. *Focus on prevention.* The focus of health planners and funding must shift from medical/dental care to prevention and health promotion.

4. *Appropriate technology.* Emphasis should be on the most appropriate technology and personnel to deal with problems.

5. *A multi-sectoral approach.* Solutions to ill-health cannot be solved only by the health sector. Social, economic, agriculture, and education sectors must co-ordinate policies that affect health.

Establishing healthy public policy is one of the five means for achieving the goal of 'Health for all by the year 2000'. The others are creating supporting environments, strengthening community action, developing personal skills, and reorienting health services (WHO 1986). The Ottawa Charter also included three process methods—mediation, enablement, and advocacy—through which people could begin to take more control over their health. 'Healthy public policy is characterized by an explicit concern for health and equity in all areas of policy and by accountability for health impact' (WHO 1988). In health care, equity is based on Aristotle's dictum that there is no greater injustice than to treat unequal cases equally. Equity requires that people who are alike in relevant respects be treated in like fashion, and people who are unlike in relevant respects be treated appropriately in unlike fashion. This corresponds to horizontal equity—like treatment of like individuals, and vertical equity—the unlike treatment of unlike individuals (Culyer 1993).

According to Whitehead (1991) the term inequity 'refers to differences which are unnecessary and avoidable but, in addition, are also considered unfair and unjust'. Reducing inequalities in health is established as one of the prime tasks of health promotion (WHO 1984). Equity is an ethical principle and it is unsurprising that the ethical principles underlying health promotion conform to the Declaration of Helsinki and include respect for persons, benefaction, non-malfeasance and justice (Beauchamp and Childress 1989). These principles are included in WHO documents concerning the ethics of health promotion (WHO 1989). Respect for persons incorporates at least two fundamental ethical considerations. The first of these is autonomy, a right to self-determination. Autonomy also includes confidentiality and respect for privacy. To make autonomous choices a person needs all relevant information, and therefore informed consent is the most important application of this principle. People who are dependent or vulnerable should be afforded security against harm or abuse.

The Ottawa Charter included the concept of healthy public policy (Table 17.2). This goes beyond the health care system. It is concerned with the health implications of all policies including economic, employment, agriculture, housing, transport, and environment policies, recognizing that improvements in health come from a multi-sectoral rather than a purely health sector approach. Milio (1987) defined healthy public policy as 'ecological in perspective, multi-sectoral in scope and participatory in strategy'. Healthy public policy stresses the need to analyze and understand the broad beliefs and cultures of the community as well as those of the professionals who act as advocates and the functioning of local and central government. Understanding the existing policy environment is central to the development of healthy public policy.

The modern health promotion movement has emerged out of the need for a fundamental change in strategy to achieve and maintain health. First, it is based on a public health philosophy that should encompass the prevention of disease

at a primary level, and secondly, the promotion of health (Milio 1986). These two concepts, when applied to developing environments which promote healthier choices for people in coping with their lives, need to be adopted in a manner that encourages those choices to be the easiest choices (Milio 1986). Health promotion can be considered 'as the combination of educational and environmental supports for actions and conditions of living conducive to health' (Green and Kreuter 1990). Strategies to change 'the range of options available to people and to make health-promoting choices easier and/or to diminish health-damaging options by making them more difficult to choose' (Milio 1986). Another definition is 'health promotion is the process of enabling individuals and communities to increase control over the determinants of health and thereby improve their health. Health promotion represents a mediating strategy between people and their environment, combining personal choice and social responsibility for health to create a healthier future'. (WHO 1984). It is directed to the underlying determinants as well as the immediate causes of health—the causes of the causes.

The social environment has become more significant for health. Because the major dental and oral diseases are chronic the persistence of health-related behaviours is important. A lifetime of simple acts related to lifestyle, becomes the target for change. Lifestyle is frequently considered a consciously chosen personal behaviour. Others interpret lifestyle as a composite expression of the social and cultural circumstances that condition and constrain behaviour in addition to the personal decisions the individual may make (Green and Kreuter 1990). But the apparent simple acts are enmeshed in more complex lifetime habits and social circumstances associated with lifestyle (Graham 1990). Living conditions provide the context in which lifestyles are sustained (Blane 1985; Graham 1990). Indeed, Blane (1985) has argued convincingly that the causative role of individual behaviours have been exaggerated. They should be seen '.... as indicators of other factors which are more straightforwardly related to the social structure, and which are the true aetiological agents' (Blane 1985).

STRATEGY FOR ORAL HEALTH PROMOTION—GENERAL PRINCIPLES

Strategies should be based on the following guiding principles (Sheiham and Plamping 1988).

1. Clearly stated goals.

2. Preventive rather than curative strategies—promote public health measures to the public and public authorities, e.g. fluoride in water.

3. A re-orientation from prescription to health promotion—redress the balance of influence and make healthier choices easier. Promote self-esteem and facilitate decision-making skills rather than be prescriptive. Combat the influence of those interests which produce and profit from ill health. That involves controls on industry—sponsored educational materials in schools, advertising, and campaigns to reduce barriers.

Table 17.2. Themes and key areas for health promotion action; the Ottawa Charter (WHO 1986)

Promoting health through public policy: by focusing attention on the impact on health of public policies from all sectors, and not just the health sector.

Creating a supportive environment: by assessing the impact on health of the environment and clarifying opportunities to make changes conducive to health.

Developing personal skills: by moving beyond the transmission of information, to promote understanding, and to support the development of personal, social, and political skills which enable individuals to take action to promote health.

Strengthening community action: by supporting concrete and effective community action in defining priorities, making decisions, planning strategies, and implementing them to achieve better health.

Reorienting health services: by refocusing attention away from the responsibility to provide curative and clinical services towards the goal of health gain.

4. Public health rather than individually focused programmes.

5. The social causes of ill health rather than a victim—blaming approach—acknowledging the limited real choices available to any individual.

6. Focus on the underlying determinants of health.

7. Tackle causes that are common to a number of chronic diseases.

8. Supportive rather than authoritarian styles of health education.

9. A commitment to distribute success equitably.

10. Community participation rather than professionally dominated activities.

11. Integration of efforts.

12. Dental workers undertaking health education should engage in activities within and beyond the health services.

Selecting a strategy is influenced by the criteria outlined above and philosophical, professional, and political perspectives. The epidemiological basis for strategy selection for health promotion is the Common Risk Factor Approach (CRFA) (Grabauskas 1987) and the Whole Population Strategy (WPS) (Rose 1992).

AN INTEGRATED COMMON RISK FACTOR APPROACH

There are basically two approaches for an equity-oriented health policy. One is to focus on actions to reduce specific diseases and the other on specific risk factors and public policies aimed at improving health conditions in general and among those at particular risk. It is within the context of the Common Risk/Health Factor Approach (CRHFA) to distinguish between actions aimed at reducing 'risk factors' and actions promoting 'health factors'. The strategy should include efforts to improve health by reducing risks, promoting health, and strengthening possibilities to cope with 'given' risk factors-creating supportive environments reducing the negative effects of certain risk factors and facilitating behaviour changes. A major benefit of the CRHFA is the focus on improving health conditions in general for the whole population and for groups at high risk. It thereby reduces social inequities.

Concepts of common risk factors must inform public health work and education. A number of chronic diseases, such as heart disease, cancer, strokes, and oral diseases, have risk factors in common and many risk factors are relevant to more than one chronic disease. Such risk factor-oriented strategies are more rational than those directed at specific diseases. Cardiovascular risk factors affect a number of diseases indicating that they have a much broader impact on health. This suggested that preventive strategies will exert a favourable effect, not only on a single disease but simultaneously on several conditions (Grabauskas 1987). The key concept

underlying the integrated common risk approach is that promoting general health by controlling a small number of risk factors may have a major impact on a large number of diseases at a lower cost than disease-specific approaches. Savings may be made by co-ordinating the work done by various specialist groups and organizations. Decision-makers and individuals will be more readily influenced by measures directed at preventing heart diseases, obesity, stroke, cancers, diabetes, and dental caries than if disease-specific recommendations are made. Three approaches may be used. If one risk factor affects several diseases the attack may be integrated across disease boundaries. Or, integrated action may affect a number of diseases. As the same group of risk factors affect a number of diseases, a policy directed at several risk factors and several diseases is more rational (Fig. 17.1) (Grabauskas 1987).

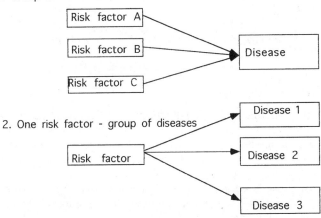

1. Group of risk factors -one disease

2. One risk factor - group of diseases

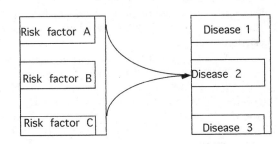

3. Group of risk factors - group of diseases

Fig. 17.1. Models of common risk factor approaches.

The same unhealthy diet affects the incidence of heart disease, cancer, and oral diseases. Working with food policy strategists to change diet to reduce the intakes of non-milk extrinsic sugars, fat, and salt and increase complex carbohydrate and/or fibre and availability and promotion of fruit, vegetables, and cereal products is more likely to succeed than one which only stresses control of sugars for caries reduction. Similarly, tobacco smoking affects heart disease and respiratory diseases as well as oral diseases. Programmes to reduce smoking for such life-threatening diseases as cancer and heart disease should be co-ordinated. Trauma to teeth affects about one in five children. Preventing tooth trauma requires a broadly based strategy to prevent accidents, especially those affecting the head.

The epidemiological basis for a common risk factor approach exists (Fig. 17.2) (Dahlgren and Diderichsen 1986).

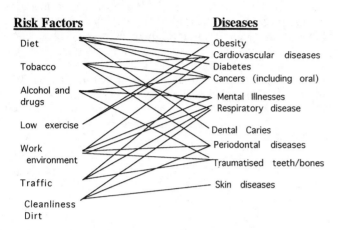

Fig. 17.2.   The common risk factor approach.

POPULATION AND HIGH-RISK STRATEGIES

The economic rationale for preventive measures depends on the prevalence of the disease: when the prevalence is very low, and the diseases not serious, the returns often do not justify the intervention. The cost per caries lesion saved increases as the level of decay decreases (Foch 1981). At the lower levels of dental caries now prevailing in most industrialized countries, the traditional preventive methods such as fluoride rinsing, professionally applied fluorides, and intensive chairside dental health education need to be justified because the cost-effectiveness is borderline (Klock 1980; Klein *et al.* 1985).

Concern for reducing disease in people with severe caries or periodontal disease rests on the assumption that those predisposed to develop many cavities and pockets are distinguishable from those at low risk. That implies some means of identifying those in special need. A High Risk Strategy (HRS) aims to identify people who may develop disease in the future by the use either of a predictive marker or of an early feature of the disease which precedes its clinical manifestation so that efforts can be focused on them. Screening is used to detect those people at high risk for close monitoring and special preventive treatment. An important purpose of risk assessment is not to categorize individuals according to a test result, but rather to identify those who have a propensity and can be helped by prevention.

One advantage of the HRS is that any preventive intervention which is undertaken is appropriate to the individual concerned, who has a high probability of future disease (Rose 1992). A corollary is that those at risk, once identified and told, are likely to be better motivated to participate in the care offered. This does, however, assume that the intervention is sensitive to the ability of the person and their social and economic circumstances. A further advantage is that those not at risk do not have to undergo preventive treatment. Finally, the

HRS conserves valuable resources by directing services where the need and potential benefits are likely to be greatest. However, this does not necessarily imply that the overall ratio of benefits to costs is favourable.

To be useful in predictive case-finding, a test must detect the majority of high risk children and at the same time identify those at low risk. To be more precise, it must have high sensitivity, otherwise many with potential caries will not be identified, as well as high specificity to prevent excessive dilution of the high risk group with subjects who are in fact at comparatively low risk. A practical way of looking at the imperfections in screening tests is to consider sensitivity and specificity in terms of screened patients whose test result is wrong. A review of the literature on the available predictors of caries found that none are of sufficient sensitivity and specificity (Sheiham and Joffe 1991). Combinations of predictors may be more effective, but none of those currently available are, despite claims to the contrary. The best indicator of future caries in individuals is past caries experience (Downer 1978) but even this is a poor basis for identifying high risk individuals. Prior disease is not a reliable predictor of future disease. Although the future course of disease is difficult to predict accurately in particular individuals, epidemiological data allow us to see what future patterns of caries in groups of children will be, if their caries status when they are young is known. This allows prediction not only of what the DMF for 10-year-olds will be when they are 18, but of which teeth will become carious and which surfaces will be attacked (Kalsbeek 1982; McDonald and Sheiham 1992). These predictions allow planning of the numbers and types of dental personnel required in the future, but not which child will need therapy.

In addition to reliability and validity, there are several factors to be considered before undertaking or advising the use of a screening test. The recommended intervention needs to be successful in reducing the incidence and/or severity of the disease. When the aim is the detection of one or more markers rather than disease itself, one must ensure that the overall effect will have more benefits than disadvantages from the point of view of the child being screened. The test itself must be acceptable to the subject in terms of inconvenience, discomfort, and risks of side-effects. Furthermore, it must be simple and capable of rapid application to large numbers of subjects (Burr and Elwood 1985).

To summarize, the HRS for preventing caries and periodontal diseases has several drawbacks, and if relied on exclusively it cannot be expected to make a major impact on the disease. The current preoccupation with markers of disease prediction is misdirected and is unlikely to produce information of use to control dental diseases.

WHOLE POPULATION STRATEGY (WPS)

Fortunately, another strategy is available which complements the use of the High Risk Strategy—this is the Whole Population Strategy. The concepts of the WPS have been adopted by the World Health Organization (WHO 1984) and incorporated as principles of health promotion:

1. Focus on whole populations rather than on disease-specific at-risk groups.

2. Action should be addressed towards the many factors influencing health in order to ensure that the 'total environment, which is beyond the control of individuals, is conducive to health'.

In many industrialized countries, compared with 20 years ago, dental health in children and young adults is today markedly better. This improvement has arisen as a result of changed norms of behaviour in the population as a whole together with an alteration in manufacturing practice and the addition of fluoride to toothpaste. The common sense view, that modern dentistry can take much of the credit by having identified the causes and methods of prevention, is only a small part of the picture (Nadanovsky 1993). The improvement of health as a result of wide social factors is not confined to caries. Concerning the major epidemic diseases which have declined dramatically during the past 100 years, McKeown examined a number of factors, including medical progress, which might have contributed to their reduction (McKeown 1979). The contribution of the medical profession, even immunization, was quite limited.

The implication of these findings is that major improvements in the prevention of disease tend to follow major social changes, whether these are alterations in social norms (dietary patterns, oral cleanliness, contraception), in the availability of key resources (fluoridated toothpaste, quality and quantity of food) or as a result of engineering (fluoridation of water supplies, clean water, effective waste disposal). There is no reason why a similar approach should not prove equally successful in the future.

Just as the HRS requires a scientific basis, both in technical matters and evaluation, the same is true of the WPS. It depends on epidemiological, sociological, and other research to identify important determinants of the disease in question, and acting to change their prevalence in the appropriate direction. In the case of caries, the determinants which are open to intervention are sugars consumption and the protective influence of fluoride: the distribution of caries (DMF) depends on the distributions of these exposures. Altering whole exposure distributions may be the most effective way of reducing the prevalence of caries, both in the population as a whole and also specifically among those who are at highest risk. Such a strategy does not exclude the use of an HRS as well, in appropriate circumstances. The scientific basis for the WPS has been eloquently discussed by Rose (1992). He draws the distinction between two kinds of aetiological question: the first seeks the causes of cases: 'Why do some *people* get caries at this time?' and the second seeks the causes of incidence: 'Why do some *populations* have much caries while in others it is uncommon?'

The first question is addressed by epidemiological research which examines the distribution of disease among the individuals of a particular population. The ability of such a study to identify risk factors depends on their distribution in the population. For example, if everyone in the country smoked cigarettes, it would be impossible to demonstrate the link with lung cancer: an epidemiological investigation conducted within the population would be reduced to studying individual susceptibility apart from exposure to tobacco smoke. This approach assumes a heterogeneity of exposure to the causative factor within the study population. The more widespread a cause, the less it explains the distribution of cases (Rose 1992). A cause which is universally present is the hardest to identify. If everyone ate similar amounts of sugars then case-control studies would lead to the false conclusion that caries was a genetic disease or that children with high caries rates have an immunological defect or different bacteriological flora.

The two approaches to aetiology, population- and individual-based, have parallels in preventive philosophy. In the latter, individuals at high risk of a disease are sought with a view to changing their risk factors and thereby their chances of developing disease. In the population strategy, the determinants of disease in the whole population are controlled (Rose 1992). The HRS seeks to protect susceptible individuals, whereas the WPS seeks to control the causes of the incidence.

Because the WPS attempts to control the determinants—removing the underlying causes—it has great benefits to all sections of the population at which it is directed. This was illustrated above in terms of the decline of caries. The approach is behaviourally appropriate. The aim is to alter social norms; when that norm is accepted and institutional changes have occurred then reinforcement of the behaviour is unnecessary. Examples of such institutional changes are the adaptation of their products on the part of industry (fluoridated toothpaste, low-sugar snacks), and government action such as a food and health policy including reduction in sugars. The more effective the basic prevention for the group the smaller will be the subgroup that will require individualized prevention and treatment.

The disadvantages of WPS are related to its long time-scale and to any possible adverse impact of its implementation. The latter might include harmful effects of fluoride, which were suggested in the past but not substantiated, and the consequences of reducing sugar consumption. The most important of these concerns employment in sugar-producing and sugar-using industries.

The WPS can be used flexibly. For example, it can be directed at a designated part of the total population such as a school, a district or part of a district—a directed population strategy. This remains different from the HRS in that it does not use screening of individual subjects for risk factors.

Rose's observations on the difference between determinants of cases and determinants of incidence can be applied to the epidemiology of caries and the intake of sugars. There is a relatively low correlation ($r = + 0.143$) between an individual's sugar intake and caries increment (Rugg-Gunn *et al.* 1984), but associations between indicators of population sugar consumption and the incidence of caries are very high—$r = + 0.72$ (Screebny 1982). Thus, although dietary sugar is the main determinant of a population's incidence of caries, measures of sugar intake generally fail to identify high risk individuals, because the variation of sugar consumption within populations is typically insufficient to have a measurable effect on caries incidence (Hackett *et al.* 1984).

Two effects of the dose-response relationship are critical for policy. How much of the burden of disease is compressed within an identifiable group where high exposure carries a high risk? Is there an exposure threshold below which risk is

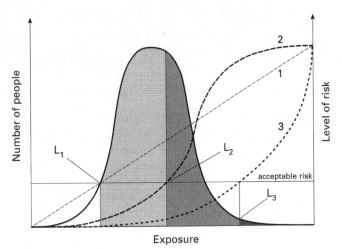

Fig. 17.3.   Three types of dose-response curves.

small. Is there a level of sugar, in the case of caries, and plaque, in the case of periodontal disease, compatible with low or no disease? That is a reverse L exposure (Fig. 17.3, curve 3), one without adverse effects until it reaches a certain level, beyond which the risk increases markedly or a S-shaped curve (Fig. 17.3, curve 2). The S-shaped curve is similar to a reverse L curve except that beyond a certain level little increase in response occurs. There is a plateau (Sheiham 1983, 1991*a*).

The dose-response curve for sugars—caries appears to be S-shaped (Sheiham 1983, 1991*a*; Rugg-Gunn 1993). At low consumption levels, sucrose leads to very little caries; increasing levels of sucrose are followed by increasing levels of disease; then the curve eventually flattens out, and further increases in sucrose do not lead to appreciable increases in caries. The rate of increase depends on the frequency of sugars consumption and the availability of fluoride. The dose-response curve rises more steeply when sucrose-containing foods are eaten frequently by children: the newly erupted teeth are less resistant to demineralization and there are more acid attacks. If the sucrose-containing foods are eaten less frequently, or if the teeth have had time to 'mature' (have been longer in the mouth), or if most of the susceptible tooth surfaces are already decayed or filled as in adults, then it may take a higher level of sucrose to cause caries and the resulting caries will be less extensive—the curve will shift to the right. Beyond a certain level of sugars intake no further increases in caries occurs—the curve flattens (Newbrun 1982, 1983; Sheiham 1991*a*). Improvements in caries will occur only when sugars levels are on the slope and not at high levels on the flat of the curve. Takeuchi (1960) found that the S-shaped dose-response curve reached a plateau at 35 kg per person per year. The benefits of prevention are larger at high levels of sugars below the 'saturation level'. At high sugars intake fluoride has little effect; even when the sugars challenge is 'strong' the topical effect of fluoride is minimal.

The dose-response relationship between non-milk extrinsic sugars consumption and dental caries is probably S-shaped. Below a consumption rate of 10 kg/person/year (27.4 g/day), the caries rate is acceptably low. At 15 kg/person/year the in-

tensity of the caries attack increases. However, where fluoride is present in drinking water at 0.7–1.0 ppm, or over 90 per cent of the toothpastes available are fluoridated, the dose-response curve may be shifted to the right. If that occurs, the permissible non-milk extrinsic sugars level could be increased to 15 kg/person/ year. Most of the world's population, predominantly in underdeveloped countries, does not have easy access to fluoride. Therefore, the 10 kg non-milk extrinsic sugars level should be adopted as a nutrient goal in such countries. The level for industrialized countries recommended by Sheiham 1991*a* is below the COMA Dietary Reference Value (DRV) for non-milk extrinsic sugars suggested by the Panel on Dietary Reference Values of the Committee on Medical Aspects of Food Policy (DoH 1991*a*). They recommended that levels should not exceed about 60 g/per/day in the UK

It is important to consider whether the adoption of a WPS might be against the interests of either high or low risk groups. One way to address this question is from historical data: in South West Avon there was an increase in the percentage of caries-free 13- to 14-year-olds from 8 per cent to 42 per cent in 8 years; the proportion of 'high risk' with 10 or more DMFT was 6.0 per cent in 1980, 2.2 per cent in 1984, and 0.5 per cent in 1988 (Dowell 1988) (Fig. 17.4). The implication is that the shift in the whole distribution had a markedly beneficial effect on those at relatively high risk, who are now eligible for far fewer restorations than the corresponding children at an earlier period. At the same time, those at intermediate and low risk have also benefited, as their prevalence of disease has similarly decreased. These data on the decline of caries in South West Avon show the change in the shape of the distribution which accompanies the fall in mean DMFT from 4.6 to 2.7 (Fig. 17.4). Caries distribution curves tend to exhibit skewness with a right tail suggesting a high risk population which could be identified. However, by decreasing the overall prevalence of caries, the position of the tail shifts to the left so that the 'high risk' population now has less disease (Fig. 17.4).

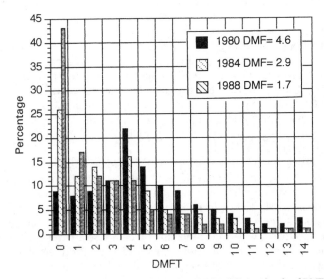

Fig. 17.4.   Percentage distributions of DMFT for different levels of DMFT in 13- to 14-year-olds. (Dowell 1988.)

The same effect can be seen even more strongly if population of high and low caries prevalence are compared. Such a comparison shows the future which is possible for populations which at present have relatively high, albeit declining, prevalence.

INDIVIDUAL CHOICE AND COLLECTIVE RESPONSIBILITY

If a small minority of people suffer from an unacceptable level of disease at current levels of consumption of a food, is there a need to get the whole population to change their eating habits? The answer is no. However, if the frequency distribution of intake is such that a high proportion have intakes which are estimated to be above the acceptable risk level, then there is a strong ethical basis for adopting a WPS. Payne and Thomson (1979) have suggested a method for deciding on strategies. Plotting the dose-response curves (Fig. 17.3, lines 1,2,3) and proposing an acceptable level of risk allows one to determine the levels of intake above the acceptable level for each of the intake-risk functions (dose-response curves). The nature of the dose-response curve is very important. This is seen when we look at them in relation to the distribution of habitual intakes of the population (Fig. 17.3). A policy aimed a getting everyone to reduce their sugars intake would be justified if the dose-response relationship is 2, as is the case, since a large percentage would benefit (those with exposure above L_2, Fig. 17.3). If the relationship is 3 the same strategy would be unjustified because only those with the highest intakes (above L_3 Fig. 17.3) would significantly benefit.

The radical approach of the Whole Population Strategy, relies heavily on intersectoral planning—involving, at the macro-level, the Ministries of Agriculture, Education, Employment, Foreign Affairs as well as the Health Ministry, and at a micro-level, interdisciplinary planning: getting teachers, primary health workers, community development, and social workers to co-ordinate their efforts. This approach sets the agenda and establishes norms. For example, the idea that excessive consumption of sugars is detrimental to health is a widely accepted belief and many food and drink manufacturers feature 'no sugar added' on their labels as a positive selling feature. Once the norm has been established, efforts should be made to institutionalize them by a reduction in subsidies to produce and promote the product, controls on advertising and on imports, by encouraging the production of low- and no-sugars alternatives, and by changing educational materials.

Policy-makers have a number of options to consider: they can accept the current option of treating cases with large numbers of dentists or stress prevention using the dental team. Both these options rely heavily on dentists and may be accepted by conservative planners because the manpower exists and the professional associations may welcome the *status quo*. A third option is a preventatively oriented High Risk Strategy which depends on behaviour change using health education/promotion methods and public health dentists with auxiliaries doing the chairside education and preventive therapy. A fourth option is the Whole Population Strategy, in the context of a risk factor approach to health

promotion. Initially, this would require a policy oriented to health-related criteria in order to establish new norms. Thus, a food policy might be implemented to support health education messages stressing the need to increase the amount of dietary fibre and decrease that of sugars, salt, and fat. Once such changes are established, they are comparatively easy to sustain.

Oral health policies are part of general health policies. The determinants and behaviours relating to the major oral diseases are common to the major chronic diseases and the preventive strategies outlined by Rose (1992) equally apply as do the principles of health promotion. Therefore, in selecting a oral strategy the following criteria and approaches apply (WHO 1984):

- the degree to which the strategy fits with general health policy and action; the strategy should be incorporated into general health strategies and tackling causes common to a number of chronic diseases
- focus on the determinants of health
- the degree to which the proposed action is compatible with oral health policies and actions
- the degree to which the strategy facilitates or establishes desirable long-term trends
- the probability of success in achieving the quantified objectives in the desired time-frame
- freedom from resource and attitude constraints now or in the foreseeable future
- the ratio between cost and effectiveness
- the degree to which desirable benefits or undesirable side-effects are anticipated
- community participation
- the level of equity.

INTERSECTORAL APPROACH

The central focus of the WHO 'Health for all by the years 2000' approach is an intersectoral approach (WHO 1981). This approach recognizes that economic, environmental, and social changes should underlie individual behaviour change. Promoting health requires the involvement not only of health professionals, but of all sectors of society, in both public and private spheres. An intersectoral approach is co-ordinated planning, implementation and evaluation of health-related and health-directed programmes and actions in order to promote a integration of health, social economic, and environmental issues in the daily life of people. The strategy should identify all groups who should be involved in creating or coping with a health problem and how their behaviour may be influenced. Exactly who is involved with a health problem will vary with the problem. Each issue requires its own analysis. Nonetheless, certain broad groupings recur in most analyses: industry, government with several ministries, quasi-autonomous agencies, and even supranational organizations, treaters, voluntary organizations, and the general population.

Another principle underlying the WHO's programme is that 'health promotion combines diverse, but complementary, methods of approaches'. Thus, while information and education are necessary and core components of health promotion, it is recognized that information alone is inadequate. Health promotion should influence all the relevant parties to more healthful forms of behaviour. In particular, the strategy should concentrate on more systematic education of policy-makers. Food and nutrition policy to reduce the consumption of non-milk extrinsic sugars will be used to illustrate an intersectoral, whole population health promotion strategy.

FOOD AND NUTRITION POLICY TO REDUCE NON-MILK EXTRINSIC SUGARS LEVELS

Since nutrition behaviour is a very complex process, a food and nutrition policy demands an intersectoral approach for implementing healthy nutrition behaviour. Considering the variety of social, cultural, economic, and physiological factors that influence dietary behaviour, an essential strategy lies in an environmental approach in which consumers, supermarkets, and professionals and food scientists from different backgrounds work together to 'make the healthy choice the easy choice'. Linking nutrition promotion to local activities also has the potential for being more easily adopted by the communities and creating social networks supporting positive behaviour change and maintenance of these changes.

The first decisions in a food policy is at what level should activities be addressed to achieve particular objectives. The policy should discriminate between activities that require changes of policy at international level, such as the Common Agriculture Policy or General Agreement on Tariffs and Trade (GATT), national, local or personal levels. With the globalization of food production and the increase in multinational companies and agreements, proposing particular changes at a local or even national level may not have any impact. A framework for identifying priorities for promotion of healthier eating is outlined in Fig. 17.5 (Sanderson 1984; Stockley (1993). It identifies which intervention should be directed at particular groups in the 'food chain'.

Many mechanisms are possible, but at least four broad strategies should be used. (1) An education strategy induces people to change their practices through the provision of education, exhortation, and instruction. (2) A pricing strategy encourages switching from harmful to healthy products by altering their relative prices. (3) A provision strategy directly affects behaviour through providing health-promoting products and not providing those detrimental to health. (4) A regulatory strategy structures options and choices through legislative and/or administrative controls.

Dietary changes which would help prevent caries have been identified by the Committee on the Medical Aspects of Food Policy (DoH 1989) and most recently in the 1991 report on Dietary Reference Values (DoH 1991a). The targets and the upper limits set represent the major elements of this advice. The Dietary Reference Value (DRV) for sugars for non-milk extrinsic (NME) sugars are 10 per cent of total energy and 11 per cent of food energy (DoH 1991a), which conform to those set by the WHO (1990, 1991) for populations worldwide. In addition to oral health reasons for reducing sugars consumption, because sugars contribute calories only, they may play a role in increasing obesity. Finally, persons who need a nutrient-dense diet—this means all 'low-energy consumers', especially the oldest and the youngest—are advised to avoid over-consumption of foods that are high in 'nutrient-free calories' (Helsing 1987). As the current levels of sucrose consumption in the UK is between 13 to 20 per cent of energy (DoH 1989; MAFF 1992) a decrease of at least 20–30 per cent is the short-term target. Soft drinks, confectionery, cakes, biscuits and cereal products account for 70 per cent of sugars in industrial products; a reduction of 50 per cent in NME sugars consumed from them will achieve a 25 per cent reduction in total NME sugars consumption.

The aim of modern food and nutrition policies is to enable, encourage, and help consumers to choose a healthy diet. The main elements of food and nutrition policy (MAFF 1992) are to:

- ensure the adequacy of the national diet in terms of its quantity, quality, and variety at affordable prices
- ensure authoritative expert advice to government
- give support to health and other professionals
- provide information about individual foods including labelling
- monitor trends in disease, health, nutritional status, and diet

	Producers	Processors	Manufacture	Intermediaries	Caterers	Consumers	Government	Pressure groups	Health service treaters
Education	✓	✓✓	✓✓✓✓✓	✓✓✓	✓✓✓✓✓	✓✓✓✓✓	✓✓✓✓	✓✓✓✓✓	✓✓✓✓✓
Pricing	✓✓✓✓✓	✓✓	✓✓✓✓✓	✓✓✓✓✓	✓✓✓✓✓✓✓		✓✓✓		
Provision	✓✓✓✓✓	✓✓✓✓✓	✓✓✓✓✓	✓✓✓✓✓	✓✓✓✓✓✓✓				✓✓✓✓✓
Regulations	✓	✓✓✓✓✓✓✓	✓✓✓✓✓	✓✓✓✓✓✓	✓✓✓✓✓		✓✓✓✓✓✓✓✓		

Fig. 17.5. The food health policy matrix—a framework for identifying priorities for promotion of healthier eating. (Sanderson 1984; Stockley 1993.)

- undertake research to establish a sound scientific basis for policy

A principal objective is to implement locally devised food and health policies (WHO 1990):

A concerted set of actions based on scientific principles and intended to ensure the safety and the nutritional quality of the food supply and the accessibility of good, affordable and properly labelled food for all population groups, as well as to encourage and facilitate the healthy use of food. Such policies are more likely to succeed where they reflect a consensus between all the parties concerned with the interest of the population in the foreground, and where there is government involvement and support.

There are a range of possible roles for government to promote health through sponsored nutrition policies and programmes (Chapman 1990):

1. Development and use of cost-efficient mass strategies in nutrition education.

2. Advocacy for regulation of food standards, nutrient labelling and advertising.

3. Formation of intersectoral mechanism between government departments, non-governmental organizations and the private sector to promote nutritional concerns in policy-making, to co-ordinate efforts/avoid duplication, and to co-ordinate desired changes.

4. Subsidies of primary food industries to encourage product development consistent with dietary guidelines.

5. Development of policy and guidelines for dietary practice in government institutions serving food (schools, hospitals, prisons, office canteens, trains):

6. 'Honest brokerage' of information: opposing misinformation.

7. Development of and participation in a national research strategy in nutrition; and

8. Training of health personnel in minimum standards of nutritional knowledge and skill.

Dental caries is a sugars-induced disease. This information must be brought to the attention of governments, industry, consumer groups and individuals. A reduction in sugar consumption to below 60 gram per person per day should be part of national food, nutrition, and agriculture policies. It is desirable to:

- discourage importation and manufacture of sugar and sugar-containing products, particularly confectionery, biscuits, baby foods, and soft drinks
- develop an agriculture policy to discourage growing sugar as a major cash crop
- remove all NME sugars from infant and baby foods, paediatric medicines, fruit juices, and vitamin preparations
- reduce the levels of NME sugars in commonly used foods and make available more sugar-free foods
- reduce the NME sugars content of confections and drinks and make available sugar-free foods, snacks, and drinks

- develop a catering policy in schools, colleges, large industries, institutions; the policy should ensure the provision of foods low in NME sugars
- introduce an education policy stressing that NME sugars are nutritionally poor and decrease the nutrient density of foods
- control advertising and misleading labels on products.

DENTAL CRITERIA FOR SELECTING AN ORAL HEALTH STRATEGY: GOALS FOR ORAL HEALTH

In the preceding sections, the general principles of strategy selection have been outlined: health promotion, healthy public policy, common risk factor approach, whole population and high risk strategies, and intersectoral approach. Here, the stages for developing policies for promoting oral health will be outlined commencing with defining oral health promotion and setting goals.

Oral health promotion can be defined as public health actions to protect or improve oral health and promote oral well-being through behavioural, educational and enabling socio-economic, legal, fiscal, environmental, and social measures. It recognizes the influence of organizations and institutions on many people's daily lives and is concerned with implementing policies which promote health. The Ottawa Declaration calls for a re-orientation of health services with a shift in emphasis from treatment and intervention services to preventive and health promotion. The role of dentists in health promotion is to organize a combination of appropriate complementary strategies including health education and to act as professional resource, raise awareness, and advocate an agenda for change to create supportive and understanding environments and help to 'make the healthy choices the easy choices'.

Clear measurable goals are prerequisites for policy. If you do not know where you want to be, you will not know when you have arrived there or by the best route. Achievable or desirable levels of health provide plausible measures for goal-setting. If a level of health has actually been achieved by some populations or segments of a population at some time or place then it can be achieved elsewhere if the risks are reduced to the levels in the 'best' population. The minimum level of disease in such a population can be considered an achievable goal that all other populations should attain. That has the added virtue of reducing inequalities. This goal indicates the maximum reduction that would follow reduction of each risk factor and the potential of prevention. The goal can be quantified using an index of unnecessary tooth deaths, determined by comparing the age-specific tooth loss in a population or subgroup with the 'best' population with levels in the other groups (Hahn *et al.* 1990).

The goals for oral health can be expressed in terms of health, disease, health education/promotion, and training (Plamping and Sheiham 1987). A oral health goal is to achieve a natural, functional, acceptable dentition dentition which enables an individual to eat, speak, and socialize without discomfort, pain or embarrassment for a lifetime, and which contributes to general well-being. In practical terms, this is the retention throughout life of a functional, aesthetic, natural dentition of not less than 20 teeth and not requiring recourse to a prosthesis (WHO 1982). Goals for acceptable levels of levels of oral health were proposed by a group of chief dental officers from northern European countries (Table 17.3).

The most important goal for periodontal health is for people to improve their oral hygiene so that they achieve levels of plaque which lead to rates of progress of periodontal destruction which is compatible with a rate of periodontal destruction which will retain teeth essential for an socially and personally acceptable dentition for a lifetime; one that does not cause handicaps (Pilot 1981; Sheiham 1991*b*).

POLICY TO IMPROVE PERIODONTAL HEALTH

The difficulties in defining periodontal health, the possibility of erratic nature of bursts of destructive disease, and the poor sensitivity and specificity of methods of predicting destructive disease suggests that screening for periodontal disease is not justified (Sheiham 1978). The prime objective of screening is to detect disease at an earlier stage than would occur with people presenting with the illness, on the assumption that earlier treatment would 'alter the natural history of the disease in a significant proportion' (Cochrane and Holland 1971). At a symposium on markers of disease susceptibility and activity for periodontal diseases Pilot (1989) concluded that '... at present no biotechnology on prognostic indicators is available for use in the practice setting. Therefore, population-screening for periodontal destruction in future life is not yet feasible'.

In addition to the problems in predicting future periodontal breakdown, the accuracy of monitoring changes in alveolar bone height with intra-oral radiographs have numerous shortcomings. Current measurement techniques are insufficiently sensitive to measure bone changes of less than 1.0 mm (Benn 1990) and are useless in diagnosis of early periodontitis. There is a very small minority of people who develop rapidly progressing periodontal disease (Johnson *et al.* 1988). At present, there is insufficient evidence to identify them. Host genotype has been implicated in certain of the more unusual forms of periodontal diseases, but together those account for only a small proportion of periodontal patients (Sofaer 1990). A relationship which has stood the test of time is that

between plaque and periodontal disease (WHO 1978). The new concepts of the progression of periodontal disease do not challenge the relationship between the quantity of plaque and the severity of periodontal diseases. The relationship does exist for groups. Indeed, the 'dose-response' relationship is S-shaped. There is a level of plaque which does not lead to progression of periodontal disease, and this level of gingival inflammation is sometimes referred to as 'contained gingivitis'. Beyond that plaque level of the dose-response relationship is a straight line up to a point where an increase in plaque does not lead to an increase in disease after which the curve flattens (Smales and Sheiham 1979). Burt *et al.* (1985) found that a level of plaque compatible with oral health throughout life was Simplified Oral Hygiene Index (OHI-S) scores of 0.3–0.6. Slightly higher OHI-S (1.3–1.7) might be compatible with acceptably low levels of periodontal disease.

The association of calculus with periodontal disease has led to the erroneous conclusion that calculus is a direct cause of the disease. Although it is assumed that the gingiva are irritated by the physical presence of calculus, the assumption awaits scientific proof (Scheffler and Rovin 1981). Calculus is inert. It does not lead to disease in germ-free animals, and epithelium attaches to it when the surface is free of plaque (Listgarten 1988). Removal of gross or obvious calculus appears to be indicated; however, what is not clear is whether it is worthwhile removing small amounts of calculus. Calculus acts as a retentive factor for plaque. Other local factors such as faulty dental restorations and prosthetic appliances, tobacco smoking, and diet also affect the accumulation of plaque.

The public health implication of the finding that there is a level of plaque which may cause gingival inflammation but not destructive periodontal diseases is that the goal of a plaque-free mouth is unnecessary, besides being unrealistic. The goal should be to achieve a level of plaque compatible with a rate of periodontal disease which will maintain a natural, functional, acceptable dentition for a lifetime. Reduction in the quantity of dental plaque will reduce the severity of gingival inflammation and the probability of destructive periodontal diseases. This change shows that the immunological and specific bacteriological factors are relatively unimportant compared to the quantity of plaque. Calculus does not have a major role in the pathogenesis of

Table 17.3. Suggestions for acceptable levels of dental health by age (WHO 1982)

Age (yrs)	Mean no. of missing teeth	DMF	Periodontal status
12	0	2	0 teeth with pockets > 3 mm
15	0	3	0 teeth with pockets > 3 mm
18	1	4	0 teeth with pockets > 3 mm
35–44	2	12	Fewer than 7 teeth with pockets > 4.5 mm
65–74	10	12	20 functional

Note: In addition, an acceptable level of oral health would include:

- Satisfactory prosthetic replacement of any missing dental unit which obviously detracts from aesthetics.
- Freedom from pain.
- No unacceptable deposits.
- No unacceptable intrinsic anomalies.
- An occlusion which is functionally and cosmetically acceptable.

periodontal diseases. Apart from social reasons, the clinical basis for calculus removal is unjustified (Manji 1988).

In a state of the science review of mechanical oral hygiene practices, Frandsen (1986) came to some important conclusions which have implications for public health aspects of periodontal disease. The conclusions are:

1. There is no scientific evidence that one specific tooth-brush type and design is more superior at removing plaque.

2. The roll technique of tooth-brushing is the least effective of removing plaque; no single method was superior to other methods.

3. Daily use of floss by children with healthy gingiva can be damaging.

4. There is no scientific justification for recommending forced irrigation devices.

5. Well-motivated and instructed people can clean their mouths adequately with most of the available oral hygiene aids and techniques.

6. The efficiency of personal, mechanical oral hygiene practices is more likely to be enhanced through an understanding of factors determining performance rather than by attempts to improve aids and techniques.

7. The optimal frequency and starting age for scaling and polishing has not been determined. The 6-month interval is unsubstantiated and is too general a recommendation.

8. Regular instrumentation and polishing should not be carried out at disease-free sites.

9. The role of root planing in preventing reinfection of the subgingival area is questionable.

10. Scaling, polishing, root planning, and surgical treatment of shallow periodontal pockets results in permanent loss of attachment.

Strategies for Controlling Periodontal Diseases

The changes mentioned have considerable implications for the future practice of dentistry in general and for community approaches to periodontal diseases in particular. The most important implication is the reassessment of periodontal diseases as a public health problem in general and a dental public health problem in particular. Although severe periodontal disease is not widespread, the fact that the costs of treating the disease are high because of the organization of dental care, does qualify it as a dental public problem. In addition, the symptoms of periodontal diseases, such as bleeding, halitosis, gingival recession, and tooth loss, have an impact on many people. Furthermore, we have sufficient information to control the common forms of the disease (Pilot 1984).

Four strategies can be considered: (1) a high risk, (2) a population, (3) a secondary prevention strategy, or (4) a combination of the three. The high risk strategy aims to truncate

the curve; bring those with unacceptably high plaque scores to below 'compatible' levels. Who are the people with the high plaque scores which will lead to rates of disease incompatible with keeping teeth for life? By and large, they are predominantly manual male workers who smoke. Their tooth-cleaning habits are not easy to change. There are high risk groups, such as those with rapidly progressing periodontal diseases, who may require antibiotic therapy. Effective periodontal care for the high risk groups is difficult to achieve and maintain and costly in time and resources. A population strategy aims to reduce the plaque level of the whole population; moving the distribution curve to the left. Such a strategy saves more teeth than a high risk one because although high risk people lose more teeth per person there are more low than high risk people. A whole population strategy, by lowering the overall plaque score, reduces the number of high risk people. A secondary prevention strategy aims to treat all persons with signs of early periodontal diseases such as gingivitis and shallow periodontal pockets. Current concepts of periodontal diseases and their treatment referred to earlier, cast serious doubts on the justification for such a strategy.

The population strategy is most likely to benefit the periodontal health of the majority of people because a small reduction overall of plaque per year will reduce the general level of periodontal disease. This should lead to the extraction of fewer teeth than if the bulk of resources is concentrated on a small number of high risk people or on treating all those with early signs of periodontal diseases.

In summary, the plan for controlling periodontal disease can include:

1. A population strategy for altering behaviour and in particular oral cleaning effectiveness to reduce the dental plaque level of the community.

2. A secondary prevention strategy of detect and treat people with destructive periodontal disease.

3. A high risk strategy for bringing preventive and therapeutic care to individuals at special risk.

4. A combined population, secondary prevention, and high risk strategy.

BUILDING HEALTHY PUBLIC POLICY

Guiding Principles

Drawing on the Ottawa Charter framework, five key strategies are identified which can be built into a model for improving oral health promotion (Dickson 1993). Governments are mainly responsible for the health of populations through conditions they permit or create. Oral health promotion policies that are the profession's and community's to recommend and the government's to legislate include:

1. A food and health policy which controls the production of non-milk extrinsic added sugars foods (Sheiham and Plamping 1988) and supports the growth and distribution of traditional foods.

2. Policy on fluoride toothpaste and water or salt fluoridation.
3. A community approach to improve body and mouth hygiene.
4. A policy to reduce cigarette smoking.
5. Policy on accident prevention to reduce trauma to teeth and jaws.
6. A national dental policy, encouraging dental workers to spend time working in such outreach programmes as school, maternal, and child health.
7. Appropriate dental care carried out in dental surgeries which will not foster the spread of hepatitis and AIDS.

CREATING SUPPORTIVE ENVIRONMENTS

The aim is to contribute to the improvement of environments which support health. Areas of attention for oral health workers to act upon include:

1. A diet and health policy to reduce non-milk extrinsic (refined) sugars consumption to below 10 per cent of total calories. The policy will include: nutritional guidelines on content of school meals (Sharp 1993). Consultation with major supermarkets to provide a wider range of low- and no-sugar confectionery, drinks, biscuits, cereals, and to introduce clear shelf- as well as product-labelling of sugars content of all sugars containing products. This work to be done in conjunction with the Coronary Prevention Group, the Maternity Alliance, the Health Visitors Association, the Community Dietitian Group of the British Dietitians Association, the National Consumer Council, and the Womens Institute.
2. Encouraging shops that are near schools to stock promote, and display sugars-free foods.
3. Periodically sampling sources of drinking water and requesting that they be analysed for contaminants and natural occurring fluoride;
4. Fostering supportive attitudes towards breast-feeding;
5. Participating in community programmes which are aimed at improving the lives of women, young children, and adolescents.
6. Monitoring all commercially sponsored materials in schools with the schools liaison teachers and district dietitians.
7. Providing minimal information necessary to act to prevent oral diseases (such as on a healthy diet, fluoride, plaque, dental care), and the skills needed to maintain their own oral health and where to obtain adequate support in maintaining health.
8. Examine misinformation emanating from vested commercial interests, e.g. decoding advertisements.
9. Establish a oral health promotion group (OHPG) to develop an action plan using the goals and strategies as their guidelines (Cohen 1990).

Strengthening community action

More people should be involved in situational analyses, programme planning, and action. Dental works can:

(1) join with community workers in networks and coalitions and work together on community issues of common concern; and

(2) organize a dental planning committee, fill half of the positions with lay members, and allow the committee to make meaningful dental decisions.

Developing coping skills

The intention is to increase people's abilities for controlling oral disease and for improving oral health (Dickson 1993); strengthening of self-confidence such that people feel they have control over the available options and, therefore, over their own oral health. To that end, dental workers can help people to:

(1) differentiate between lay beliefs and practices that are good and worth keeping and those that are harmful and need to be changed;

(2) be role models to family members and neighbours in terms of food that is eaten, and practices of oral hygiene;

(3) examine at home the mouths of younger children, recognize developing problems, and know where and when to get help;

(4) choose toothpastes that contain fluoride.

Reorientating dental services

The desire is twofold (Dickson 1993): to nurture a more holistic practice of dentistry and oral health promotion, recognising the importance of people's emotional, cultural, and social well-being; and to challenge the professional status quo such that strategies of care include restructuring established delivery systems (Hobdell and Sheiham 1981; Sheiham and Plamping 1988).

Change is possible when dental decision-makers accept the principles of primary health care and prepare dental workers, through training and support in the field, to (Dickson 1993):

- Make their services more accessible and acceptable to groups that are disadvantaged.
- Solicit public opinion about their work in order to be accountable to the people they serve.
- Focus on prevention instead of only cure, promote practices of self-care, and prepare others to become informal teachers for oral health;
- Function in association with other community health and development workers and their programmes.

CONCLUSIONS

- The main reasons for the dramatic decline in dental caries in industrialized countries are related more to health promotion than to dental services (Nadanovsky 1993).

- All preventive measures require economic, social, and political strategies to ensure their acceptance, implementation, and effectiveness. The acceptance of water fluoridation, fluoride rinsing, and sealants have all involved public health strategies.

- A public oral health strategy directed at reducing the consumption of sugars and promoting water fluoridation and fluoridated toothpaste will reduce the prevalence of dental caries to a level where it will be an insignificant problem.

- The policies and community health promotion presented here have been widely accepted by international, national, and local groups as well as public and community health practitioners.

- By adopting a health promotion, common risk/health factor approach and integrating oral health with general health policies, policies to promote oral health should become more effective and efficient. What is more, oral health will cease to be marginalized.

- Dentists must become team members in advocacy and education with other organizations, government sectors, and with community organizations.

REFERENCES

Beachamp, T.L. and Chidress, J.F. (1989). *Principles of biomedical ethics*, (3rd edn). Oxford University Press.

Benn, D.K. (1990). A review of the reliability of radiographic measurements in estimating alveolar bone changes. *J. Clin. Perio.*, **17**, 14–21.

Blane, D. (1985). An assessment of the Black Report's 'explanations of health inequalities'. *Soc. Hlth Ill*, **7**, 423–45.

Burr, M. L. and Elwood, P. C. (1985). Research and development of health promotion services—screening. In *Oxford textbook of public health*, Vol III, (ed. W.W. Holland, R. Detels, and G. Knox), pp. 373–84. Oxford University Press.

Burt, B.A. Ismail, A.I., and Eklund, S.A. (1985). Periodontal disease, tooth loss and oral hygiene among older Americans. *Communi. Dent. oral Epidemiol.* **13**, 93–6.

Castle, P. (1987). *The politics of fluoridation*. John Libbey, London.

Chapman, S. (1990). Intersectoral action to improve nutrition: the roles of the state and private sector. A case study from Australia. *Hlth Prom. Int.*, **5**, 35–44.

Cochrane A.L. and Holland, W.W. (1971). Validation of screening procedure. *Br. med. Bull.* **27**, 3–8.

Cohen, L.K. (1990). Promoting oral health: guidelines for dental associations. *Int. dent. J.*, **40**, 79–102.

Cowell, C.R. and Sheiham, A. (1981). *Promoting dental health*. King Edward's Hospital Fund for London.

Croucher, R. (1993). General dental practice, health education, and health promotion: a critical approach. In *Oral health promotion*, (ed. L. Schou and A.S. Blinkhorn), pp. 153–68. Oxford University Press.

Culyer, A.J. (1993). *Equity and health care policy*. A discussion paper. Research and Policy Group, Premier's Council on Health, Well-being and Social Justice, Ontario (Mimeo).

Cushing, A.M., Sheiham, A. and Maizels, J. (1986). Developing socio-dental indicators—the social impact of dental disease. *Commun. dent Health*, **3**, 3–17.

Dahlgren, G. and Diderichsen, F. (1986). Strategies for equity in health: Report from Sweden. *Int. J. Hlth Serv.* **4**, 1–21.

Dickson, M. (1993). Oral health promotion in developing countries. In *Oral health promotion*, (ed. L. Schou and A.S. Blinkhorn), pp. 233–47. Oxford University Press.

DoH (Department of Health) (1989). *Dietary sugars and human disease*. Report of the Panel on Dietary Sugars of the Committee on Medical Aspects of Food Policy. Report No. 37, HMSO, London.

DoH (Department of Health) (1991a). *Dietary reference values for food energy and nutrients for the United Kingdom*. Report of the Panel on Dietary Reference Values of the Committee on Medical Aspects of Food Policy. Report No. 41, HMSO, London.

DoH (Department of Health) (1991b). *The health of the nation: a consultative document for health in England*. HMSO, London.

Dowell, T.B. (1988). *Dental care for children in South West Avon*. Report to Regional Dental Committee, South Western Health Authority, 24 May 1988, Bristol.

Downer, M.C. (1978). Caries prediction from epidemiologic data. In *Methods of caries prediction*, (ed. B.G. Bibby and R.J. Shern), pp. 37–42. Information Retrieval Inc, Washington, DC.

Dror, Y. (1974). *Public policymaking reexamined*. Leonard Hill, Bedfordshire.

Foch, C.B. (1981). *The costs, effects, and benefits of preventive dental care: a literature review*. Report N-1732-RWJF. Rand Corporation, Santa Monica.

Frandsen, A. (1986). Mechanical oral hygiene practises. In *Dental plaque control measures and oral hygiene practices*, (ed. H. Loe and D.V. Kleinman), pp. 93–116. IRL Press, Oxford.

Grabauskas, V.J. (1987). Integrated programme for community health in noncommunicable disease (Interhealth). In *The prevention of non-communicable diseases: experiences and prospects*, (ed. E. Leparski), pp. 285–310. World Health Organization Regional Office for Europe, Copenhagen.

Graham, H. (1990). Behaving well: Women's health behaviour in context. In *Women's health counts*, (ed. H. Roberts). London, Routledge.

Green, L.W. and Kreuter, M. (1990). Health promotion as a public health strategy for the 1990s. *Ann. Rev. Publ. Health*, **11**, 319–34.

Hackett, A.F., Rugg-Gunn, A.J., Appleton, D.R., Allinson, M., and Eastoe, J.E. (1984). Sugar eating habits of 405 11- to 14-year-old English Children. *Br. J. Nutr.*, **51**, 347–356.

Hahn, R.A., Teutsch, S.M., Rothenberg, R.B., and Marks, J.S. (1990). Excess deaths from nine chronic diseases in the United States, 1986. *J. Am. med. Ass.*, **264**, 2654–9.

Helsing, E. (1987). Healthier nutrition in Europe—what can be done? In *The prevention of non-communicable diseases: experiences and prospects*, (ed. E. Leparski), pp. 43–69. World Health Organization Regional Office for Europe, Copenhagen.

Hobdell, M.H. and Sheiham, A. (1981). Barriers to the promotion of dental health in developing countries. *Soc. Sci. Med.*, **15A**, 817–23.

Johnson, N.W., *et al.* (1988). Detection of high risk groups and individuals for periodontal diseases: Evidence for the existence of high risk groups and approaches to their detection. *J. Clin. Perio.* **15**, 276–82.

Kalsbeek, H. (1982). Evidence of decrease in prevalence of dental caries in the Netherlands: an evaluation of epidemiological caries surveys on 4–6 and 11–15-year-old children, performed between 1965 and 1980. *J. dent. Res.* **61** (Special issue), 1321–6.

Klein, S.P., Bohannan, H.M., Bell, R.M., Disney, J.A., Foch, C.B., and Graves, R.C. (1985). *The cost and effectiveness of school-based preventive dental care.* Rand Corporation, Santa Monica.

Klock, B. (1980). Economic aspects of a caries preventive program. *Commun. Dent. oral Epidemiol.* **8**, 97–102.

Labonte R. (1989). Community health promotion. In *Readings for a new public health,* (ed. C.L. Martin and D.V. McQueen), pp. 235–49. Edinburg University Press.

Lalonde, M. (1974). *A new perspective in the health of Canadians.* Government Printing Office, Ottawa.

Lindblom, C.E. (1965). *The intelligence of democracy: Decision-making through mutual adjustment.* Free Press of Glencoe, New York.

Listgarten, M.A. (1988): Why do epidemiological data have no diagnostic value? In *Perodontology today,* (ed. B. Guggenheim), pp. 59–67. Karger, Basel.

Locker, D. (1988). Measuring oral health—A conceptual framework. *Commun. dent. Health,* **5**, 3–18.

Locker, D. (1988). *An introduction to behavioural science and dentistry,* pp. 73–87. Routledge, London.

Manji, F. (1988). Epidemiology of periodontal diseases—summary of session. In *Periodontology today,* (ed. B. Guggenheim). Karger, Basel.

MAFF (Ministry of Agriculture Fisheries and Food) (1992). *United Kingdom Country Paper.* International Conference on Nutrition, Rome December 1992. Ministry of Agriculture Fisheries and Food, London, (mimeo).

McDonald, S.P. and Sheiham, A. (1992). The distribution of caries on different tooth surfaces at varying levels of caries—a compilation of data from 18 previous studies. *Commun. dent. Health,* **9**, 39–48.

McKeown, T. (1979). *The role of medicine.* Basil Blackwell, Oxford.

McKinlay, J.B. (1974). A case for refoccussing upstream—the political economy of illness. In *Proceedings of the American Heart Association,* pp. 7–17. Conference on applying behavioral sciences to cardiovascular risk. Seattle.

Milio, N. (1986). *Promoting health through public policy.* Canadian Public Health Association, Ottawa.

Milio, N. (1987). *Healthy public policy: issues and scenarios.* Symposium on Health Public Policy, Yale University.

Milio, N. (1988). Making healthy public policy. *Hlth Prom.* **2**, 263–74.

Nadanovsky, P. (1993). The relative contribution of dental services to changes in dental caries status of children in some industrialized countries since the 1970s. Ph.D. thesis. University of London.

National Advisory Committee on Nutrition Education (NACNE) (1983). *Proposals for nutritional guidelines for health education in Britain.* The Health Education Council, London.

Newbrun, E. (1982). Sugar and dental caries: a review of human studies. *Science* **217**, 418–23.

Newbrun, E. (1983). *Cariology,* (2nd edn), p. 102. Williams & Wilkins, London.

Oral Health Coordinating Committee of the USA Public Health Service (OHCC) (1993). Toward improving the oral health of Americans: an overview of oral health status, resources, and care delivery. *Publ. Hlth. Rep.,* **108**, 657–72.

Ottawa Charter for Health Promotion (1986). Department of Health and Welfare, Ottawa.

Plamping, D. and Sheiham, A. (1987). *Strategies for improving oral health in Britain.* Department of Community Dental Health, University College London.

Payne, P. and Thomson, A. (1979). Food health: individual choice and collective responsibility. *J. Roy. Soc. Health,* **5**, 185–9.

Pilot, T. (1981). Analysis of the overall effectiveness of treatment of periodontal disease. In *Efficacy of treatment procedures in periodontics,* (ed. D. Shanley), pp. 213–30. Quintessence, Chicago.

Pilot, T. (1984). Implementation of preventive periodontal programmes at a community level. In *Public health aspects of periodontal disease,* (ed. A. Frandsen), pp. 181–96. Quintessence, Chicago.

Pilot, T. (1989). Implications for health screening and public health planning. In *Markers of disease susceptibility and activity for periodontal diseases,* (ed. N.W. Johnson). Cambridge University Press.

Rose, G. (1992). *The strategy of preventive medicine.* Oxford University Press.

Rugg-Gunn A J. (1993). *Nutrition and dental health,* pp. 177–179. Oxford University Press.

Rugg-Gunn, A.J., Hackett, A.F., Appleton, D.R., Jenkins, G.N., and Estoe, J.E. (1984). Relationship between dietary habits and caries increment assessed over two years in 405 English school children. *Arch. oral Biol.* **29**, 983–92.

Rugg-Gunn J.A., Carmichael C.L. and Ferrell R.S., (1988). Effect of fluoridation and secular trend in caries in 5-year-old children living in Newcastle and Northumberland. *Br. dent. J.* **165**, 359–64.

Sanderson, M.E. (1984). Strategies for implementing NACNE recommendations. *Lancet,* **ii**, 1352–6.

Sharp, I. (1993). *Nutrition guidelines for schools.* The Caroline Walker Trust, London.

Scheffler, R.M. and Rovin, S. (1981). Periodontal disease: assessing the effectiveness and costs of the Keyes technique. In *The implications of cost-effectiveness analysis of medial technology.* Case Study No. 5, pp. 3–33. Office of Technology Assessment, Congress of the United States, Washington, DC.

Sheiham, A. (1978). Screening for periodontal disease. *J. clin. Perio.,* **5**, 237–45.

Sheiham, A. (1983). Sugars and dental decay. *Lancet,* **i**, 282–4.

Sheiham, A. (1991*a*). Why sugar consumption should be below 15 kg per person per year in industrialized countries; the dental evidence. *Br. dent. J.,* **171**, 63–5.

Sheiham, A. (1991*b*). Public health aspects of periodontal diseases in Europe. *J. clin. Perio.* **18**, 362–9.

Sheiham, A. and Joffe, M. (1991). Public dental health strategies for identifying and controlling dental caries in high and low risk populations. In *Risk markers for oral diseases. Vol. 1, Dental caries: markers of high and low risk groups and individuals,* (ed. N.W. Johnson), pp. 445–8. Cambridge University Press.

Sheiham, A. and Plamping, D. (1988). Strategies for improving oral health and reforming oral health care systems. *Afric. Dent. J.* **2**, 2–7.

Smales, F.C. and Sheiham, A. (1979). Some results from a computer model for predicting the long term effects of periodontal therapy upon tooth loss in large populations. *J. perio. Res.,* **14**, 248–9.

Sofaer, J.A. (1990). Genetic approaches in the study of periodontal diseases. *J. clin. Perio.,* **17**, 401–8.

Sreebny, L.M. (1982). Sugar availability, sugar consumption and dental caries. *Commun. Dent. oral Epidemiol.,* **10**, 1–7.

Stockley, L. (1993). *The promotion of healthier eating. A basis for action.* Health Education Authority, London.

Takeuchi, M. (1960). Epidemiological study of the relationship between dental caries incidence and sugar consumption. *Bull. Tokyo dent. Coll.*, **1**, 58–70.

Weaver, R. (1950). Fluorine and wartime diet. *Br. dent. J.*, **88**, 231–9.

WHO (World Health Organization) (1978). *Alma-Ata 1978: Primary health care.* Report of the Internaitonal Conference on Primary Health Care, Alma-Ata, USSR, September 1978. WHO, Geneva.

WHO (World Health Organization) (1978). *Primary health care, Alma Ata 1978,* Health for All Series, No. 1. WHO, Geneva.

WHO (World Health Organization) (1981). *Global strategy for health for all by the year 2000.* WHO, Health for All Series, No. 3. WHO, Geneva.

WHO (World Health Organization) (1982). *A review of current recommendations for the organization and administration of community oral health services in Northern and Western Europe.* Report of a WHO Workshop. WHO regional Office for Europe, Copenhagen.

WHO (World Health Organization) (1984). *Health promotion. A discussion document on the concept and principles* WHO Regional Office for Europe, Copenhagen.

WHO (World Health Organization) (1986). *The Ottawa Charter for Health Promotion. Hlth Prom.* **1**, iii–v. WHO, Geneva.

WHO (World Health Organization) (1988). *The Adelaide recommendations, healthy public policy,* WHO Regional Office for Europe, Copenhagen.

WHO (World Health Organization) (1989). *Ethics and health promotion. A report from the Health Promotion programme.* WHO Regional Office for Europe, Copenhagen.

WHO (World Health Organization) (1990). *Food and nutrition policy for Europe.* Report of a WHO Conference, Budapest 1990, p. 12. EUR/ICP/NUT 133. WHO Regional Office for Europe, Copenhagen.

WHO (World Health Organization) (1991). *Diet, nutrition, and the prevention of chronic diseases. Technical Report Series 797.* WHO, Geneva.

Whitehead, M. (1991). The concepts and principles of equity and health. *Hlth Prom.*, **6**, 217–28.

18.   The changing pattern of dental disease

J.J. MURRAY

INTRODUCTION

Dental disease very rarely causes death and is widely accepted by the public at large as something they all get and have to live with. However, dental disease is not static and the dental health of the population depends on the amount of disease, on the attitude of the patient, and on the type of treatment offered by the dental profession. Important changes have been noted in the caries experience of children, particularly over the last 10 or 15 years in many developed countries, and this reduction in disease should eventually result in a changing type of dental treatment in adulthood.

THE CHANGING PATTERN OF CARIES EXPERIENCE IN CHILDREN

Jackson (1974) summarized the results of over 70 published and unpublished surveys of caries experience in English children and young adults during the period from 1947 to 1972. With regard to 5-year-old children (Table 18.1), he concluded that there had been little change in the mean dmf between 1947 and 1960 and 1960 and 1972. In the permanent dentition an apparent *increase* in mean DMF values for 12-year-old children was reported according to the Ministry of Education quinquennial surveys (HMSO 1958–68; Table 18.2) between 1948 and 1968, and this trend was supported by results from other studies (Jackson 1974). However the available evidence with regard to 15-year-old English schoolchildren between 1950 and 1977 (Table 18.3) suggested that little or no *increase* in caries had occurred. In contrast, one year later, an opposing view, that the dental health of children was improving, was cautiously put forward by Palmer (1980), who suggested that the dental health of children in Somerset had improved in recent years. His view was based on personal observations and the comments of practitioners in both the general and community dental service. Data for both 5- and 14-year-old children showed a downward trend between 1975 and 1979 (Table 18.4).

The weakness in the type of analysis put forward by Jackson (1974) is that the studies are not strictly comparable, having been carried out by different investigators, all with different standards of diagnosis. Palmer recognized the problem, even from his own area, because he acknowledged that his records did not satisfy strict epidemiological requirements in that the methods were not calibrated nor standardized. Nevertheless, his samples were large and included virtually all children attending state-maintained

schools in Somerset, in particular age bands. Shortly afterwards there followed a steady stream of papers, by research workers using strict epidemiological techniques, confirming Palmer's assertion that caries experience in English children was declining (Table 18.5). Similar findings were reported in pre-school children (Table 18.6).

The theme of a decline in dental caries took on an international flavour when the first international conference devoted to this topic was held in Boston in June 1982. Speakers from Denmark, Eire, the Netherlands, New Zealand, Norway, Scotland, Sweden, and the United States all confirmed that a downward trend in dental caries in children and young adults had occurred in the 1970s (Glass 1982; Table 18.7).

Data from various surveys in the Netherlands was given in the form of a diagram for 6- and 12-year-old children (Figs 18.1 and 18.2); Kalsbeek 1982. These data suggested a gradual decline in caries in the 1970s. A report from Australia (Burton *et al.* 1984) suggested that caries experience of 12-year-old children had declined by 84 per cent from 1963 to 1982 (Table 18.8)

This downward trend was confirmed by a Working Group of the FDI (1985) and WHO who had access to figures from the WHO Global Oral Data Bank (Fig. 18.3). They concluded that the most probable reasons for the decrease in dental caries in children in the developed countries were considered to be associated with:

(1) the widespread exposure to fluoridated water and/or fluoride supplements, especially the regular use of fluoride toothpaste;

(2) the provision of preventive oral health services;

(3) the increased 'dental awareness' through organized oral health education programmes;

(4) the ready availability of dental resources.

The factor common to all countries with a substantial reduction in caries was fluoride, either as fluoridated water or toothpaste.

NATIONAL DENTAL HEALTH SURVEYS OF CHILD DENTAL HEALTH IN ENGLAND AND WALES 1973–83

The first national survey of children's dental health in England and Wales was carried out in 1973. The Office of Population Censuses and Surveys was responsible for drawing

Table 18.1. Caries experience of 5-year-old English children: 1947–72 (references in Jackson 1974)

Year of survey	Author	Area	No. of children	Mean dmf
1947	Miller (1950)	Manchester	128	4.80
1947	Mellanby and Mellanby (1948)	London	1590	4.06
1948	HSC (1958–59)[1]	7 areas, England	15 158	4.29
1948	Miller (1950)	Manchester	42	6.07
1949	Miller (1950)	Manchester	109	5.39
1949	Weaver (1950)	North Shields	500	4.45
1949	Mellanby and Mellanby (1950)	London	692	5.34
1950	Miller (1950)	Manchester	74	5.50
1950	Jackson (1952)	Accrington	142	4.16
1960	Sanderson (1960)	West Riding	521	4.60
1961	Sanderson (1961)	West Riding	534	4.19
1962	Bulman *et al.* (1968)	Darlington	66	4.80
1962	Bulman *et al.* (1968)	Salisbury	101	4.90
1962	Dodd (1965)	Cheshire	300	5.74
1963	HSC (1962–63)	7 regions, England	16 390	5.10
1964	Smyth *et al.* (1964)	Gloucestershire	90	2.98
1966	Millward (1967)	Maidstone	45	4.29
1967	Murray (1969a)	York	527	4.09
1967	Beal and James (1970)	Balsall Heath	257	5.24
1967	UKF Studies (1969)	Sutton	119	2.80
1967	Beal and James (1971)	Dudley	329	5.24
1967	Beal and James (1970)	Sutton Coldfield	304	3.27
1967	Beal and James (1971)	Northfield	335	5.02
1968	BES (1972)	Leicestershire	1757	4.07
1968	BES (1972)	Lincolnshire	409	4.06
1968	Beal and James (1971)	Dudley	274	4.80
1968	HSC (1966–68)	7 regions, England	15 781	4.50
1969	Clayton (1969)	West Riding	403	5.10
1969	Timmis (1971)	Essex	959	4.19
1969	BES (1972)[2]	Scunthorpe	196	4.28
1969	BES (1972)	Corby	205	4.28
1969	Beal and James (1971)	Dudley	255	5.04
1969	Hesterman (1969)	Shropshire	542	5.09
1969	Bride (1969)	Manchester	390	3.89
1970	Beal and James (1971)	Dudley	229	5.09
1970	BES (1972)	Devon	1150	4.70
1970	Teasdale (1972)	Huddersfield	224	4.17
1970	Awath-Behari (1970)	Wolverhampton	100	4.47
1970	Whitehouse (1970)	Nottinghamshire	193	3.82
1970	Gordon (1973)	6 areas, England	1909	4.26
1972	Lowery (1972)	West Riding	257	4.58
		Total	63 586	4.59

[1] HSC = Health of the School Child.

[2] BES = Birmingham Epidemiological Studies.

up a stratified random sample of over 12 000 children, aged 5–15 years, attending over 500 schools in the two countries. Dental examinations were undertaken at the schools by 70 dentists who had been specially trained and calibrated for the study. In addition, parents of children aged 5, 8, 12, and 14 years were visited in their homes by Social Survey Interviewers, to obtain information on social class, patterns of dental attendance, and other issues.

The second national survey was held 10 years later, in 1983; this time Scotland and Northern Ireland were included, and the sample size was increased to over 20 000 to enable data from the four countries in the United Kingdom to be presented separately. Seventy-six dentists, many of whom had been involved in the previous survey, carried out the examinations at school, after participating in a training and calibration exercise. In order to reduce costs, information from parents was obtained mainly from a postal questionnaire. In both surveys the level of co-operation was very high—between 88 and 95 per cent of selected children were examined successfully. For the purposes of this review the state of children's dental health for England and Wales between 1973 and 1983 will be compared.

Table 18.2. Caries experience of 12-year-old children (*Source: Health of the school child. Quinquennial Surveys.* HMSO 1954–68)]

Area	1948	1953	1958	1963	1968
Manchester	3.7	3.5	4.1	4.4	4.5
Middlesex	–	4.6	5.1	5.8	5.4
Northumberland	2.5	3.6	5.6	5.6	5.3
Nottinghamshire	4.2	3.0	3.8	4.1	4.9
Somerset	2.7	4.3	5.6	5.4	5.0
West Riding	2.9	4.2	6.1	6.1	6.3
West Sussex	2.7	3.2	–	–	–
East Sussex	–	–	4.5	5.3	5.1
All areas	2.9	3.8	5.5	5.3	5.5

Table 18.4. Somerset Area Health Authority statistics (Palmer 1980)

Year	5-year-olds		14-year-olds	
	No. of children	Mean def	No. of children	Mean DMF
1975	3022	2.6	2294	7.2
1976	3369	2.5	2259	6.4
1977	3426	2.1	3402	6.3
1978	3279	1.8	2612	5.8
1979	3528	1.7	3149	5.3

Table 18.3. Caries experience in 15-year-old English children; 1950–77. (Jackson 1974)

Year of survey	Author	Area	No. of children	Mean DMF
1950	Jackson (1952)	Accrington	148	7.9
1957–59	Starkey (1966)	Naval recruits	4795	10.8
1958–59	Jackson (1961)	Leeds	94	9.5
1963–65	Starkey (1966)	Naval recruits	5156	11.2
1964	Bulman *et al.* (1968)	Salisbury	22	9.8
1964	Bulman *et al.* (1968)	Darlington	58	8.5
1956	HSC (1969–71)*	England	14 025	9.8
1967	Murray (1969)	York	381	8.9
1968	Bristow (1975)	Portsmouth	437	9.5
1973	Todd (1975)	England	576	8.0
1974	Papyanni (1974)	Halifax	300	8.0
1977	Crossland (1977)	Bury	309	9.6
1977	Jackson (1978)	Yorkshire	2827	9.7
1977	Fairpo (1978)	Harrogate	208	7.5
1977	Williams (1978)	York	174	9.1

*HSC = Health of the School Child.

Table 18.5. Changes in caries experience in England

Author	Date	Age of children (yrs)	Place	Year of examination	Mean DMF
Anderson	1981a	12	Somerset	1963	5.4
		12	Somerset	1978	3.4
Anderson	1981b	12	Shropshire	1970	4.5
		12	Shropshire	1980	3.1
Anderson	1981c	12	Gloucestershire	1964	4.5
		12	Gloucestershire	1979	4.2
Andlaw *et al.*	1982	11	Bristol	1970	4.6
		11	Bristol	1979	2.9
		14	Bristol	1973	9.5
		14	Bristol	1979	6.7

Table 18.6. Changes in caries experience of pre-school children

Author	Date	Age of children (yrs)	Place	Year of examination	Mean def
Winter *et al.*	1971	3	London	1967	1.4
Holt *et al.*	1982	3	London	1981	0.7
Silver	1982	3	Hertfordshire	1973	1.5
Silver	1982	3	Hertfordshire	1981	0.6

Table 18.7.   Declining dental caries in various (references in Glass 1982)

Author	Country	Age of subjects (yrs)	Year of examination	Mean DMFT
Fejerskov *et al.*	Denmark	20	1972	16.6
Fejerskov *et al.*	Denmark	20	1982	11.8
O'Mullane	Eire	8–9	1961	2.8
O'Mullane	Eire	8–9	1979	1.3
O'Mullane	Eire	13–14	1961	8.0
O'Mullane	Eire	13–14	1979	4.4
Brown	New Zealand	12–13	1950	7.9
Brown	New Zealand	12–13	1982	4.1
Von der Fehr	Norway	15	1970	32.0*
Von der Fehr	Norway	15	1979	15.0*
Downer	Scotland	10	1970	5.0
Downer	Scotland	10	1980	3.6
Carlos	USA	6–11	1971–74	1.7
Carlos	USA	6–11	1979–80	1.1
Carlos	USA	12–17	1971–74	6.2
Carlos	USA	12–17	1979–80	4.6

* DMFS values.

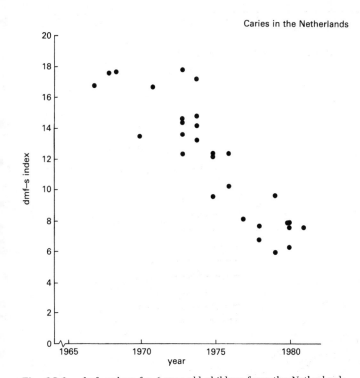

Fig. 18.1.   dmfs values for 6-year-old children from the Netherlands. (Kalsbeek 1982.)

Table 18.8.   Changes in caries experiences of 12-year-old Sydney children (Burton *et al.* 1984)

1963		1982	
No. of children	Mean DMFT	No. of children	Mean DMFT
426	8.5	736	1.4

Table 18.9.   Caries experience in 5-year-old children in England and Wales: 1973–83

	1973	1983
Per cent caries-free	28.0	51.0
Mean dmft	4.0	1.8

the number of untreated carious deciduous teeth over the 10-year period.

(i) Dental caries in deciduous teeth

Dramatic reductions in caries in 5-year-old children were observed (Table 18.9) over the 10-year period. The proportion of children with untreated decay in deciduous teeth was much less in 1983 compared with 1973 (Fig. 18.4), and more importance was being placed on the preservation of deciduous teeth through restorative treatment among the older children than was the case in 1973 (Fig. 18.5). There was therefore a considerable reduction in

(ii) Dental caries in permanent teeth

A similar general trend was observed in the permanent dentition. The proportion of children with decay was lower for every age group. In 1973, 50 per cent of 7-year-olds had some decay in their permanent teeth, but in 1983 this point was not reached until children were 9 years of age (Fig. 18.6). The mean DMFT had fallen from 8.4 to 5.6 for 15-year-old children, a reduction of approximately 33 per cent (Fig. 18.7).

The DMFT values for England and Wales in 1983 are compared with those reported in the survey of United States children in 1979–80 in Fig. 18.8 (Miller *et al.* 1981).

(iii) Periodontal disease in children

In contrast to the good news on dental caries, there was virtually no change in gum inflammation and calculus

Caries in the Netherlands

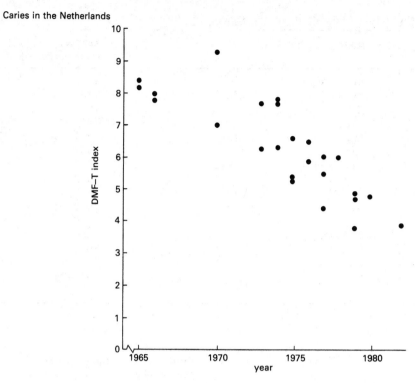

Fig. 18.2. DMFT values for 12-year-old children from the Netherlands. (Kalsbeek 1982.)

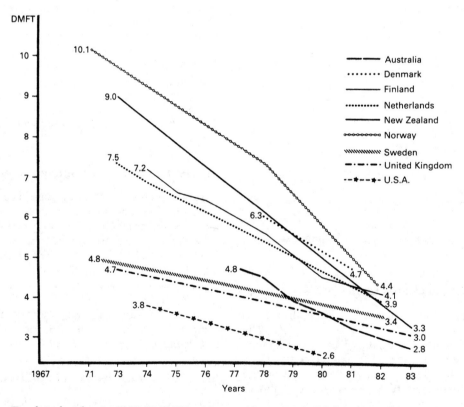

Fig. 18.3. Trends in dental caries 1967–83 DMFT as 12 years. (*Source*: WHO Global Oral Data Bank; Renson *et al.* 1986.)

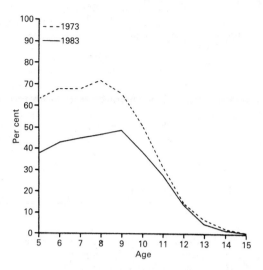

Fig. 18.4. The proportion of children with some decayed deciduous teeth in England and Wales in 1973 and 1983 (Todd 1985). (Reproduced by kind permission of Miss Todd and OPCS.)

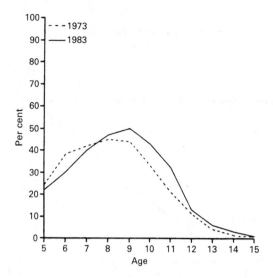

Fig. 18.5. The proportion of children with some filled deciduous teeth in England and Wales in 1973 and 1983 (Todd 1985). (Reproduced by kind permission of Miss Todd and OPCS.)

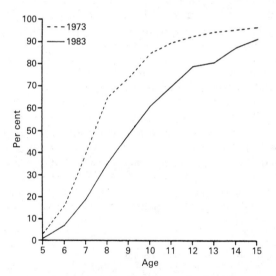

Fig. 18.6. The proportion of children with known decay experience of permanent teeth in England and Wales in 1973 and 1983 (Todd 1985). (Reproduced by kind permission of Miss Todd and OPCS.)

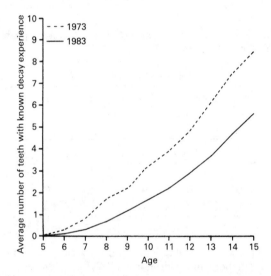

Fig. 18.7. The average number of permanent teeth with known decay experience (DMFT) in England and Wales in 1973 and 1983 (Todd 1985). (Reproduced by kind permission of Miss Todd and OPCS.)

between 1973 and 1983 (Table 18.10). There was a slight trend towards less debris in 1983, although this still meant that half the children from the age of 7 years had debris present on the day of the examination.

Table 18.10. Proportions of children with gum inflammation, calculus, and debris in England and Wales: 1973–83

Age (yrs)	Gum inflammation		Calculus		Debris	
	1973	1983	1973	1983	1973	1983
5	26	18	5	3	39	29
8	56	47	15	13	67	55
12	57	50	28	21	64	49
15	51	49	34	33	51	47

(iv) Orthodontic condition of children

The orthodontic assessment in 1983 was not identical to that carried out 10 years earlier, but incisor problems, crowding and orthodontic treatment and need could be compared. Very little change in 'incisor problems' was observed (Table 18.11). In contrast the prevalence of crowding had increased substantially between 1973 and 1983. This may be related at least in part to a sharp decrease in proportion of children who had teeth extracted for decay reasons (Table 18.12). During the dental examination in both 1973 and 1983 the dentist asked the children whether they had ever worn a brace and also recorded whether each child was wearing a brace at the time of the examination. In addition, an assessment was made by the dentist as to whether orthodontic treatment was needed (Table 18.13). Despite the difference between the

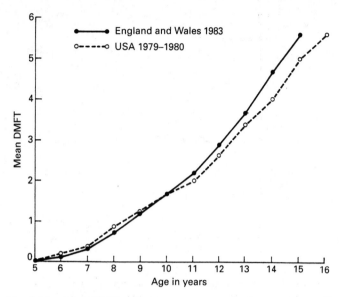

Fig. 18.8. Mean DMFT values in permanent teeth of 5- to 16-year-old children from the USA (1979–80) and England and Wales (1983).

Table 18.11. The prevalence of specific occlusal problems in children in England and Wales: 1973–83

| | Proportion (per cent) of children with | | | | | |
| | Instanding or edge-to-edge incisors | | Overjet 5–6 mm | | Overjet 7 mm or more | |
Age (yrs)	1973	1983	1973	1983	1973	1983
8	12	9	11	16	7	8
12	9	10	11	13	7	8
15	9	13	11	12	3	4

Table 18.12. Crowding, orthodontic extractions, and decay extractions in children in England and Wales: 1973–83

| | Per cent children with | | | | | |
| | crowding | | orthodontic extractions | | decay extractions | |
Age (yrs)	1973	1983	1973	1983	1973	1983
8	65	70	—	—	4	2
12	55	65	13	15	23	13
15	53	66	21	29	33	22

orthodontic examinations of 1973 and 1983, it is clear that orthodontic extractions increased, appliance therapy increased (although not apparently statistically significantly) but there was still almost one-third of 15-year-old children who were regarded by the survey dentists as in need of orthodontic treatment. Parents were asked some questions about what they thought about the appearance of their

Table 18.13. Proportions of children who had had appliance therapy and who were in need of orthodontic treatment

| | Per cent who | | | | | |
| | had a brace at the examination | | had had a brace | | were in need of orthodontic treatment | |
Age (yrs)	1973	1983	1973	1983	1973	1983
8	—	—	1	1	57	56
12	5	7	7	7	37	41
15	1	3	16	20	27	31

child's teeth, especially whether they thought the teeth were crooked or protruding, and they were asked whether they would like their child to have their teeth straightened. Among children whom the dentist assessed as not needing any orthodontic treatment for crowding about four out of five parents said their child's teeth were not crooked. However, among those for whom the dentist said there was an orthodontic treatment need for reasons for crowding, fewer than half the parents said their child's teeth were crooked. The results showed that crowding that was of dental significance to the examiner was not recognized as being a problem by over half of the parents.

These findings raise an interesting point with regard to aesthetics and the need for treatment, which was referred to in the Schanschieff Report into Unnecessary Dental Treatment (DHSS 1986). Are dentists over-emphasizing the problem and advocating treatment when parents do not perceive an aesthetic problem? The alternative explanation is that the general public are not aware of crowding, especially in the premolar and canine regions, and that dentists are using their professional judgement to score crowding which parents had not appreciated.

(v) Trauma to anterior teeth

By the age of 15 years over a quarter of children in England and Wales had suffered accidental damage to their front teeth. The prevalence was much higher in boys than in girls (Table 18.14). These findings were much higher than in 1973, probably because there had been very large reported increase in the number of incisors with fracture of the enamel only (the least serious traumatic injury). In the vast majority of cases the damaged incisors received no treatment (Table 18.15). Among 12-year-olds for example, only 10 per cent of incisors with traumatic injury had been treated. When the information from the questionnaire to the parents relating to

Table 18.14. Prevalence (per cent) of accidental dental damage among children in the UK: 1983

Age (yrs)	Males	Females	Both sexes
8	12	7	10
12	29	16	23
15	33	19	26

Table 18.15. Proportion (per cent) of children in the UK with damaged incisors that have not been treated in 1983

Age (yrs)	Males	Females	Both sexes
8	89	84	88
12	89	93	90
15	85	81	84

damage to the incisors was correlated with the clinical findings, it was obvious that parents were not as aware of accidental damage to the teeth as were the dental examiners. For example, among 15-years-olds, the dentist recorded 26 per cent with traumatic injury whilst the parents felt only 16 per cent had damaged a permanent incisor.

CHILDREN'S DENTAL HEALTH IN THE UK IN 1993

The preliminary results from the 1993 survey of over 17 000 children in the UK ages 5–15 years, gave information on dental caries (OPCS Monitor 1994). The full report (O'Brien 1994) was published in December 1994. There has been a fall in the proportion of 5-year-old children with at least one decayed deciduous tooth in the UK as a whole, from 52 per cent in 1983 to 47 per cent in 1993. The change in England was only four percentage points over the 10-year interval between the surveys, from 48 to 44 per cent, and the UK figure masks much greater falls in the other UK countries, from 67 to 54 per cent in Wales, from 75 to 58 per cent in Scotland and from 78 to 67 per cent in Northern Ireland (Fig. 18.9). The mean dmf also fell, from 2.1 to 2.0 in the UK, with no improvements in England (1.9 compared with 1.8 in 1983) but with substantial improvements in Wales (2.3 compared with 3.1 in 1983), Scotland (3.0 as against 3.9), and Northern Ireland (3.3 as against 4.5). Marked improvements were noted at all ages from 6 to 15 years in the condition of permanent teeth. In 1993, 40 per cent of 15-year-olds were caries-free and the mean DMF had declined from 5.6 to 2.1.

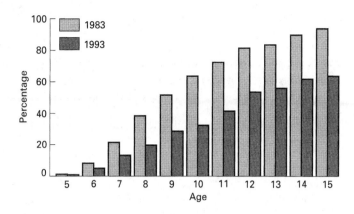

Fig. 18.10. Proportion of children with decay experience in the permanent dentition by age (UK 1983, 1993).

A comparison, over 20 years, of the DMF values for permanent teeth in England and Wales in 1973, and the United Kingdom in 1993, using the same scale, is given in Fig. 18.11a, b). The difference in total decay experience is dramatic, but the proportion of untreated decay (D/DMF) has hardly changed at all over the 20 year period.

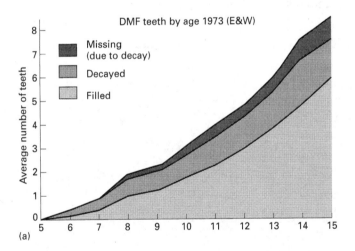

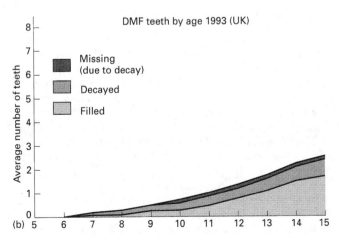

Fig. 18.11. Comparison of the DMF values for permanent teeth in (a) England and Wales in 1973, and (b) the UK in 1993.

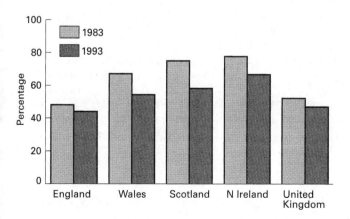

Fig. 18.9. Estimated proportion of 5-year-olds with deciduous decay experience by year and country (UK 1983, 1993).

SECULAR DECLINE IN CARIES: INTERNATIONAL COMPARISONS

Epidemiological studies in the early 1970's showed tremendous inter-country variations in caries experience. Figure 18.3 shows, that for 12-year-olds, the mean DMF could vary from 3.8 to 10.1.

Data presented at the Second International Conference on Declining Caries held in London in 1994 showed a marked convergence in results of recent surveys from many parts of the world.

Information on 5- to 6-year-old children came from 11 countries. The sample sizes and methodology varied considerably and this must be taken into account when comparing results. For example, the data for England and Wales came from the latest national survey carried out in 1993, when over 17 000 children aged 5–15 years, from 500 schools were examined. Other studies, although labelled, for example, 'Canada' or 'Belgium', were local surveys and did not claim to be truly representative of that country. Nevertheless, the range for dmft values from 11 countries was from 1.3 (Canada) to 2.1 (Norway). (Table 18.16). The proportion caries free varied from 55–72 per cent.

Table 18.16. Data from 11 countries providing dmft values for 5- to 6-year old children: 1987–93 (Murray 1994)

Country	Year	Mean dmf	% caries-free
Australia*	1992	2.0	
Belgium*	1990	?	59
Canada	1990	1.3	65
Denmark	1992	1.5	61
England and Wales	1993	1.8	55
Finland	1991	1.4	60
Iceland	1988	2.9	40
Netherlands	1993	?	55
Norway	1991	2.1	63
Sweden	1991	?	72
USA	1987	2.0	

* Six-year-olds.

Data from only one country, Iceland, fell outside this range (mean dmf 2.9, 40 per cent caries free). The countries are listed in the order of the presentations at the Conference. Information on 12-year-old children was provided from 14 countries (Table 18.17). The mean DMF varied from 1.1 (Switzerland and England and Wales) to 2.7 (Belgium). All countries were well below the WHO goal of a mean DMF value of less than 3 by the year 2000. The percentage caries-free varied from 25 per cent (Belgium) to 60 per cent (the Netherlands) with many studies showing that about 50 per cent of 12-year-olds were caries-free.

Seven studies provided data for 15-year-old children (Table 18.18). In six studies the mean DMF varied from 2.1 to 3.6. In four studies, those caries-free was 23–40 per cent, but the study from Sweden reported that 70 per cent of 15-year-olds were caries-free, even though this country had the highest

Table 18.17. Data from 14 countries providing DMFT values for 12-year-old children (Murray 1994)

Country	Year	Mean DMF	% caries-free
Australia	1992	1.2	55
Belgium	1990	2.7	25
Canada	1990	1.5	
China	1992	1.3	50
Denmark	1991	1.3	49
Eire GHB	1992	1.5	
WHBF	1992	1.6	
WHB non F	1992	2.1	
England and Wales	1993	1.1	50
Finland	1991	1.2	30
Germany	1993	2.5	
Iceland	1991	2.5	23
Netherlands			60
Norway	1991	2.2	36
Sweden	1991	1.6	43
Switzerland	1992	1.1	

Table 18.18. Data from 7 studies providing DMFT values for 15-year-old children (Murray 1994)

Country	Year	Mean DMF	% caries-free
China		2.1	29
Denmark	1991	3.1	25
England and Wales	1993	2.1	40
Finland	1991	3.1	23
Iceland	1991	5.3	9
Sweden	1991	3.6	70
Switzerland		2.2	

mean DMF (3.6). This suggests that considerable caries is concentrated in 30 per cent of their population. Iceland was the exception with only 9 per cent of 15-year-olds caries free and a mean DMF of 5.3.

One other aspect which was covered in the Conference was the standard of dental health of the adult dentate population. More variation was evident here, particularly in the age groups reported on (28-year-olds in Finland, and up to 45- to 54-year-olds in the Netherlands and Germany). Nevertheless, apart from 35-year-olds in Norway, who had a mean DMF of 25, all the other results reported were clustered between 16.7 and 19.0 (Table 18.19).

In round figures, the average dentate of 40-year-old from nine countries around the world has a mean DMFT value of 18, but the 'average' 15-year-old, in 1991–3, had a mean DMFT value of less than 3. The question for the future is will the present 15-year-old deteriorate by 15 DMFT in 25 years, or will the low caries experience of present-day teenagers ensure a much healthier dentate population when they reach middle age?

THE NEED FOR TREATMENT IN CHILDREN AND ITS EFFECT ON TREATMENT NEEDS IN LATER LIFE

The results of these surveys show clearly the direction in which the dental services should move in order to provide a

Table 18.19. Mean DMFT values for adult dentate populations from 9 countries (Murray 1994)

Country	Year	Age	Mean DMF
Australia		35–44	18.8
Denmark		30–39	17.8
England and Wales	1988	35–44	19.0
Finland		28	16.7
Germany		35–44	16.7
		45–54	18.4
Netherlands		35–44	17.4
		45–54	18.4
New Zealand	1988	35–44	18.3
Norway		35	25.0
Sweden		30	17.5

better standard of dental health for children. Although great emphasis has been placed on the welcome reduction in caries in many Western countries, there has not been the same reduction in the prevalence of periodontal disease. As parental awareness increases there will be an increasing demand for orthodontic treatment, and for the treatment and prevention of trauma to anterior teeth. Experience in the United States has shown that, in spite of the substantial decrease in the prevalence of dental caries, the demand for dental services by children aged between 5 and 17 years did

not decline. There was an increase in the ratio of filled teeth to total caries experience, and an extension of dental care to a large proportion of the population, together with more complete maintenance care and a growing awareness of the need for programmes for prevention of all dental diseases (Waldman 1987).

The prevention of dental caries by a combination of public health and individual preventive measures gives us the opportunity to ensure that the whole dental environment for children is improved so that their future dental needs are reduced and simplified. It may be a gross simplification and generalization to say that by the age range 12–14 years the future dental needs of a patient are largely determined, but consider the following examples.

The first, a 13-year-old boy, had his first permanent molars extracted some years ago (Fig. 18.12). He was referred for orthodontic treatment of misplaced maxillary canines. The failure to manage the space created by extraction of first molars some years previously means that complex orthodontic treatment will be necessary and more teeth may have to be extracted in the upper arch in order to provide him with a reasonable occlusion. The next patient has fared so much better (Fig. 18.13). She has very good oral hygiene, well-aligned incisor and canine teeth, and an excellent upper arch. All second permanent molars have been fissure sealed, three first permanent molars have been restored but, for some reason, the lower left first permanent molar was extracted

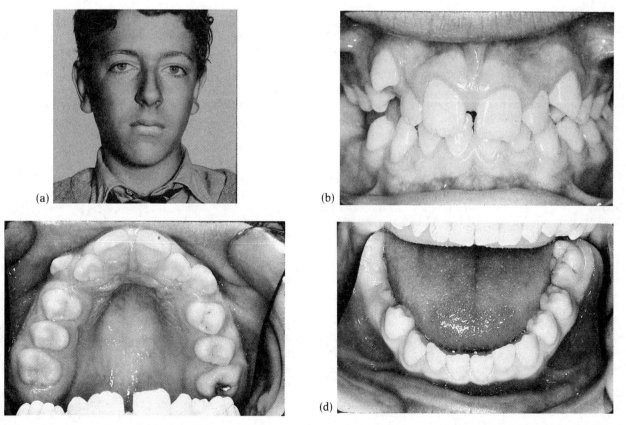

Fig. 18.12. (a) Facial appearance of a 13-year-old patient. (b) View of anterior teeth showing upper canines crowded out of the arch. (c) Occlusal view of upper arch showing lack of space in the upper canine region. First permanent molars had been extracted and second permanent molars had moved forward closing the space. (d) Occlusal view of the lower arch showing the poor alignment of second permanent molars, following the extraction of first permanent molars.

260   *The changing pattern of dental disease*

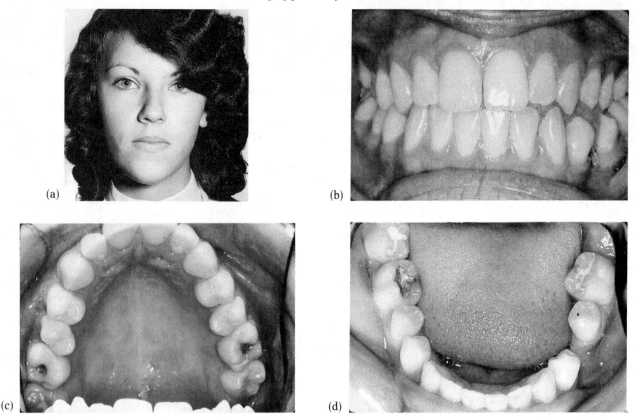

Fig. 18.13. (a) Facial appearance of a 14-year-old patient. (b) View of anterior teeth showing incisor and canine teeth well aligned. (c) Occlusal view of upper arch: teeth are well aligned; the upper first permanent molars have been restored with amalgam and the upper second molars have been fissure sealed. (d) Occlusal view of the lower arch showing fissure sealants on both lower second molars, and occlusal restoration in the lower right first permanent molar, but a poor occlusion on the left side because the lower left first permanent molar has been extracted some years ago.

shortly after eruption. The resulting occlusion in that quadrant is poor, the contact points non-existent, and she will have to concentrate more effort in that quadrant to ensure that periodontal disease is kept to a minimum in later life.

The next patient (Fig. 18.14) also has a beautiful smile and good oral hygiene. Her upper arch shows true prevention, with all four permanent molars fissure sealed. The lower arch has been preserved by amalgam restorations in the occlusal and buccal surfaces. Which arch will require further dental attention in future years? How often will those amalgams be replaced and extended in the next 50 years? Why were we able to prevent caries in the upper arch but only 'manage' caries in the lower arch? The bitewing radiographs (Fig. 18.14) (e), (f) certainly suggest that some of the occlusal amalgams are minimal and might have been obviated by a more preventive approach.

This preventive philosophy can be illustrated by the next case (Fig. 18.15). If one sees a small brown line or the earliest of decalcification in first permanent molars in a 7-year-old child, it is very easy to feel that caries will inevitably occur in all first permanent molars, and that the patient is caries-susceptible. However, if by fissure sealing and oral hygiene instruction those same surfaces can be kept free from amalgams, the same child when 13 years of age, with all premolar and second molar teeth in occlusion, is labelled caries-immune. The bitewings show a caries-free dentition (Fig.

18.15) (e), (f) and with reasonable oral hygiene it can be predicted that this patient will keep his teeth for life with the minimum of restorative treatment being required.

NATIONAL SURVEYS OF ADULT DENTAL HEALTH

(i) PREVALENCE OF EDENTULOUSNESS

The standard of dental health in a country depends in part on the attitude of the population to dental care, and the resources available for dental treatment. There is also a historical perspective in that treatment available to a population in the past often makes itself felt in the statistics of the present. For example, the 'management' of periodontal disease during the 1930s to 1950s in the UK by the extraction of teeth and the provision of dentures has resulted in a high prevalence of edentulousness. The finding in the first national survey in England and Wales carried out in 1968 (Gray *et al.* 1970), that 37 per cent of adults over the age of 16 years had no natural teeth, certainly focused attention on the dental needs of adults. Even if the pattern of dental treatment changed immediately from extraction towards restoration and prevention, those already rendered edentulous will feature in the statistics until they die. A summary of edentulousness in various European countries

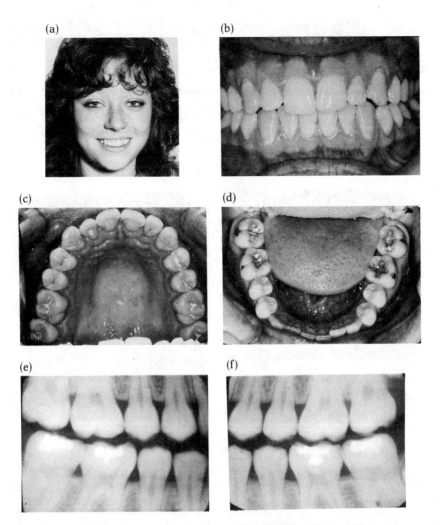

Fig. 18.14. Facial appearance of 17-year-old patient. (b) View of anterior teeth showing good alignment of incisor and canine teeth. (c) Occlusal view of upper arch showing a caries-free arch with all molars fissure sealed. (d) Occlusal view of lower arch showing amalgam restoration in all four permanent molar teeth. (e, f) Bitewing radiographs of this patient showing shallow amalgam restorations.

(WHO 1986) shows the United Kingdom almost at the bottom of the list in terms of edentulousness at two age groups (Table 18.20).

Edentulousness has continued to decline in the UK. The proportion of adults aged 16 and over in this category fell to 19 per cent in 1978 and 21 per cent in 1988. It is heavily influenced by age. The latest results show that only 4 per cent of 35- to 44-year-olds are edentulous. Because the age profile of the British population is well known, it can be predicted that the prevalence of edentulous will fall to 10 per cent by 2008 (Table 18.21). About half those aged 75 and over will be edentulous, but very few adults under 50 years of age will have no natural teeth.

(ii) THE DENTATE POPULATION

Two factors, regional variations and dental attendance, were found to affect the dental health of dentate adults in the 1968 survey in England and Wales (Gray *et al.* 1970). Considering the 16- to 34-year-olds with some natural teeth, the best

group, in terms of the number of standing teeth, was from London and the south-east, who attended regularly at the dentist. The worst group were those from the North, who attended only when having trouble. However, there was a higher proportion of people in the North with sound and untreated teeth, compared with those in London and the South East, who had many more restored teeth, particularly in premolar region (Fig. 18.16). The report found no evidence to suggest that there were major differences in the occurrence of tooth decay among the regions of England and felt that the reasons for the variations found between London and the North, regular and irregular attenders, was due partly to a difference in the attitudes of patients to dental health and treatment, and partly to a different in treatment given by dentists.

Ten years later, the 1978 survey (Todd and Walker 1980) again enabled a comparison to be made between the same groups of regular and irregular attenders. These data are also reproduced in Fig. 18.16. Comparing these two subgroups, 10 years apart, it can be seen that relatively little has

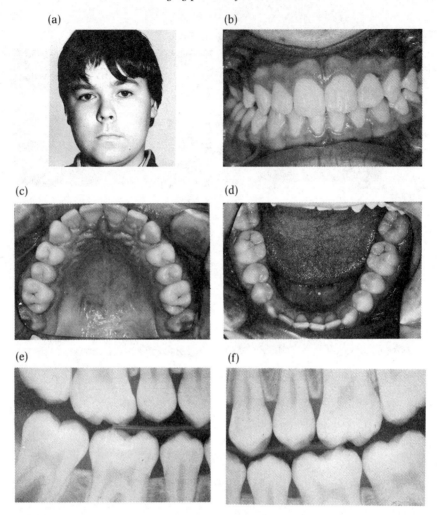

Fig. 18.15. (a) facial appearance of a 13-year-old patient. (c) View of anterior teeth showing anterior teeth well aligned. (c) Occlusal view of upper arch: a small amount of staining is evident in the fissures of the upper first permanent molars, but these teeth have been fissure-sealed. (d) Occlusal view of lower arch: the lower first permanent molars have been fissure-sealed with a clear sealant. (e) Bitewing radiographs of this patient showing a caries-free dentition.

changed in the pattern of dental care for dentate adults. In the London and South-East regular attenders there is a slightly higher proportion of sound, untreated teeth and a small decrease in the proportion of filled teeth among premolars and wisdom teeth. In the 'worst-group'—young dentate adults in the North who only go to the dentist when they are having trouble, the level of untreated decay was still very high, but there was a slight increase in the number of molar teeth that had been filled rather than extracted. Overall, very little change had occurred in the mean number of sound, decayed and treated teeth among adults with some natural teeth in England and Wales between 1968 and 1978 (Table 18.22).

The position of the United Kingdom in comparison to the rest of Europe in terms of missing teeth in dentate adults, aged 35–44 years, is shown in Table 18.23. The worst figure (15.0) was found in Finland and the best figure (4.5) in Denmark. On the basis of this table the UK is in the middle band with respect to missing teeth in dentate adults.

The third decennial survey of adult dental health in the UK was carried out in 1988 (Todd and Lader 1991). It showed

that the secular decline in dental caries in children in the 1970s was now having an effect on the dental needs of adults. The distribution of tooth conditions for 16- to 24-year-olds showed many more sound teeth and far fewer filled teeth than for the 25- to 34-year-old age group (Fig. 18.17). One indication of 'low disease' in adults is the proportion with 18 or more sound untreated teeth (Table 18.24). The improvement for 16- to 24-year-olds with this dental attribute has been dramatic over the last 20 years (44 per cent in 1968 to 83 per cent in 1988). The 16- to 24-year-olds in 1968 were equivalent to the 35- to 44-year-olds in 1988. The deterioration over time for this indication of 'low disease' has been from 44 to 23 per cent in 20 years, or approximately 10 percentage points for every 10 years. If this rate of deterioration were to be maintained, then in 1998 about 75 per cent of 25- to 34-year-olds would have 18 or more sound and untreated teeth. However, it is likely that the dental health of 16- to 24-year-olds in 1988 will not deteriorate as quickly as in the past, leading to more positive attitudes to the preservation of teeth of older adults in the future.

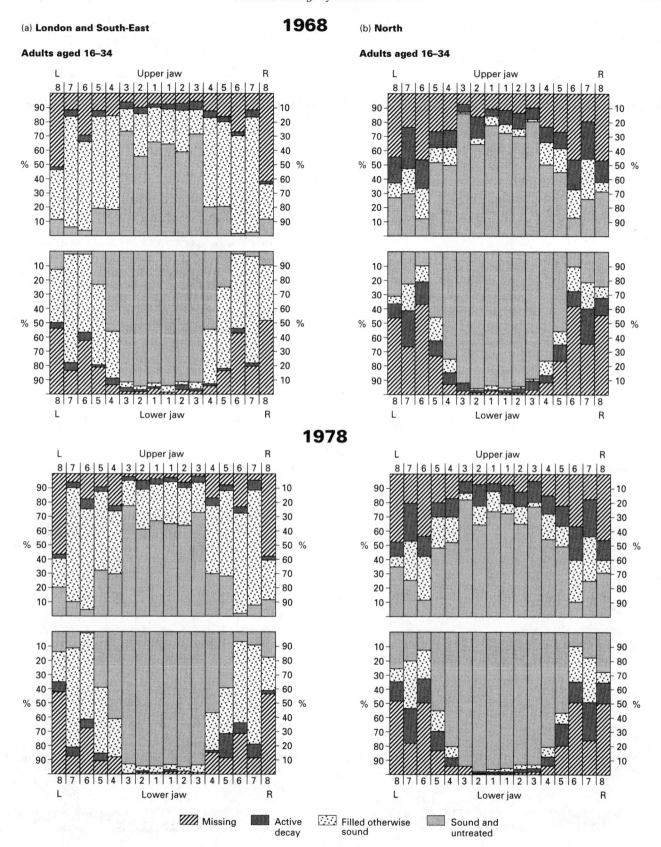

Fig. 18.16. The distribution of tooth conditions (missing, active decay, filled otherwise sound, sound and untreated) around the mouth for adults, aged 16–34 years, with some natural teeth. A comparison of two subgroups, those from (a) London and south-east, who attend for a regular check up and (b) those from the north, who attend only when having trouble, for 1968 and 1978. (Reproduced by kind permission of Miss Todd and OPCS.)

Table 18.20. Prevalence of edentulousness in various European countries (WHO 1986)

Country	Per cent edentulous	
	35–44 yrs	65+ yrs
Austria	—	30
Denmark	8.0	60
Finland	15.0	65
GDR	0.5	58
Hungary	—	18
Ireland	12.0	72
Malta	—	50
Morocco	2.8	—
Netherlands	18.0	70
Poland	13.5	—
Portugal	2.0	—
Sweden	1.0	20
Switzerland	—	25
United Kingdom	13.0	79

One measure of 'considerable restorative care' was the proportion of adults with 12 or more filled teeth (Table

Table 18.21. Predictions of tooth loss to 2008 (Todd and Lader 1991)

Age (yrs)	1988	1998	2008
16–24	0.1	0.1	0.1
25–34	1	1	1
35–44	4	2	2
45–54	17	7	5
55–64	37	22	12
65–74	57	41	26
75+	80	64	48
Total	21	14	10

18.25). In 1968, 32 per cent of 16- to 24-year-olds had 12 or more filled teeth. Ten years later, 40 per cent of the 25- to 34-year-olds had 12 or more filled teeth and this figure increased to 49 per cent for 35- to 44-year-olds in 1988. Thus, the picture is of a consistent increase in the provision of restorations as the population reached middle age. However, in 1988 only 7 per cent of 16- to 24-year-olds had 12 or more filled teeth. It is very unlikely that this age group will require considerable restorative care in 20 years time.

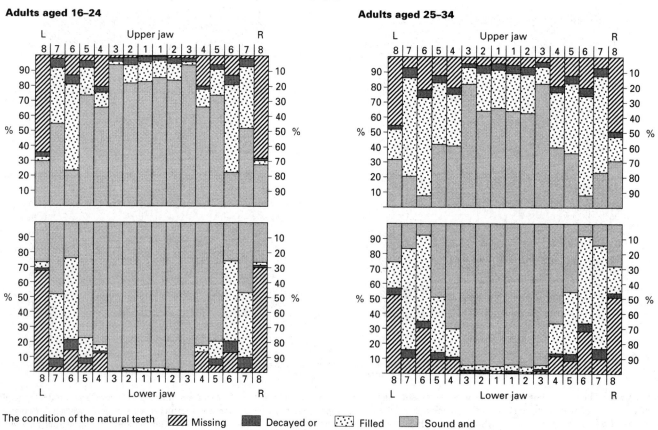

Fig. 18.17. The distribution of tooth conditions around the mouth for dentate adults in the UK different age groups: 1988.

Table 18.22. Mean number of sound, decayed and treated teeth among adults with some natural teeth in England and Wales (Todd and Walker 1980)

Tooth condition	1968	1978
Sound and untreated	12.8	13.2
Crowned or bridged	0.1	0.3
Filled (otherwise sound)	6.8	7.8
Filled, and decayed, or not restorable	2.2	1.9
Missing	10.1	8.8

Table 18.23. Missing teeth per person, age 35–44 years (WHO 1986)

Czechoslovakia	8.0
Denmark	4.5
Finland	15.0
GDR	5.0
Hungary	13.0
Ireland	10.6
Malta	6.5
Morocco	7.3
Netherlands	9.9
Portugal	6.7
Spain	5.6
Sweden	5.0
Switzerland	5.0
United Kingdom	9.2

CONCLUSIONS

- The important reduction in caries observed in children should now begin to be seen in statistics for young adults. This will only occur if both dentists' and patients' attitudes to dental health and treatment change.

- If caries is declining, real improvements in the number of sound teeth should be seen. This change will be accelerated if emphasis can be directed onwards from restoration to prevention.

REFERENCES

Anderson, R.J. (1981a). The changes in dental health of 12-year-old school children in two Somerset schools. A review after an interval of 15 years. *Br. dent. J.* **150**, 354–6.

Anderson, R.J., Bradnock, C., and James, P.M.C. (1981b). The change in dental health of 12-year-old school children in Shropshire. A review after an interval of 15 years. *Br. dent. J.* **150**, 278–81.

Anderson, R.J. (1981c). The changes in the dental health of 12-year-old school children resident in a naturally fluoridated area of Gloucestershire. A review after an interval of 15 years. *Br. dent. J.* **150**, 354–6.

Andlaw, R.J., Burchell, C.K., and Tucker, G.J. (1982). Comparison of dental health of 11-year-old children in 1970 and 1979 and of 14-year-old children in 1973 and 1979; studies in Bristol, England. *Caries Res.* **16**, 257–64.

Burton, V.J., Rob, M.I., Craig, G.G., and Lawson, J.S. (1984). Changes in the caries experience of 12-year-old Sydney school children between 1963 and 1982. *Med. J. Australia* **140**, 405–7.

Table 18.24. The proportion (%) of dentate adults with 18 or more sound and untreated teeth in England and Wales: 1968–88.

Age (yrs)	1968	1978	1988
16–24	44	53	83
25–34	23	28	42
35–44	19	20	23

Table 18.25. The proportion (%) of dentate adults with 12 or more filled teeth in England and Wales: 1968–88

Age	1968	1978	1988
16–24	32	23	7
25–34	36	40	40
35–44	24	34	49
45–54	15	21	41
55+	9	9	19
All ages	25	27	31

DHSS (Department of Health and Social Security) (1986)

FDI (Federation Dentaire Internationale) (1985). *Changing patterns of oral health*, Commission on Oral Health, Research and Epidemiology, Joint FDI/WHO Working Group 5, 72nd Annual World Dental Congress, Helsinki, Finland (August 1984).

Glass, R.I. (ed). (1982). *The first international conference on the declining prevalence of dental caries. J. dent. Res.* **61** (special issue), 1301–83.

Gray, P.G., Todd, J.E., Slack, G.I., and Bulman, J.S. (1970). *Adult dental health in England and Wales in 1968.* HMSO, London.

HMSO (1954). *Health of the school child.* Report of the Chief Medical Officer of the Ministry of Education for the years 1952 and 1953. London.

HMSO (1958). Health of the school child, Report of the Chief Medical Officer of the Ministry of Education for the years 1956 and 1957. London.

HMSO (1960). Health of the school child, Report of the Chief Medical Officer of the Ministry of Education for the years 1958 and 1958. London.

HMSO (1962). Health of the school child, Report of the Chief Medical Officer of the Ministry of Education for the years 1960 and 1961. London.

HMSO (1964). Health of the school child, Report of the Chief Medical Officer of Department of Education and Science for the years 1962 and 1963. London.

Holt, R.D., Joels, D., and Winter, G.B. (1982). Caries in pre-school children. *Br. dent. J.* **153**, 107–9.

Jackson, D. (1974). Caries experience in English children young adults during the years 1947–1972. *Br. dent. J.* 137,91–8.

Kalsbeek, H. (1982). Evidence of decrease in prevalence of dental caries in the Netherlands: an evaluation of epidemiological caries survey on 4–6 and 11–15 year old children between 1965 and 1980. *J. dent. Res.* **61** (special issue), 1321–6.

Miller, A.J., Brunelle, J.A., Carlos, J.P., and Scott, D.B. (1981). *The prevalence of dental caries in United States children 1979–80.* National Institute of Dental Research, U.S. Department of Health and Human Services, Public Health Service, National Institutes of Health.

Murray, J.J. (1994). Comments on results reported at the Second International Conference: changes in caries prevalence. *Int. dent. J.* **44**, 457–8.

O'Brien, M. (1994). *Children's dental health in the United Kingdom 1993*. OPCS. HMSO, London.

Palmer, J.D. (1980). Dental health in children–an improving picture? *Br. dent. J.* **149**, 48–50.

Renson, C.E. (1986). Changing patterns of dental caries: a survey of 20 countries. *Ann. Acad. Med. Singagpore*, **15**, 284–98.

Schanschieff Report (1986). Report of the Committee of Enquiry into Unnecessary Dental Treat, HMSO, London.

Silver, D.H. (1982). Improvements in the dental health of 3-year Hertfordshire children after 8 years. *Br. dent. J.* **153**, 179–82.

Todd, J.E. (1975). *Children's dental health in England and Wales 1973*, HMSO, London.

Todd, J.E. and Walker, A.M. (1980). *Adult dental health, Vol., 1, England and Wales 1968–1978*. HMSO, London.

Todd, J.E. and Dodd, T. (1985). *Children's dental health in the United Kingdom in 1988*. HMSO, London.

Todd, J.E. and Lader, (1991). *Adult dental health in the United Kingdom in 1988*. OPCS. HMSO, London.

Waldman, B.H. (1987). Increasing use of dental services by very young children. *J. dent. Child.* **54**, 248–50.

Winter, G.B., Rule, D.C., Marker, G.P., James, P.M.C. and Gordon, P.J. (1971). The prevalence of dental caries in pre-school children aged 1 to 4 years. *Br. dent. J.* **130**, 271–7; 434–6.

WHO (World Health Organization) (1986). *Country profiles on oral health in Europe 1986*. WHO, Geneva.

19. Resources, treatment, and prevention

J.J. MURRAY

THERE is a dynamic relationship between the natural history of any disease and the response by society in trying to combat the problem. As far as dental disease is concerned, in Britain and in many other countries, the original response to a carious tooth was to extract it. Historically, this was usually a painful and hazardous procedure performed by poorly trained operators. Society's response was to encourage the development of professional skills and to allow the practice of dentistry to be limited to those who had received appropriate professional training. As knowledge and skill increased, attention turned to the preservation of teeth and the treatment of caries by restoration rather than extraction. This trend from extraction to restoration depended not only on the skill of the dental profession but also on the reaction of society with respect to the economic, resources that individuals and government were prepared to commit to dental treatment, and the attitude of individuals to the advice proffered by professionals. Real improvements in health can only occur when both the community at large and the health professionals share the same objectives, which surely should be the primary prevention of disease.

Simplistically, the progress of dentistry can be represented as one in which there is movement from extraction to restoration and onwards to prevention (Fig. 19.1). The main thrust of this book has been to gather together information on diet, fluoridation, preventive measures for the individual, and oral hygiene, all of which would have an effect on the prevention of the two main dental diseases, caries and periodontal disease. But it would be facile to assume that these measures alone can exert a beneficial effect without appreciating that they can only work within a favourable framework agreed by society. Patient's attitude, dentist's attitude,

remuneration and manpower all have a crucial role to play in the prevention of dental disease.

In the 1940s the major dental treatment option in the United Kingdom was extraction, but in the 1950s and 1960s there was a definite shift towards restoration. A number of factors were responsible for this change in direction. The introduction of high-speed rotor cutting instruments revolutionized restorative dentistry and, in particular, enabled more complex restorative procedures, crowns, and bridgework to be completed more quickly, and with less discomfort to the patient. The attitude of the patient has certainly changed—to give just one example, in 1968 27 per cent of adults with some teeth found the thought of full dentures very upsetting, (Gray *et al.* 1970), whereas in 1978 the figure had almost doubled to 48 per cent (Todd and Walker 1980).

The interaction between dentists' attitude and remuneration can be seen by examining the changes in the pattern of dental treatment carried out in the general dental services in England and Wales over the last 35 years. The uptake of more complex restorative procedures—crowns, bridges, endodontics treatment—has occurred partly because of the increasing technical skills acquired by the dental profession and partly because the regulations of the Dental Estimates Board (DEB) have expanded so that more complex restorative procedures have been allowed within the National Health Service. Graphs showing the trends in various aspects of dental treatment were included in the second edition. These have been upgraded by including figures for 1992–93 prepared by the Dental Practice Board (Fig. 19.2). The number of permanent teeth extracted in the general dental services has fallen from nearly 18 million in 1950 to 3.7 million in 1985, and down to 3.8 million in 1992. The number of general

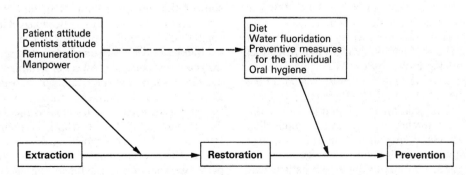

Fig. 19.1. Factors affecting changes in dental treatment and prevention.

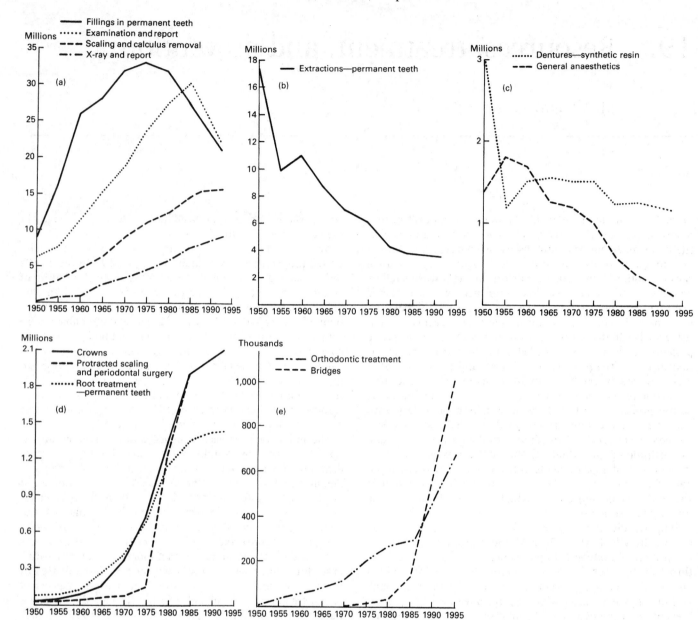

Fig. 19.2. The changing pattern of dental treatment in the general dental services of the National Health Service in England and Wales, 1950–1995. (By kind permission of the Chairman of the Dental Estimates Board 1985 and Dental Practice Board 1994.)

anaesthetics has fallen at a similar rate, from 1.5 million in 1955 to 433 000 in 1986 and to 141 000 in 1992–93. The provision of dentures (and this includes remaking dentures for those rendered edentulous many years ago) has fallen from its high point of almost 3 million in 1950 to a plateau of approximately 1.25 million in the 1980s.

The habit of regular attendance at the dentist was one of the factors reported by the Adult Dental Health Surveys to be of significance to the dental conditions of adults. Since the inception of the NHS, the number of dental examinations (Fig. 19.2) has increased steadily each year and, in 1985, reached 30 million (this examination, until changes in regulations by the Government in 1988, was free as far as the patient was concerned). The number of amalgam and synthetic restorations increased extremely rapidly in the 1950s and 1960s,

reaching a peak of 32 million in 1975. Figures for 1992–93 showed that no fewer than 21 million fillings were placed in permanent teeth of adults. Because of the introduction of capitation, the number of fillings placed in the permanent teeth of children under 18 years of age is not recorded. Over the last 10 years this particular aspect of treatment has reduced. What are the reasons for this? Could it be that the fall in caries noticed in children is coming through with young adults and so fewer teeth need to be restored? Is there a change of attitude on the part of the dentist, who is becoming more aware that the 'repair of repair'—replacing fillings with new fillings—is not as vitally important as it may have been thought in the past? Are patient charges having an effect in that as patients have to pay an increasing amount for NHS dental treatment, they are beginning to resist simple restorative treatment?

Elderton and Davies (1984), in their follow-up study of dental treatment provided in the General Dental Service for 720 randomly selected dentate adults in Scotland, showed that overall 66 per cent of the surfaces restored over a 5-year period were replacement restorations. They also reported that 12 per cent of the sample were recipients of half of all the restorative treatment and commented: 'It seems that once a person has a number of teeth filled, he tends to have an ever increasing commitment to receiving further restorative treatment. It would seem that the 12 per cent are a high risk group—at high risk of having their teeth re-filled'. They concluded that owing to the general decline in caries prevalence it may well be that many morphologically imperfect restorations do not now warrant replacement. If dentists and the dental service understood the characteristics of restorative care provided, it might be possible to slow down the cycle of replacement restorations by employing a more selective approach when deciding which restorations should be placed.

More complex restorative treatment in the general dental services increased very slowly in the 1950s, and 1960s but the rate of change increased dramatically in the 1970s and 80s (Fig. 19.2). Over 2 million teeth were crowned 1.4 million teeth were root-treated, and 156 000 bridges were placed in 1986. By 1992–3 over 1 million bridges were placed in the general dental services. How much are these increases due to changing patient attitudes so that they are now demanding a more sophisticated service, or to dentist realizing that it is more profitable and satisfying to provide more complex restorative treatment?

The emphasis on restoration of teeth has, in a sense, overshadowed the need for the treatment of malocclusion, especially in children. It has been suggested that about 50 per cent of British children have malocclusions sufficiently severe as to warrant orthodontic treatment, but only about half of these children receive treatment (Todd 1975; Todd and Dodd 1985). Although the total cost of orthodontic treatment in the General Dental Services was £23 million in 1986 or 3 per cent of the total (see Chapter 1), the vast majority of this treatment is completed by the time children have reached 15 years of age. A summary of the cost of the service to children, aged 0–15 years, in the General Dental Services only (Table 19.1) shows that, in 1980, 35 per cent of the fees were for the treatment of caries, compared with 19 per cent

for the treatment of malocclusion, whereas in 1986, the restoration of teeth accounted for 25.6 per cent of the cost and orthodontic treatment had increased slightly to 21.2 per cent of the total cost in this age group.

Government financial policy may also have an impact on dental treatment. The number of dental examinations in the general dental services in England and Wales has risen steadily every year since the inception of the National Health Service. In 1986 dentists were paid for 30.6 million 'examinations and report' by the DEB. This part of dental treatment was free as far as the patient was concerned. In 1987 the Government announced in its White Paper *Promoting better health* (HMSO) 1987) that the dental examination was now to be included in fees paid for by the patient, although children, expectant nursing mothers, and those receiving social security payments, would still receive all their dental treatment free. The patient will now pay a proportion of the total cost of dental examination and treatment. In the 1990s capitation for children and continuing care arrangements for adults were introduced and the Bloomfield Report considered major changes to dental remuneration. Alterations in remuneration may affect the quality of child and adult dental health in the long term. The introduction of capitation for children has caused some commentators to raise the spectre of 'supervised neglect' (watching caries develop rather than treating it) and the possibility that more complex restorative procedures for adults, especially crowns, bridges, and endodontics treatment may cost more under the NHS in a post-Bloomfield scenario, may force some of the less well-off to opt for extraction rather than restorations.

Much more emphasis is now placed on the management of periodontal disease. Scaling and calculus removal approached the 15 million mark in 1985, and protracted scaling and periodontal surgery has rocketed from 1975 (100 000) to almost 2 million courses of treatment 10 years later, helped by changes in the narrative of the DEB (Fig. 19.2).

The changes in the DEB regulations, which gave dental practitioners greater opportunity to engage in more complex restorative and periodontal procedures, certainly helped to emphasize the importance of preservation as against extraction. The statistics reflect a situation where the dentist's attitude and remuneration, and the patient's attitude or acceptance of the treatment suggested, react together to

Table 19.1. Cost of various items of dental treatment in the general dental services of the NHS in England and Wales for children aged 0–15 years (DEB Annual Report 1980/1986)*

	1980		1986	
	£m	per cent	£m	per cent
Examination and X-rays	19.4	31.0	34.1	33.9
Restoration of teeth				
(i) deciduous	6.0	10.0	9.0	8.9
(ii) permanent	16.0	26.0	16.8	16.7
Dentures	0.3	0.5	0.3	0.3
Periodontal treatment	4.6	7.5	11.6	11.5
Extractions, other surgical treatment (except periodontal), and general anaesthetics	3.8	6.0	7.5	7.5
Orthodontics	12.0	19.0	21.3	21.2
Total	62.1	100.0	100.6	100.0

*Now the Dental Practice Board (DPB).

Table 19.2. Cost of some items of treatment (Fig. 19.2) and cost of all treatment (DPB 1992–3)

	1992–3 Age < 18	1992–3 Age 18+	Total
	£m	£m	£m
Exam and Report*	6.3	109.3	115.6
Fillings in permanent teeth*	1.2	187.0	188.2
Scaling and calculus removal*	0.1	134.4	134.5
X-ray and report*	7.5	31.9	39.4
Extraction: permanent teeth	4.5	19.6	24.1
Dentures: synthetic resin	0.3	108.2	108.5
General anaesthetics + sedation	2.5	3.4	5.9
Crowns + Inlays	3.7	168.1	171.8
Root treatment	1.8	42.7	44.5
Orthodontic treatment	34.5	1.4	35.19
Bridges	0.6	42.2	42.8
Other items	35.1	73.7	—
Total	98.1	921.9	1020.0

*Because of the introduction of capitation, information on children for items covered under capitation is not included in the Digest of Statistics, so complete comparison with previous years is not possible.

produce change. In addition, manpower and the availability of dental services also play an important part in helping to promote the trend from extraction to restoration. The number of dental practitioners in the general dental services in England and Wales has grown from 9359 in 1955 to 15 076

in 1985. More dentists serving a community should allow more time to be spent on the preservation of the dentition rather than extracting teeth.

The cost of treatment in the general dental services in 1992–3 was just over £1billion (Table 19.2), of which almost 50 per cent was paid for fillings, crowns, bridges, and root canal therapy. This is apparently a very significant increase on the sum of £40 million for 1980. Four points should, however, be borne in mind: first, the rate of inflation; second, the fact that increasingly sophisticated treatment means higher laboratory costs; third, the number of dentists had increased by more than 2000 (from 13 039 to 15 256) between 1980 and 1986; fourth, patient charges contribute substantially to the total sum.

The number of dentists in the general dental services, total treatment cost, patient contributions, and the net amount received by GDPs, having been standardized for inflation, from 1950 to 1987, are given in Table 19.3. These data show that although the total treatment cost has increased from £40.6 million in 1950 to over £800 million in 1987, the real cost per GDP, that is, the mean annual sum each dental practitioner receives from the DEB, has not changed a great deal in real terms over the last 27 years. The number of dentists working in the General Dental Service in England and Wales appears to have stabilized at about 16 300 for the years 1990–94 (Table 19.4). Gross expenditure peaked at £1.38 billion in 1992/3. Data for 1993/4 show that, for the first time since 1955, the total cost of treatment in the General Dental Services, of the National Health Service, has decreased. Constraints on the public expenditure mean that any new initiative in health has to be looked at carefully, but how will the next movement, from restoration onwards to prevention, be achieved?

First, dental attitudes to the management of the dentition need to change. Anderson (1981) reported the changes in dental health of 12-year-old children from two Somerset

Table 19.3. Studies concerning the general dental services in England and Wales (D. Scarrott, personal communications 1988)

Year	Number of dentists	Total treatment cost £m	Patients' contributions £m	Treatment cost for exchequer £m	1987 (4) £m	Average cost per GDP at 1987 prices £m
1950	9657 (1)	40.6 (2)	–(3)	40.6	492.5	51 000
1955	9788	33.3	7.1	26.1	241.8	24 700
1960	10 254	50.6	9.2	41.4	337.5	32 900
1965	10 405	59.0	11.2	47.8	329.1	31 600
1970	10 843	90.3	16.5	73.8	406.5	37 500
1975	11 737	191.4	32.2	159.2	474.3	40 400
1980	13 039	410.2	93.9	316.3	481.8	37 000
1985	15 076	667.6	198.1	469.5	505.7	33 500
1987	15 545	811.7	244.2	567.5	567.5	36 500

(1) At end of year, to 1960; at 30 September from 1965.
(2) Treatment fees only—that is, the total cost of the general dental services apart from employers' superannuation contributions and (from 1970) seniority payments.
(3) Contributions actually paid, net of remitted charges for low-income patients.
(4) Exchequer cost at 1987 prices inflating by the retail prices index (all items).

Table 19.4. Expenditure in the General Dental Services NHS in England and Wales, 1991–4 (*Source:* Department of Health)

	No. of dentists*	Gross Expenditure (£000s)	Net Expenditure (£000s) (excluding patient charges)
1990/1	16 281	1 097 051	699 190
1991/2	16 283	1 315 483	891 426
1992/3	16 242	1 379 673	964 419
1993/4	16 403	1 289 686	903 623

*Dentists include Principals, Assistants, and Vocational Trainees and are the numbers at 30th September, 1994.

schools over a 15-year period. Dental caries prevalence had fallen by 35 per cent. One interesting finding from the survey of the two schools was that the DMF had fallen much more in one school than the other, the difference was most marked in the DMF values for first permanent molars (Fig. 19.3). In both schools the amount of untreated decay had fallen dramatically and the need for extracting first permanent molars had been reduced almost to zero, but the number of fillings had increased slightly in one school and virtually doubled in the other school. In the first school, dental treatment was provided by the same practitioners as 15 years ago, but there had been a marked change in the provision of general dental services in the catchment area of the second school, with the opening of new multi-practitioner surgeries. Anderson (1981) pointed out that if carious lesions have been prevented, the dental profession must not spoil the situation by continuing to fill occlusal surfaces in teeth which may not become carious. He suggested that dentists' attitudes should change and that the maxim 'If in doubt fill' should be changed to 'if in doubt, wait', especially for occlusal fissures of the permanent dentition of younger children. It is now known that dental caries is not simply a process of demineralization but an alternating process of destruction and repair. Once a

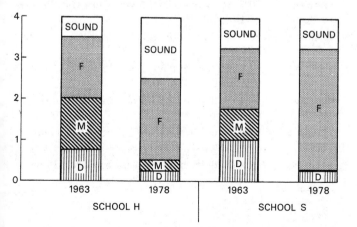

Fig. 19.3. The average number of decayed, missing, filled, and sound first permanent molars of 12-year-old children from two schools examined in 1963 and 1978. (With permission of the Editor, *British Dental Journal*.)

cavity has formed, repair will not 'fill up the hole', but if caries can be detected in its earliest stage, clinician and educated patient can then combine their efforts to ensure that operative intervention is not required. Unless practitioner and informed patient have the courage to 'watch the early lesion' they will never know whether prevention would have been preferable to restoration (see Chapter 6, p. 99).

Second, just as restorative dentistry gained an increasing share of the general dental services' cake in the 1970s and 80s, so measures aimed to prevent disease need to be given more resources in the next phase of the development of dental services. Until 1986, GDPs received no payment for applying topical fluorides or fissure sealants. Now a fee is allowed for topical fluoride therapy and fissure sealants may be applied, having received prior approval, for children with special needs. The introduction of a capitation scheme will give practitioners the opportunity to practise preventive measures and so help to tip the balance from restoration to prevention. The provision of resources is essential if the goal to reduce dental caries still further is to be realized.

What is a realistic objective to aim for with respect tot he prevention of dental disease? The World Health Organization and the International Dental Federation have proposed that the following indicators of improved oral health should be adopted, covering the young, the mature, and the elderly (WHO 1982):

The following global goals for the year 2000 are proposed:

Goal 1. 50 per cent of 5- to 6-year-olds will be caries free.

Goal 2. The global average will be no more than 3 DMF teeth at 12 years of age.

Goal 3. 85 per cent of the population should retain all their teeth at age 18.

Goal 4. A 50 percent reduction in present levels of edentulousness at age 35 to 44 will be achieved.

Goal 5. A 25 per cent reduction in present levels of edentulousness at age 65 and over will be achieved.

Goal 6. A data-based system for monitoring changes in oral health will be established.

According to the Child Dental Health Survey figures for England (Todd 1985), about 51 per cent of 5-year-olds are caries-free, and the mean DMF for 12-year-olds is 2.9 teeth. This means that the first two goals suggested by the Federation Dentaire Internationale (FDI) for the year 2000 had already been reached in England. However, there is still no room for complacency. Even with the reduction in caries noted in the 1983 survey, the impact of dental caries on British children is still unacceptable. By the age of 8 years, 27 per cent of children were reported to have had teeth extracted under a general anaesthetic, and by the age of 15 the figure had risen to 49 per cent. Even accepting that some of these in the 8- to 15-year age group were orthodontic extractions, the stigma of caries is still casting far too long a shadow over a large proportion of our children. By the year 2000, 90 per cent of our 5-year-old children should be caries-free, and the mean DMF rate for 12-year-old children should be no higher than 1.0 DMFT. These objectives would be better than the first two global goals suggested by the FDI and would enable more resources to be allocated to the treatment of traumatized anterior teeth, the management of malocclusion, and the prevention of periodontal disease in children. However, if the decline in the prevalence of dental caries is to continue, more emphasis on the prevention of dental disease will be required. Two recent studies (Holt *et al.* 1988; Rugg-Gunn *et al.* 1988) have reported little change in caries levels in young English children between 1980 and 1986.

The next three goals suggested by the FDI depend very heavily on the successful prevention of periodontal breakdown. The prospect of absolute periodontal health on a large scale is remote as it requires the widespread adoption of meticulous plaque control. A more realistic objective is the reduction in the rate of progress of periodontal disease to a level compatible with tooth survival for life. The success of standardized programmes of professional tooth cleaning and oral hygiene education, such as that described by Suomi *et al.* (1971), show that this may be achieved when resources are made available to interested patients. The benefits of this approach, however, can only apply to individuals who present themselves to a dentist who recognizes the value of a plaque-control programme. A further drawback to the dentist-based approach to periodontal care is the excessive consumption of time and resources involved. These factors, therefore, suggest that a satisfactory community-based strategy of periodontal care must be developed before the benefits will be enjoyed by the population as a whole.

An Oral Health Strategy for England was published by the Department of Health in 1994. It proposed eight objectives specifically for England (see Table 19.5).

These objectives are based on the results of the National Surveys of Children and Adult Dental Health that have been carried out in the UK over the last 25 years, and local studies carried out by the British Association for the Study of Community Dentistry. Three of the objectives refer to children and are stiffer targets than those proposed by the World Health Organization. The objective with regard to periodontal disease is concerned with reducing the proportion of the population with deep pocketing, and the remaining four objectives are concerned with the dentate population, particularly targets for the elderly dentate population.

In the UK there has been a welcome reduction in the percentage of the adult population who are edentulous. In the 20-year period between 1968 and 1988 the proportion of the population in England and Wales age 16 years and over who had no natural teeth fell from 37 per cent to 21 per cent. This was in part due to changing attitudes on the part of the public and the dental profession, and the increased opportunity to carry out restorative and periodontal treatment in the general dental service. Nevertheless, there is still a long way to go before the prevalence of edentulousness in the UK falls to the levels enjoyed by other countries, for example, Scandinavia, Japan, and America.

The impact of prevention on the need for dental treatment can be shown diagrammatically by comparing the results of national surveys in England and Wales over a 20-year period (Fig. 19.4a–f). The treatment needs of 5-year-olds has been affected by the rise in the proportion who were caries-free

Table 19.5. The objectives set in the Goal for Oral Health Strategy (DoH 1994)

Caries prevalence in children by the year 2003

Objective:	**70% of 5-year-old children should have had no caries experience.**
Baseline:	Proportion of caries-free children ranged from 43 to 69%.
Objective:	**On average, 5-year-old children should have no more than one decayed, missing, or filled primary tooth.**
Baseline:	dmft between 1.04 and 2.67
Objective	**On average, 12-year-old children should have no more than one decayed, missing or filled permanent tooth.**
Baseline:	DMFT of 1.2

Periodontal diseases by the year 1998

Objective:	**The percentage of dentate adults over 45 years old with at least one deep periodontal pocket, (greater than 6 mm), should be reduced to 10%.**
Baseline:	17% of adults in the UK aged 45–54 had some deep pockets.

Tooth loss in adults by the year 1998

Objective:	**50% of 30-year-olds should have more than 20 teeth which are sound and unfilled.**
Baseline:	23% of dentate adults in the UK aged 30 had more than 20 sound and untreated teeth in 1988.
	63% of dentate adults in the UK aged 20 had more than 20 sound and untreated teeth in 1988.
Objective:	**75% of 50-year-olds should have more than 20 teeth.**
Baseline:	60% of adults in UK aged between 45 and 54 had more than 20 teeth in 1988.
Objective:	**33% of adults over 75 years old should have teeth.**
Baseline:	20% of adults in the UK aged over 75 had teeth in 1988.
	63% of adults in the UK aged between 55 and 64 had teeth in 1988.
Objective:	**10% of adults over 75 years old should have more than 20 teeth.**
Baseline:	3% of adults in the UK aged over 75 had more than 20 teeth in 1988.
	11% of adults in the UK aged between 65 and 74 had more than 20 teeth in 1988.

(from 28 to 55 per cent). Even in 1993 a considerable proportion of decay was left untreated or was treated by extractions. Dental health of 14-year-olds has improved markedly, again because the proportion of caries-free teeth has risen

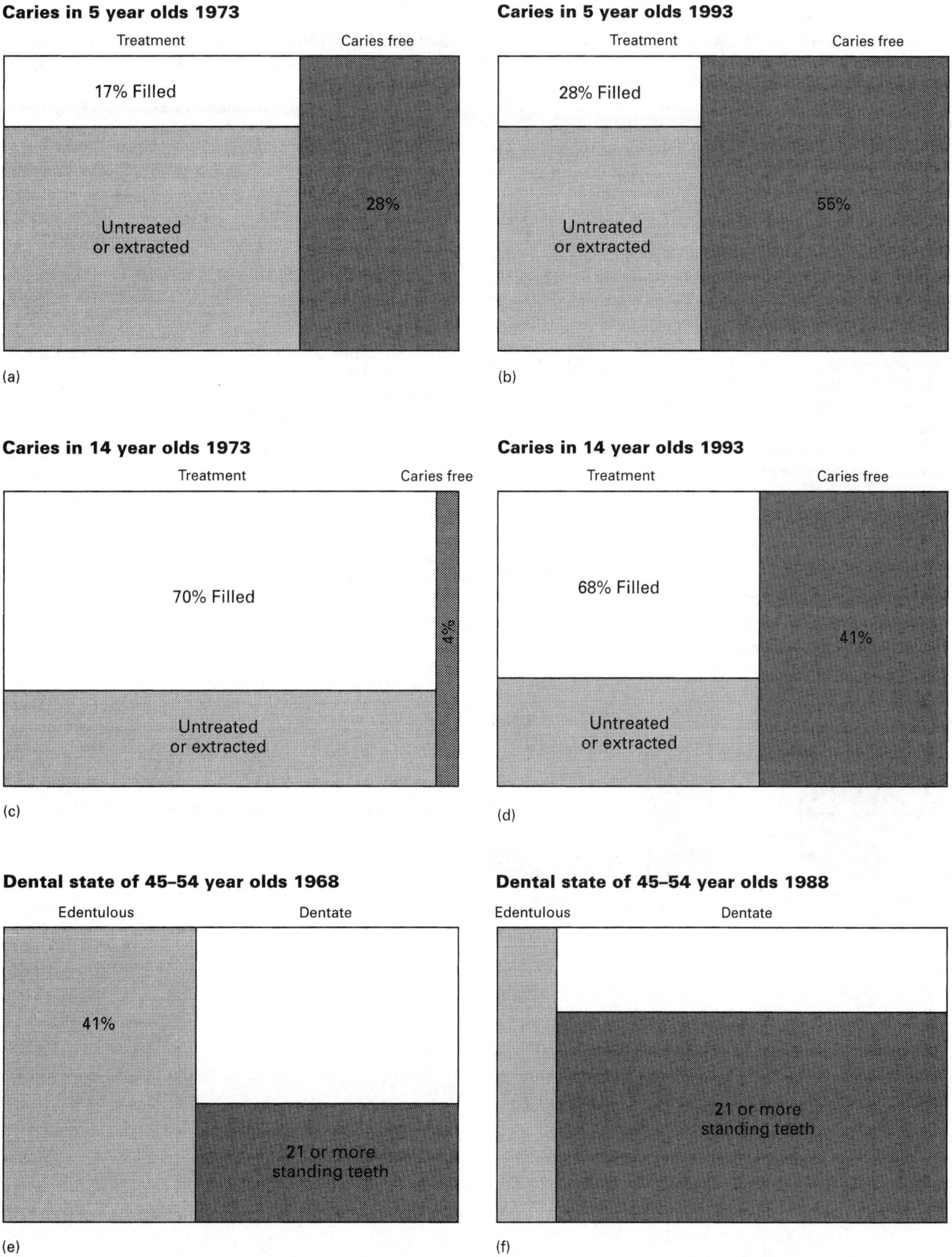

Caries in 5 year olds 1973

Treatment   Caries free

17% Filled

Untreated
or extracted

28%

(a)

Caries in 5 year olds 1993

Treatment   Caries free

28% Filled

Untreated
or extracted

55%

(b)

Caries in 14 year olds 1973

Treatment   Caries free

70% Filled

Untreated
or extracted

4%

(c)

Caries in 14 year olds 1993

Treatment   Caries free

68% Filled

Untreated
or extracted

41%

(d)

Dental state of 45–54 year olds 1968

Edentulous   Dentate

41%

21 or more
standing teeth

(e)

Dental state of 45–54 year olds 1988

Edentulous   Dentate

21 or more
standing teeth

(f)

Fig. 19.4. Impact of preventive treatment in England and Wales: 1973–93.

from 4 to 41 per cent, but still about one-third of caries presented is not treated, or the carious teeth are extracted. Dental Health of 45- to 54-year-olds has also changed. Far fewer are edentulous (41 per cent in 1968 down to 12 per cent in 1988) and a far higher proportion of the dentate population have 21 or more standing teeth. This in itself is not a sufficient goal—if we consider the requirement of the WHO goal of a shortened dental arch (the retention throughout life of a functional aesthetic natural dentition of not less than 20 teeth—shortened dental arch—and not requiring recourse to a prosthesis) then only 29 per cent of the 45- to 54-year-old dentate population were in this category in 1988.

Figure 19.5 is a diagrammatic representation of dental health in Britain for 1988–93, using the results of the latest national surveys for 5-, 14-, and 45–54-year-olds. The dark rectangles represent either no clinical caries (5- and 14-year-olds) or a shortened dental arch (45–54-year-olds). The grey rectangles represent untreated caries or extracted teeth (children) or the proportion edentulous (45–54-year-olds). The light rectangles are a measure of restorative treatment. Presenting the data in this way shows how the effect of prevention has its greatest impact in childhood, and the effect of restorative treatment becomes prominent in the 45–54-year age group.

CONCLUSIONS

● The dental profession must continue to provide good treatment for those affected by oral disease.

● The profession and the public must increase emphasis on prevention, which is the only way to reduce the burden of disease, particularly untreated disease.

Dental Health   **1988–1993**

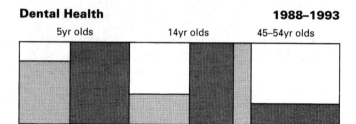

Fig. 19.5. Impact of treatment from childhood to middle age: 1988–93.

REFERENCES

Anderson, R.J. (1981). The changes in the dental health of 12-year-old school children in two Somerset schools. *Br dent. J.* **150**, 218–21.

Annual Reports, Dental Estimates Board 1950–1986.

DEB (Dental Extractions Board) (1980/1986). Annual Report.

DPB (Dental Practice Board) (1992–3). *Digest of statistics.*

DoH (Department of Health) (1994). An *Oral health strategy for England.*

Elderton, R.J. and Davies, J.A. (1984). Restorative dental treatment in the general dental service in Scotland. *Br. dent. J.* **157**, 196–200.

FDI (Fédération Dentaire Internationale (19??)

Gray, P.G., Todd, J.E., Slack, G.L., and Bulman, J.S. (1970). *Adult dental health in England and Wales 1968.* HMSO, London.

HMSO (1987). *Promoting better health.* White Paper. The Government's programme for improving primary health care. HMSO, London.

Holt, R.D., Joels, D., Bulman, J., and Maddick, I.H. (1988). A third study of caries pre-school aged children in Camden. *Br. dent. J.* **165**, 87–91.

Rugg-Gunn, A.J., Carmichael, C.L., and Ferrell, R.S. (1988). Effect of fluoridation and secular trend in caries in 5-year-old children living in Newcastle and Northumberland. *Br. dent. J.* 165, 359–64.

Suomi, J.D., Greene, J.C., Vermillion, J.R., Doyle, J., Chang, J.J., and Leatherwood, E.C. (1971). The effect of controlled oral hygiene procedures on the progression of periodontal disease in adults: results after third and final year. *J. Perio.* 42, 152.

Todd, J.E. (1975). *Children's dental health in England and Wales 1973.* HMSO, London.

Todd, J.E. and Dodd, T. (1985). *Children's dental health in England and Wales 1983.* HMSO, London.

Walker, A.M. and Dodd, P. (1980). *Adult dental health United Kingdom 1978,* Vol. 2. HMSO, London.

WHO (World Health Organization) Goal for oral health in the year 2000. *Br. dent. J.* **152**, 21–2.

WHO (World Health Organization) (1987). *Alternative systems of oral care delivery.* Technical Report Series 750. Geneva.

20. Oral health for the 21st century

J.J. MURRAY

ALTHOUGH some aspects of this book have discussed prevention mainly in the UK context, most of the information in this book applies to dental disease world-wide. The reports of a fall in caries and improvement in the level of gingivitis in North America, the UK, and much of northern Europe and in Australasia indicates that dental disease is preventable on a country-wide scale. More disturbing are the reports of the increase in dental caries prevalence in the developing countries of the world, and it is obligatory that information on prevention of dental disease is available to those in charge of their dental services. The delivery of dental care to the community was considered by a World Health Organization expert committee in 1985 (WHO 1987). In their document they pointed out that all the member states of WHO have adopted the goal of health for all by the year 2000, and all national oral health care systems must take their share of responsibility in efforts to meet this goal. In their view, most oral health services, while providing acceptable treatment-orientated service care financed by various direct or third-party payment systems, are now faced with difficulties when a change is needed in order to provide a preventive-orientated service and different restorative care to deal with rapidly changing levels of oral disease, social patterns, and priorities.

Profound changes are needed not only in the type of care offered and in the way it is provided, but also in the way providers are trained, employed, supervised and supported. Yet in all the major industrialized countries, as well as a number of developing countries, there now exist deeply entrenched systems which have evolved over many decades and which represent security and continuity to those working within them. There is therefore an understandable reluctance to change even when the need for change is overwhelmingly evident.

They concluded that there is a need to revise financing systems so as to improve rewards for effective prevention and care, and to facilitate access and coverage.

The WHO recently considered the present global situation of oral diseases that occur in and affect the oral cavity, in a document *Oral health for the 21st century*, and also in a Technical Report *Recent advances in oral health* (1992). It examined the trends and advances in oral health research, delivery of oral care, education of personnel for oral care related to changes in the attitudes and demands of members of the community. It concluded that oral health services and education of personnel will need to be radically transformed. Less technical/manual skills will be needed, due in part to new technology, and more special skills in diagnosis,

pathophysiology, disease risk, assessment and management, and communication will be required. The Expert Group identified 12 guiding principles.

1. Oral health is an essential part of human function and the quality of life.

2. Oral health status should be improved and maintained in the most economical manner consistent with quality and access.

3. Prevention is preferable to treatment as a general rule.

4. Individuals should do as much as possible for themselves to achieve and maintain oral health.

5. Caries and periodontal diseases can be prevented and controlled.

6. Community methods of prevention should be supportive of individual and personal care, and in some situations is more efficient.

7. Oral health care should be provided in the context of comprehensive care.

8. Oral health care providers should be prepared and motivated to consider general health, and should participate in the provision of general health care.

9. The type, number, and distribution of oral health care personnel should be maintained at levels consistent with need, quality, cost, and access necessary to achieve desired oral health status.

10. Planning, health care practices, and educational programmes should be appropriate for the population or situation in question.

11. Research, evaluation, and education are essential for the continued advancement of oral health.

12. Learning must continue throughout the career of the health professional.

The Expert Group recognized that dramatic successes in prevention have results in the major changes in the epidemiology of the most common oral diseases, dental caries, and periodontal diseases, in many parts of the world in the past two decades.

The aim of this book has been to draw together the available evidence concerning the prevention of oral diseases.

There is no doubt that, even on the basis of our present knowledge concerning the pathogenesis of dental diseases, if this information were put into practice, a vast amount of dental disease afflicting the Western world in particular could be eliminated and much unnecessary suffering could be prevented. If this is to be achieved, the dental profession must extend its horizons beyond the traditional role of clinical, diagnostic, and technical expertise for individual patients in the surgery, and become more aware of the psychological and social factors relevant to the prevention of dental disease.

We hope this book helps to stimulate, foster and guide changes in all sectors of the oral health community, as outlined by the 1993 WHO Report so that major improvements in oral health are achieved.

REFERENCES

World Health Organization (1987). *Alternative systems of oral care delivery*. Technical Report Series 750, Geneva.

World Health Organization (1992). *Recent advances in oral health*. Report of a WHO Expert Committee. Technical Report Series 826, Geneva.

World Health Organization (1993). *Oral health for the 21st century*. Oral Health Unit Geneva, Switzerland.

Index

acesulfame K   28
acid-etch retained materials   78–9
acidogenicity of meals   18
acidulated carbonated beverages   15
acidulated phosphate fluoride (APF) gels   179, 180
acquired pellicle   122
Actinomyces   122
Actinomyces viscossus   16, 178–9
Adult Dental Health Surveys   268
Africa   6
ageing dentition   173–85
  periodontal disease   174
  salivary composition   173
  structural changes   173
  surface maturation of enamel   173
ageing patients
  acceptable levels of dental health   244
  oral health in   189–99
  see also oral health, in older adults
alcohol use   160–1
amalgam
  comparison with fissure sealants   87–9
  corrosion products around restorations   104
  ditched restorations   103
  versus fissure sealing   87–9
amalgam/dental tissue interface   102
animal studies
  bacterial aetiology of caries   107–8
  fruits   22
  starchy foods   20–1
  sugar and dental caries   15–17
  vaccination   111–13
anterior teeth, restorative material in   103
antibodies
  in the mouth   109
  to *Strep. mutans*   111
antigens of oral bacteria   109
aphthae   166–7
aspartame   28
average caries figure (ACF)   4

bacterial aetiology of caries, animal studies   107–8
bacterial infections   166
benzydamine-hydrochloride mouth wash   167
betel quid   161
betel use   161
biopsy, oral mucosal lesions   163–4
bis-(glycidyl-methacrylate) (GMA) resins   79
bitewing radiographs   99, 100, 104
Bloomfield Report   269
breakfast cereals   15
British Association for the Study of Community
  Dentistry   272
British Dental Association   88
British Society of Paediatric Dentistry   88

calcium to phosphorus ratio   5
calculus
  and periodontal disease   244
  and plaque accumulation   123
  formation   123, 128
  removal   269
Candida albicans   164, 165

candidiasis   164, 165
carbohydrate consumption   69
cariogenicity testing   108
cast gold inlays   102
cellular immune responses   110
cerebral palsy   203
  dental caries   203
  malocclusion   203
  periodontal disease   203
cheese   25
chewing gums   28–9
child dental health surveys   250–7, 271
chlorhexidine
  administration   130–2
  clinical applications   132
  mode of action   130
  as mouthwash   130
  oral irrigation   130
  safety and side-effects   131–2
  spray application   131
  tooth gel   131
  toothpaste   131
chlorhexidine gluconate aqueous mouth rinse   167
chronic gingivitis   118, 119
chronic periodontitis   118
cocoa factor   25–6
Colorado stain   32–3, 61
Committee on Medical Aspects of Food Policy   234
Common Risk/Health Factor Approach (CRHFA)
  237
Community Dental Service   204
Community Periodontal Index of Treatment Needs
  (CPITN)   121
composite resin materials   102–3
confectionery workers   8
coronal decay   178
corrosion products around amalgam restorations
  104
cost of primary dental care   1
Critical Fall height (CFH)   147
Crohn's disease   167–8
cyano-acrylate resins   79

debridement, repair following   118
Declaration of Alma Ata   235
defective margin   103
dental attendance   145
dental caries   1
  animal experiments   15–17
  in cerebral palsy   203
  changing pattern in children   250
  in children   225–6, 250–7, 271
  in deciduous teeth   253
  in developing countries   2
  and diet   3–31
  in Down's syndrome   202
  epidemiological studies   258
  impact of preventive treatment   273
  international comparisons   258
  and malnutrition   3–4
  in mental handicap   201–2
  in permanent teeth   253
  prevalence   1

  secular decline in   258
  and sugar consumption   19
dental disease, changing pattern of   250–65
Dental Estimates Board (DEB)   267
dental floss   125
dental fluorosis   60–1
dental handicap   200–16
  classification   200–1
  terminology   200
dental health
  adult national surveys   260–4
  in children
    national surveys   250–7, 271
    need for treatment and effect on treatment needs
      in later life   258–60
  dentate adults   261–3
  impact of preventive treatment from childhood to
    middle age   274
dental health education   123–4
  assessment of   145
  current messages   143–4
  effectiveness of   144–5
  importance of correct message   143
  principles of   142–3
  and social factors   227–30
  target groups   142–3
Dental Health Programme Planning Group   143
Dental Health Promotion Units   141
dental injuries
  aetiology of   147
  associated with sports   148–50
dental manpower, maldistribution in   226
Dental Practice Board   267
dental services
  planning   226
  reorienting   246
Dental Strategy Review Group   204
dental trauma
  anterior teeth in children   256–7
  prevention of   147–52
  primary protection   147–51
  secondary prevention   151
dental treatment
  changing pattern of   267, 268
  cost of various items of   269–70
  factors affecting changes in   267
  impact of prevention on need for   272
dentine   97
dentine-enamel junction   97, 104
dentures and social class   219
diet
  and dental caries   3–31
  and natural cleansing   127
  and plaque accumulation   127
  post-eruptive effect   3, 5
  pre-eruptive effect   3
  quality of   11
  war-time   8
  see also meals
digit-sucking habits   154
disabled children
  dental health   204–9
  inadequate dental care   209

need for prevention   209
need for special dental care   209
preventive programmes   209–10
ditched amalgam restoration   103
ditching   102
Down's syndrome   202
    dental caries   202
    malocclusion   203
    periodontal disease   202

edentulousness, prevalence of   260–1
electric tooth-brush   125
electron microscopy, white spot lesions   97–8
enamel carious lesions   95–106
    approximal surfaces   100
    arrested lesions   98
    body   96–7
    clinical detection   99–100
    clinical relevance of arrest and remineralization
        99
    dark zone   96
    in deciduous teeth   97
    free smooth surfaces   99
    macroscopic features   95
    management of   100–1
    microscopic features   95–8
    and organic matrix   98
    pits and fissures   99–100
    remineralization   99–100
    subsurface demineralization   97
    surface zone   97
    translucent zone   96
enamel-dentine junction   97, 104
enamel slab experiments   17
    starchy foods   21
epidemiological surveys   6
erythema multiforme   169
erythroplasia   163
Eskimos   6
essential minerals and oral cancer   162
ethnic origin and dental health   224–5

Federation Dentaire Internationale (FDI)   147, 271
fibre   26
fissure caries   97
fissure sealants   78–94
    application technique   79–84
    comparisons with amalgam   87–9
    cost-effectiveness   86–7
    early materials   78–9
    further clinical trials   84
    new developments   88–9
    and preventive resin restoration   88
    questionnaire surveys   85–6
    results of clinical trials   79
    use of   85–6
fluoridated salt   50–2
fluoridation of water supplies   141, 144
    social factors   226
fluoride dentifrices   53–60, 68, 144
    combining more than one fluoride agent   56–7
    comparisons of different formulations   57–9
    effect of additives   59
    effect on root caries   59
    fluoride concentration in   54–6
    formulation   54–60
    and tooth-brushing habits   75–6
fluoride-releasing cements   89
fluoride supplementation   9, 10, 61
    see also fluoride tablets and drops
fluoride tablets and drops
    compared with other methods   48
    dosage   49–50

effect on permanent teeth   45
effect on primary teeth   45
effectiveness in caries prevention   44–9
effects on deciduous teeth   46
effects on permanent teeth   47–8
prenatal effect   45–8
summary of effectiveness   48–9
fluoride–vitamin combination   48
fluorides   32–68
    administration methods   50–4
    applied by dentist   53
    and cancer   44
    compounds   48
    effect of cessation of fluoridation   42–3
    effect of varying concentrations in drinking water
        35–6
    historical background   32–5
    incorporated into resins   89
    legislation   43–4
    lesion progression delay   99
    and patterns of caries in 15- to 16-year-old
        children in low fluoride areas   38–40
    pre-eruptive caries preventive effect   5
    pre-eruptive effect   41–2
    secular changes in caries   40–1
    self-applied agents   53–4
    topical therapy   53, 101
    WHO reports   61–2
    work of H. Trendley Dean   34–5
    world-wide studies   36–8
fluoridized fruit juice   52–3
fluoridized milk   52–3
fructose
    intolerance   8
    Turku studies   13
fruit flavoured drinks   23
fruit juices
    and dental caries   23
    fluoridized   52–3
fruits   21–3
    animal studies   22
    incubation experiments   22
fungal infections   165

General Dental Services   1, 269
    cost studies   270
    expenditure   271
genetic fingerprinting techniques   108
gingival hyperplasia   169
gingival inflammation and plaque levels   244
gingivitis
    epidemiology   119
    improvements in   122
    prevalence and severity   119
glass ionomer cements   89, 103
glass ionomer sealant restoration   88
glossitis   169
glucosyltransferase (GTF)   109, 110, 112–14
Goals for Oral Health Strategy   271–2

Handbook on policies and priorities   204
handicapped children   201
Head Injury Criteria (HIC)   146
health education
    and health protection   142
    positive   142
    preventive   141
    for preventive health protection   141
    see also dental health; oral health
Health for all by the year 2000   235, 241
health promotion   235–6
    basic concept   141–3
    preventive services and facilities   141

Tannahill model   140
health protection
    and health education   142
    positive   142
    preventive   141
herpesvirus infections   164–6
High Risk Strategy (HRS)   238
HIV   164, 165
Hopewood House   7, 68
human cytomegalovirus (HCMV)   166
hydrogenated glucose syrup, cariogenicity   27
hypodontia   158
hypoplasia   3, 4

iatrogenic oral disease   169
immune responses   110–11
immune systems   107
immunoglobulins   111
    IgA   109–10
    IgG   110, 114
    s-IgA   109–10, 112
immunological microenvironments in the mouth   110
immunology of oral cavity   109–10
incubation experiments   18–19
    fruits   22
    starchy foods   21
interdental brush (bottle brush)   126
interdental cleaning   125
International Dental Federation   271
interspace tooth-brush   125
iron deficiency   169
    in carcinogenesis   162
irrigation devices   127
isomalt, cariogenicity   27

J-chain   109

lactitol, cariogenicity   27–8
lactobacilli   10, 179
legislation, fluoridation   43–4
leukoplakia   163
lichen planus   167
lichenoid reactions   167
liquorice   25–6
listerine   133
Lycasin   15, 27

major recurrent aphthous stomatitis (MaRAS)
        166–7
malignant lesions   162–3
malnutrition and dental caries   3–4
malocclusion
    abnormalities of tooth position   157–8
    aetiology   153–4
    anterior crossbites   156
    balancing and compensating extractions   155
    cerebral palsy   203
    in cerebral palsy   203
    dento-alveolar factors   154, 156
    dilaceration of incisors   158
    in Down's syndrome   203
    early loss of primary molar teeth   155
    hypodontia   158
    interceptive measures   154–7
    malpositioned maxillary canine teeth   157–8
    in mental handicap   202
    mixed dentition   155
    planned loss of first permanent molar teeth   157
    posterior crossbites   156–7
    prevention of   153–9
    primary dentition   154–5
scope and limitations of interceptive orthodontics
        159

malocclusion—contd.
  screening 158–9
  serial extractions 155–6
  skeletal factors 153–4
  soft tissue form and function in 154
  sucking habits in 154
  supernumerary teeth 157
  transposition of teeth 158
  treatment of 269
mannitol, cariogenicity 27
marijuana use 161–2
meals
  acidogenicity 18
  and plaque pH 18
  see also diet
medically compromized children 204–9
mental handicap 201–3
  dental caries in 201–2
  malocclusion in 202
  periodontal disease in 202
microbial specificity in caries 107–8
microradiography 97
milk 24–5
  fluoridized 52–3
minor recurrent aphthous stomatitis (MiRAS)
    166–7
mottled enamel
  aetiological factors 33–4
  and fluoride concentration 34
mottled teeth, endemic areas of 33
mouth protection
  for special groups 150–1
  in sports 148–50
mouthguards
  care of 150
  construction criteria 149
  custom-made 150
  design 149, 150
  functions of 149
  life of 150
  materials 150
  mouth-formed 150
  stock 150
  types 150
mouthwash
  chlorhexidine as 131
  remineralizing 180
  use in oral cancer 161
mucosal disorders, immunologically mediated
    166–9
mucosal infections 164–6
mucosal lesions in nutritional deficiencies 169
muscular dystrophy 204

nicotinic acid deficiency 169
non-milk extrinsic (NME) sugars 242
nutrition policy 242–3
nutritional deficiencies, mucosal lesions in 169

occlusal development 153
oral bacteria, antigens of 109
oral cancer 1, 160–4
  and fluorides 44
  occupation and oral health status in 162
  prevention 163
oral carcinoma-*in situ* 163–4
oral care habits in adolescents 59–60
oral cavity, immunology of 109–10
oral cleanliness and dental caries 68–77
oral diseases, public health importance of 235
oral health
  biological element 140
  determinants of 139–40

environmental factors 140
goals for 271–2
in older adults 189–99
  cost as limiting factor 195
  dental non-attendance as limiting factor 194
  limiting factors 192–5
  long-term changes in 189–90
  management concepts 195–7
  medical and physical limitations 193–4
  minimum dentition consistent with function and
      satisfaction 191–2
  possibilities for 190–2
  see also ageing dentition; ageing patients
lifestyle factors 140
optimum 190–1
policy 234–9
  creating supportive environments 246
  developing coping skills 246
  guiding principles 245–6
promotion 140–6
  general principles 236–41
  integrated common risk factor approach
      237–8
  strategy 271
  dental criteria for 243–5
  21st century 275–6
oral hygiene 9, 10
  education 123
  mechanical practices 245
  promotion of 230
  role of commerce and politics 230
oral mucosal disease 160–72
oral mucosal lesions, biopsy 163–4
oral squamous carcinomas 160
oro-facial granulomatosis 167–8
orthodontic condition of children 255–6
orthodontic treatment 269
  see also malocclusion
Ottawa Charter 235–6, 245
overjets, early (mixed dentition) treatment 148

partial dentures and plaque formation 123
patient education and review 103
Patients first 204
periodontal disease 1, 118–38
  aetiology 123–4
  ageing effects 174
  and calculus 244
  in cerebral palsy 203
  in children 253–5
  control strategies 245
  in dentate adults 219
  in Down's syndrome 202
  epidemiology 119–22
  factors affecting prevalence and severity of 119
  factors modifying inflammatory response 123
  intra-oral distribution 121
  in mental handicap 202
  pathogenesis of 118–19
  preventive policy 244
  public health aspects of 245
  rate of destruction 121–2
  rationale for prevention and management 123–7
  treatment needs 121
  trends in 122
periodontitis
  adult 120
  age of onset 120
  forms of 120
  juvenile 120
  pre-pubertal 120
  prevalence and severity 119–20
  rapidly progressive 120

periodontium, appearance of normal healthy 118
pharyngeal cancer 162
phenolic compounds 132
phenylketonuria 8
physical handicap 203–4
plant products, protective factors derived from 25–6
plaque 122–3
  and calculus 123
  effect of diet on accumulation 127
  factors predisposing to 123
  microbial make-up 108
  mineralization 123
  subgingival 129
  supragingival 129
plaque control 102
  chemical 129–32
  in immunocompromised patient 166
  preventive programmes 127–9
plaque formation and partial dentures 123
plaque levels and gingival inflammation 244
plaque pH
  different sugars and concentrations 18
  fruits 22
  and meals 18
  methods of measuring 17–18
  and snack foods 18
  starchy foods 21
playground surfaces in tooth injury 147
Plummer–Vinson syndrome 162
point-prevalence surveys 68–70
polishing 125
polymorphonuclear leukocytes (PMNLs) 110, 114
polyurethane
  fissure sealants 79
  mouthguards 150
polyvinyl acetate-polyethylene copolymer (PVAc-PE)
      mouthguards 150
posterior teeth, restorative material in 102–3
preventive programmes 127–9
  in adults 128–9
  in children 127–8
preventive resin restoration
  and fissure sealants 88
  results of clinical trials 88
primary health care 235–6
professional tooth-cleaning 73–4
Promoting better health 268
prospective studies 72–4

radiographic examination, frequency of 101
Recent advances in oral health 275
recurrent aphthous stomatitis (RAS) 166–7
Registrar General's Social Class 217
remineralization of carious lesions 99
remineralizing mouth wash 180
residual caries in cavities 103
residual demineralization 104
restorations
  and plaque accumulation 123
  replacement of 101
  and treatment for malocclusions 267
restorative material
  in anterior teeth 103
  in posterior teeth 102–3
restorative technique 102
restored teeth, diagnosis of caries in 103–4
retrospective longitudinal studies 70–1
risk factors 101
root caries
  distribution within the mouth 177
  histology 178
  incidence 175–7
  management 181

root caries—contd.
  microbiology 178
  prevalence 174–5
  prevention 179–81
  risk factors 177, 178
root caries index 176
root planing 125
root surface caries, incidence rates 176
root surface lesions 179
Roslagen Study 15

saccharin 28
salivary composition, ageing dentition 173
salivary flow, treatment options 180
scaling 124, 128, 269
scanning electron microscope 97
Scientific basis of dental health education, The 143
screening, malocclusion 158–9
secondary caries 101
  histological features of early lesion 101
  prevention of 101–2
self-cleansing 72–3, 102
self-inflicted injuries 150–1
shortened dental arch (SDA) treatment planning
    philosophy 196–7
Skoal Bandits 142
smokeless tobacco 161
snack foods and plaque pH 18
social class 217–31
  and decay experience of 5-year-old children 219
  and dental disease 218–19
  and dental health 223
  and dental knowledge, attitudes, and behaviour
      221–3
  and dental treatment 219–21
  and dental treatment in 5-year-old children 221
  and disease 218
  and full or partial dentures 219
  and medical treatment 219
social factors 217–33
  and dental health education 227–30
  and fluoridation of water supplies 226–7
social status 217
sodium monofluorophosphate dentifrices 56
sorbitol, cariogenicity 27
spina bifida
  dental caries in 204
  periodontal disease in 204
sports, dental injuries associated with 148–50
stains 123
starchy foods 19
  animal experiments 20–1
  animal studies 20–1
  enamel slab experiments 21

human interventional studies 20
human observational studies 19–20
incubation experiments 21
plaque pH 21
stomatitis 169
Strathclyde fluoridation case 43–4
Streptococcus mutans 10, 16, 27, 107–14, 122,
    178, 179
Streptococcus sanguis 110, 122
subgingival débridement 124
sucrose
  in dental caries 3
  Turku studies 13
sugar and sugar products 3, 6, 230
  animal experiments 15–17
sugar-cane chewers 8
sugar-containing food and drink 143–4
sugar consumption 6–7
  and dental caries 19
  cross-sectional observational studies 9–11
  high 8–9
  low 7–8
sugar levels 242–3
supernumerary teeth 157
supragingival plaque accumulation 119
surgical pocket therapy 124–5
sweeteners 3, 26–9
  cariogenicity 27
  intense 28
  role in caries prevention 28
  types of 26
sweets, restrictions of sales 8
syphilitic leukoplakia 163
syrup medicines 9

Tannahill model 140
T-cells 110
thaumatin 28
T-lymphocytes 110
tobacco 160–1
tooth-brush, electric 125
tooth-brushing 125
  frequency 71–2
  habits 75–6
tooth-cleaning
  duration and technique 126–7
  frequency of 126
  professional 73–4
tooth gel, chlorhexidine 131
tooth injury, *see* dental trauma
tooth malalignment and plaque accumulation
    123
tooth mortality statistics 121
tooth retention in ageing population 177

tooth wear 181–5
  abrasion 184, 185
  aetiology 182
  attrition 183–5
  erosion 182–5
  management 184–5
  prevalence 182
  prevention 184–5
toothpaste 127
  chlorhexidine 132
  fluoride 145
toothpicks (woodpoints) 125
Towards better dental health 204
trace elements 5
transmission electron microscope 98
trauma, *see* dental trauma
triclosan 133
Tristan da Cunha 6, 68
Turku sugar studies 13–15

vaccination 111–14
  animal studies 111–13
  prospects for human caries 113–14
Vanguard electronic caries detector 100
varicella-zoster virus (VZV) infections 166
Vipeholm study 11–13, 25
viral infections 165
virulence factors 108
vitamin B$_2$ deficiency 169
vitamin B$_{12}$ deficiency 169
vitamin D 3, 4–5
vitamins and oral cancer 162
Von der Fehr short-term caries experiments 15

water, hardness and calcium content 5
water supplies
  fluoridation 35–6, 42–3, 142, 145
    social factors 226
    see also fluorides
white spot lesions 95, 99
  electron microscopy 97–8
  multiple 101
Whole Population Strategy (WPS) 237–41
woodpoints (toothpicks) 126
World Health Organization (WHO) 235, 238, 241,
    271, 275

xerostomia 169
xylitol
  cariogenicity 27
  Turku studies 13

zinc deficiency 169